Cancer Genome and Tumor Microenvironment

Andrei Thomas-Tikhonenko

Editor

Cancer Genome and Tumor Microenvironment

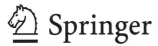 Springer

Editor
Andrei Thomas-Tikhonenko
University of Pennsylvania
Children's Hospital of Philadelphia
3615 Civic Center Blvd.
Philadelphia PA 19104
USA
andreit@mail.med.upenn.edu

ISBN 978-1-4419-0710-3   e-ISBN 978-1-4419-0711-0
DOI 10.1007/978-1-4419-0711-0
Springer New York Dordrecht Heidelberg London

Library of Congress Control Number: 2009934786

Printed on acid-free paper

Springer is part of Springer Science+Business Media (www.springer.com)

Acknowledgments

The idea to put this book together has emerged after years of thought-provoking conversations with numerous members of the cancer research community at the University of Pennsylvania and well beyond its ivied walls. I am particularly grateful to faculty and students of the CAMB512 Cancer Biology and Genetics course, which I co-directed for a number of years with Drs. Frederic Barr, Warren Pear, Martin Carroll, Costas Koumenis, and Carlo Maley. Their contributions to this volume would not show up in PubMed (save for Carlo Maley's) but nonetheless are highly significant. Very special thanks to my assistant Kate Wurges (née Simmermon), who dealt with the contributors and their submissions with utmost patience, diligence, and can-do spirit. On the personal level, my parents, Tomas and Irina, are gratefully acknowledged for their determination to have a second-generation biologist in their household. Finally, I am indebted to my immediate family for being so understanding and supportive of this time-consuming undertaking. So, thank you Nicolas, Alexander, and Elizabeth!

Contents

Contributors

Jamie K. Alan Department of Pharmacology, University of North Carolina at Chapel Hill, Chapel Hill, NC, jalan@med.unc.edu

Alfonso Bellacosa Fox Chase Cancer Center, Philadelphia, PA, alfonso.bellacosa@fccc.edu

Subbarao Bondada University of Kentucky, Lexington, KY, bondada@email.uky.edu

Donita C. Brady Department of Pharmacology, University of North Carolina at Chapel Hill, Chapel Hill, NC, dbrady@med.unc.edu

Adrienne D. Cox Departments of Radiation Oncology & Pharmacology, University of North Carolina at Chapel Hill, Chapel Hill, NC, adrienne_cox@med.unc.edu

Chi V. Dang The Sidney Kimmel Comprehensive Cancer Center, Johns Hopkins University School of Medicine, Baltimore, MD, cvdang@jhmi.edu

Greg H. Enders Department of Medicine, Fox Chase Cancer Center, Philadelphia, PA, greg.enders@fccc.edu

Sara K. Evans University of Massachusetts, Program in Molecular Medicine, Worcester, MA, sara.evans@umassmed.edu

Himabindu Gaddipati The Wistar Institute, Philadelphia, PA, hbg125@yahoo.com

JG Garcia Department of Medicine, University of Chicago, Chicago, IL, jgarcia@medicine.bsd.uchicago.edu

Laura F. Gibson Mary Babb Randolph Cancer Center, West Virginia University Health Sciences Center, Morgantown, WV, lgibson@hsc.wvu.edu

Michael R. Green University of Massachusetts, Program in Molecular Medicine, Worcester, MA, michael.green@umassmed.edu

Murali Gururajan Department of Pathology – DSB, Emory University, Atlanta, GA, mgurura@emory.edu

Meenhard Herlyn The Wistar Institute, Philadelphia, PA, herlynm@wistar.org

Luisa Iruela-Arispe Biomedical Research Building, UCLA, 615 Charles E. Young Drive South, Los Angeles, CA, USA, arispe@mbi.ucla.edu

Michele Jacob The Wistar Institute, Philadelphia, PA, mjacob@wistar.org

Rajeev Kaul Abramson Comprehensive Cancer Center, University of Pennsylvania School of Medicine, Philadelphia, PA, rkaul@mail.med.upenn.edu

Chand Khanna Head, Tumor and Metastasis Biology Section, Pediatric Oncology Branch, National Cancer Institute, Bethesda, MD, khannac@mail.nih.gov

Pankaj Kumar Abramson Comprehensive Cancer Center, University of Pennsylvania School of Medicine, Philadelphia, PA, pankajk@mail.med.upenn.edu

Lionel Larue UMR 146 CNRS – Institut Curie, Orsay 91405, France, lionel.larue@curie.fr

Wen-Hui Lien Division of Human Biology, Fred Hutchinson Cancer Research Center, Seattle, WA, wlien@mail.rockefeller.edu

John P. Lynch Division of Gastroenterology/650 CRB, 415 Curie Blvd., Philadelphia, PA, lynchj@mail.med.upenn.edu

Carlo C. Maley Department of Cellular and Molecular Oncology, Wister Institute, Philadelphia, PA, cmaley@alum.mit.edu

Masanao Murakami Abramson Comprehensive Cancer Center, University of Pennsylvania School of Medicine, Philadelphia, PA, masanao@mail.med.upenn.edu

Heather O'Leary Mary Babb Randolph Cancer Center, West Virginia University Health Sciences Center, Morgantown, WV, holeary@hsc.wvu.edu

Boris Pasche Division of Hematology/Oncology, Department of Medicine & UAB Comprehensive Cancer Center, The University of Alabama at Birmingham, Birmingham, Al, boris.pasche@ccc.uab.edu

Ellen Puré The Wistar Institute, Philadelphia, PA, pure@wistar.org

Janusz Rak Montreal Children's Hospital Research Institute, Montreal, QC, Canada, janusz.rak@mcgill.ca

Mandira Ray Department of Medicine, University of Chicago, Chicago, IL, mandira.ray@uchospitals.edu

Ling Ren Pediatric Oncology Branch, National Cancer Institute, Bethesda, MD, renl@mail.nih.gov

Erle S. Robertson Department of Microbiology and Tumor Virology Program, Abramson Comprehensive Cancer Center, University of Pennsylvania School of Medicine, Philadelphia, PA, erle@mail.med.upenn.edu

Ravi Salgia Department of Medicine, University of Chicago, 5841 South Maryland Ave. Chicago, IL, rsalgia@medicine.bsd.uchicago.edu

Gregg L. Semenza Departments of Pediatrics, Medicine, Oncology, and Radiation Oncology, The Johns Hopkins University School of Medicine, Broadway Research Building, Suite 671, Baltimore, MD, gsemenza@jhmi.edu

Antonia R. Sepulveda, Hospital of the University of Pennsylvania, Philadelphia, PA, asepu@mail.med.upenn.edu

Kathleen Sprouffske Genomics & Computational Biology Graduate Group, University of Pennsylvania, Philadelphia, PA, sprouffk@mail.med.upenn.edu

Prema Sundaram Department of Pathology and Laboratory Medicine, University of Pennsylvania, Philadelphia, PA, sundaramp@email.chop.edu

Jose G. Teodoro McGill Cancer Centre and Department of Biochemistry,McGill University, Montreal, Quebec, Canada, jose.teodoro@mcgill.ca

Andrei Thomas-Tikhonenko University of Pennsylvania and the Children's Hospital of Philadelphia, 516H Abramson Research Center, Philadelphia, PA, andreit@mail.med.upenn.edu

Antoni Xavier Torres-Collado Department of Molecular, Cell and Developmental Biology and Molecular Biology Institute UCLA, Los Angeles, CA, axtorres@gmail.com

Valeri Vasioukhin Division of Human Biology, Fred Hutchinson Cancer Research Center, C3-168, Seattle, WA, vvasiouk@fhcrc.org

Lin Wang Department of Tissue Morphogenesis, Max-Planck Institute for Molecular Biomedicine, Germany, lin.wang@mpi-muenster.mpg.de

Qinghua Zeng. Division of Hematology/Oncology, Department Of Medicine & UAB Comprehensive Cancer Center, The University of Alabama at Birmingham, Birmingham, Al, qzeng@uab.edu

Huafeng Zhang The Johns Hopkins University School of Medicine, Baltimore, MD, hzhang22@jhmi.edu

Part I
Opening Remarks

Chapter 1
Hardwiring Tumor Progression

Andrei Thomas-Tikhonenko

Oncogenes and tumor suppressor genes were traditionally studied in the context of cell proliferation, differentiation, senescence, and survival, four relatively cell-autonomous processes. Consequently, in the late 1980s–mid-1990s, neoplastic growth was described largely as a net imbalance between cell accumulation and loss, brought about through mutations in cancer genes (Evan and Littlewood, 1998). In the last 10 years, a more holistic understanding of cancer slowly emerged, stressing the importance of interactions between neoplastic and various stromal components: extracellular matrix, basement membranes, fibroblasts, endothelial cells of blood and lymphatic vessels, tumor-infiltrating lymphocytes, etc. (Hanahan and Weinberg, 2000). Nevertheless, the commonly held view is that changes in tumor microenvironment are "softwired," i.e., epigenetic in nature and often reversible. Yet, there exists a large body of evidence suggesting that well-known mutations in cancer genes profoundly affect tumor milieu. In fact, these cell-extrinsic changes might be one of the primary reasons such mutations are preserved in late-stage tumors. This book will review how tumor microenvironment and progression can be "hardwired," i.e., genetically controlled.

These "Opening Remarks" (Part 1) will be followed by Part 2 entitled "Breaking Away: Epithelial–Mesenchymal Transition." As stated in Chapter 2 by Drs. Alfonso Bellasco and Lionel Larue, EMT is "a major developmental process during which epithelial cells develop mesenchymal, fibroblast-like properties, increased motility, and reduced intercellular adhesion." Furthermore, "EMT-like events are central to tumor progression and malignant transformation, endowing the incipient cancer cell with invasive and metastatic properties." Their chapter focuses on the PI3 kinase, one of the most frequently mutated genes in human cancers, and its inhibitor PTEN, which is mutated with very high frequency in endometrial cancer, glioblastomas, and some other malignancies. Although the PI3K–Pten–Akt axis closely controls cell proliferation and death, deregulation of this pathway has important implications for the epithelial–mesenchymal transition as well.

A. Thomas-Tikhonenko (✉)

Department of Pathology and Laboratory Medicine, University of Pennsylvania, and Department of Pathology, The Children's Hospital of Philadelphia, Philadelphia, PA, USA

e-mail: andreit@mail.med.upenn.edu

A. Thomas-Tikhonenko (ed.), *Cancer Genome and Tumor Microenvironment*,
DOI 10.1007/978-1-4419-0711-0_1, © Springer Science+Business Media, LLC 2010

Chapter 3 by Drs. Wen-Hui Lien and Valeri Vasioukhin zeroes in on one particular downstream effector of the Akt pathway, E-cadherin. Since E-cadherin is a component of the cell–cell adhesion system dubbed adherens junctions, its loss is the key event in epithelial–mesenchymal transition. While epigenetic downregulation of E-cadherin is a well-known consequence of aberrant Akt signaling, discussion here focuses on inactivating mutations in the E-cadherin gene itself, which are frequently found in gastrointestinal and mammary cancers of epithelial origin.

Parallel to the PI3K pathway – and sometimes intertwining with it – lies the receptor tyrosine kinase pathway transmitting the signal from the plasma membrane to Ras, an enzyme capable of converting GTP to GDP and in the process undergoing conformational changes that trigger downstream signaling events. Ras family members work in conjunction with other small GTPases, of which Rho GTPases are a subclass. The latter and their role in cell motility are described in Chapter 4 co-written by Drs. Donita Brady, Jamie Alan, and Adrienne Cox. Interestingly, at least one of these enzymes, RhoH (or ARHH) is affected by mutations in multiple myelomas and diffuse large B-cell and other non-Hodgkin's lymphomas, warranting their inclusion in this book.

Drs. Ling Ren and Chand Khanna follow with Chapter 5 on the classical (in the strict Knudsen's sense) NF2 tumor suppressor and related ERM proteins. While these proteins have a multitude of functions, one of their well-recognized properties is to serve as linkers between plasma membrane and cytoskeleton and thus contribute to cell movement. Moreover, the authors point out that "ERM proteins function both upstream and downstream of Rho-[GTPases] which are known regulators of tumor cell motility and invasion."

It is now well-recognized that in addition to the invasive growth, tumors must acquire access to blood vasculature; hence the following Part 3 entitled "Coming up for Air: Hypoxia and Angiogenesis."

Chapter 6 co-authored by Drs. Huafeng Zhang and Gregg Semenza focuses on hypoxia-induced factor 1. This transcription factor is an important regulator of many a gene responsible for tumor neovascularization, including vascular endothelial growth factor, or VEGF. While the role of HIF-1 in spontaneous tumors is well-recognized, nowhere is its importance more obvious than in Von Hippel–Lindau (VHL) disease, an autosomal dominant, familial cancer syndrome. The VHL protein, of course, is the ubiquitin ligase responsible for degradation of the alpha subunit of HIF-1, and the loss of this enzyme sets in motion a complex set of events culminating in tumor angiogenesis.

If tumor suppressors inhibit angiogenesis, oncogenes certainly aspire to do just the opposite. Not to be outdone by HIF-1, Ras family members, upon being touched by activating mutations, devised their own ways to contribute to the tumor-vascular interface. Chapter 7 by Dr. Rak details how "expression of mutant H-ras leads to ... the exuberant production of VEGF" – and to other important events in tumor angiogenesis.

Still, there are strong hints that in "real" tumors Ras cannot do it alone, or at least would rather not. Either way, it definitely benefits from coactivation of another oncogene, c-Myc, which was first shown to cooperate with Ras more than 25 years ago (Land et al., 1983). Chapter 8 by Drs. Prema Sundaram, Chi Dang, and myself describes how Myc influences and is influenced by hypoxia and how in the end it turns off expression of thrombospondin-1, an endogenous inhibitor of angiogenesis, to yield tumors with robust vascularization.

Yet even when acting together, Ras and Myc might need to go back to tumor suppressors for help. Chapter 9 by Drs. Jose Teodoro, Sara Evans, and Michael Green delineate the contribution of p53 loss to tumor neovascularization. They state that retention of p53 inhibits angiogenesis in at least three ways: through "inhibition of hypoxia-sensing systems, downregulation of pro-angiogenesis genes, and up-regulation of anti-angiogenesis pathways," including but not limited to thrombospondins. Given that "the overall combination of these effects ... tilts the tumor microenvironment in the host substantially towards angiogenesis suppression," it comes as little surprise that loss of p53 is the most common inactivating mutation in human neoplasm (Vogelstein and Kinzler, 2004).

It is equally unsurprising that another tumor suppressor, ink4a, which profoundly influences p53 activity (if the *TP53* gene happens to be retained), also has important cell-extrinsic effects. Chapter 10 by Dr. Greg Enders describes how GI cancer-susceptible APC-deficient mice develop significantly more vascular tumors if ink4a is concomitantly lost. In an interesting twist, of the two ink4a-encoded proteins, the anti-angiogenic effects appear to be linked to p16, which negatively regulates not p53 but another tumor suppressor Rb. The conclusion is that this cell cycle-controlling, cdk-inhibiting protein "appears, directly and/or indirectly, to repress certain extracellular signaling, such as expression of VEGF, with substantial non-cell-autonomous impact."

Even highly vascular tumors do not generally become life threatening (save for neoplasms arising in confined spaces such as the cranium) unless they undergo metastatic spread and learn to survive in and productively interact with the new organ. These interactions are the subject of Part 4 on "Gaining New Ground: Metastasis and Stromal Cell Interactions."

It opens with the discussion of NM23 as a metastasis inhibitor. Chapter 11 by Drs. Rajeev Kaul, Masanao Murakami, Pankaj Kumar, and Erle Robertson describes the gene "first cloned from a murine melanoma cell line wherein its expression correlated inversely with metastatic potential." How this intracellular nucleoside-binding protein suppresses metastatic spread is still incompletely understood. However, consistent with the mouse model studies, the allelic deletions of the nm23-H1 variant "have been associated with a more aggressive behavior in colorectal cancers."

We have a somewhat better understanding of another long-known metastasis gene, c-MET, which is the receptor tyrosine kinase activated by hepatocyte growth factor (HGF) a.k.a. Scatter Factor (SF). The HGF/SF-Met axis, described in detail in Chapter 12 by Drs. Mandira Ray, JG Garcia, and Ravi Salgia, appears to be genetically altered in papillary renal carcinomas (a relative of the von Hippel-Lindau disease). Interestingly, its role in metastasis in vivo is not limited to literally promoting tumor cell "scattering." One additional example is the involvement of c-Met signaling in tumor angiogenesis; hence the renewed interest in therapeutic targeting of this pathway in renal cell carcinomas, lung cancers, and other solid and hematopoietic tumors.

In addition to properties intrinsic to tumor cells (e.g., enhanced motility), extracellular milieu has to be conducive to metastatic spread as well. Drs. Antoni Xavier Torres-Collado and Luisa Iruela-Arispe, in Chapter 13, point out that "tumor expansion requires...destruction of parenchyma and remodeling of the extracellular matrix...[which] is greatly assisted by the catalytic activity of extracellular proteases." Chapter 13 focuses on the proteases of the adamalysin family: the membrane-anchored ADAMs (a disintegrin and metalloprotease) and the secreted ADAMTSs (a disintegrin and metalloprotease with thrombospondin repeats). The rather counterintuitive finding of recent years was the identification of inactivating mutations in adamalysin family members in various tumors. However, this discovery is consistent with the realization that ADAM and ADAMTS protein play several inhibitory roles in cancer progression, which are reviewed by Torres-Collado and Iruela-Arispe.

Chapters 14 and 15 of Part 4 deal directly with the interactions between tumor and stromal cells. Chapter 14 by Drs. Michele Jacob and Ellen Puré states that platelet-derived growth factor, or PDGF, "is one of the most potent chemoattractants and activators of fibroblasts, stimulating their differentiation into myofibroblasts, which represent a prominent stromal cell type in carcinomas." Not surprisingly, PDGF is affected by mutations in dermatofibrosarcoma protuberans and aberrant PDGF signaling in carcinomas is a well-recognized phenomenon. While it definitely assists in recruitment of tumor-associated fibroblasts (TAFs), mechanisms of tumor promotion by TAFs are diverse and at times non-linear. The chapter ends with the discussion of the topic of considerable controversy: whether TAFs themselves accumulate specific mutations, for example in the TP53 gene.

The complementary contribution by Drs. Qinghua Zeng and Boris Pasche in Chapter 15 is concerned with alterations in TGFβ signaling in both neoplastic and stromal cells. While mutations in TGFβ itself do not appear to occur in cancer, "type I and II TGFβ receptors and their downstream effectors SMADs are often targeted by oncogenic events." The authors present compelling evidence (much of it coming from their own laboratory) that at least in mice abrogation of TGFβ signaling within the stromal fibroblasts is accompanied by changes in the epithelial compartment and the development of invasive squamous cell carcinomas. Moreover, to the extent that TGFβ signaling is a potent negative regulator of the immune system, its loss in the immune cells can lead to chronic inflammation and thus create a pro-tumorigenic environment.

This logically brings us to Part 5 entitled "Getting Attention: Immune Recognition and Inflammation." Drs. Antonia Sepulveda and John Lynch in Chapter 16 pick up where Zeng and Pasche in Chapter 15 left off and most thoroughly review the connection between inflammation and cancer using as a model colon carcinomas with microsatellite instability, owing to defects in DNA mismatch repair.

The authors ask not only "how the induction of MSI leads to the increased inflammatory response," but also "how chronic inflammatory processes provoke genetic instabilities that lead to the development of cancer."

The second key aspect of the interplay between cancer and immunity is that tumors readily arise in the immune system itself. Still, they often remain dependent on normal stroma for both antigenic stimulation and microenvironmental cues. Chapter 17 by Drs. Murali Gururajan and Subbarao Bondada reviews the evidence that stimulation of the B-cell receptor (BCR) in B-lymphomas substantively contributes to tumor cell proliferation. This idea is supported by several lines of evidence. One is the existence of gain-of-function mutations in the Pax5 gene, which is required for BCR signaling. Another is the retention of somatically hypermutated, high-affinity BCR alleles even when the other allele is inactivated due to oncogenic translocations (e.g., IgH-Myc).

In parallel, chronic myelogonous and acute lymphoblastic leukemias are known to carry the so-called Philadelphia chromosome (Ph), with its characteristic gain-of-function translocation resulting in the expression of the Bcr-Abl fusion protein. Drs. Lin Wang, Heather O'Leary, and Laura Gibson in Chapter 18 demonstrate that "while high, constitutive Abl kinase activity is thought to be the driving force in initiation and progression of leukemic disease, the bone marrow microenvironment also plays a pivotal role in maintaining Ph+ leukemic stem cells. The salient example of this interplay is the propensity of Bcr-Abl "to drive expression of VE-cadherin expression at the hemangioblast stage from which both tumor and endothelial populations may be derived."

As editor, I envisioned that Part 6, "Putting it all together," would deal with the following two notions. The first one is that while individual mutations described in this book can profoundly alter tumor milieu on their own, the naturally occurring tumors tend to utilize multiple strategies that complement and sometimes duplicate each other. Hence, Chapter 19 by Drs. Himabindu Gaddipati and Meenhard Herlyn demonstrates what it takes to "construct" a malignant melanoma. Melanoma microenvironment-related genes under review in their submission (or at least their close relatives) have all been featured in the preceding chapters: the receptor tyrosine kinase c-Kit, N-Ras, B-Raf, β-catenin, PI3 kinase, Akt3, Ink4a, Arf, and Pten.

The second notion, amply illustrated in Chapter 20 by Drs. Kathleen Sprouffske and Carlo Maley, is that while mutations in microenvironment-friendly genes like PDGFB, CDH1, TGFBR1, KRAS might have arisen independently, they certainly function together and co-evolve, to yield the final product called the malignant tumor. To wit, "these interactions could increase the rate of progression to malignancy if two clones may independently acquire different hallmarks of cancer rather than waiting for one clone to accumulate all the hallmarks itself." On the therapeutic side, the authors envision that "decreasing the heterogeneity of the tumor environment will slow the evolution of new clones and the opportunities for tumorigenesis." Our shared hope is that this book will assist current and future researchers in achieving this goal.

References

Evan G, Littlewood T (1998) A matter of life and cell death. *Science* 281:1317–1322

Hanahan D, Weinberg RA (2000) The hallmarks of cancer. *Cell* 100:57–70

Land H, Parada LF, Weinberg RA (1983) Tumorigenic conversion of primary embryo fibroblasts requires at least two cooperating oncogenes. *Nature* 304:596–602

Vogelstein B, Kinzler KW (2004) Cancer genes and the pathways they control. *Nat Med* 10: 789–799

Part II
Breaking Away:
Epithelial-Mesenchymal Transition

Chapter 2
PI3K/AKT Pathway and the Epithelial–Mesenchymal Transition

A. Bellacosa and L. Larue

Cast of Characters

The catalytic subunit of the phosphatidylinositol 3-kinase (*PIK3*; EC 2.7.1.137) is one of the most frequently mutated gene in human cancers, as is its inhibitor *PTEN*. By some estimates, *PIK3CA* carries gain-of-function mutations in 32% of colorectal cancers, 36% of hepatocellular carcinomas, 36% of endometrial carcinomas, 25% of breast carcinomas, 15% of anaplastic oligodendrogliomas, and 5% of medulloblastomas and anaplastic astrocytomas (recently reviewed in Velculescu, 2008). Similarly, spontaneous mutations in *PTEN* are found in 50% of endometrial cancers, 30% of glioblastomas, 10% of prostate, and 5% of breast carcinomas. Moreover, inherited mutations in *PTEN* lead to a variety of conditions, such as Cowden syndrome, which are associated with an increased risk of cancer (recently reviewed in Keniry and Parsons, 2008). In addition, frequent alterations and hyperactivation of AKT kinases have been described in almost every tumor type studied (reviewed in Bellacosa et al., 2005; Brugge et al., 2007). While many of the downstream effectors of the AKT pathway are involved in cell autonomous processes (i.e., cell cycle and apoptosis), the following chapter will focus on the implications of aberrant AKT signaling for epithelial–mesenchymal transition, in particular on the PI3K–AKT–NF-κB–Snail pathway with emphasis on E-cadherin regulation.

Introduction

Epithelial–mesenchymal transition (EMT) is a major developmental process during which epithelial cells develop mesenchymal, fibroblast-like properties, increased motility, and reduced intercellular adhesion. There is growing evidence that

A. Bellacosa (✉)
Human Genetics Program, Epigenetics and Progenitor Cells Program, Fox Chase Cancer Center, Philadelphia PA, USA; Laboratory of Developmental Therapeutics, Regina Elena Cancer Center, Rome, Italy
e-mail: alfonoso.bellacosa@fccc.edu

A. Thomas-Tikhonenko (ed.), *Cancer Genome and Tumor Microenvironment*,
DOI 10.1007/978-1-4419-0711-0_2, © Springer Science+Business Media, LLC 2010

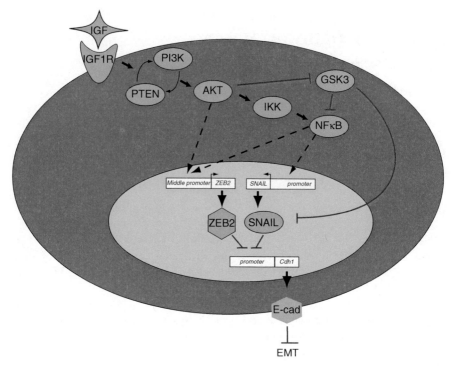

Fig. 2.1 Model of the regulation of E-cadherin transcription by the PI3K/AKT signaling pathway

EMT-like events are central to tumor progression and malignant transformation, endowing the incipient cancer cell with invasive and metastatic properties. Several oncogenic pathways (peptide growth factors, Src, Ras, Ets, integrin, Wnt/β-catenin, and Notch) induce processes characteristic of EMT, such as downregulation of the cell adhesion molecule and obligate epithelial marker E-cadherin. EMT also now appears to involve activation of the IGF/IGF-1R–phosphatidylinositol 3′-kinase (PI3K)/AKT–NF-κB–Snail–E-cadherin axis (Fig. 2.1), which is discussed in the following pages and also Chapter 3.

EMT Definition

EMT was first defined based on morphological features, but currently, morphological, cellular, and molecular factors are also included. Any analysis of EMT requires consideration of the defining features of epithelium and mesenchyme, the start and endpoints of the transition. One fundamental issue is whether the transition involves an abrupt or a gradual passage from one state to the other. Deployment of EMT certainly requires and involves several modifications of the cells, so the transition may appear to be abrupt or gradual depending on the degree of accuracy or precision that is applied, for technical or other reasons.

Epithelial cellular characteristics as determined in various in vivo or in vitro systems can be classified into five groups: (a) cohesive interactions among cells, allowing the formation of continuous cell layers; (b) presence of three types of membrane domains (apical, lateral, and basal); (c) presence of tight junctions between apical and lateral domains; (d) polarized distribution of the various organelles and components of the cytoskeleton; and (e) near immobility of cells in the local epithelial microenvironment. Based on these properties, epithelia perform three types of function: they form large surfaces for exchange (e.g., the alveolar epithelium in the lung for gaseous exchange), and this includes the creation of cavities by epithelial layer folding (e.g., the intestine and the neural tube); the separation of biological compartments with the selective permeability of the cells, ensuring different ionic compositions of the compartments; and trafficking macromolecules by absorption, transcytosis, and vectorial secretion.

A major property allowing the formation and the maintenance of an epithelium is adhesion: cell–cell adhesion, between the sides of the cells, and cell–matrix adhesion, mostly involving the basal surfaces of the cells. Cell–cell adhesion is a defining characteristic of epithelia, ensuring tissue cohesiveness, whereas other cell types, including mesenchymal cells, may also express cell–matrix adhesion. Epithelial cell–cell adhesion systems are multiple – gap junctions, adherens junctions, desmosomes, and tight junctions – and involve different families of proteins.

Mesenchymal architecture is unlike the supracellular epithelial organization and in fact mesenchymal cells have various characteristics: (a) loose or no interaction between cells, and consequently no continuous cell layer is formed; (b) there are no apical and lateral membranes; (c) the distribution of the cytoskeletal organelles and components is not polarized; and (d) the cells are motile and in some cases invasive. Mesenchymal functions include support and nutrient supply; also mesenchymes may be transitory intermediates during the formation of an epithelial structure from another epithelial structure – mesenchymal to epithelial transition or MET – during development and cancer progression. Nevertheless, mesenchymal architecture can be durable.

In summary, it is the tightness of cell–cell junctions that determines epithelial organization. Cell–cell adhesion is dependent on transmembrane glycoproteins, including E-cadherin, a typical epithelial marker. If cells do not have an epithelial status, they are, by default, mesenchymal.

EMT During Development and Cancer

During early mammalian embryonic development, there are interconversions between epithelium and mesenchyme, the first MET being the formation of the trophectoderm during preimplantation and the first EMT being the formation of the mesoderm during gastrulation. Mouse mutants have been largely uninformative with regard to PI3K/AKT signaling during early development, but cadherin regulation is clearly involved in early development (Larue et al., 1996). There are further EMT conversions during subsequent embryonic development, some associated with major developmental milestones: the formation of neural crest cells from the neural tube on embryonic day 8 (E8); the formation of the atrial and ventricular mesenchymal septa from the endothelium during heart development on E8; the formation of the sclerotome from somites on E9; the formation of coronary vessel progenitor cells from the epicardium around E10–11; the formation of palate mesenchymal cells from the oral epithelium on E13.5; and the formation of mesenchymal cells during regression of the Mullerian tract on E15. Although regulated differently, these EMT are associated with common events, but the role of PI3K and AKT in these processes remains unclear.

Normal development involves highly regulated spatial and temporal master plans, whereas pathological processes, and in particular transformation, are characterized by stochastic and time-independent sequences of events and some events failing to occur. EMT associated with tumorigenesis may increase the motility and invasiveness of cancer cells, and malignant transformation may involve activation of signaling pathways promoting EMT (Boyer et al., 2000). During tumor progression, there is activation of various processes associated with EMT and resembling those occurring in normal development. Nevertheless, normal EMT and physiopathological EMT differ in important ways. The molecular program leading to EMT during tumor progression is based on amplification of a restricted set of the components of complete developmental EMT. This may be because oncogenic signaling associated with tumorigenesis involves fewer signal transduction pathways.

IGF and EMT

General Functions of IGF

Insulin-like growth factors (IGFs) are peptide ligands that bind to the insulin receptor (IR), the IGF-I receptor (IGF-1R), and the IGF-II receptor (IGF-2R). IR and IGF-1R are both receptor protein tyrosine kinases (RPTK) with intrinsic tyrosine kinase activity and structures similar to that of the classic epidermal growth factor receptor. Structurally related, secreted proteins called IGF-binding proteins (IGFBPs) modulate the biological effects of IGF ligands (but not insulin) and are found in the blood and extracellular spaces. IGFBPs bind to IGFs with affinities similar to those for their receptors. Thus, IGFBPs regulate the bioavailability of IGFs by increasing their longevity, facilitating their transport, and promoting/inhibiting IGF binding to their receptors.

IGFs contribute to various cellular mechanisms including cell growth and cell division, antiapoptotic signaling, invasion, differentiation, migration, and EMT. In particular, phenotypic analysis of genetically engineered mice showed that IGFs are involved in growth control: the relevant mutant mice display somatic undergrowth. Disruption of the *IGF-II* gene results in a birth weight that is only 60% of that of wild-type mice. Disruption of the *IGF-1R* gene results in a birth weight that is 45% of that of wild-type littermates. The embryo birth weight of *IGF-II* and *IGF-1R* gene double mutants is 30% of that of wild-type littermates. Phenotypic analysis suggests that *IGF-II* signals through an alternative receptor, also an IR.

IGFs have powerful mitogenic effects on many cell types, and this may explain, at least in part, these phenotypes. IGFs stimulate cell growth and cell division of numerous cell types both in vivo and in vitro (granulosa, granulosa-luteal cells, Sertoli, Leydig, prostate epithelial, bladder urothelial, smooth and skeletal muscle cells, and also spermatogonia, astrocytes, and osteoblasts). IGFs also regulate apoptosis and thereby cell number; most IGFs are antiapoptotic and are consequently classified as survival factors. IGFs are thus generally mitogenic and IGF signaling is dysregulated in various cancer cells; these observations have led to the view that inappropriate activation of the IGF pathway may be central to carcinogenesis. IGFs are also implicated in physiological invasion mechanisms during development, such as trophoblast invasion of the endometrium during implantation (Rosenfeld and Roberts, 1999).

Surprisingly, IGF promotes the acquisition or the maintenance of the differentiated state of some cell types; it stimulates differentiation of skeletal muscle cells and Leydig cells, modulates androgen production by Sertoli and Leydig cells, and promotes neuronal differentiation and myelinization of the central and peripheral neural systems. Therefore, although proliferation and differentiation are widely considered to be two mutually exclusive cellular states, both are stimulated by IGF. Note that these activities are not incompatible with induction of EMT by IGFs.

IGFs Induce EMT

Various in vitro models, notably NBT-II, MDCK, and MCF7 cell lines and embryonic stem cells, have been used to study the effects of IGFs on cell–cell adhesion.

If not stimulated by IGFs and insulin, NBT-II, MDCK, and MCF7 cells have standard epithelial cell morphology: polarized and tightly attached to each another. Treatment of NBT-II, MDCK, and MCF7 cells with IGF results in loss of cell–cell contacts, and the cells flatten and spread. Embryonic stem (ES) cells, which are tightly cohesive, undergo the same morphological changes upon IGF treatment, whereas mesenchymal NIH-3T3 cells do not. These morphological modifications appear rapidly after exposure to IGF (typically within 1 h) and are not associated with cell division.

Various molecular events accompany the loss of cell–cell contacts: (i) the rapid internalization of E-cadherin and desmoplakin, leading to the disruption of junctional complexes (adherens junctions, desmosomes, and particularly gap junctions) and (ii) the expression of the mesenchymal-specific marker vimentin after 4 days of IGF treatment. The cellular and molecular modifications caused by IGF are thus typical of standard EMT. If IGF is removed, NBT-II cells revert to an epithelial morphology within 24 hours, and E-cadherin relocalizes to cell–cell contacts (Morali et al., 2001); in other words, the IGF-induced transition is reversible.

Minimally, EMT is characterized by tightly attached and polarized epithelial cells becoming a set of loosely attached and nonpolarized mesenchymal cells. Full-blown EMT also involves cell motility. IGF can induce migration of some epithelial cells, for example, MCF7 (Guvakova et al. 2002) and melanoma cells (Li et al., 1994), but not others, for example, NBT-II cells (Morali et al., 2001). Whether IGFs induce minimal or complete EMT seems therefore to depend on the cell type.

IGF-1R and EMT

IGF-1R is a RPTK (for reviews, see Ullrich and Schlessinger, 1990; Schlessinger, 2000; Favelyukis et al., 2001) that binds IGF; such binding activates several signaling pathways (see below), and the diversity of the biological effects of IGFs may be a consequence of this multiplicity of signaling pathways. Five families of cytoplasmic proteins interact with IGF-1R and transmit the outside signal to the cytoplasm: (1) the large Grb family of adaptor proteins containing SH2 (Src homology 2) and SH3 domains; (2) the adaptor protein SHC, with SH2 domains and also numerous tyrosines susceptible to phosphorylation by IGF-1R; (3) the Crk family (Crk-I, Crk-II, and Crk-L) of adaptor proteins, containing both SH2 and SH3 domains; (4) the IRS family of adaptor proteins containing a PTB (phosphotyrosine binding) domain, a tyrosine-rich C-terminal region, and a PH domain, but no SH2 domain (note that IRS-1 and IRS-2 are rapidly phosphorylated by activated IGF-1R); and (5) class I PI3K, a heterodimer consisting of a regulatory subunit, p85, and a lipid kinase catalytic subunit, p110.

A constitutively activated IGF-1R (CD8-IGF-1R) has been expressed in MCF10A breast carcinoma cells, and as expected in view of the activities described above, caused EMT (Kim et al., 2007); in wound-healing and trans-well chamber assays, these cells migrated efficiently and, as assessed using a BD Matrigel invasion chamber, were highly invasive.

Downstream of IGFR

PRL-3 and EMT

Tyrosine phosphatase 4a3 (Ptp4a3 or PRL-3), a 22-kDa protein, is expressed in various tissues both during development and in the adult. Its primary function concerns cell growth (Matter et al., 2001). Two lines of evidence have implicated PRL-3 in EMT: its interaction with integrin α1 and its regulation by growth factors and growth factor receptors (Peng et al., 2006). However, induction of IGF-1R by IGF has not been demonstrated to regulate PRL-3. PRL-3 expression is high in various metastatic cancers (colorectal, breast, ovary, melanoma) and higher in metastatic vs. nonmetastatic tumors of colon, liver, lung, brain, and ovary (Saha et al. 2001; Bardelli et al. 2003). PRL-3 expression promotes cell migration, tumor angiogenesis, invasion, and metastasis in cell culture models, such as the Chinese hamster ovary cancer (CHO), human breast cancer (MCF-7), and murine B16 melanoma (Zeng et al., 2003; Wu et al., 2004). Inversely, the growth of ovarian cancer cells is inhibited by RNA interference-mediated downregulation of PRL-3 (Polato et al., 2005).

Thus, PRL-3 is a metastasis-associated phosphatase that may acts as an upstream regulator of PTEN (Wang et al., 2007a).

PTEN and EMT

Phosphatase and tensin homolog (PTEN) is a lipid and protein phosphatase that inhibits diverse signaling pathways and biological processes via its lipid phosphatase activity on the $3'$ phosphate of phosphatidylinositol (PtdIns)(3,4,5)P3 and PtdIns(3,4)P2. PtdIns(3,4,5)P3 and PtdIns(3,4)P2 are elements of the PI3K/AKT signaling pathway and have various cellular functions (see below).

PTEN is involved in proliferation, angiogenesis, and cell survival (Stambolic et al., 1998; Sun et al., 1999; Hamada et al., 2005). Although there is no direct evidence for a major contribution of PTEN to EMT in mammals, it affects cell migration. Indeed, murine embryonic fibroblasts (MEFs) migrate faster in vitro in the absence of PTEN (Liliental et al., 2000). Expression of exogenous PTEN in PTEN-null MEFs, or in aggressive colon or prostate carcinoma cell lines, substantially inhibits migration (Tamura et al. 1998; Liliental et al. 2000; Chu and Tarnawski 2004).

AKT is the best known downstream target of PTEN and may be its main effector in EMT; however, the specific molecular mechanisms connecting PTEN to AKT in mammals have not been investigated. PTEN mutants have been used in an elegant study demonstrating the importance of PTEN and its lipid and protein phosphatase activities in chicken, at the gastrulation stage of development (Leslie et al. 2007). During gastrulation, some ectodermal cells in the primitive streak undergo EMT and migrate away to produce mesodermal cells. These cells then migrate back toward the midline. Cells from the primitive streak can be grafted into a different embryo before outward migration. Consequently, the donor cells can be manipulated genetically after initial and appropriate electroporation of donor chicken embryos and before grafting. This allowed the demonstration that the protein–phosphatase activity, but not the lipid–phosphatase activity, of PTEN in these cells was involved in EMT during early gastrulation. The lipid–phosphatase activity may affect cell polarity and directional cell migration later during gastrulation. If AKT is regulated by the lipid–phosphatase activity, but not the protein–phosphatase activity, of PTEN, it is presumably not involved in early mesodermal EMT in chicken. However, work with other model systems suggests that AKT is involved in EMT.

PI3K and AKT

Biochemical Mechanisms

Direct binding of p85, the regulatory subunit of PI3K, to the tyrosine-phosphorylated forms of IGF-1R and IRS-1 triggers tyrosine phosphorylation and consequently a conformational change of p85, activating p110, the PI3K catalytic subunit. It should be noted that Ras-GTP can activate p110 directly (Kodaki et al. 1994; Rodriguez-Viciana et al. 1996).

Active PI3K phosphorylates the 3'-OH group of the inositol ring of phosphatidylinositol (PtdIns), PtdIns(4)P, and Ptd(4,5)P to produce Ptd(3)P, PtdIns(3,4)P_2, and PtdIns(3,4,5)P3 (also called D3-phosphorylated phosphoinositides), respectively. Amphipathic PtdIns(3,4)P_2 and PtdIns(3,4,5)P3 molecules bind to proteins containing a pleckstrin homology (PH) domain. Serine/threonine kinases, including AKT1, -2, and -3 (also known as PKB alpha, beta, and gamma, respectively), and PDK1 (phosphatidylinositol-dependent kinase 1), translocate to the cell membrane upon binding to these D3-phosphorylated phosphoinositides. AKT is then appropriately localized for phosphorylation of its threonine 308 by PDK1 and serine 473 by PDK2. The identity of PDK2, the kinase(s) responsible for Ser-473/474 phosphorylation, has been the subject of debate (Chan and Tsichlis, 2001). AKT phosphorylated on T308 and S473 is fully active.

AKT kinases phosphorylate diverse molecules at threonine or serine residues with different functional outcomes, stimulatory or inhibitory. For instance, AKT family members regulate the activity of several transcription factors, notably CREB (cAMP-response element-binding protein), members of Forkhead family, and Ets-2. AKT phosphorylation of CREB stimulates CREB-dependent transcription (Du and Montminy, 1998), whereas AKT phosphorylation of FKHR (Forkhead in rhabdomyosarcoma) and FKHRL1 (Forkhead in rhabdomyosarcoma-like 1) inhibits CREB-dependent transcription (Brunet et al. 1999; Tang et al. 1999). Ets-2-dependent transcription is activated when Ets-2 is phosphorylated by JNK-2 in cells in which AKT is also activated (Smith et al. 2000).

Ras-mediated reorganization of the actin cytoskeleton and cell migration also depends on PI3K. Indeed, some membrane lipid targets of PI3K regulate (i) the activity and structure of actin-binding proteins and (ii) the GTPase Rac, thereby controlling membrane folding.

General Functions of AKT

AKT promotes cell cycle progression, cell survival, and tumor cell invasion (Testa and Bellacosa 2001). Interestingly, it also phosphorylates and inhibits GSK-3β, thereby, presumably, linking IGF and Wnt pathways.

Activated AKT kinases phosphorylate numerous substrates associated with cell proliferation, survival, intermediary metabolism, and cell growth. The consensus sequence for AKT phosphorylation, RXRXXS/T, is found in most but not all these substrates.

AKT stimulates proliferation in various ways. It phosphorylates and inhibits glycogen synthase kinase 3β (GSK3β; the first AKT substrate identified) (Cross et al. 1995) and thereby inhibits the degradation of cyclin D1 (Diehl et al. 1998); it also simultaneously upregulates translation (see below) of the cyclin D1 and D3 mRNAs (Muise-Helmericks et al. 1998). AKT phosphorylates the cell cycle inhibitors p21^{WAF1} and p27^{Kip1} near their nuclear localization signal such that they are retained in the cytoplasm, remaining inactive. In contrast, Mdm2 requires AKT phosphorylation for translocation to the nucleus, where it complexes with p53 promoting its ubiquitin/proteasome-mediated degradation (Testa and Bellacosa 2001). Thus, several tumor suppressors, including p21^{WAF1}, p27^{Kip1}, and p53, are inhibited by AKT, and this is specular to inhibition of the oncogenic PI3K/AKT axis by the tumor suppressor PTEN. Inhibition of p53 function is particularly relevant to the control of cell cycle checkpoints associated with DNA damage.

AKT also acts through various mechanisms to generate survival signals that prevent programmed cell death (Testa and Bellacosa 2001; Franke et al. 2003). It phosphorylates the proapoptotic factor BAD, and thereby stops cytochrome c from being released from mitochondria, and also phosphorylates (pro)caspase 9, thereby inhibiting the consequences of cytochrome c release. PED/PEA15, a cytosolic inhibitor of caspase-3, is also phosphorylated and stabilized by AKT (Trencia et al. 2003). AKT kinases deliver antiapoptotic signals involving positive and negative transcriptional mechanisms. AKT phosphorylation restricts nuclear entry of transcription factors of the Forkhead family, as it does for p21^{WAF1} and p27^{Kip1}, preventing transcription of proapoptotic genes: *Fas ligand*, *BIM*, *TRAIL*, and *TRADD*. It phosphorylates and activates IκB kinase (IKK), causing degradation of IκB, and consequently stimulates translocation of NF-κB to the nucleus and transcription of *BFL1*, *cIAP1*, *cIAP2*, all antiapoptotic genes. AKT also phosphorylates and inactivates the apoptosis signal-regulating kinase, ASK1.

AKT kinases are also involved in intermediary metabolism, and in particular glucose metabolism. It phosphorylates and inactivates GSK3, resulting in increased glycogen synthesis. Note that GSK3 is also involved in the Wnt/wingless pathway that includes β-catenin and the tumor suppressor APC. Although AKT may thus interact with this pathway, any such interaction is probably indirect and very complex (Grille et al. 2003). Following insulin stimulation, glucose transport is increased by AKT phosphorylation of the glucose transporters GLUT1 and GLUT4, and their translocation to the membrane (Kohn et al. 1996), whereas AKT phosphorylation of phosphofructokinase stimulates glycolysis (Deprez et al. 1997). The relationship between the metabolic consequences of AKT activation and its antiapoptotic functions is complex (Gottlob et al. 2001; Plas et al. 2002), and AKT regulation of cell growth also reveals interplay between different AKT functions.

Work with animal models implicated AKT kinases in the control of cell growth. Cells grow (defined here as an increase in cell size rather than cell number) in response to increased availability of nutrients, energy, and mitogens. mTOR, the mammalian target of rapamycin, is a kinase downstream from PI3K that mediates cell growth pathways by stimulating protein synthesis. mTOR phosphorylates directly or indirectly two targets with immediate effects on translation: p70 ribosomal protein S6 kinase (p70 S6K) and eukaryotic initiation factor 4E-binding protein 1 (4E-BP1). p70 S6K phosphorylates the ribosomal protein S6, thereby increasing translation of mRNAs containing 5′-terminal oligopolypyrimidine (5′TOP) tracts. In contrast, phosphorylation of 4E-BP1 relieves inhibition of the initiation factor eIF4E such that the efficiency of cap-dependent translation is increased (Ruggero and Pandolfi, 2003).

mTOR is clearly activated downstream from AKT, but the activation mechanism has not been established. Although mTOR is a direct target of AKT in vitro, mTOR activation by AKT in vivo may be very complex. The tuberous sclerosis (TSC) 2 protein is one of the numerous targets of AKT signaling. Tuberous sclerosis complex, a hereditary disorder characterized by the formation of hamartomas in various organs, is a consequence of mutations in either *TSC1* or *TSC2* tumor suppressor genes. The TSC1 and TSC2 proteins form a complex in vivo, and the complex inhibits signaling by mTOR, possibly through TSC2 GTPase-activating protein (GAP) activity toward the Ras family small GTPase Rheb. TSC2 – one of many tumor suppressors antagonized by AKT – is phosphorylated and inhibited by AKT signaling (Inoki et al. 2002; Potter et al. 2002); this destabilizes TSC2 and disrupts its interaction with TSC1, leading to the activation of the mTOR/p70 S6 kinase/eIF4E pathways. Consequently, mTOR is a potential target for chemopreventive or chemotherapeutic treatment of tuberous sclerosis patients.

The mTOR pathway is activated in many human tumors, suggesting that tumorigenesis is associated with abnormal regulation of nutrient availability. However, cell size in tumors is rarely larger than that in normal tissues. Consequently, the abnormal activation of the AKT/mTOR pathway in tumors may be further evidence of interplay between different functions. Indeed, there is recent evidence that the mTOR/eIF4E pathway can provide an antiapoptotic signal, in addition to growth/translation control. It is also plausible that mTOR promotes chromosomal instability which is then selected during tumorigenesis (Aoki et al. 2003).

AKT phosphorylates and activates other targets implicated in cancer, including nitric oxide synthase (that promotes angiogenesis) and the reverse transcriptase subunit of telomerase (that stimulates unlimited replicative potential).

The number of known AKT substrates is growing but it is still not clear whether each of the various members of the AKT family has their own substrates or whether the specificities of AKT1, -2 and -3 are determined by their tissue distribution, temporal expression, or upstream activation. However, work on AKT activation using human cancer and animal models suggests that the family members are not completely redundant and may be differentially activated/inactivated in various physiological and disease states.

AKT and EMT

It has become evident that EMT is one of the many cellular processes subject to AKT kinase regulation. EMT driven by activated AKT (Grille et al. 2003) involves loss of cell–cell adhesion, morphological changes, loss of apico-basolateral cell polarization, induction of cell motility, reduced cell–matrix adhesion, and changes in the production or the distribution of various proteins. For example, desmoplakin, a protein involved in the formation and maintenance of desmosomes, is internalized, and vimentin, an intermediate filament protein found in many mesenchymal cells, is induced. AKT also induces production of metalloproteinases and cell invasion (Kim et al. 2001; Park et al. 2001; Irie et al. 2005).

GSK3 and EMT

Glycogen synthase kinase-3 (GSK-3) is a ubiquitously expressed protein serine kinase. It participates in glycogen metabolism and in both the Wnt/β-catenin and the PI3K/AKT signaling pathways; it has antiapoptotic and proliferative activities (Hoeflich et al. 2000) and is involved in differentiation and morphogenesis (Hoeflich et al. 2000; Tang et al. 2003).

GSK3 is also involved in EMT (Bachelder et al. 2005): treatment with a specific GSK3 inhibitor (SB415286) causes an EMT in human epithelial breast cancer cells (MCF10). Genetic inhibition of GSK3 activates Snail transcription in both MCF10 and human keratinocyte cells (HaCaT) (Zhou et al. 2004; Bachelder et al. 2005); pharmacological inhibition of GSK3 in HaCaT cells leads to the activation of NF-κB through IκB

From AKT to NF-κB

General Functions of NF-κB

The protein NF-κB is a transcription factor that binds to the DNA sequence gggACTTTCC that was originally found in the intronic enhancer of the immunoglobulin κ light chain in B cells. Through its stimulation of the transcription of various genes, including *c-myc*, *Ras*, and *p53*, NF-κB participates in numerous aspects of cell growth, survival, differentiation, and proliferation. However, one of its major known functions is in stress, injury, and especially immune responses. NF-κB is central to tumorigenesis, mainly in solid tumors, in which it is constitutively active and controls the expression and function of a number of pertinent genes (Pacifico and Leonardi, 2006). Active NF-κB switches on the expression of genes that promote proliferation and protect cells from proapoptotic conditions that would otherwise cause them to die. NF-κB can be constitutively active, and this is the consequence of mutations in genes encoding the NF-κB transcription factors themselves and in genes that control NF-κB activity (such as IκB genes) or is a consequence of constitutive and abnormal secretion of NF-κB-activating factors.

NF-κB and EMT

NF-κB can induce EMT in breast, bladder, and squamous carcinoma cell lines (Huber et al. 2004; Chua et al. 2007; Julien et al. 2007; Wang et al. 2007b), and the induction is either indirect (Wang et al. 2007a) or direct (Chua et al. 2007; Julien et al. 2007). Indirect activation of EMT by NF-κB has been described in estrogen receptor (ERα)-negative breast cancer cells, and in particular MDA-MB-231 cells. In association with c-Jun/Fra-2, p50–p65 NF-κB stimulated the expression of RelB, and this induction of RelB led to the induction of Bcl-2; Bcl-2 then suppressed radiation-induced apoptosis and induced EMT. More direct activation of EMT by NF-κB is found in various cell lines, although the pathways involved, while sharing the same end target – the E-cadherin gene, were not all based on the induction of the same intermediate transcription factor (Snail or ZEB-1/ZEB-2).

Snail and Related Transcription Factors in EMT

Snail is a zinc finger transcription factor and the Snail family also includes Slug (also called Snai2) and Smuc (or Snai3 or Zfp293). Snail is best known as a repressor of transcription and it was identified as being essential for *Drosophila* development and, in particular, correct gastrulation.

Snail and Slug (encoded by Snai1 and Snai2 genes, respectively) together with the transcription factor Twist are involved in mesoderm formation. Snail and E-cadherin expressions are inversely correlated. Abnormal Snail production in numerous cell lines and primary tumors is associated with aggressiveness and loss of E-cadherin expression (Birchmeier and Behrens 1994; De Craene et al. 2005).

Snail or Slug overproduction in vitro induces EMT (Batlle et al. 2000); and repression of Snail RNA production is associated with E-cadherin upregulation and MET. E-cadherin is subject to an interesting positive–negative regulation (Palmer et al. 2004): it is positively regulated by $1,25(OH)_2D3$ via the vitamin D receptor and Snail can repress both E-cadherin and vitamin D receptor, so the balance between vitamin D receptors and Snail may regulate E-cadherin levels (Palmer et al. 2004). Phosphorylation of Snail by the p21-activated kinase PAK1 causes it to be retained in the nucleus and stimulates its repressor activity (Yang et al. 2005). These various observations indicate the complexity of E-cadherin regulation during EMT.

Sip1 (also known as ZFHX1B or SMADIP1) is a member of the delta EF1/Zfh1 family of two-handed zinc finger/homeodomain proteins. It contains a Smad-binding domain through which it interacts with full-length Smad proteins and may therefore modulate EMT induction by the TGFβ signaling pathway. Many patients with mega-colon or Hirschsprung disease carry mutations in the *Sip1* gene (Amiel and Lyonnet, 2001; Cacheux et al. 2001; Wakamatsu et al. 2001; Yamada et al. 2001; Van de Putte et al. 2003). Mice with targeted inactivation of Sip1 have been obtained. These mice present clinical features of Hirschsprung disease–mental retardation syndrome: they fail to develop postotic vagal neural crest cells – the precursors of the enteric nervous system affected in patients with Hirschsprung disease – and display arrest in the delamination of cranial neural crest cells, which form the skeletal muscle elements of the vertebral head; in the absence of Sip1, the neural crest cells are not correctly delaminated. The delamination of neural crest cells is a good example of EMT requiring cadherin downregulation.

E-cadherin and EMT

E-cadherin is one of the main effectors of EMT, and many details of the regulation of E-cadherin signaling during EMT have been described. E-cadherin participates in both EMT and MET, and cells undergoing EMT necessarily downregulate E-cadherin.

E-cadherin and Epithelial Cells

The detailed overview of this system is provided in Chapter 3. Briefly, this cell–cell adhesion molecule is a calcium-dependent transmembrane glycoprotein. In particular, cadherin molecules associate at the cell surface in a Ca^{2+}-dependent manner through homophilic interactions, thus mediating cell–cell adhesion. It is found in most epithelial cells in both embryonic and adult tissues, and is essential for normal embryonic development and homeostasis. Consequently, there has been substantial interest in its regulation. Generally, both the transcription and the translation of cadherins are regulated, and the mechanisms include changes in subcellular distribution, translational and transcriptional events, and degradation. E-cadherin is classified as a tumor suppressor for two reasons: its gene is silent in various carcinomas, and re-expression of a native form of E-cadherin in carcinomas in vitro reduces the aggressiveness of tumor cells (Vleminckx et al. 1991). Further supporting its classification as a tumor suppressor, germline mutations of the E-cadherin gene (called *CDH1*) are associated with a syndrome of hereditary gastric and colorectal cancer (Guilford et al. 1998; Suriano et al. 2003).

The loss of E-cadherin function observed in some human carcinomas is associated with the production of a defective protein or transcriptional silencing due to promoter hypermethylation. Gene mutations, abnormal post-translational modifications (phosphorylation or glycosylation), and protein degradation (proteolysis) can all lead to the production of a defective E-cadherin protein. Cases of E-cadherin upregulation in tumor progression have also been reported (Kang and Massague 2004; Thiery and Morgan 2004) but only during intravasation and seeding of metastatic cells.

Alternatively, E-cadherin transcriptional repression may result from the activation of the repressors Snail, Slug, Sip1, and Ets. It is still not known how E-cadherin is internalized/sequestered or the E-cadherin gene repressed, but it has been demonstrated that AKT regulates E-cadherin mRNA and protein abundance (Grille et al. 2003). Two main types of consensus-binding sites have been shown to downregulate E-cadherin expression: Ets sites and palindromic E-boxes (E-pal).

Moreover, the loss of expression of E-cadherin during development and transformation is often associated with increased expression of N-cadherin. The molecular mechanisms underlying this widespread switch remain unclear.

E-cadherin Function Is Modulated by IGF

As mentioned above, IGF affects cell–cell adhesion. The cadherin/catenin complex is undoubtedly a critical determinant for cell–cell adhesion and, as a consequence, there has been substantial work on the signaling pathways that may link IGF-1R and the cadherin/catenin complex.

IGF-1R Interacts Indirectly with E-cadherin and β-catenin

As mentioned above, E-cadherin forms the physical link, resulting in cell–cell adhesion by binding adjacent cell surfaces, thus allowing the formation of large cellular networks and tissues. The cytoplasmic domain of cadherin binds to β-catenin, which binds to α-catenin. As a result, the cadherin/catenin complex is linked to the actin-based cytoskeleton. IGF-1R and E-cadherin are coexpressed in most epithelial cells; they also appear to form a membrane-associated complex as assessed by coimmunoprecipitation experiments (Guvakova and Surmacz 1997; Morali et al. 2001). Immunoprecipitation experiments also indicate that the interaction of IGF-1R with E-cadherin, β-catenin, and α-catenin does not impede the binding of cadherins to catenins. Presumably, there is a supra-molecular complex composed of IGF-1R/E-cadherin/β-catenin/α-catenin on the surface of various cells.

Only the cytoplasmic domain of E-cadherin is required to interact with the cytoplasmic domain of the IGF-1Rβ subunit (Morali et al. 2001). However, protein–protein interaction assays reveal that IGF-1R does not interact directly with either E-cadherin or β-catenin (Morali et al. 2001). The molecules linking members of the complex together have not been identified.

IGFs Redistribute Proteins of Adherens Junctions

Most E-cadherin and β-catenin are found at cell–cell contacts in epithelial cells not exposed to IGFs, and IGF-1R is present both at cell–cell contacts and in the cytoplasm. Treatment with IGFs results in the redistribution of E-cadherin and IGF-1R from the membrane to the cytoplasm, and E-cadherin becomes concentrated in a halo around the nucleus. It has been demonstrated that E-cadherin constantly cycles from the cytoplasm to the cell membrane and back (Bauer et al. 1998; Le et al.

1999). If IGFs are extremely abundant, this equilibrium may be perturbed, and E-cadherin is internalized more rapidly than it is readdressed to the membrane.

These various in vitro observations suggest that the expression of each IGF-II, IGF-1R, and E-cadherin is correlated during gastrulation. At this stage, IGF-II is mainly expressed by mesenchymal cells (mesoderm), E-cadherin is generally absent from murine mesodermal cells (Butz and Larue, 1995), and IGF-1R is found at the membrane of epithelial cells (ectoderm and endoderm) and in the cytoplasm of mesodermal cells.

It has also been suggested that E-cadherin degradation, despite not being extensive, is associated with IGF treatment (Morali et al. 2001). Indeed, a subset of E-cadherin molecules partially colocalize with LAMP1 (lysosomal-associated protein 1), an endosomal and lysosomal marker, consistent with E-cadherin being degraded in LAMP1-positive organelles. Thus, it appears that IGFs cause rapid internalization of E-cadherin, leading to some degradation and sequestration in vesicles near nucleus (Morali et al. 2001). This allows a simple model explaining the reversibility of the EMT: as soon as IGFs are removed from the medium, stored E-cadherin is rapidly readdressed to the membrane.

IGFs also determine the distribution of β-catenin. β-Catenin participates in cell–cell adhesion and in signal transduction through the Wnt signaling pathway. In the absence of Wnt, β-catenin is part of a complex containing GSK-3β (glycogen synthase kinase-3β), APC (adenomatous polyposis coli), and axin. GSK-3β phosphorylates β-catenin, which is then ubiquitinated and degraded by proteasomes (Yost et al. 1996; Aberle et al. 1997). Wnt binding to Frizzled, its cell surface receptor, activates the serine–threonine kinase Dishevelled (Dsh) (Yanagawa et al. 1995; Axelrod et al. 1998; Karasawa et al. 2002). Dsh then phosphorylates GSK-3β and thereby inhibits its activity. Unphosphorylated β-catenin (which cannot be degraded) accumulates in the cytoplasm and is translocated into the nucleus (for review, see Novak and Dedhar 1999). In the nucleus, a complex of β-catenin with TCF/LEF (T-cell factors/lymphoid enhancer factors) can induce or repress the expression of numerous genes including *Cyclin D1, c-Myc, T-Brachyury, c-Jun, Fra-1, Matrix-Metalloprotease-7 (MMP-7), Fibronectin, Cyclo-oxygenase-2, m-Mitf* (melanocyte-specific microphthalmia transcription factor), receptors *EphB2* and *EphB3*, and *ephrin-B1* (He et al. 1998; Brabletz et al. 1999; Crawford et al. 1999; Gradl et al. 1999; Howe et al. 1999; Mann et al. 1999; Shtutman et al. 1999; Arnold et al. 2000; Takeda et al. 2000; Batlle et al. 2002). Some of these genes are expressed ubiquitously (e.g., *cyclin D1*) and others only in certain cell types (e.g., *m-Mitf* in the melanocyte lineage) (Amae et al. 1998; Fuse et al. 1999). IGF treatment results in the translocation of β-catenin from the cell membrane to the nucleus and of TCF3 from the cytoplasm to the nucleus (Morali et al. 2001). No single gene known to be activated/repressed by β-catenin can induce an EMT. Note that not all gene targets of β-catenin have been identified; some as yet unidentified target gene(s) may be involved in EMT. Also, the IGF signaling pathway may induce the expression of genes involved in EMT.

To conclude, IGFs induce a reversible EMT based on reducing the cell–cell adhesion involving E-cadherin and the redistribution of the proteins associated with it.

Indeed, IGF treatment causes (i) rapid delocalization of E-cadherin from cell–cell contacts, (ii) disruption of the interaction between E-cadherin and β-catenin by phosphorylation, (iii) induction of limited degradation of E-cadherin, (iv) activation of genes via β-catenin/TCF, and, self-evidently (v) induction of the IGF signaling pathway.

Other Regulators of E-cadherin

Ets-Binding Sites in the E-cadherin Promoter

An Ets-binding site has been identified at position -97 in the E-cadherin promoter, and indeed, the expression of c-ets-1 in breast carcinoma cell lines induces EMT, partly due to repression of the E-cadherin gene (Gilles et al. 1997; Rodrigo et al. 1999). Ets binding to this region downregulates E-cadherin promoter activity in keratinocyte cell lines (Rodrigo et al. 1999). Ets factors, in addition to being repressors of E-cadherin transcription, upregulate key mediators of invasiveness, including matrilysin, matrix metalloprotease, collagenase, heparanase, and urokinase (reviewed in Shepherd and Hassell, 2001; Hsu et al. 2004).

E-cadherin E-boxes

E-boxes are widespread in genomic sequences. The human E-cadherin promoter contains three E-box consensus sequences (CANNTG). Two are upstream from the coding sequence and one is in exon 1. Snail, Slug, Sip1/Zeb2, and Zeb1 bind to these E-boxes and repress E-cadherin transcription. Presumably, the E-cadherin gene is tightly regulated by the binding of these various transcription factors to its E-boxes.

Conclusions

There has been substantial work on EMT over the last 20 years, and some of the key molecular and cellular events involved have been identified. Also, the signaling pathways mediating the critical events that make up EMT have been described. Our improved insight into these molecular processes leading to and constituting EMT provides the basis for clinical application. In particular, novel therapies involving inhibition of EMT could be developed to prevent the various manifestations of cancer, and particularly local invasion and metastasis. A detailed understanding of the EMT pathways, and their involvement in cell physiology in general, would undoubtedly be beneficial for rational development of therapies with minimal effects on other cellular functions, and therefore minimal toxicity.

Acknowledgments We would like to thank the staff at the Bellacosa and Larue laboratories for constructive discussions and rigorous dedication to this field of research. We apologize to colleagues whose work is not cited – despite its value – due to space constraints. This work was supported by NIH grants CA78412, CA105008, and CA06927. Additional support was provided by an appropriation from the Commonwealth of Pennsylvania to the Fox Chase Cancer Center. The Ligue Contre le Cancer – comité de l'Oise, INCa, cancéropole IdF and Institut Curie also provided support.

References

Aberle, H., Bauer, A., Stappert, J., Kispert, A. and Kemler, R. (1997) Beta-catenin is a target for the ubiquitin-proteasome pathway. Embo J 16: 3797–804.

Amae, S., Fuse, N., Yasumoto, K., Sato, S., Yajima, I., Yamamoto, H., Udono, T., Durlu, Y. K., Tamai, M., Takahashi, K. and Shibahara, S. (1998) Identification of a novel isoform of microphthalmia-associated transcription factor that is enriched in retinal pigment epithelium. Biochem Biophys Res Commun 247: 710–15.

Amiel, J. and Lyonnet, S. (2001) Hirschsprung disease, associated syndromes, and genetics: A review. J Med Genet 38: 729–39.

Aoki, K., Tamai, Y., Horiike, S., Oshima, M. and Taketo, M. M. (2003) Colonic polyposis caused by mTOR-mediated chromosomal instability in Apc+/Delta716 Cdx2+/– compound mutant mice. Nat Genet 35: 323–30.

Arnold, S. J., Stappert, J., Bauer, A., Kispert, A., Herrmann, B. G. and Kemler, R. (2000) Brachyury is a target gene of the Wnt/beta-catenin signaling pathway. Mech Dev 91: 249–58.

Axelrod, J. D., Miller, J. R., Shulman, J. M., Moon, R. T. and Perrimon, N. (1998) Differential recruitment of Dishevelled provides signaling specificity in the planar cell polarity and Wingless signaling pathways. Genes Dev 12: 2610–22.

Bachelder, R. E., Yoon, S. O., Franci, C., de Herreros, A. G. and Mercurio, A. M. (2005) Glycogen synthase kinase-3 is an endogenous inhibitor of Snail transcription: Implications for the epithelial–mesenchymal transition. J Cell Biol 168: 29–33.

Bardelli, A., Saha, S., Sager, J. A., Romans, K. E., Xin, B., Markowitz, S. D., Lengauer, C., Velculescu, V. E., Kinzler, K. W. and Vogelstein, B. (2003) PRL-3 expression in metastatic cancers. Clin Cancer Res 9: 5607–15.

Batlle, E., Sancho, E., Franci, C., Dominguez, D., Monfar, M., Baulida, J. and Garcia De Herreros, A. (2000) The transcription factor snail is a repressor of E-cadherin gene expression in epithelial tumour cells. Nat Cell Biol 2: 84–9.

Batlle, E., Henderson, J. T., Beghtel, H., van den Born, M. M., Sancho, E., Huls, G., Meeldijk, J., Robertson, J., van de Wetering, M., Pawson, T. and Clevers, H. (2002) Beta-catenin and TCF mediate cell positioning in the intestinal epithelium by controlling the expression of EphB/ephrinB. Cell 111: 251–63.

Bauer, A., Lickert, H., Kemler, R. and Stappert, J. (1998) Modification of the E-cadherin-catenin complex in mitotic Madin-Darby canine kidney epithelial cells. J Biol Chem 273: 28314–21.

Bellacosa A, Kumar CC, Di Cristofano A, Testa JR (2005) Activation of AKT Kinases in Cancer: Implications for Therapeutic Targeting. Adv Cancer Res 94:29–86.

Birchmeier, W. and Behrens, J. (1994) Cadherin expression in carcinomas: Role in the formation of cell junctions and the prevention of invasiveness. Biochim Biophys Acta 1198: 11–26.

Boyer, B., Valles, A. M. and Edme, N. (2000) Induction and regulation of epithelial–mesenchymal transitions. Biochem Pharmacol 60: 1091–9.

Brabletz, T., Jung, A., Dag, S., Hlubek, F. and Kirchner, T. (1999) Beta-catenin regulates the expression of the matrix metalloproteinase-7 in human colorectal cancer. Am J Pathol 155: 1033–8.

Brugge J, Hung MC, Mills GB (2007) A new mutational aktivation in the PI3K pathway. Cancer Cell 12:104–7.

Brunet, A., Bonni, A., Zigmond, M. J., Lin, M. Z., Juo, P., Hu, L. S., Anderson, M. J., Arden, K. C., Blenis, J. and Greenberg, M. E. (1999) AKT promotes cell survival by phosphorylating and inhibiting a Forkhead transcription factor. Cell 96: 857–68.

Butz, S. and Larue, L. (1995) Expression of catenins during mouse embryonic development and in adult tissues. Cell Adhes Commun 3: 337–52.

Cacheux, V., Dastot-Le Moal, F., Kaariainen, H., Bondurand, N., Rintala, R., Boissier, B., Wilson, M., Mowat, D. and Goossens, M. (2001) Loss-of-function mutations in SIP1 Smad interacting protein 1 result in a syndromic Hirschsprung disease. Hum Mol Genet 10: 1503–10.

Chan, T. O. and Tsichlis, P. N. (2001) PDK2: A complex tail in one Akt. Sci STKE 2001: E1.

Chu, E. C. and Tarnawski, A. S. (2004) PTEN regulatory functions in tumor suppression and cell biology. Med Sci Monit 10: RA235–41.

Chua, H. L., Bhat-Nakshatri, P., Clare, S. E., Morimiya, A., Badve, S. and Nakshatri, H. (2007) NF-kappaB represses E-cadherin expression and enhances epithelial to mesenchymal transition of mammary epithelial cells: potential involvement of ZEB-1 and ZEB-2. Oncogene 26: 711–24.

Crawford, H. C., Fingleton, B. M., Rudolph-Owen, L. A., Goss, K. J., Rubinfeld, B., Polakis, P. and Matrisian, L. M. (1999) The metalloproteinase matrilysin is a target of beta-catenin transactivation in intestinal tumors. Oncogene 18: 2883–91.

Cross, D. A., Alessi, D. R., Cohen, P., Andjelkovich, M. and Hemmings, B. A. (1995) Inhibition of glycogen synthase kinase-3 by insulin mediated by protein kinase B. Nature 378: 785–9.

De Craene, B., Gilbert, B., Stove, C., Bruyneel, E., van Roy, F. and Berx, G. (2005) The transcription factor snail induces tumor cell invasion through modulation of the epithelial cell differentiation program. Cancer Res 65: 6237–44.

Deprez, J., Vertommen, D., Alessi, D. R., Hue, L. and Rider, M. H. (1997) Phosphorylation and activation of heart 6-phosphofructo-2-kinase by protein kinase B and other protein kinases of the insulin signaling cascades. J Biol Chem 272: 17269–75.

Diehl, J. A., Cheng, M., Roussel, M. F. and Sherr, C. J. (1998) Glycogen synthase kinase-3beta regulates cyclin D1 proteolysis and subcellular localization. Genes Dev 12: 3499–511.

Du, K. and Montminy, M. (1998) CREB is a regulatory target for the protein kinase Akt/PKB. J Biol Chem 273: 32377–9

Favelyukis, S., Till, J. H., Hubbard, S. R. and Miller, W. T. (2001) Structure and autoregulation of the insulin-like growth factor 1 receptor kinase. Nat Struct Biol 8: 1058–63.

Franke, T. F., Hornik, C. P., Segev, L., Shostak, G. A. and Sugimoto, C. (2003) PI3K/AKT and apoptosis: Size matters. Oncogene 22: 8983–98.

Fuse, N., Yasumoto, K., Takeda, K., Amae, S., Yoshizawa, M., Udono, T., Takahashi, K., Tamai, M., Tomita, Y., Tachibana, M. and Shibahara, S. (1999) Molecular cloning of cDNA encoding a novel microphthalmia-associated transcription factor isoform with a distinct amino-terminus. J Biochem (Tokyo) 126: 1043–51.

Gilles, C., Polette, M., Birembaut, P., Brunner, N. and Thompson, E. W. (1997) Expression of c-ets-1 mRNA is associated with an invasive, EMT-derived phenotype in breast carcinoma cell lines. Clin Exp Metastasis 15: 519–26.

Gottlob, K., Majewski, N., Kennedy, S., Kandel, E., Robey, R. B. and Hay, N. (2001) Inhibition of early apoptotic events by Akt/PKB is dependent on the first committed step of glycolysis and mitochondrial hexokinase. Genes Dev 15: 1406–18.

Gradl, D., Kuhl, M. and Wedlich, D. (1999) The Wnt/Wg signal transducer beta-catenin controls fibronectin expression. Mol Cell Biol 19: 5576–87.

Grille, S. J., Bellacosa, A., Upson, J., Klein-Szanto, A. J., van Roy, F., Lee-Kwon, W., Donowitz, M., Tsichlis, P. N. and Larue, L. (2003) The protein kinase AKT induces epithelial mesenchymal transition and promotes enhanced motility and invasiveness of squamous cell carcinoma lines. Cancer Res 63: 2172–8.

Guilford, P., Hopkins, J., Harraway, J., McLeod, M., McLeod, N., Harawira, P., Taite, H., Scoular, R., Miller, A. and Reeve, A. E. (1998) E-cadherin germline mutations in familial gastric cancer. Nature 392: 402–5.

Guvakova, M. A. and Surmacz, E. (1997) Overexpressed IGF-I receptors reduce estrogen growth requirements, enhance survival, and promote E-cadherin-mediated cell–cell adhesion in human breast cancer cells. Exp Cell Res 231: 149–62.

Guvakova, M. A., Adams, J. C. and Boettiger, D. (2002) Functional role of alpha-actinin, PI 3-kinase and MEK1/2 in insulin-like growth factor I receptor kinase regulated motility of human breast carcinoma cells. J Cell Sci 115: 4149–65.

Hamada, K., Sasaki, T., Koni, P. A., Natsui, M., Kishimoto, H., Sasaki, J., Yajima, N., Horie, Y., Hasegawa, G., Naito, M., Miyazaki, J., Suda, T., Itoh, H., Nakao, K., Mak, T. W., Nakano, T. and Suzuki, A. (2005) The PTEN/PI3K pathway governs normal vascular development and tumor angiogenesis. Genes Dev 19: 2054–65.

He, T. C., Sparks, A. B., Rago, C., Hermeking, H., Zawel, L., da Costa, L. T., Morin, P. J., Vogelstein, B. and Kinzler, K. W. (1998) Identification of c-MYC as a target of the APC pathway. Science 281: 1509–12.

Hoeflich, K. P., Luo, J., Rubie, E. A., Tsao, M. S., Jin, O. and Woodgett, J. R. (2000) Requirement for glycogen synthase kinase-3beta in cell survival and NF-kappaB activation. Nature 406: 86–90.

Howe, L. R., Subbaramaiah, K., Chung, W. J., Dannenberg, A. J. and Brown, A. M. (1999) Transcriptional activation of cyclooxygenase-2 in Wnt-1-transformed mouse mammary epithelial cells. Cancer Res 59: 1572–7.

Hsu, Y. S., Wang, J. S. and Wu, T. T. (2004) E-cadherin expression in prostate adenocarcinomas in Chinese and its pathological correlates. Urol Int 73: 36–40.

Huber, M. A., Azoitei, N., Baumann, B., Grunert, S., Sommer, A., Pehamberger, H., Kraut, N., Beug, H. and Wirth, T. (2004) NF-kappaB is essential for epithelial–mesenchymal transition and metastasis in a model of breast cancer progression. J Clin Invest 114: 569–81.

Inoki, K., Li, Y., Zhu, T., Wu, J. and Guan, K. L. (2002) TSC2 is phosphorylated and inhibited by AKT and suppresses mTOR signalling. Nat Cell Biol 4: 648–57.

Irie, H. Y., Pearline, R. V., Grueneberg, D., Hsia, M., Ravichandran, P., Kothari, N., Natesan, S. and Brugge, J. S. (2005) Distinct roles of Akt1 and Akt2 in regulating cell migration and epithelial–mesenchymal transition. J Cell Biol 171: 1023–34.

Julien, S., Puig, I., Caretti, E., Bonaventure, J., Nelles, L., van Roy, F., Dargemont, C., de Herreros, A. G., Bellacosa, A. and Larue, L. (2007) Activation of NF-kappaB by AKT upregulates Snail expression and induces epithelium mesenchyme transition. Oncogene 26: 7445–56.

Kang, Y. and Massague, J. (2004) Epithelial–mesenchymal transitions: Twist in development and metastasis. Cell 118: 277–9.

Karasawa, T., Yokokura, H., Kitajewski, J. and Lombroso, P. J. (2002) Frizzled-9 is activated by Wnt-2 and functions in Wnt/beta-catenin signaling. J Biol Chem 277: 37479–86.

Keniry M, Parsons R (2008) The role of PTEN signaling perturbations in cancer and in targeted therapy. Oncogene 27:5477–85.

Kim, D., Kim, S., Koh, H., Yoon, S. O., Chung, A. S., Cho, K. S. and Chung, J. (2001) Akt/PKB promotes cancer cell invasion via increased motility and metalloproteinase production. Faseb J 15: 1953–62.

Kim, H. J., Litzenburger, B. C., Cui, X., Delgado, D. A., Grabiner, B. C., Lin, X., Lewis, M. T., Gottardis, M. M., Wong, T. W., Attar, R. M., Carboni, J. M. and Lee, A. V. (2007) Constitutively active type I insulin-like growth factor receptor causes transformation and xenograft growth of immortalized mammary epithelial cells and is accompanied by an epithelial-to-mesenchymal transition mediated by NF-kappaB and snail. Mol Cell Biol 27: 3165–75.

Kodaki, T., Woscholski, R., Hallberg, B., Rodriguez-Viciana, P., Downward, J. and Parker, P. J. (1994) The activation of phosphatidylinositol 3-kinase by Ras. Curr Biol 4: 798–6.

Kohn, A. D., Summers, S. A., Birnbaum, M. J. and Roth, R. A. (1996) Expression of a constitutively active AKT Ser/Thr kinase in 3T3-L1 adipocytes stimulates glucose uptake and glucose transporter 4 translocation. J Biol Chem 271: 31372–8.

Larue, L., Antos, C., Butz, S., Huber, O., Delmas, V., Dominis, M. and Kemler, R. (1996) A role for cadherins in tissue formation. Development 122: 3185–94.

Le, T. L., Yap, A. S. and Stow, J. L. (1999) Recycling of E-cadherin: A potential mechanism for regulating cadherin dynamics. J Cell Biol 146: 219–32.

Leslie, N. R., Yang, X., Downes, C. P. and Weijer, C. J. (2007) PtdIns(3,4,5)P(3)-dependent and -independent roles for PTEN in the control of cell migration. Curr Biol 17: 115–25.

Li, Y., Bhargava, M. M., Joseph, A., Jin, L., Rosen, E. M. and Goldberg, I. D. (1994) Effect of hepatocyte growth factor/scatter factor and other growth factors on motility and morphology of non-tumorigenic and tumor cells. In Vitro Cell Dev Biol Anim 30A: 105–10.

Liliental, J., Moon, S. Y., Lesche, R., Mamillapalli, R., Li, D., Zheng, Y., Sun, H. and Wu, H. (2000) Genetic deletion of the Pten tumor suppressor gene promotes cell motility by activation of Rac1 and Cdc42 GTPases. Curr Biol 10: 401–4.

Mann, B., Gelos, M., Siedow, A., Hanski, M. L., Gratchev, A., Ilyas, M., Bodmer, W. F., Moyer, M. P., Riecken, E. O., Buhr, H. J. and Hanski, C. (1999) Target genes of beta-catenin-T cell-factor/lymphoid-enhancer-factor signaling in human colorectal carcinomas. Proc Natl Acad Sci U S A 96: 1603–8.

Matter, W. F., Estridge, T., Zhang, C., Belagaje, R., Stancato, L., Dixon, J., Johnson, B., Bloem, L., Pickard, T., Donaghue, M., Acton, S., Jeyaseelan, R., Kadambi, V. and Vlahos, C. J. (2001) Role of PRL-3, a human muscle-specific tyrosine phosphatase, in angiotensin-II signaling. Biochem Biophys Res Commun 283: 1061–8.

Morali, O. G., Delmas, V., Moore, R., Jeanney, C., Thiery, J. P. and Larue, L. (2001) IGF-II induces rapid beta-catenin relocation to the nucleus during epithelium to mesenchyme transition. Oncogene 20: 4942–50.

Muise-Helmericks, R. C., Grimes, H. L., Bellacosa, A., Malstrom, S. E., Tsichlis, P. N. and Rosen, N. (1998) Cyclin D expression is controlled post-transcriptionally via a phosphatidylinositol 3-kinase/Akt-dependent pathway. J Biol Chem 273: 29864–72.

Novak, A. and Dedhar, S. (1999) Signaling through beta-catenin and Lef/Tcf. Cell Mol Life Sci 56: 523–37.

Pacifico, F. and Leonardi, A. (2006) NF-kappaB in solid tumors. Biochem Pharmacol 72: 1142–52.

Palmer, H. G., Larriba, M. J., Garcia, J. M., Ordonez-Moran, P., Pena, C., Peiro, S., Puig, I., Rodriguez, R., de la Fuente, R., Bernad, A., Pollan, M., Bonilla, F., Gamallo, C., de Herreros, A. G. and Munoz, A. (2004) The transcription factor SNAIL represses vitamin D receptor expression and responsiveness in human colon cancer. Nat Med 10: 917–19.

Park, B. K., Zeng, X. and Glazer, R. I. (2001) Akt1 induces extracellular matrix invasion and matrix metalloproteinase-2 activity in mouse mammary epithelial cells. Cancer Res 61: 7647–53.

Peng, L., Jin, G., Wang, L., Guo, J., Meng, L. and Shou, C. (2006) Identification of integrin alpha1 as an interacting protein of protein tyrosine phosphatase PRL-3. Biochem Biophys Res Commun 342: 179–83.

Plas, D. R., Rathmell, J. C. and Thompson, C. B. (2002) Homeostatic control of lymphocyte survival: Potential origins and implications. Nat Immunol 3: 515–21.

Polato, F., Codegoni, A., Fruscio, R., Perego, P., Mangioni, C., Saha, S., Bardelli, A. and Broggini, M. (2005) PRL-3 phosphatase is implicated in ovarian cancer growth. Clin Cancer Res 11: 6835–9.

Potter, C. J., Pedraza, L. G. and Xu, T. (2002) AKT regulates growth by directly phosphorylating Tsc2. Nat Cell Biol 4: 658–65.

Rodrigo, I., Cato, A. C. and Cano, A. (1999) Regulation of E-cadherin gene expression during tumor progression: the role of a new Ets-binding site and the E-pal element. Exp Cell Res 248: 358–71.

Rodriguez-Viciana, P., Warne, P. H., Vanhaesebroeck, B., Waterfield, M. D. and Downward, J. (1996) Activation of phosphoinositide 3-kinase by interaction with Ras and by point mutation. Embo J 15: 2442–51.

Rosenfeld, R. G. and Roberts, C. T. (1999). The IGF system: Molecular Biology, Physiology, and Clincial Applications (Contemporary Endocrinology). Humana Press, Towanda, NJ.

Ruggero, D. and Pandolfi, P. P. (2003) Does the ribosome translate cancer? Nat Rev Cancer 3: 179–92.

Saha, S., Bardelli, A., Buckhaults, P., Velculescu, V. E., Rago, C., St Croix, B., Romans, K. E., Choti, M. A., Lengauer, C., Kinzler, K. W. and Vogelstein, B. (2001) A phosphatase associated with metastasis of colorectal cancer. Science 294: 1343–6.

Schlessinger, J. (2000) Cell signaling by receptor tyrosine kinases. Cell 103: 211–25.

Shepherd, T. and Hassell, J. A. (2001) Role of Ets transcription factors in mammary gland development and oncogenesis. J Mammary Gland Biol Neoplasia 6: 129–40.

Shtutman, M., Zhurinsky, J., Simcha, I., Albanese, C., D'Amico, M., Pestell, R. and Ben-Ze'ev, A. (1999) The cyclin D1 gene is a target of the beta-catenin/LEF-1 pathway. Proc Natl Acad Sci U S A 96: 5522–7.

Smith, J. L., Schaffner, A. E., Hofmeister, J. K., Hartman, M., Wei, G., Forsthoefel, D., Hume, D. A. and Ostrowski, M. C. (2000) ets-2 is a target for an akt (Protein kinase B)/jun N-terminal kinase signaling pathway in macrophages of motheaten-viable mutant mice. Mol Cell Biol 20: 8026–34.

Stambolic, V., Suzuki, A., de la Pompa, J. L., Brothers, G. M., Mirtsos, C., Sasaki, T., Ruland, J., Penninger, J. M., Siderovski, D. P. and Mak, T. W. (1998) Negative regulation of PKB/Akt-dependent cell survival by the tumor suppressor PTEN. Cell 95: 29–39.

Sun, H., Lesche, R., Li, D. M., Liliental, J., Zhang, H., Gao, J., Gavrilova, N., Mueller, B., Liu, X. and Wu, H. (1999) PTEN modulates cell cycle progression and cell survival by regulating phosphatidylinositol 3,4,5,-trisphosphate and Akt/protein kinase B signaling pathway. Proc Natl Acad Sci U S A 96: 6199–204.

Suriano, G., Oliveira, C., Ferreira, P., Machado, J. C., Bordin, M. C., De Wever, O., Bruyneel, E. A., Moguilevsky, N., Grehan, N., Porter, T. R., Richards, F. M., Hruban, R. H., Roviello, F., Huntsman, D., Mareel, M., Carneiro, F., Caldas, C. and Seruca, R. (2003) Identification of CDH1 germline missense mutations associated with functional inactivation of the E-cadherin protein in young gastric cancer probands. Hum Mol Genet 12: 575–82.

Takeda, K., Takemoto, C., Kobayashi, I., Watanabe, A., Nobukuni, Y., Fisher, D. E. and Tachibana, M. (2000) Ser298 of MITF, a mutation site in Waardenburg syndrome type 2, is a phosphorylation site with functional significance. Hum Mol Genet 9: 125–32.

Tamura, M., Gu, J., Matsumoto, K., Aota, S., Parsons, R. and Yamada, K. M. (1998) Inhibition of cell migration, spreading, and focal adhesions by tumor suppressor PTEN. Science 280: 1614–17.

Tang, E. D., Nunez, G., Barr, F. G. and Guan, K. L. (1999) Negative regulation of the forkhead transcription factor FKHR by Akt. J Biol Chem 274: 16741–6.

Tang, Q. Q., Otto, T. C. and Lane, M. D. (2003) Mitotic clonal expansion: a synchronous process required for adipogenesis. Proc Natl Acad Sci U S A 100: 44–9.

Testa, J. R. and Bellacosa, A. (2001) AKT plays a central role in tumorigenesis. Proc Natl Acad Sci U S A 98: 10983–5.

Thiery, J. P. and Morgan, M. (2004) Breast cancer progression with a Twist. Nat Med 10: 777–8.

Trencia, A., Perfetti, A., Cassese, A., Vigliotta, G., Miele, C., Oriente, F., Santopietro, S., Giacco, F., Condorelli, G., Formisano, P. and Beguinot, F. (2003) Protein kinase B/AKT binds and phosphorylates PED/PEA-15, stabilizing its antiapoptotic action. Mol Cell Biol 23: 4511–21.

Ullrich, A. and Schlessinger, J. (1990) Signal transduction by receptors with tyrosine kinase activity. Cell 61: 203–12.

Van de Putte, T., Maruhashi, M., Francis, A., Nelles, L., Kondoh, H., Huylebroeck, D. and Higashi, Y. (2003) Mice lacking ZFHX1B, the gene that codes for Smad-interacting protein-1, reveal a role for multiple neural crest cell defects in the etiology of Hirschsprung disease-mental retardation syndrome. Am J Hum Genet 72: 465–70.

Velculescu VE (2008) Defining the blueprint of the cancer genome. Carcinogenesis 29:1087–91.

Vleminckx, K., Vakaet, L., Jr., Mareel, M., Fiers, W. and van Roy, F. (1991) Genetic manipulation of E-cadherin expression by epithelial tumor cells reveals an invasion suppressor role. Cell 66: 107–19.

Wakamatsu, N., Yamada, Y., Yamada, K., Ono, T., Nomura, N., Taniguchi, H., Kitoh, H., Mutoh, N., Yamanaka, T., Mushiake, K., Kato, K., Sonta, S. and Nagaya, M. (2001) Mutations in SIP1, encoding Smad interacting protein-1, cause a form of Hirschsprung disease. Nat Genet 27: 369–70.

Wang, H., Quah, S. Y., Dong, J. M., Manser, E., Tang, J. P. and Zeng, Q. (2007a) PRL-3 down-regulates PTEN expression and signals through PI3K to promote epithelial–mesenchymal transition. Cancer Res 67: 2922–6.

Wang, X., Zheng, M., Liu, G., Xia, W., McKeown-Longo, P. J., Hung, M. C. and Zhao, J. (2007b) Kruppel-like factor 8 induces epithelial to mesenchymal transition and epithelial cell invasion. Cancer Res 67: 7184–93.

Wu, X., Obata, T., Khan, Q., Highshaw, R. A., De Vere White, R. and Sweeney, C. (2004) The phosphatidylinositol-3 kinase pathway regulates bladder cancer cell invasion. BJU Int 93: 143–50.

Yamada, K., Yamada, Y., Nomura, N., Miura, K., Wakako, R., Hayakawa, C., Matsumoto, A., Kumagai, T., Yoshimura, I., Miyazaki, S., Kato, K., Sonta, S., Ono, H., Yamanaka, T., Nagaya, M. and Wakamatsu, N. (2001) Nonsense and frameshift mutations in ZFHX1B, encoding Smad-interacting protein 1, cause a complex developmental disorder with a great variety of clinical features. Am J Hum Genet 69: 1178–85.

Yanagawa, S., van Leeuwen, F., Wodarz, A., Klingensmith, J. and Nusse, R. (1995) The dishevelled protein is modified by wingless signaling in Drosophila. Genes Dev 9: 1087–97.

Yang, Z., Rayala, S., Nguyen, D., Vadlamudi, R. K., Chen, S. and Kumar, R. (2005) Pak1 phosphorylation of snail, a master regulator of epithelial-to-mesenchyme transition, modulates snail's subcellular localization and functions. Cancer Res 65: 3179–84.

Yost, C., Torres, M., Miller, J. R., Huang, E., Kimelman, D. and Moon, R. T. (1996) The axis-inducing activity, stability, and subcellular distribution of beta-catenin is regulated in Xenopus embryos by glycogen synthase kinase 3. Genes Dev 10: 1443–54.

Zeng, Q., Dong, J. M., Guo, K., Li, J., Tan, H. X., Koh, V., Pallen, C. J., Manser, E. and Hong, W. (2003) PRL-3 and PRL-1 promote cell migration, invasion, and metastasis. Cancer Res 63: 2716–22.

Zhou, B. P., Deng, J., Xia, W., Xu, J., Li, Y. M., Gunduz, M. and Hung, M. C. (2004) Dual regulation of Snail by GSK-3beta-mediated phosphorylation in control of epithelial–mesenchymal transition. Nat Cell Biol 6: 931–40.

Chapter 3
Loss of Cadherin–Catenin Adhesion System in Invasive Cancer Cells

Wen-Hui Lien and Valeri Vasioukhin

Cast of Characters

As described in the previous chapter, the loss of E-cadherin is the key event in epithelial–mesenchymal transition. While downregulation of E-cadherin could occur via aberrant Akt signaling, direct somatic mutations in *E-cadherin* are frequent in epithelial tumors such as diffuse-type gastric and lobular breast cancers, where they can be found in up to 50% of primary neoplasms (Berx et al. 1998). *E-cadherin* mutations were also observed in primary endometrial and ovarian carcinomas, albeit with a lower frequency (Risinger et al. 1994; Muta et al. 1996). The consequences of these mutations for EMT and tumor cell invasion are discussed below.

Introduction

Properly organized intercellular adhesion is critical for the assembly of all metazoan organisms. Cell–cell adhesion is especially prominent in all epithelial tissues, where it helps to seal the membranes of neighboring cells to generate a tissue that provides a barrier function separating organisms from the environment and different compartments within the organism from each other. The majority of human tumors arise in epithelial tissues and one of the most noticeable hallmarks of epithelial tumors is the loss of highly ordered cellular organization. This is usually accompanied by an abnormal focal increase in cell number and formation of a primary tumor. Most of the tumors at this stage can be cured by surgical removal. However, when cancer cells spread beyond the primary tumor and establish metastatic foci in distant organs, the cancer becomes essentially incurable. Thus, understanding of how and why cancer cells disseminate throughout the body is one of the central questions of cancer biology. Detailed knowledge of this process can result in development of efficient targeted therapies that can prevent tumor metastasis and save lives.

V. Vasioukhin (✉)
Division of Human Biology, Fred Hutchinson Cancer Research Center, C3-168, Seattle, WA, USA
e-mail: vvasiouk@fhcrc.org

A. Thomas-Tikhonenko (ed.), *Cancer Genome and Tumor Microenvironment*,
DOI 10.1007/978-1-4419-0711-0_3, © Springer Science+Business Media, LLC 2010

Metastasis is an extraordinarily complex process which involves such physiologically dissimilar processes as breakage from the tumor mass, local migration and invasion, intravasation into blood or lymphatic vasculature, survival in circulation, extravasation, survival in the distant organs, angiogenesis, and growth of the distant metastatic foci. This chapter concentrates on the role of cell–cell adhesion mechanisms in epithelial tumor metastasis. Disruption or modification of intercellular adhesion appears to be critical for initial stages of tumor metastasis, especially during primary cell tumor invasion. In general, well-differentiated, low-grade tumors display prominent cell–cell adhesion and are less likely to metastasize. In contrast, the high-grade tumors contain less-differentiated cells that often show disruption of cell–cell adhesion. This can happen either focally at the invasive front of the tumor or throughout the extensive regions of the primary tumor. Activation of many pro-tumorigenic signaling pathways results in disruption of epithelial organization and acquisition of a migratory cellular phenotype that facilitates tumor cell migration and invasion. In cultured cells the process may be so dramatic that it results in a complete loss of epithelial differentiation and acquisition of a mesenchymal cell phenotype (epithelial to mesenchymal transition, EMT). While it is still debated whether such a dramatic transition takes place in the primary tumors in cancer patients, it appears that at least some elements of decreased epithelial and increased mesenchymal phenotypes indeed occur and in fact are responsible for the local cancer cell invasion, as well as intravasation and extravasation. We will discuss the evidence implicating changes in cell–cell adhesion mechanisms in tumor progression and metastasis.

Overview of Cadherin–Catenin Adhesion System

Epithelial cells can form different types of cell–cell adhesion structures. One of these structures, the adherens junction (AJ), has been heavily implicated in human cancer. Cadherins and catenins are the essential core molecules of the AJs (Fig. 3.1). Cadherin is a transmembrane protein directly involved in homophilic adhesive interactions. Cadherins are a large family of a rather diverse transmembrane proteins that carry extracellular domain containing several 110 amino acids-long cadherin repeats. Based on the overall domain structure of the proteins and the number of cadherin domain repeats, cadherin superfamily can be subdivided into classical, protocadherins, and atypical cadherins. The classical cadherins include well-known E(epithelial)-, P(placental)-, VE(vasculo-endothelial)-, and N(neural)-cadherins. This is the most studied cadherin family that can bind to catenins through their cytoplasmic domain and confer strong adhesive interactions. In this chapter, we will concentrate on the role and significance of classical cadherins in cancer progression. While nonclassical and atypical cadherins may play an important role in cancer (for example, the atypical cadherin Fat is a tumor suppressor in Drosophila), their role in mammalian cancer is still not well understood.

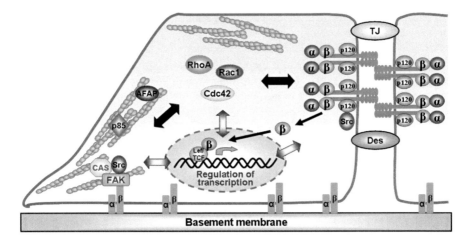

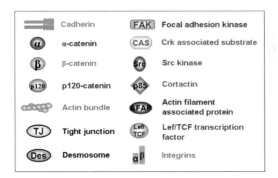

Fig. 3.1 Cadherin–catenin adhesion system. Cadherin-catenin complexes are clustered by actin cytoskeleton at the sites of cell–cell contacts and promote strong adhesive interaction. Dynamics of the actin cytoskeleton at the cadherin–catenin complexes, focal contacts, and the leading edge are regulated by the family of small GTPases including RhoA, Rac1, and Cdc42. In addition to its role in intercellular adhesion, β-catenin is also a critical part of the Lef/TCF-mediated canonical Wnt signaling pathway

The cytoplasmic domain of classical cadherins binds to β- and p120-catenins. p120-catenin is necessary for delivery and stabilization of cadherins at the plasma membrane (Chen et al. 2003b; Davis et al. 2003). In addition, p120-catenin is a major regulator of RhoA and Rac1 small GTPases and the actin cytoskeleton (Noren et al. 2000; Anastasiadis and Reynolds 2001). β-Catenin and its cousin, plakoglobin, are critical for connecting cadherins with α-catenin. In addition to its role in AJs, β-catenin is also a central part of the canonical Wnt signaling pathway, which plays pivotal roles in both normal development and cancer. β-Catenin can bind to Lef/TCF family of transcription factors and activate transcriptional program resulting in the upregulation of cell-type-specific morphogenetic and cell proliferation programs. The role of β-catenin-mediated Wnt signaling in human cancer has been recently covered by several excellent reviews (Clevers 2006; Huang and He 2008) and will not be discussed in this chapter.

α-Catenin is principally responsible for the linkage of the cadherin–catenin complex at the membrane to the actin cytoskeleton. There are three α-catenin genes, αE(epithelial), αN-(neural), and αT(testicular), with αE-catenin being the most abundant α-catenin expressed in normal epithelial tissues. Mediated by α-catenin, connection between cadherin–catenins and the actin cytoskeleton is very dynamic and it involves focal regulation of actin polymerization (Vasioukhin et al. 2000; Kobielak et al. 2004; Drees et al. 2005), as well as a direct linkage to f-actin through actin-binding protein EPLIN (Abe and Takeichi 2008).

In mammalian cells, all core AJ molecules are essential for AJ formation and maintenance; however, it is important to remember that many of these proteins may have partially redundant functions due to a frequent presence of additional and rather similar family members that can often compensate for the loss of one specific molecule.

Loss of Cadherin–Catenin Adhesion System in Human Cancer and Cancer Prognosis

The overwhelming majority of human tumors are carcinomas, which arise from a variety of epithelial cell types. While these cells normally show prominent intercellular adhesion, invasion of primary epithelial tumor cells into surrounding tissues is accompanied by marked decrease in cell–cell adhesion. Since cadherin–catenin protein complexes play an important role in intercellular adhesion, soon after their discovery, changes in expression and localization of these proteins were analyzed in multiple tumor types. We will now discuss the available information concerning specific changes in cadherin–catenin adhesion system and prognostic value of these changes for tumor progression and patient survival.

Breast Cancer

Ductal and lobular carcinomas are the two major types of breast cancer that significantly differ with respect to expression of cadherin–catenin proteins. While junctional E-cadherin, β-catenin, and α-catenin are expressed at high levels in both normal ductal and lobular luminal breast epithelia, their expression is lost in >85% of invasive lobular breast tumors (Cowin et al. 2005). Moreover, primary lobular tumors that retain E-cadherin expression display its mislocalization, indicating that disruption of cadherin–catenin-mediated cell–cell adhesion is almost a completely penetrant event in lobular breast cancer (Moll et al. 1993; Berx et al. 1995; Berx and Van Roy 2001). Since critical cadherin molecules are missing in lobular breast carcinoma, cancer cells in these tumors are unable to form AJs and display characteristic disruption of normal epithelial cell–cell adhesion and invasion of the stromal cell compartment. Loss of E-cadherin is an early event in development of lobular breast tumors, because even carcinoma in situ frequently lacks E-cadherin (Vos et al. 1997;

Rieger-Christ et al. 2001). Since almost all lobular tumors lose cadherin-mediated expression, the predictive value of this phenotypic change is not obvious; however, the high penetrance of this event strongly suggests that loss of cadherin–catenin adhesion plays an important role in lobular cancer development.

Unlike lobular cancer, more frequent and surprisingly more aggressive ductal breast carcinoma usually retains expression of E-cadherin in low-grade lesions. In this tumor type, the levels of E-cadherin and associated catenins are often reduced in advanced tumors (Oka et al. 1993; Nagae et al. 2002; Pedersen et al. 2002; Rakha et al. 2005; Jeschke et al. 2007; Park et al. 2007). Most studies revealed a correlation between the reduction in expression of E-cadherin and associated catenins and tumor size, invasiveness, distant metastasis, and unfavorable patient outcome (Asgeirsson et al. 2000; Heimann et al. 2000; Nakopoulou et al. 2002; Pedersen et al. 2002; Rakha et al. 2005; Dolled-Filhart et al. 2006; Park et al. 2007).

While it is generally believed that β-catenin signaling is involved in breast cancer, β-catenin is rarely mutated in breast carcinomas. One study reported prominent nuclear β-catenin localization in breast carcinomas and significant correlation between nuclear β-catenin and poor patient outcome (Lin et al. 2000). In dissent, many subsequent studies report that nuclear β-catenin is a very rare event in human breast cancer (Gillett et al. 2001; Pedersen et al. 2002; Wong et al. 2002). A recent large study utilized tissue microarray technology and analyzed 600 samples of human breast cancers. Only 10 out of 600 samples displayed presence of nuclear β-catenin (Dolled-Filhart et al. 2006). Thus, while β-catenin is likely to play an important role in breast cancer cell proliferation and survival, it is still not clear whether β-catenin signaling is playing a prominent role in human breast cancer initiation and progression.

Gastrointestinal Cancer

Gastric cancer (GC) is the second most deadly cancer worldwide. There are two major types of gastric cancer: intestinal type and diffuse type. Diffuse GC is characterized by noncohesive tumor cells that infiltrate the gastric wall. Loss of cell–cell adhesion in diffuse GC is a direct outcome of disruption of cadherin–catenin-mediated adhesion. Expression of E-cadherin is downregulated or lost in 70–76% of diffuse GC and in 40–46% of the intestinal GC (Shun et al. 1998). In another study, decrease in expression of E-cadherin was found in 92% of GCs, and loss of E-cadherin correlated with tumor recurrence and mortality (Mayer et al. 1993). About 28–50% of sporadic diffuse GCs carry genetic alterations in E-cadherin (Becker et al. 1994; Ascano et al. 2001). Interestingly, 48% of all families with hereditary diffuse GC carry one allele with a germ line mutation in E-cadherin (Brooks-Wilson et al. 2004). In addition to E-cadherin, α-catenin is also often absent (41%) or decreased (29%) in GCs (Zhou et al. 2005). Analysis of β-catenin expression and localization in 111 cases of GCs revealed a frequent loss of membrane staining (59%) and nuclear accumulation in 17.5% of primary tumors (Jung et al. 2007). Alterations in β-catenin localization often correlate with changes in E-cadherin expression. Overall, presence of nuclear β-catenin and loss of E-cadherin correlates with poor patient survival (Jawhari et al. 1997; Joo et al. 2000; Zhou et al. 2002; Jung et al. 2007). This conclusion is not universally shared by other studies that found no correlation between the loss of membranous β-catenin, presence of nuclear β-catenin, and patients' outcome (Grabsch et al. 2001). Overall, inactivation of E-cadherin is one of the very early events in diffuse GC and loss of cadherin-mediated adhesion is likely to be involved in development of this cancer.

Thyroid Cancer

Diffuse sclerosing variant (DSV) of papillary thyroid carcinoma (PTC) is a rare and highly invasive variant of PTC in which tumor cells display prominent loss of intercellular adhesion. Almost all DSV of PTC display loss of membranous cadherin–catenin expression (Rocha et al. 2001). Classic PTC also displays decreased E-cadherin–catenin expression, but these events are more common in advanced tumors displaying poor differentiation (Rocha et al. 2001; Kato et al. 2002; Rocha et al. 2003; Wiseman et al. 2006; Mitselou et al. 2007). In general, it is believed that poorly differentiated anaplastic thyroid tumors arise from preexisting well-differentiated foci. Comparison of differentiated foci with adjacent anaplastic tumors revealed that E-cadherin/β-catenin expression was present in a majority of well-differentiated foci (92% for E-cadherin, 67% for β-catenin), but was maintained only in a minority of anaplastic tumors (17% for E-cadherin, 50% for β-catenin) (Wiseman et al. 2006). In addition to E-cadherin and β-catenin, abnormal cytoplasmic expression of α-catenin is also found in papillary thyroid carcinomas (78%) and anaplastic thyroid carcinomas (100%) (Baloch et al. 2001). Therefore, disruption of E-cadherin–catenin complex is associated with transformation of differentiated thyroid carcinoma into anaplastic tumor. Analysis of potential causal connections between changes in cadherin–catenin expression and patients survival revealed a statistically significant correlation between reduced E-cadherin–catenin expression and lymph node metastasis as well as poor patient prognosis (von Wasielewski et al. 1997; Böhm et al. 2000; Naito et al. 2001; Brecelj et al. 2005). Analysis of β-catenin signaling revealed presence of nuclear β-catenin in 42% of advanced anaplastic thyroid carcinomas and 61% of tumors had alterations in β-*catenin* gene, suggesting that activation of β-catenin signaling may be causally involved in late-stage thyroid carcinoma (Garcia-Rostan et al. 1999).

Basal and Squamous Cell Carcinoma (BCC and SCC)

Two major cancer types BCC and SCC arise from malignant transformation of skin, oral, esophageal, and vaginal epithelia. Both BCC and SCC display changes in cadherin–catenin expression pattern. While normal skin epidermis displays prominent expression and cell–cell junctional localization of E-cadherin, β-catenin, and α-catenin, skin tumors often show decreased or complete absence of junctional staining. These changes are especially prominent in human SCCs. While well-differentiated, low-grade SCCs of the head and neck express detectable E-cadherin, moderately differentiated SCCs express variable levels of E-cadherin, and poorly differentiated SCCs are E-cadherin negative (Schipper et al. 1991). Similar phenotypes were observed in oral, esophageal, and cervical SCCs (Nakanishi et al. 1997; Saito et al. 1998; Carico et al. 2001; Brouxhon et al. 2007). In general, while the percentage of SCC tumors showing low or absent levels of E-cadherin varied between different studies, up to 50% of primary tumors display low and up to 25% of tumors show absent expression of E-cadherin (Fuller et al. 1996; Tada et al. 1996). The differences were even more dramatic in studies on α-catenin. Up to 50% of primary SCCs display absent α-catenin and an additional 30% of primary tumors show decreased levels of expression (Kadowaki et al. 1994; Nakanishi et al. 1997; Sakaki et al. 1999; Setoyama et al. 2007). Decreased or absent levels of E-cadherin and especially α-catenin inversely correlate with invasive phenotype, lymph node metastasis, recurrence of the disease, and patient outcome (Schipper et al. 1991; Mattijssen et al. 1993; Kadowaki et al. 1994; Tamura et al. 1996; Nakanishi et al. 1997; Dursun et al. 2007; Setoyama et al. 2007). Stainings for β-catenin and p120-catenin, in general, show the phenotypes similar to E-cadherin. They are often downregulated in poorly differentiated, malignant SCCs (Nakanishi et al. 1997; Carico et al. 2001; Ishizaki et al. 2004; Chung et al. 2007; Fukumaru et al. 2007). Since abnormal activation of β-catenin signaling has been implicated in human cancer, several studies analyzed potential nuclear localization and/or activating mutations in β-*catenin*. No mutations in β-*catenin* were detected in SCCs; however, a fraction of tumors displayed abnormal cytoplasmic and nuclear localization of β-catenin (Lo Muzio et al. 2005; Odajima et al. 2005; Kudo et al. 2007).

In addition to SCCs, advanced BCCs also display somewhat decreased levels of E-cadherin and α-catenin expression; however, differences in expression levels are not as prominent and expression of E-cadherin and α-catenin is usually preserved in BCCs (Pizarro et al. 1994; Pizarro et al. 1995; Fuller et al. 1996; Tada et al. 1996; Kooy et al. 1999). A fraction of BCCs (23–67%) display presence of nuclear β-catenin; however, no mutations in β-*catenin* were found in these tumors (Yamazaki et al. 2001; El-Bahrawy et al. 2003; Saldanha et al. 2004).

Overall, while both advanced SCCs and BCCs display a decrease in expression of cell–cell junctional cadherin–catenin proteins, these changes are significantly more prominent in SCC tumors, which often show a complete absence of E-cadherin or α-catenin.

Prostate Cancer

Significant attention to the expression of cadherin–catenin proteins was devoted to human prostate cancer. The results obtained by different studies display significant differences, which can be potentially explained by differences in the staining protocols, tissue processing, and definitions of aberrant expression. In a majority of the studies, expressions of E-cadherin and α-catenin were found to be decreased in 45–90% of primary prostate tumors (Umbas et al. 1994; Richmond et al. 1997; Loric et al. 2001; Koksal et al. 2002; Wehbi et al. 2002; Wu et al. 2003; Jaggi et al. 2005; van Oort et al. 2007). Abnormal decrease in expression of α-catenin was found in 19–42% of primary prostate tumors and 3% of tumors were α-catenin negative (Richmond et al. 1997; Aaltomaa et al. 1999; Aaltomaa et al. 2005). Aberrant expression of E-cadherin and especially α-catenin was significantly correlated with tumor grade and patient survival (Umbas et al. 1992; Umbas et al. 1994; Richmond et al. 1997; Aaltomaa et al. 1999; Loric et al. 2001; Koksal et al. 2002; Wu et al. 2003; Aaltomaa et al. 2005; Gravdal et al. 2007; van Oort et al. 2007). More advanced tumors were more likely to express lower levels of E-cadherin and α-catenin. In other studies, abnormal expression of E-cadherin was seen only in 18–20% of primary tumors and E-cadherin was well expressed in 90% of hormone refractory prostate tumors (Rubin et al. 2001).

Changes in junctional β-catenin expression often parallel the changes in expression of E-cadherin and α-catenin (Aaltomaa et al. 2005; Jaggi et al. 2005). Nuclear β-catenin was found in up to 20% of advanced high-grade primary prostate tumors and it was a biomarker of aggressive disease (Chesire et al. 2002; Jaggi et al. 2005). Activating mutations in β-catenin were found in 5% of primary prostate tumors (Voeller et al. 1998; Chesire et al. 2000). However, in a different study, which analyzed 232 radical prostatectomy specimens from patients with clinically localized prostate cancer (PC) and 20 cases of advanced PC, nuclear β-catenin was found to be decreased in PCs and even more so in the advanced tumors (Horvath et al. 2005). Moreover, decreased nuclear β-catenin was associated with a poorer prognosis in localized PCs. Only a small proportion of β-catenin exists in the nucleus at any given time and this may potentially account for discrepancies in these studies.

Overall, it appears that some decreased E-cadherin and α-catenin expression is evident in about a half of advanced primary prostate cancers and decrease in expression of these proteins correlates with unfavorable prognosis. Complete loss of E-cadherin and α-catenin are not frequent events in human prostate cancer. While activation of β-catenin may play a role in human prostate cancer progression, direct mutations in β-catenin or APC are not frequent in prostate cancer cells.

Lung Cancer

In human lung cancer, E-cadherin and α- and β-catenins are present in low-grade well-differentiated tumors; however, expression of these genes is reduced in more advanced poorly differentiated tumors. In general, reduced expression of E-cadherin is noted in 42–60% of primary non-small cell lung cancer (NSCLC) tumors and it is associated with poor differentiation (Bohm et al. 1994; Toyoyama et al. 1999; Kase et al. 2000; Kimura et al. 2000; Stefanou et al. 2003; Salon et al. 2005; Nozawa et al. 2006). A subset of tumors showing reduced expression of E-cadherin also display reduced expression of α-catenin (30–50% of all NSCLC) (Toyoyama et al. 1999;

Kimura et al. 2000). Immunohistochemical analysis of tissue microarray containing primary NSCLCs from 193 patients with stages I to III cancer revealed reduced expression of E-cadherin, α-, β-, γ-, and p120-catenins in 10, 17, 8, 31, and 61% of the cases, respectively (Bremnes et al. 2002).

Loss of membrane staining for cadherin and catenins in lung cancer often correlates with advanced tumors, metastasis, and poor patient prognosis. Analysis of NSCLC tumors reported correlation between positive E-cadherin, α-catenin, and β-catenin staining and tumor differentiation, longer time to progression, and overall better survival (Kimura et al. 2000; Bremnes et al. 2002; Stefanou et al. 2003; Deeb et al. 2004; Nozawa et al. 2006; Miyanaga et al. 2008). While some studies found that among AJ proteins, reduction in α-catenin appeared to reflect most strikingly the presence of lymph node metastasis and the short survival periods of NSCLC patients (Kimura et al. 2000), other studies reported high junctional E-cadherin staining as the best prognostic marker of survival (Bremnes et al. 2002). In yet another study, which used 331 lung cancer tissues, reduced expression of β-catenin, but not E-cadherin, was found to be the most accurate prognostic marker of poor survival (Kase et al. 2000). In contrast, only few studies on NSCLCs report no correlation between E-cadherin, α- and β-catenin levels, tumor differentiation, lymph node metastasis, and patient survival (Ramasami et al. 2000).

While NSCLC is the most common type of lung cancer, neuroendocrine tumors (NETs) represent up to 20% of lung cancers. Impaired cadherin–catenin expression was found in NETs of the lung. Immunohistochemical analyses on 102 NET tumors revealed aberrant expression of E-cadherin and β-catenin in 78 and 72% of NETs, correspondingly (Salon et al. 2004). Impaired expression of the E-cadherin and β-catenin molecules correlated with lymph node metastasis and with advanced stage disease.

Overall, a massive amount of published data show that cadherin–catenin expression is affected in most human epithelial tumors. Disruption of the cadherin–catenin adhesion system is an early event in such tumor types as diffuse stomach carcinoma, breast lobular carcinoma, and diffuse sclerosing variant of papillary thyroid carcinoma. Loss of intercellular adhesion in these tumors results in infiltration of the tissue by masses of isolated tumor cells. This phenotype has such a profound effect on tumor histology that it helps to define the tumor type and to differentiate it from other types of epithelial tumors in these organs. An early onset and a complete disruption of cadherin–catenin adhesion system, as well as an *E-cadherin*-dependent genetic predisposition for these tumors, strongly suggest that cadherin–catenin adhesion system plays a tumor suppressor role in these tumor types. In contrast, in the overwhelming majority of other epithelial tumors, the cadherin–catenin adhesion system is usually maintained in low-grade, well-differentiated tumors; however, it is often decreased or severely disrupted in advanced, poorly differentiated tumors and this usually correlates with tumor metastasis and poor patient outcome. These findings suggest that in these epithelial tumors the cadherin–catenin system is likely to function as a metastasis suppressor that attenuates the spread of the primary tumor (Fig. 3.2A).

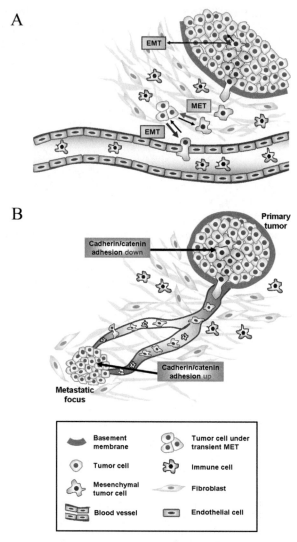

Fig. 3.2 Role of inactivation of cadherin–catenin-mediated adhesion in epithelial tumor spread and metastasis. (**A**) Loss of cadherin–catenin function results in epithelial–mesenchymal transition (EMT), invasion of surrounding tissues, and intravasation. Downregulation of epithelial E-cadherin and upregulation of mesenchymal N-cadherin on tumor cells undergoing EMT may promote local invasion by decreasing the affinity for epithelial cells and increasing the affinity for mesenchymal stromal cells, which surround the tumor. Note that EMT may be transient and it can be reversed by mesenchymal–epithelial transition (MET). (**B**) Tumor cells disperse throughout the body via blood and lymphoid systems, extravasate in the distant organs, and establish metastatic foci. Cadherin–catenin adhesion system may promote attachment and survival of tumor cells in the foreign microenvironment

Switch from Epithelial to Mesenchymal Cadherin Expression and Its Role in Tumor Invasion

E-cadherin is the most prominent cadherin molecule expressed in normal epithelial tissues. Interestingly, a decrease in expression of E-cadherin in epithelial carcinomas often coincides with an increase in expression of other cadherin types, most notably N-cadherin (Wheelock et al. 2008). This phenomenon has major significance in the progression of epithelial tumors and it is known as "cadherin switching." EMT takes place often during normal mammalian development and it is characterized by phenotypical and functional transition of epithelial cells into mesenchymal cells, which are usually more invasive and migratory. This process is driven by changes in expression of cadherin molecules and replacement of E-cadherin in epithelial cells by N-cadherin, which is normally expressed in neuronal and mesenchymal cells. Similar process was observed in many cultured cancer cell lines, and at least some elements of cadherin switching and EMT may take place during tumor progression in vivo (Hugo et al. 2007). During EMT, expression of E-cadherin is decreased and expression of N-cadherin is upregulated. Presently, it is not clear whether upregulation of N-cadherin during EMT is simply a response to the cell fate change and acquisition of a mesenchymal cell phenotype or it represents the driving event in cancer progression. Experiments in cell lines show that forced expression of even low levels of N-cadherin in epithelial cells expressing E-cadherin results in major changes in cell morphology and stimulates cell migration and invasion (Nieman et al. 1999; De Wever et al. 2004). Mechanistically, N-cadherin may stimulate cell migration by binding and potentiation of the activity of the FGF receptor and also by activation of Rac1 and Cdc42 small GTPases via p120-catenin (Wheelock et al. 2008). Expression of N-cadherin has been documented in human tumors and there is a correlation between tumor progression and cadherin switching events (Cavallaro et al. 2002). Experiments with cancer model systems demonstrated that the role of N-cadherin expression in tumors is likely to be cancer-type specific. Overexpression of N-cadherin in normal mammary gland or NEU-induced mammary gland tumors did not produce discernable phenotype (Knudsen et al. 2005). However, overexpression of N-cadherin in polyomavirus middle T-antigen-induced mammary tumors led to enhanced extracellular signal-regulated kinase activation and increased metastasis (Hulit et al. 2007). It is possible that upregulation of N-cadherin in epithelial cells results in changes in specific signaling pathways and, depending on the nature of the oncogenic insult, N-cadherin may or may not promote tumor progression and metastasis. A critical question that will have to be addressed is whether increase in endogenous N-cadherin in primary tumors is playing an important role in tumor progression. Future experiments with conditional knockouts of endogenous N-cadherin in the context of developing epithelial tumors will help to answer this question.

Paradoxical Re-emergence of the Cadherin–Catenin-Mediated Adhesion System in Metastatic Lesions

Analyses of primary epithelial tumors almost universally show decrease or complete absence of E-cadherin in the advanced stages of the disease. Moreover, this loss of cadherin expression usually correlates with the probability of metastasis and poor overall prognosis. Nevertheless, analyses of metastatic lesions, often from the same patients that showed loss of E-cadherin in the primary tumors, revealed the re-emergence of E-cadherin-mediated adhesion in metastatic cells (Bukholm et al. 2000; Imai et al. 2004; Hung et al. 2006). This could be considered as rather surprising. Indeed, if disruption of adhesion favors tumor progression and metastasis, would not one expect to see no adhesion in the final product of the metastatic process? After all, many studies analyze metastatic lesions and consider the transcriptional phenotype of these cells as the phenotype that promotes metastasis. Clearly this would not be the case for E-cadherin, which is present in metastatic lesions, but often absent in the advanced primary tumors. Applying the same type of reasoning, we would have to consider E-cadherin as a metastasis promoter, which is contrary to all that we know about E-cadherin in human cancer. So how can the re-establishment of cadherin–catenin adhesion in metastatic lesions be explained?

The process of metastasis is very complex and it is comprised of several different stages. The breaking from the primary tumor mass, local invasion, intravasation are more easily achieved by tumor cells that undergo complete or partial EMT. In contrast, survival in the blood or lymph systems, re-establishment in the foreign microenvironment may be more easily achieved by cells that increase intercellular adhesion, which can provide cell survival signals in the environment when integrin-based adhesion is minimal or does not exist (blood stream). In this scenario, the most favorable course of events for efficient metastasis would be the loss of adhesion and EMT in the primary tumors and re-emergence of cell–cell adhesion in the distant sites (Fig. 3.2B). A remarkably similar course of events is observed in human cancer.

Causal Evidence Implicating Cadherin–Catenin System in Cancer Progression and Metastasis

While the studies on cadherins in primary epithelial tumors and tumor metastasis certainly implicate cadherin–catenin complex in epithelial tumor initiation and progression, the evidence generated by this approach is rather circumstantial in nature and, as such, it does not allow for establishing a causal relationship between loss of cadherin–catenin-mediated adhesion and tumor initiation and progression. We will now discuss results from the studies that attempted to address the role and significance of cadherin–catenin proteins in cancer using experimental loss-of-function and gain-of-function approaches.

Causal Evidence from Studies on Cell Lines In Vitro and on Xenograft Tumors

Advanced epithelial tumors and cell lines generated from these malignancies often lose E-cadherin–catenin-mediated adhesion. Thus, restoration of cadherin–catenin expression provided a simple but powerful tool, which was utilized to understand the significance of the loss of cadherin–catenin-mediated adhesion in cancer. Experimental inactivation of cadherin–catenin adhesion in cancer cell lines that maintained this system provided a complementary approach to analyze the role of cadherin–catenin adhesion. These two approaches have been employed in multiple studies that utilized cancer cell lines derived from a variety of tumor types (Behrens et al. 1989; Vleminckx et al. 1991; Watabe et al. 1994). In general, loss of E-cadherin resulted in the increase in cell invasion and decrease in cell differentiation, while restoration of E-cadherin led to suppression of invasive phenotype both in vitro and in mouse xenograft tumors in vivo (Behrens et al. 1989; Chen and Obrink 1991; Frixen et al. 1991; Vleminckx et al. 1991). Restoration of α-catenin expression in cancer cell lines missing this protein had even more dramatic phenotypes. For example, expression of α-catenin in the lung carcinoma cell line PC9 or prostate carcinoma cell line PC3, which both expressed E-cadherin, but lacked α-catenin, resulted not only in the restoration of polarized epithelial phenotype but also in significantly decreased rates of cell proliferation (Watabe et al. 1994; Ewing et al. 1995). Re-establishing of α-catenin expression in ovarian carcinoma cell line Ov2008 restored the epithelial morphology of these cells and also attenuated their proliferation and ability to form tumors in immunocompromised mice (Bullions et al. 1997). Overall, these data provide causal evidence suggesting that cadherin–catenin-mediated adhesion system plays a role of invasion suppressor in epithelial cancer-derived cell lines and it may regulate not only cell invasion and metastasis but also cell proliferation. While analysis of established cancer cell lines in culture or in nude mice is very informative, it usually models the final stages of metastatic process, which includes cancer cell survival and proliferation at the distant sites and secondary metastasis. Experimental analysis of the initial stages of tumor formation and progression in properly three-dimentionally (3-D) organized organs became possible via analyses of genetically engineered mice.

Evidence from Genetically Engineered Mice

Similar to human epithelial tumors, loss of E-cadherin expression is often observed in genetically induced tumors in mice. For example, the transition from well-differentiated adenoma to invasive carcinoma in a transgenic mouse model of pancreatic β-cell carcinogenesis (Rip1Tag2 mice) coincides with transcriptional decrease in endogenous E-cadherin (Perl et al. 1998). Intercrossing Rip1Tag2 mice with transgenic mice that expressed E-cadherin under the control of exogenous promoter, which was not affected in Rip1Tag2 tumors, resulted in arrest of tumor development at the adenoma stage. Alternatively, expression of a dominant-negative form of E-cadherin in this model system induces early invasion and metastasis (Perl et al. 1998). Similar experiments in mouse models of non-small-cell lung cancer induced by C-Raf overexpression demonstrated that disruption of *E-cadherin* promotes β-catenin-dependent upregulation of VEGF-A and VEGF-C, massive formation of intratumoral vessels, rapid growth of primary tumors, and micrometastasis (Ceteci et al. 2007).

Loss of E-cadherin is a critical hallmark of human lobular breast carcinoma. Conditional deletion of E-cadherin in breast epithelial cells was not sufficient to induce tumor development; however, it significantly accelerated the development of invasive and metastatic mammary carcinomas induced by inactivation of *p53* (Derksen et al. 2006). Perhaps not surprisingly, these tumors showed strong resemblance to human invasive lobular carcinoma. Loss of E-cadherin in this model system induced resistance to anoikis and facilitated angiogenesis, thus promoting metastatic disease.

The role of α-catenin in vivo in the context of a cancer model has not been analyzed; however, deletion of epithelial α*E-catenin* in mouse embryonic neuroepithelial and skin progenitors cells resulted in the loss of tissue organization, hyperplasia, and early postnatal death (Vasioukhin et al. 2001; Lien et al. 2006). In contrast, loss of α*E-catenin* in breast epithelial cells resulted in increased epithelial cell death and failure of proper mammary gland development (Nemade et al. 2004).

While a significant amount of data concerning the role of β-catenin in mammalian cancer has been accumulated in the recent years, most of the in vivo experiments analyzed the function of β-catenin in the canonical Wnt signaling rather than its role in the AJs, because junctional loss of β-catenin is usually well compensated by the presence of plakoglobin. In general, stabilization of β-catenin in vivo results in constitutive activation of the canonical Wnt signaling pathway and development of tumors in a variety of epithelial organs (Clevers. 2006). Since the canonical Wnt signaling pathway is necessary for proper maintenance of stem and progenitor cell populations in many organs and tissues, conditional loss of β-*catenin* usually results in quick depletion of these cell populations and severe problems with organ development and maintenance (Machon et al. 2003; Zechner et al. 2003; Fevr et al. 2007).

Overall, genetic loss-of-function experiments demonstrated that loss of E-cadherin–catenin adhesion system is playing a causal role in epithelial tumor progression. While disruption of the AJs usually is not sufficient for tumor initiation, loss of cadherin-mediated adhesion cooperates with other pro-tumorigenic pathways to facilitate tumor angiogenesis, progression to locally invasive carcinoma, and metastasis. We will now discuss potential mechanisms that may be responsible for the tumor-suppressor function of cadherin–catenin system.

Cadherin–Catenin Function in Cancer Progression

Adhesive Function of Cadherin–Catenin System as an Inhibitor of Invasion

One of the primary functions of epithelial cells is the formation of a barrier that separates different compartments within the organism. This function is mediated by an active process of cell–cell adhesion orchestrated by the cadherin–catenin complexes, which use the forces generated by the underlying actin cytoskeleton to drive epithelial cells together (Vasioukhin et al. 2000; Perez-Moreno et al. 2003). This process will ensure that epithelial cells are connected to each other as tightly as possible to function as an epithelial barrier.

During epithelial tumor progression, the forces generated by the cadherin–catenin-mediated adhesion will continue to function to keep tumor cells together. Therefore, it could be very difficult for tumor cells with a functional cadherin–catenin system to break from the bulk of the tumor. Thus, downregulation of cadherin–catenin adhesion is necessary for epithelial tumor cell invasion into the surrounding tissues and subsequent metastasis (Fig. 3.3A). While this purely adhesive role may appear dull and unexciting, this function of cadherin–catenin-mediated adhesion is probably one of the most significant mechanisms that prevents invasion and spread of epithelial tumors.

Cadherin–Catenin System as Regulator of Growth Factor Receptor Signaling

In addition to their purely adhesive role, cadherin–catenin complexes may impact tumor initiation and progression by regulation of a variety of growth factor receptor signaling pathways. Indeed, cadherin–catenin complexes directly or indirectly bind to a variety of growth factor receptors and exercise potent influence on their activity (Fig. 3.3B). Probably one of the most cancer relevant effects is the potent negative influence of E-cadherin on the activity of several receptor tyrosine kinases (RTKs) (Takahashi and Suzuki 1996; Qian et al. 2004). E-cadherin interferes with their function through direct or indirect complex formation and inhibition of their ligand-dependent activation (Qian et al. 2004). Interestingly, mutations in E-cadherin that are found in human tumors result in decreased complex formation between E-cadherin and EGFR and enhanced activation of EGF-mediated signaling (Bremm et al. 2008). Since E-cadherin can induce formation of cell–cell junctions that engage multiple protein complexes, some of the cadherin–catenin effects on regulation of RTKs activity could have been indirect. This possibility was addressed by engaging E-cadherin complexes on the surface of isolated epithelial cells by using functionally active recombinant E-cadherin protein attached to microspheres (Perrais et al. 2007). Such engagement inhibited cell proliferation and this effect

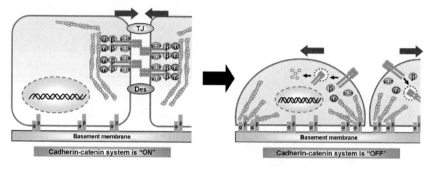

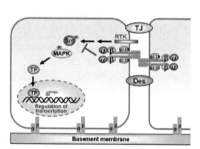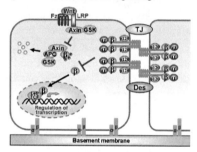

Fig. 3.3 Potential mechanisms of cadherin–catenin system in suppression of tumor invasion and metastasis. (**A**) Cadherin-catenin system uses the force of the actin cytoskeleton to pull neighboring epithelial cells together and prevent tumor cell dissemination. (**B**) Epithelial cadherin-catenin complexes negatively regulate signaling by receptor tyrosine kinases. (**C**) Cadherin-catenin complexes may sequester β-catenin away from the nucleus and attenuate β-catenin/TCF signaling. RTK, receptor tyrosine kinase. TF, transcription factor. MAPK, mitogen-activated protein kinase

was dependent on EGFR-mediated activation of signal transducers and activator of transcription 5 (STAT5).

In contrast to attenuation of RTKs signaling toward the MAPK pathway and activation of cell proliferation, cadherin–catenin adhesion system can potentiate RTKs signaling toward the PI3K pathway and cell survival (Carmeliet et al. 1999; Kang et al. 2007). This function is probably important for pro-survival role of cadherin–catenin in tumor cells when integrin-mediated signaling is downregulated in the soft agar and, potentially, in the blood stream during tumor metastasis. This pro-survival function of cadherin–catenin complexes may potentially explain the re-emergence of E-cadherin in the metastatic lesions.

As previously discussed, many advanced epithelial tumors switch their expression of cadherin molecules from E-cadherin to N-cadherin. N-cadherin also associates with a variety of growth factor receptors; however, its impact on RTK signaling is very different, since it potentiates rather than inhibits RTK signaling cascades. For example, interaction between N-cadherin and fibroblast growth factor receptor (FGFR) resulted in the prevention of ligand-mediated internalization of FGFR-1 and caused sustained activation of the MAPK–ERK pathway, leading to MMP-9 gene transcription and cellular invasion (Suyama et al. 2002). Similarly, N-cadherin in complex with the platelet-derived growth factor-receptor β (PDGFRβ) promotes PDGF-dependent cell migration (Theisen et al. 2007). These activities of N-cadherin may explain the significance of the cadherin switch phenomenon in epithelial tumor progression and paradoxical increase in cell motility and invasion in epithelial cells that express large amounts of E-cadherin and only small amounts of N-cadherin.

Cadherin–Catenin System as a Regulator of β-Catenin Signaling

β-Catenin is a critical regulator of the canonical Wnt signaling pathway and sustained activation of this pathway by overexpression of Wnts, mutation of β-catenin or mutation of the proteins involved in its degradation results in cancer development (Clevers 2006). It is logical to hypothesize that disruption of cadherin–catenin complexes may result in liberation of β-catenin, which can then translocate to the nucleus and activate its transcriptional program (Fig. 3.3C). Indeed, it has been demonstrated that sequestration of β-catenin by overexpressed E-cadherin and α-catenin in a variety of model systems results in attenuation of β-catenin signaling activities (Sehgal et al. 1997; Simcha et al. 1998; Orsulic et al. 1999; Giannini et al. 2000; Gottardi et al. 2001; Merdek et al. 2004; Onder et al. 2008). Since loss of endogenous E-cadherin or α-catenin was observed in human epithelial tumors, it was important to analyze whether deletion of endogenous E-cadherin or α-catenin in vivo can activate β-catenin signaling pathway.

This has been analyzed using several model systems and results of these studies indicate that the connection between the loss of E-cadherin or α-catenin and activation of β-catenin signaling is rather complex and probably tissue specific. Conditional deletion of *E-cadherin* and epithelial α*E-catenin* in mice does not result in significant changes in β-catenin signaling pathway (Young et al. 2003; Lien et al. 2008). One of the earliest genetic demonstrations of the role of E-cadherin as an inhibitor of tumor progression and metastasis was performed in an SV40 T-antigen-driven transgenic mouse model of β-cell carcinogenesis (Rip1Tag2 mice). Remarkably, subsequent analysis of the mechanisms responsible for E-cadherin-mediated metastasis suppression in this model did not reveal activation of β-catenin signaling (Herzig et al. 2007). Therefore, pathways other than β-catenin/Tcf-mediated Wnt signaling are induced by the loss of E-cadherin during tumor progression in Rip1Tag2 transgenic mice. Deletion of *E-cadherin* in a mouse model of breast and skin carcinoma (conditional *p53-/-* mice) promoted tumor progression and angiogenesis via inhibition of apoptosis; however, activation of β-catenin signaling was not reported in this model (Derksen et al. 2006). E-cadherin-dependent activation of β-catenin signaling was reported in a Raf-driven murine lung cancer model; however, it appears that most of the β-catenin signaling analysis in this study was performed in the animals overexpressing dominant-negative

E-cadherin, rather than mice with deletion of *E-cadherin* gene (Ceteci et al. 2007). It will be interesting to know whether the loss of endogenous *E-cadherin* also resulted in activation of β-catenin in this cancer model.

Overall, it appears that cadherin–catenin adhesion system attenuates epithelial tumor progression and metastasis by engaging several mechanisms ranging from the classic glue-like adhesion, to regulation of the growth factor-mediated and Wnt signaling pathways. While a significant amount of information has been accumulated, many questions regarding the molecular mechanisms remain unanswered. What are the molecular mechanisms of cadherin–catenin-mediated adhesion that drive epithelial cells together? How cadherins modulate signaling by growth factor receptors in such a way that promotes survival, but inhibits proliferation? What is the role of cadherin–catenin adhesion in the classic Wnt signaling pathway? These exciting questions will be addressed in the future. However, the mechanisms that are responsible for inactivation of cadherin–catenin adhesion system in human epithelial tumors are currently well understood.

Mechanisms of Cadherin–Catenin System Inactivation in Human Tumors

Inactivation of Cadherin–Catenin System by Mutations in Cadherins and Catenins

Germ line homozygous loss-of-function mutations in *E-cadherin*, *β-catenin*, and *αE-catenin* are embryonic lethal in mice and it is likely that similar genetic alterations also result in embryonic lethality in humans (Larue et al. 1994; Haegel et al. 1995; Torres et al. 1997; Huelsken et al. 2000). Although heterozygous mutants in these critical AJs genes do not show prominent phenotype in mice, heterozygous germ line mutation in *E-cadherin* strongly predispose humans to diffuse-type gastric cancer (see above). Interestingly, while E-cadherin is also lost in lobular breast carcinomas, an increase in the probability of lobular breast cancer in individuals with germ line mutation in E-cadherin is much less certain than increase in gastric cancer. While individuals heterozygous for *β-catenin* and *αE-catenin* are likely to be present in the general human population, presently, it is not known whether these genetic alterations predispose to development of any diseases.

Somatic mutation in *E-cadherin* is a frequent event in epithelial tumors. The highest incident rate is documented in diffuse-type gastric and lobular breast cancers, where up to 50% of primary tumors contain mutations in *E-cadherin*. In addition, mutations in *E-cadherin* were also observed in primary endometrial, ovarian, and signet-cell stomach carcinomas; however, this happens at a much lower frequency (Risinger et al. 1994; Muta et al. 1996). Inactivating mutations in α- and β-*catenins* have been observed in a variety of epithelial cancer cell lines; however, very little information exists concerning the presence of mutations in these genes in primary epithelial tumors. Gene sequencing of a very limited sample of breast and colon tumors identified mutations in αE- and αN-*catenins* and a number of cadherin genes; however, the frequency of these mutations did not allow to conclude that they may play a causal role in cancer initiation (Wood et al. 2007).

Inactivation of Cadherin–Catenin System by Transcriptional Repression

While genetic inactivation of E-cadherin occurs relatively often in the diffuse gastric and lobular breast carcinoma and endometrial cancer, by far the most frequent mechanism responsible for inactivation of cadherin–catenin system in human epithelial tumors is epigenetic decrease in transcription of *E-cadherin*. *E-cadherin* can be downregulated via promoter hypermethylation and/or changes in the transcription factors that regulate *E-cadherin* promoter activity.

Hypermethylation of *E-cadherin* promoter and decrease in *E-cadherin* expression is a widespread phenomenon in human epithelial cancers. In fact, even in tumors in individuals with hereditary diffuse gastric cancers that contain mutations in *E-cadherin*, a second allele is often maintained, but silenced via hypermethylation in the CpG island in the promoter region of *E-cadherin* (Grady et al. 2000). Hypermethylation of *E-cadherin* promoter has been reported in primary gastric, breast, prostate, non-small-cell lung, cervical, thyroid, bladder, esophageal, renal, hepatocellular, colorectal, and many other cancer types (Graff et al. 1995; Yoshiura et al. 1995; Graff et al. 1998; Tamura et al. 2000; Matsumura et al. 2001; Nojima et al. 2001; Si et al. 2001; Garinis et al. 2002; Ribeiro-Filho et al. 2002; Chen et al. 2003a; Kim et al. 2007). Hypermethylation of *E-cadherin* is erased and expression of *E-cadherin* is restored in many E-cadherin-negative cancer cell lines treated with demethylating agent 5-azacytidine (Nam et al. 2004). In some cases, the correlation between *E-cadherin* promoter hypermethylation and E-cadherin expression is not perfect, and treatment with demethylating agents does not restore expression of E-cadherin (Hajra et al. 1999; Fearon. 2000). Downregulation of E-cadherin expression in some of these cases can be explained by the action of transcriptional factors regulating *E-cadherin* promoter activity.

Analysis of *E-cadherin* promoter activity in somatic cell hybrids indicated that *E-cadherin* transcription in epithelial cancer cell lines is extinguished by factors acting on the E-box element within the *E-cadherin* promoter (Giroldi et al. 1997). Subsequent studies identified several transcription factors that can bind to the E-box of the *E-cadherin* promoter and repress its transcription. These include zinc-finger transcriptional repressors SNAIL (Batlle et al. 2000; Cano et al. 2000), SLUG (Savagner et al. 1997), delta EF1/ZEB1 (Grooteclaes and Frisch 2000), SIP1/ZEB2 (Comijn et al. 2001), and the basic helix–loop–helix factors E12/E47 (Perez-Moreno et al. 2001) and Twist (Yang et al. 2004). The transcriptional repressors of *E-cadherin* are utilized in normal development for quick downregulation of *E-cadherin* and suppression of the epithelial phenotype and EMT. EMT can be induced by important developmental pathways including Notch, Wnt, BMP, and

RTKs (Thiery and Sleeman 2006; Leong et al. 2007). Epithelial tumors often upregulate the expression of transcription repressors of *E-cadherin* and this results in prominent stimulation of tumor cell invasion and metastasis (Yang et al. 2004; Peinado et al. 2007). Interestingly, some of E-cadherin repressors can be controlled by endogenous microRNAs. For example, miR-141, mir-200b, and mir-205 miR-NAs directly repress ZEB1 and ZEB2 (Gregory et al. 2008; Park et al. 2008). Knockdown of these miRNAs in epithelial cell lines reduces E-cadherin expression, indicating that decrease in expression of these endogenous miRNAs may be involved in promotion of EMT and metastasis in human cancer.

Inactivation of Cadherin–Catenin System by Post-transcriptional Regulation

In addition to a decrease in the expression of crucial AJ proteins, cadherin–catenin-mediated adhesion can be disrupted via multiple post-translational mechanisms. Usually, the normal function of AJs completely depends on the formation of ternary complex containing cadherin, β- or γ-catenin, and α-catenin. Any cellular signaling mechanisms that can result in disruption of this complex will inactivate AJs and impact cell–cell adhesion. Since normal development and adult tissue homeostasis often require quick disassembly of cell–cell junctions to generate EMT and activate cell movement, cells have developed multiple mechanisms that can be used to disassemble the cadherin–catenin complexes.

Cadherins and β- and α-catenins can be phosphorylated by tyrosine and serine–threonine kinases and this phosphorylation can result in major changes in their binding affinities and overall stability. E-cadherin–catenin complexes can directly or indirectly bind to EGFR, ErbB2, Met, and IGF1R (Ochiai et al. 1994; Hiscox and Jiang. 1999; Reshetnikova et al. 2007; Canonici et al. 2008). In general, sustained activation of RTKs results in disassembly of the cadherin–catenin complexes (Behrens et al. 1993; Hamaguchi et al. 1993). Increase in tyrosine phosphorylation of E-cadherin upon activation of RTKs and/or Src-kinases results in its monoubiquitination by Hakai, binding to monoubiquitine-interacting protein Hrs, internalization, and subsequent lysosome-mediated degradation (Fujita et al. 2002; Palacios et al. 2005; Toyoshima et al. 2007; Shen et al. 2008). In addition to Hakai, E-cadherin can also be ubiquitinated by MDM2, which is often overexpressed in certain types of human cancers (Yang et al. 2006). Tyrosine phosphorylation of β-catenin by Src-family, BCR-Abl, MET, and RET RTKs results in decreased affinity for both E-cadherin and α-catenin, stabilization of β-catenin in the cytoplasm, and activation of β-catenin-specific transcriptional program (Roura et al. 1999; Brembeck et al. 2004; Lilien and Balsamo 2005; Coluccia et al. 2006; Zeng et al. 2006; Coluccia et al. 2007; Gujral et al. 2008).

In addition to tyrosine kinases, serine–threonine kinases can also influence cadherin–catenin interactions. Phosphorylation of cadherin cytoplasmic tail by casein kinase I results in disassembly of cadherin–catenin complexes (Ochiai et al. 1994). β-Catenin phosphorylation by AKT and cyclic AMP-dependent protein kinase also results in activation of β-catenin-mediated signaling (Hino et al. 2005; Fang et al. 2007). Phosphorylation of β-catenin by GSK3β results in rapid destruction of β-catenin by the proteasome-mediated degradation pathway (Aberle et al. 1997). GSK3β is constitutively active in the cytoplasm, where β-catenin is efficiently degraded, and only in the cells receiving the Wnt signal, GSK3β is unable to phosphorylate β-catenin, which escapes degradation, accumulates in the nucleus, and activates the canonical Wnt transcriptional program (Clevers 2006).

In addition to phosphorylation, cadherin–catenin complex formation can be influenced by the activity of small Rho-family GTPases. Indeed, cadherin–catenin clustering is completely dependent on the activity of the actin cytoskeleton (Hirano et al. 1987; Angres et al. 1996). Since Rho-family GTPases regulate the dynamics of the actin cytoskeleton, they play a pivotal role in AJs assembly and disassembly and their activities have been implicated in tumor cell migration and invasion (Ellenbroek and Collard 2007). p120-Catenin is a critical regulator of Rho-family GTPases, which activates Rac1, inactivates RhoA, and promotes AJs assembly and stabilization (Reynolds 2007). Literature on the roles of particular members of Rho-family GTPases may be a little confusing, as the same molecules are often implicated in either promoting or disrupting the intercellular adhesion. For example, activation of RhoA results in disassembly of the AJs; however, destruction of RhoA induces EMT (Zhong et al. 1997; Sahai and Marshall 2002; Ozdamar et al. 2005; Fang et al. 2008). It is likely that carefully regulated actin cytoskeleton dynamics is required for the formation of the AJs; however, induced by the oncogenic signaling hyperactivation of either RhoA or Rac1 may result in destabilization of the contacts and stimulation of migration and invasion (Zhong et al. 1997; Gimond et al. 1999; Lozano et al. 2008).

While actin cytoskeleton regulators can influence cadherin function inside the cells, several mechanisms that function on the cell surface can negatively regulate cell–cell adhesion and contribute to tumor development and progression. Proteolytic cleavage of cadherin molecules by matrix metalloproteinases (MMPs), a disintegrin and metalloproteases (ADAMs), or γ-secretase is another mechanism that may be involved in transient downregulation of cadherin function in primary epithelial tumors (Lochter et al. 1997; Marambaud et al. 2002; Maretzky et al. 2005; Ferber et al. 2008). MMPs and ADAMs are often upregulated in human tumors, where they may perform multiple functions including promotion of tumor cell invasion and metastasis. Generated by cleavage extracellular fragment of E-cadherin can function as a dominant-negative pseudo-ligand that will inactivate cadherin–catenin-mediated adhesion on cells that are not directly exposed to the proteases (Damsky et al. 1983). In addition to the cell surface cleavage of the extracellular domain of E-cadherin, E-cadherin-mediated adhesion can be negatively regulated by the cell membrane glycoprotein dysadherin (Nam et al. 2007). It can impair adhesion and stimulate metastasis by several mechanisms including downregulation of E-cadherin-mediated adhesion and activation of production of chemokines.

Conclusions

Overall, an enormous amount of evidence documents disruption and disorganization of cadherin–catenin adhesion system in human epithelial tumors. While disruption of cadherin–catenin adhesion is an early and tumor-type-defining event in diffuse gastric cancer, lobular breast carcinoma, and diffuse sclerosing variant of papillary thyroid tumor, in other types of epithelial tumors loss of cell–cell adhesion usually happens in high-grade tumors. In general, disruption of cadherin–catenin adhesion system correlates with higher probability of tumor metastasis and poor rates of survival. Importantly, the causal relation between loss of cadherin-mediated adhesion and epithelial tumor progression and metastasis has been well documented not only in tumor-derived cell lines but also in mouse cancer models.

One of the major challenges that lie ahead is to understand how exactly disruption of cell–cell adhesion contributes to tumor progression. Significant progress has already been made in this direction. While simple loss of attractive forces that keep epithelial cells together is undeniably one of the important mechanisms responsible for tumor cell dispersion and invasion, the potential role of cadherin in negative regulation of β-catenin signaling activities and an already well-defined role of cadherin–catenin complexes in modulation of various growth factor receptor pathways open a completely different perspective at the role of cadherin–catenin system in tumor progression. Future research is likely to uncover novel mechanisms that will explain and clarify the role and the mechanisms of cadherin–catenin-mediated adhesion system in human cancer.

References

Aaltomaa S., Lipponen P., Ala-Opas M., Eskelinen M., Kosma VM. (1999) Alpha-catenin expression has prognostic value in local and locally advanced prostate cancer. Br J Cancer 80:477–82.

Aaltomaa S., Kärjä V, Lipponen P, Isotalo T, Kankkunen JP, Talja M, Mokka R. (2005) Reduced alpha-and beta-catenin expression predicts shortened survival in local prostate cancer. Anticancer Res 25:4707–12.

Abe K., Takeichi M. (2008) EPLIN mediates linkage of the cadherin catenin complex to F-actin and stabilizes the circumferential actin belt. Proc Natl Acad Sci U S A 105:13–19.

Aberle H., Bauer A., Stappert J., Kispert A., Kemler R. (1997) Beta-catenin is a target for the ubiquitin proteasome pathway. Embo J 16:3797–804.

Anastasiadis PZ, Reynolds AB. (2001) Regulation of Rho GTPases by p120-catenin. Curr Opin Cell Biol 13:604–10.

Angres B, Barth A, Nelson WJ. (1996) Mechanism for transition from initial to stable cell-cell adhesion: Kinetic analysis of E-cadherin-mediated adhesion using a quantitative adhesion assay. J Cell Biol 134:549–57.

Ascano JJ, Frierson H Jr, Moskaluk CA, Harper JC, Roviello F, Jackson CE, El-Rifai W, Vindigni C, Tosi P, Powell SM. (2001) Inactivation of the E-cadherin gene in sporadic diffuse-type gastric cancer. Mod Pathol 14:942–49.

Asgeirsson KS, Jónasson JG, Tryggvadóttir L, Olafsdóttir K, Sigurgeirsdóttir JR, Ingvarsson S, Ogmundsdóttir HM. (2000) Altered expression of E-cadherin in breast cancer. Patterns, mechanisms and clinical significance. Eur J Cancer 36:1098–106.

Baloch ZW, Pasha T, LiVolsi VA. (2001) Cytoplasmic accumulation of alpha-catenin in thyroid neoplasms. Head Neck 23:573–78.

Batlle E, Sancho E, Francí C, Domínguez D, Monfar M, Baulida J, García De Herreros A. (2000) The transcription factor snail is a repressor of E-cadherin gene expression in epithelial tumour cells. Nat Cell Biol 2:84–9.

Becker KF, Atkinson MJ, Reich U, et al. (1994) E-cadherin gene mutations provide clues to diffuse type gastric carcinomas. Cancer Res 54:3845–52.

Behrens J, Mareel MM, Van Roy FM, Birchmeier W. (1989) Dissecting tumor cell invasion: Epithelial cells acquire invasive properties after the loss of uvomorulin-mediated cell-cell adhesion. J Cell Biol 108:2435–47.

Behrens J, Vakaet L, Friis R, Winterhager E, Van Roy F, Mareel MM, Birchmeier W. (1993) Loss of epithelial differentiation and gain of invasiveness correlates with tyrosine phosphorylation of the E-cadherin/beta-catenin complex in cells transformed with a temperature-sensitive v-SRC gene. J Cell Biol 120:757–66.

Berx G, Cleton-Jansen AM, Nollet F, de Leeuw WJ, van de Vijver M, Cornelisse C, van Roy F. (1995) E-cadherin is a tumour/invasion suppressor gene mutated in human lobular breast cancers. Embo J 14:6107–15.

Berx G, Becker KF, Hofler H, van Roy F. (1998) Mutations of the human E-cadherin (CDH1) gene. Hum Mutat 12:226–37.

Berx G and Van Roy F. (2001) The E-cadherin/catenin complex: An important gatekeeper in breast cancer tumorigenesis and malignant progression. Breast Cancer Res 3:289–93.

Böhm J, Niskanen L, Kiraly K, Kellokoski J, Eskelinen M, Hollmen S, Alhava E, Kosma VM. (2000) Expression and prognostic value of alpha-, beta-, and gamma-catenins indifferentiated thyroid carcinoma. J Clin Endocrinol Metab 85:4806–11.

Bohm M, Totzeck B, Birchmeier W, Wieland I. (1994) Differences of E-cadherin expression levels and patterns in primary and metastatic human lung cancer. Clin Exp Metastasis 12:55–62.

Brecelj E, Frkovic Grazio S, Auersperg M, Bracko M. (2005) Prognostic value of E-cadherin expression in thyroid follicular carcinoma. Eur J Surg Oncol 31:544–8.

Brembeck FH, Schwarz-Romond T, Bakkers J, Wilhelm S, Hammerschmidt M, Birchmeier W. (2004) Essential role of BCL9-2 in the switch between beta-catenin's adhesive and transcriptional functions. Genes Dev 18:222530.

Bremm A, Walch A, Fuchs M, Mages J, Duyster J, Keller G, Hermannstädter C, Becker KF, Rauser S, Langer R, von Weyhern CH, Höfler H, Luber B. (2008) Enhanced activation of epidermal growth factor receptor caused by tumor-derived E-cadherin mutations. Cancer Res 68: 707–14.

Bremnes RM, Veve R, Gabrielson E, Hirsch FR, Baron A, Bemis L, Gemmill RM, Drabkin HA, Franklin WA. (2002) High-throughput tissue microarray analysis used to evaluate biology and prognostic significance of the E-cadherin pathway in non-small-cell lung cancer. J Clin Oncol 20:2417–28.

Brooks-Wilson AR, Kaurah P, Suriano G, Leach S, Senz J, Grehan N, Butterfield YS, Jeyes J, Schinas J, Bacani J, Kelsey M, Ferreira P, MacGillivray B, MacLeod P, Micek M, Ford J, Foulkes W, Australie K, Greenberg C, LaPointe M, Gilpin C, Nikkel S, Gilchrist D, Hughes R, Jackson CE, Monaghan KG, Oliveira MJ, Seruca R, Gallinger S, Caldas C, Huntsman D. (2004) Germline E-cadherin mutations in hereditary diffuse gastric cancer: Assessment of 42 new families and review of genetic screening criteria. J Med Genet 41:508–17.

Brouxhon S, Kyrkanides S, O'Banion MK, Johnson R, Pearce DA, Centola GM, Miller JN, McGrath KH, Erdle B, Scott G, Schneider S, VanBuskirk J, Pentland AP. (2007) Sequential down-regulation of E-cadherin with squamous cell carcinoma progression: Loss of E-cadherin via a prostaglandin E2-EP2 dependent posttranslational mechanism. Cancer Res 67: 7654–64.

Bukholm IK, Nesland JM, Borresen-Dale AL. (2000) Re-expression of E-cadherin, alpha-catenin and beta-catenin, but not of gamma-catenin, in metastatic tissue from breast cancer patients [see comments]. J Pathol 190:15–19.

Bullions LC, Notterman DA, Chung LS, Levine AJ. (1997) Expression of wild-type alpha-catenin protein in cells with a mutant alpha-catenin gene restores both growth regulation and tumor suppressor activities. Mol Cell Biol 17:4501–8.

Cano A, Pérez-Moreno MA, Rodrigo I, Locascio A, Blanco MJ, del Barrio MG, Portillo F, Nieto MA. (2000) The transcription factor snail controls epithelial-mesenchymal transitions by repressing E-cadherin expression. Nat Cell Biol 2:76–83.

Canonici A, Steelant W, Rigot V, Khomitch-Baud A, Boutaghou-Cherid H, Bruyneel E, Van Roy F, Garrouste F, Pommier G, André F. (2008) Insulin-like growth factor-I receptor, E-cadherin and alpha v integrin form a dynamic complex under the control of alpha-catenin. Int J Cancer 122:572–82.

Carico E, Atlante M, Bucci B, Nofroni I, Vecchione A. (2001) E-cadherin and alpha-catenin expression during tumor progression of cervical carcinoma. Gynecol Oncol 80:156–61.

Carmeliet P, Lampugnani MG, Moons L, Breviario F, Compernolle V, Bono F, Balconi G, Spagnuolo R, Oosthuyse B, Dewerchin M, Zanetti A, Angellilo A, Mattot V, Nuyens D, Lutgens E, Clotman F, de Ruiter MC, Gittenberger-de Groot A, Poelmann R, Lupu F, Herbert JM, Collen D, Dejana E. (1999) Targeted deficiency or cytosolic truncation of the VE-cadherin gene in mice impairs VEGF-mediated endothelial survival and angiogenesis. Cell 98:147–57.

Cavallaro U, Schaffhauser B, Christofori G. (2002) Cadherins and the tumour progression: Is it all in a switch? Cancer Lett 176:123–8.

Ceteci F, Ceteci S, Karreman C, Kramer BW, Asan E, Götz R, Rapp UR. (2007) Disruption of tumor cell adhesion promotes angiogenic switch and progression to micrometastasis in RAF-driven murine lung cancer. Cancer Cell 12:145–59.

Chen WC, Obrink B. (1991) Cell-cell contacts mediated by E-cadherin (uvomorulin) restrict invasive behavior of L-cells. J Cell Biol 114:319–27.

Chen CL, Liu SS, Ip SM, Wong LC, Ng TY, Ngan HY. (2003a) E-cadherin expression is silenced by DNA methylation in cervical cancer cell lines and tumours. Eur J Cancer 39:517–23.

Chen X, Kojima S, Borisy GG, Green KJ. (2003b) p120 catenin associates with kinesin and facilitates the transport of cadherin-catenin complexes to intercellular junctions. J Cell Biol 163:547–57.

Chesire DR, Ewing CM, Sauvageot J, Bova GS, Isaacs WB. (2000) Detection and analysis of beta-catenin mutations in prostate cancer. Prostate 45:323–34.

Chesire DR, Ewing CM, Gage WR, Isaacs WB. (2002) In vitro evidence for complex modes of nuclear beta-catenin signaling during prostate growth and tumorigenesis. Oncogene 21:2679–94.

Chung Y, Lam AK, Luk JM, Law S, Chan KW, Lee PY, Wong J. (2007) Altered E-cadherin expression and p120 catenin localization in esophageal squamous cell carcinoma. Ann Surg Oncol 14:3260–7.

Clevers H. (2006) Wnt/beta-catenin signaling in development and disease. Cell 127:469–80.

Coluccia AM, Benati D, Dekhil H, De Filippo A, Lan C, Gambacorti-Passerini C. (2006) SKI-606 decreases growth and motility of colorectal cancer cells by preventing pp60(c-Src)-dependent tyrosine phosphorylation of beta-catenin and its nuclear signaling. Cancer Res 66:2279–86.

Coluccia AM, Vacca A, Duñach M, Mologni L, Redaelli S, Bustos VH, Benati D, Pinna LA, Gambacorti-Passerini C. (2007) Bcr-Abl stabilizes beta-catenin in chronic myeloid leukemia through its tyrosine phosphorylation. Embo J 26:1456–66.

Comijn J, Berx G, Vermassen P, Verschueren K, van Grunsven L, Bruyneel E, Mareel M, Huylebroeck D, van Roy F. (2001) The two-handed E box binding zinc finger protein SIP1 downregulates E-cadherin and induces invasion. Mol Cell 7:1267–78.

Cowin P, Rowlands TM, Hatsell SJ. (2005) Cadherins and catenins in breast cancer. Curr Opin Cell Biol 17:499–508.

Damsky CH, Richa J, Solter D, Knudsen K, Buck CA. (1983) Identification and purification of a cell surface glycoprotein mediating intercellular adhesion in embryonic and adult tissue. Cell 34:455–66.

Davis MA, Ireton RC, Reynolds AB. (2003) A core function for p120-catenin in cadherin turnover. J Cell Biol 163:525–34.

De Wever O, Westbroek W, Verloes A, Bloemen N, Bracke M, Gespach C, Bruyneel E, Mareel M. (2004) Critical role of N-cadherin in myofibroblast invasion and migration in vitro stimulated by colon-cancer-cell-derived TGF-beta or wounding. J Cell Sci 117:4691–703.

Deeb G, Wang J, Ramnath N, Slocum HK, Wiseman S, Beck A, Tan D. (2004) Altered E-cadherin and epidermal growth factor receptor expressions are associated with patient survival in lung cancer: A study utilizing high-density tissue microarray and immunohistochemistry. Mod Pathol 17:430–9.

Derksen PW, Liu X, Saridin F, van der Gulden H, Zevenhoven J, Evers B, van Beijnum JR, Griffioen AW, Vink J, Krimpenfort P, Peterse JL, Cardiff RD, Berns A, Jonkers J. (2006) Somatic inactivation of E-cadherin and p53 in mice leads to metastatic lobular mammary carcinoma through induction of anoikis resistance and angiogenesis. Cancer Cell 10:437–49.

Dolled-Filhart M, McCabe A, Giltnane J, Cregger M, Camp RL, Rimm DL. (2006) Quantitative in situ analysis of beta-catenin expression in breast cancer shows decreased expression is associated with poor outcome. Cancer Res 66:5487–94.

Drees F, Pokutta S, Yamada S, Nelson WJ, Weis WI. (2005) Alpha-catenin is a molecular switch that binds E-cadherin-beta-catenin and regulates actin-filament assembly. Cell 123:903–15.

Dursun P, Yuce K, Usubutun A, Ayhan A. (2007) Loss of epithelium cadherin expression is associated with reduced overall survival and disease-free survival in early-stage squamous cell cervical carcinoma. Int J Gynecol Cancer 17:843–50.

El-Bahrawy M, El-Masry N, Alison M, Poulsom R, Fallowfield M. (2003) Expression of beta-catenin in basal cell carcinoma. Br J Dermatol 148:964–70.

Ellenbroek SI, Collard JG. (2007) Rho GTPases: Functions and association with cancer. Clin Exp Metastasis 24:657–72.

Ewing CM, Ru N, Morton RA, Robinson JC, Wheelock MJ, Johnson KR, Barrett JC, Isaacs WB. (1995) Chromosome 5 suppresses tumorigenicity of PC3 prostate cancer cells: Correlation with re-expression of alpha-catenin and restoration of E-cadherin function. Cancer Res 55: 4813–17.

Fang D, Hawke D, Zheng Y, Xia Y, Meisenhelder J, Nika H, Mills GB, Kobayashi R, Hunter T, Lu Z. (2007) Phosphorylation of beta-catenin by AKT promotes beta-catenin transcriptional activity. J Biol Chem 282:11221–9.

Fang WB, Ireton RC, Zhuang G, Takahashi T, Reynolds A, Chen J. (2008) Overexpression of EPHA2 receptor destabilizes adherens junctions via a RhoA-dependent mechanism. J Cell Sci 121:358–68.

Fearon ER. (2000) BRCA1 and E-cadherin promoter hypermethylation and gene inactivation in cancer-association or mechanism? J Natl Cancer Inst 92:515–17.

Ferber EC, Kajita M, Wadlow A, Tobiansky L, Niessen C, Ariga H, Daniel J, Fujita Y. (2008) A Role for the Cleaved Cytoplasmic Domain of E-cadherin in the Nucleus. J Biol Chem 283:12691–700.

Fevr T, Robine S, Louvard D, Huelsken J. (2007) Wnt/beta-catenin is essential for intestinal homeostasis and maintenance of intestinal stem cells. Mol Cell Biol 27:7551–9.

Frixen UH, Behrens J, Sachs M, Eberle G, Voss B, Warda A, Löchner D, Birchmeier W. (1991) E-cadherin-mediated cell-cell adhesion prevents invasiveness of human carcinoma cells. J Cell Biol 113:173–85.

Fujita Y, Krause G, Scheffner M, Zechner D, Leddy HE, Behrens J, Sommer T, Birchmeier W. (2002) Hakai, a c-Cbl-like protein, ubiquitinates and induces endocytosis of the E-cadherin complex. Nat Cell Biol 4:222–31.

Fukumaru K, Yoshii N, Kanzaki T, Kanekura T. (2007) Immunohistochemical comparison of beta-catenin expression by human normal epidermis and epidermal tumors. J Dermatol 34: 746–53.

Fuller LC, Allen MH, Montesu M, Barker JN, Macdonald DM. (1996) Expression of E-cadherin in human epidermal non-melanoma cutaneous tumours. Br J Dermatol 134:28–32.

Garcia-Rostan G, Tallini G, Herrero A, D'Aquila TG, Carcangiu ML, Rimm DL. (1999) Frequent mutation and nuclear localization of beta-catenin in anaplastic thyroid carcinoma. Cancer Res 59:1811–15.

Garinis GA, Menounos PG, Spanakis NE, Papadopoulos K, Karavitis G, Parassi I, Christeli E, Patrinos GP, Manolis EN, Peros G. (2002) Hypermethylation-associated transcriptional silencing of E-cadherin in primary sporadic colorectal carcinomas. J Pathol 198:442–9.

Giannini AL, Vivanco M, Kypta RM. (2000) Alpha-catenin inhibits beta-catenin signaling by preventing formation of a beta-catenin*T-cell factor*DNA complex. J Biol Chem 275: 21883–8.

Gillett CE, Miles DW, Ryder K, Skilton D, Liebman RD, Springall RJ, Barnes DM, Hanby AM. (2001) Retention of the expression of E-cadherin and catenins is associated with shorter survival in grade III ductal carcinoma of the breast. J Pathol 193:433–41.

Gimond C, van Der Flier A, van Delft S, Brakebusch C, Kuikman I, Collard JG, Fässler R, Sonnenberg A. (1999) Induction of cell scattering by expression of beta1 integrins in beta1-deficient epithelial cells requires activation of members of the rho family of GTPases and downregulation of cadherin and catenin function. J Cell Biol 147:1325–40.

Giroldi LA, Bringuier PP, de Weijert M, Jansen C, van Bokhoven A, Schalken JA. (1997) Role of E boxes in the repression of E-cadherin expression. Biochem Biophys Res Commun 241:453–8.

Gottardi CJ, Wong E, Gumbiner BM. (2001) E-cadherin suppresses cellular transformation by inhibiting beta-catenin signaling in an adhesion-independent manner. J Cell Biol 153:1049–60.

Grabsch H, Takeno S, Noguchi T, Hommel G, Gabbert HE, Mueller W. (2001) Different patterns of beta-catenin expression in gastric carcinomas: Relationship with clinicopathological parameters and prognostic outcome. Histopathology 39:141–9.

Grady WM, Willis J, Guilford PJ, Dunbier AK, Toro TT, Lynch H, Wiesner G, Ferguson K, Eng C, Park JG, Kim SJ, Markowitz S. (2000) Methylation of the CDH1 promoter as the second genetic hit in hereditary diffuse gastric cancer. Nat Genet 26:16–17.

Graff JR, Herman JG, Lapidus RG, Chopra H, Xu R, Jarrard DF, Isaacs WB, Pitha PM, Davidson NE, Baylin SB. (1995) E-cadherin expression is silenced by DNA hypermethylation in human breast and prostate carcinomas. Cancer Res 55:5195–9.

Graff JR, Greenberg VE, Herman JG, Westra WH, Boghaert ER, Ain KB, Saji M, Zeiger MA, Zimmer SG, Baylin SB. (1998) Distinct patterns of E-cadherin CpG island methylation in papillary, follicular, Hurthle's cell, and poorly differentiated human thyroid carcinoma. Cancer Res 58:2063–6.

Gravdal K, Halvorsen OJ, Haukaas SA, Akslen LA. (2007) A switch from E-cadherin to N-cadherin expression indicates epithelial to mesenchymal transition and is of strong and independent importance for the progress of prostate cancer. Clin Cancer Res 13:7003–11.

Gregory PA, Bert AG, Paterson EL, Barry SC, Tsykin A, Farshid G, Vadas MA, Khew-Goodall Y, Goodall GJ. (2008) The miR-200 family and miR-205 regulate epithelial to mesenchymal transition by targeting ZEB1 and SIP1. Nat Cell Biol 10:593–601.

Grooteclaes ML, Frisch SM. (2000) Evidence for a function of CtBP in epithelial gene regulation and anoikis. Oncogene 19:3823–8.

Gujral TS, van Veelen W, Richardson DS, Myers SM, Meens JA, Acton DS, Duñach M, Elliott BE, Höppener JW, Mulligan LM. (2008) A novel RET kinase-beta-catenin signaling pathway contributes to tumorigenesis in thyroid carcinoma. Cancer Res 68:1338–46.

Haegel H, Larue L, Ohsugi M, Fedorov L, Herrenknecht K, Kemler R. (1995) Lack of beta-catenin affects mouse development at gastrulation. Development 121:3529–37.

Hajra KM, Ji X, Fearon ER. (1999) Extinction of E-cadherin expression in breast cancer via a dominant repression pathway acting on proximal promoter elements. Oncogene 18:7274–9.

Hamaguchi M, Matsuyoshi N, Ohnishi Y, Gotoh B, Takeichi M, Nagai Y. (1993) p60v-src causes tyrosine phosphorylation and inactivation of the N-cadherin-catenin cell adhesion system. Embo J 12:307–14

Heimann R, Lan F, McBride R, Hellman S. (2000) Separating favorable from unfavorable prognostic markers in breast cancer: The role of E-cadherin. Cancer Res 60:298–304.

Herzig M, Savarese F, Novatchkova M, Semb H, Christofori G. (2007) Tumor progression induced by the loss of E-cadherin independent of beta-catenin/Tcf-mediated Wnt signaling. Oncogene 26:2290–2298.

Hino S, Tanji C, Nakayama KI, Kikuchi A. (2005) Phosphorylation of beta-catenin by cyclic AMP-dependent protein kinase stabilizes beta-catenin through inhibition of its ubiquitination. Mol Cell Biol 25:9063–72.

Hirano S, Nose A, Hatta K, Kawakami A, Takeichi M. (1987) Calcium-dependent cell-cell adhesion molecules (cadherins): Subclass specificities and possible involvement of actin bundles. J Cell Biol 105:2501–10.

Hiscox S, Jiang WG. (1999) Association of the HGF/SF receptor, c-met, with the cell-surface adhesion molecule, E-cadherin, and catenins in human tumor cells. Biochem Biophys Res Commun 261:406–11.

Horvath LG, Henshall SM, Lee CS, Kench JG, Golovsky D, Brenner PC, O'Neill GF, Kooner R, Stricker PD, Grygiel JJ, Sutherland RL. (2005) Lower levels of nuclear beta-catenin predict for a poorer prognosis in localized prostate cancer. Int J Cancer 113:415–22.

Huang H, He X. (2008) Wnt/beta-catenin signaling: New (and old) players and new insights. Curr Opin Cell Biol 20:119–25.

Huelsken J, Vogel R, Brinkmann V, Erdmann B, Birchmeier C, Birchmeier W. (2000) Requirement for beta-catenin in anterior-posterior axis formation in mice. J Cell Biol 148:567–78.

Hugo H, Ackland ML, Blick T, Lawrence MG, Clements JA, Williams ED, Thompson EW. (2007) Epithelial–mesenchymal and mesenchymal–epithelial transitions in carcinoma progression. J Cell Physiol 213:374–83.

Hulit J, Suyama K, Chung S, Keren R, Agiostratidou G, Shan W, Dong X, Williams TM, Lisanti MP, Knudsen K, Hazan RB. (2007) N-cadherin signaling potentiates mammary tumor metastasis via enhanced extracellular signal-regulated kinase activation. Cancer Res 67:3106–16.

Hung KF, Chang CS, Liu CJ, Lui MT, Cheng CY, Kao SY. (2006) Differential expression of E-cadherin in metastatic lesions comparing to primary oral squamous cell carcinoma. J Oral Pathol Med 35:589–94.

Imai T, Horiuchi A, Shiozawa T, Osada R, Kikuchi N, Ohira S, Oka K, Konishi I. (2004) Elevated expression of E-cadherin and alpha-, beta-, and gamma-catenins in metastatic lesions compared with primary epithelial ovarian carcinomas. Hum Pathol 35:1469–76.

Ishizaki Y, Omori Y, Momiyama M, Nishikawa Y, Tokairin T, Manabe M, Enomoto K. (2004) Reduced expression and aberrant localization of p120 catenin in human squamous cell carcinoma of the skin. J Dermatol Sci 34:99–108.

Jaggi M, Johansson SL, Baker JJ, Smith LM, Galich A, Balaji KC. (2005) Aberrant expression of E-cadherin and beta-catenin in human prostate cancer. Urol Oncol 23:402–6.

Jawhari A, Jordan S, Poole S, Browne P, Pignatelli M, Farthing MJ. (1997) Abnormal immunoreactivity of the E-cadherin-catenin complex in gastric carcinoma: Relationship with patient survival. Gastroenterology 112:46–54.

Jeschke U, Mylonas I, Kuhn C, Shabani N, Kunert-Keil C, Schindlbeck C, Gerber B, Friese K. (2007) Expression of E-cadherin in human ductal breast cancer carcinoma in situ, invasive carcinomas, their lymph node metastases, their distant metastases, carcinomas with recurrence and in recurrence. Anticancer Res 27:1969–74.

Joo YE, Park CS, Kim HS, Choi SK, Rew JS, Kim SJ. (2000) Prognostic significance of E-cadherin/catenin complex expression in gastric cancer. J Korean Med Sci 15:655–66.

Jung IM, Chung JK, Kim YA, Kim JE, Heo SC, Ahn YJ, Hwang KT, Kim BG, Lee KL, Kim CW, Kim WH, Chang MS. (2007) Epstein-Barr virus, beta-catenin, and E-cadherin in gastric carcinomas. J Korean Med Sci 22:855–61.

Kadowaki T, Shiozaki H, Inoue M, Tamura S, Oka H, Doki Y, Iihara K, Matsui S, Iwazawa T, Nagafuchi A, et al. (1994) E-cadherin and alpha-catenin expression in human esophageal cancer. Cancer Res 54:291–6.

Kang HG, Jenabi JM, Zhang J, Keshelava N, Shimada H, May WA, Ng T, Reynolds CP, Triche TJ, Sorensen PH. (2007) E-cadherin cell-cell adhesion in ewing tumor cells mediates suppression of anoikis through activation of the ErbB4 tyrosine kinase. Cancer Res 67:3094–105.

Kase S, Sugio K, Yamazaki K, Okamoto T, Yano T, Sugimachi K. (2000) Expression of E-cadherin and beta-catenin in human non-small cell lung cancer and the clinical significance. Clin Cancer Res 6:4789–96.

Kato N, Tsuchiya T, Tamura G, Motoyama T. (2002) E-cadherin expression in follicular carcinoma of the thyroid. Pathol Int 52:13–18.

Kim DS, Kim MJ, Lee JY, Kim YZ, Kim EJ, Park JY. (2007) Aberrant methylation of E-cadherin and H-cadherin genes in nonsmall cell lung cancer and its relation to clinicopathologic features. Cancer 110:2785–92.

Kimura K, Endo Y, Yonemura Y, Heizmann CW, Schafer BW, Watanabe Y, Sasaki T. (2000) Clinical significance of S100A4 and E-cadherin-related adhesion molecules in non-small cell lung cancer. Int J Oncol 16:1125–31.

Knudsen KA, Sauer C, Johnson KR, Wheelock MJ. (2005) Effect of N-cadherin misexpression by the mammary epithelium in mice. J Cell Biochem 95:1093–107.

Kobielak A, Pasolli HA, Fuchs E. (2004) Mammalian formin-1 participates in adherens junctions and polymerization of linear actin cables. Nat Cell Biol 6:21–30.

Koksal IT, Ozcan F, Kilicaslan I, Tefekli A. (2002) Expression of E-cadherin in prostate cancer in forma-lin-fixed, paraffin-embedded tissues: Correlation with pathological features. Pathology 34:233–8.

Kooy AJ, Tank B, de Jong AA, Vuzevski VD, van der Kwast TH, van Joost T. (1999) Expression of E-cadherin, alpha-& beta-catenin, and CD44V6 and the subcellular localization of E-cadherin and CD44V6 in normal epidermis and basal cell carcinoma. Hum Pathol 30:1328–35.

Kudo J, Nishiwaki T, Haruki N, Ishiguro H, Shibata Y, Terashita Y, Sugiura H, Shinoda N, Kimura M, Kuwabara Y, Fujii Y. (2007) Aberrant nuclear localization of beta-catenin without genetic alterations in beta-catenin or Axin genes in esophageal cancer. World J Surg Oncol 5:21.

Larue L, Ohsugi M, Hirchenhain J, Kemler R. (1994) E-cadherin null mutant embryos fail to form a tro-phectoderm epithelium. Proc Natl Acad Sci U S A 91:8263–7.

Leong KG, Niessen K, Kulic I, Raouf A, Eaves C, Pollet I, Karsan A. (2007) Jagged1-mediated Notch activation induces epithelial-to-mesenchymal transition through Slug-induced repression of E-cadherin. J Exp Med 204:2935–48.

Lien WH, Klezovitch O, Fernandez TE, Delrow J, Vasioukhin V. (2006) alpha E-catenin controls cerebral cortical size by regulating the hedgehog signaling pathway. Science 311:1609–12.

Lien WH, Klezovitch O, Null M, Vasioukhin V. (2008) {alpha}E-catenin is not a significant regulator of {beta}-catenin signaling in the developing mammalian brain. J Cell Sci 121 (Pt 9): 1357–62.

Lilien J, Balsamo J. (2005) The regulation of cadherin-mediated adhesion by tyrosine phosphory-lation/dephosphorylation of beta-catenin. Curr Opin Cell Biol 17:459–65.

Lin SY, Xia W, Wang JC, Kwong KY, Spohn B, Wen Y, Pestell RG, Hung MC. (2000) Beta-catenin, a novel prognostic marker for breast cancer: Its roles in cyclin D1 expression and cancer progression. Proc Natl Acad Sci U S A 97:4262–66.

Lo Muzio L, Goteri G, Capretti R, Rubini C, Vinella A, Fumarulo R, Bianchi F, Mastrangelo F, Porfiri E, Mariggiò MA. (2005) Beta-catenin gene analysis in oral squamous cell carcinoma. Int J Immunopathol Pharmacol 18:33–8.

Lochter A, Galosy S, Muschler J, Freedman N, Werb Z, Bissell MJ. (1997) Matrix metal-loproteinase stromelysin-1 triggers a cascade of molecular alterations that leads to stable epithelial-to-mesenchymal conversion and a premalignant phenotype in mammary epithelial cells. J Cell Biol 139:1861–72.

Loric S, Paradis V, Gala JL, Berteau P, Bedossa P, Benoit G, Eschwège P. (2001) Abnormal E-cadherin expression and prostate cell blood dissemination as markers of biological recurrence in cancer. Eur J Cancer 37:1475–81.

Lozano E, Frasa MA, Smolarczyk K, Knaus UG, Braga VM. (2008) PAK is required for the disruption of E-cadherin adhesion by the small GTPase Rac. J Cell Sci 121:933–8.

Machon O, van den Bout CJ, Backman M, Kemler R, Krauss S. (2003) Role of beta-catenin in the developing cortical and hippocampal neuroepithelium. Neuroscience 122:129–43.

Marambaud P, Shioi J, Serban G, Georgakopoulos A, Sarner S, Nagy V, Baki L, Wen P, Efthimiopoulos S, Shao Z, Wisniewski T, Robakis NK. (2002) A presenilin-1/gamma-secretase cleavage releases the E-cadherin intracellular domain and regulates disassembly of adherens junctions. Embo J 21:1948–56.

Maretzky T, Reiss K, Ludwig A, Buchholz J, Scholz F, Proksch E, de Strooper B, Hartmann D, Saftig P. (2005) ADAM10 mediates E-cadherin shedding and regulates epithelial cell-cell adhesion, migration, and beta-catenin translocation. Proc Natl Acad Sci U S A 102:9182–87.

Matsumura T, Makino R, Mitamura K. (2001) Frequent down-regulation of E-cadherin by genetic and epigenetic changes in the malignant progression of hepatocellular carcinomas. Clin Cancer Res 7:594–9.

Mattijssen V, Peters HM, Schalkwijk L, Manni JJ, van 't Hof-Grootenboer B, de Mulder PH, Ruiter DJ. (1993) E-cadherin expression in head and neck squamous-cell carcinoma is associated with clinical outcome. Int J Cancer 55:580–5.

Mayer B, Johnson JP, Leitl F, Jauch KW, Heiss MM, Schildberg FW, Birchmeier W, Funke I. (1993) E-cadherin expression in primary and metastatic gastric cancer: Down-regulation correlates with cellular dedifferentiation and glandular disintegration. Cancer Res 53:1690–5.

Merdek KD, Nguyen NT, Toksoz D. (2004) Distinct activities of the alpha-catenin family, alpha-catulin and alpha-catenin, on beta-catenin-mediated signaling. Mol Cell Biol 24:2410–22.

Mitselou A, Ioachim E, Peschos D, Charalabopoulos K, Michael M, Agnantis NJ, Vougiouklakis T. (2007) E-cadherin adhesion molecule and syndecan-1 expression in various thyroid patholo-gies. Exp Oncol 29:54–60.

Miyanaga A, Gemma A, Ando M, Kosaihira S, Noro R, Minegishi Y, Kataoka K, Nara M, Okano T, Miyazawa H, Tanaka T, Yoshimura A, Kobayashi K, Iwanami H, Hagiwara K, Tsuboi E, Kudoh S. (2008) E-cadherin expression and epidermal growth factor receptor mutation status predict outcome in non-small cell lung cancer patients treated with gefitinib. Oncol Rep 19:377–383.

Moll R, Mitze M, Frixen UH, Birchmeier W. (1993) Differential loss of E-cadherin expression in infiltrating ductal and lobular breast carcinomas. Am J Pathol 143:1731–42.

Muta H, Noguchi M, Kanai Y, Ochiai A, Nawata H, Hirohashi S. (1996) E-cadherin gene mutations in signet ring cell carcinoma of the stomach. Jpn J Cancer Res 87:843–8.

Nagae Y, Kameyama K, Yokoyama M, Naito Z, Yamada N, Maeda S, Asano G, Sugisaki Y, Tanaka S. (2002) Expression of E-cadherin catenin and C-erbB-2 gene products in invasive ductal-type breast carcinomas. J Nippon Med Sch 69:165–71.

Naito A, Iwase H, Kuzushima T, Nakamura T, Kobayashi S. (2001) Clinical significance of E-cadherin expression in thyroid neoplasms. J Surg Oncol 76:176–80.

Nakanishi Y, Ochiai A, Akimoto S, Kato H, Watanabe H, Tachimori Y, Yamamoto S, Hirohashi S. (1997) Expression of E-cadherin, alpha-catenin, beta-catenin and plakoglobin in esophageal carcinomas and its prognostic significance: Immunohistochemical analysis of 96 lesions. Oncology 54:158–65.

Nakopoulou L, Gakiopoulou-Givalou H, Karayiannakis AJ, Giannopoulou I, Keramopoulos A, Davaris P, Pignatelli M. (2002) Abnormal alpha-catenin expression in invasive breast cancer correlates with poor patient survival. Histopathology 40:536–46.

Nam JS, Ino Y, Kanai Y, Sakamoto M, Hirohashi S. (2004) 5-aza-2'-deoxycytidine restores the E-cadherin system in E-cadherin-silenced cancer cells and reduces cancer metastasis. Clin Exp Metastasis 21:49–56.

Nam JS, Hirohashi S, Wakefield LM. (2007) Dysadherin: A new player in cancer progression. Cancer Lett 255:161–9.

Nemade RV, Bierie B, Nozawa M, Bry C, Smith GH, Vasioukhin V, Fuchs E, Hennighausen L. (2004) Biogenesis and function of mouse mammary epithelium depends on the presence of functional alpha-catenin. Mech Dev 121:91–9.

Nieman MT, Prudoff RS, Johnson KR, Wheelock MJ. (1999) N-cadherin promotes motility in human breast cancer cells regardless of their E-cadherin expression. J Cell Biol 147:631–44.

Nojima D, Nakajima K, Li LC, Franks J, Ribeiro-Filho L, Ishii N, Dahiya R. (2001) CpG methylation of promoter region inactivates E-cadherin gene in renal cell carcinoma. Mol Carcinog 32:19–27.

Noren NK, Liu BP, Burridge K, Kreft B. (2000) p120 catenin regulates the actin cytoskeleton via Rho family GTPases. J Cell Biol 150:567–80.

Nozawa N, Hashimoto S, Nakashima Y, Matsuo Y, Koga T, Sugio K, Niho Y, Harada M, Sueishi K. (2006) Immunohistochemical alpha-and beta-catenin and E-cadherin expression and their clinicopathological significance in human lung adenocarcinoma. Pathol Res Pract 202: 639–50.

Ochiai A, Akimoto S, Kanai Y, Shibata T, Oyama T, Hirohashi S. (1994) c-erbB-2 gene product associates with catenins in human cancer cells. Biochem Biophys Res Commun 205:73–8.

Odajima T, Sasaki Y, Tanaka N, Kato-Mori Y, Asanuma H, Ikeda T, Satoh M, Hiratsuka H, Tokino T, Sawada N. (2005) Abnormal beta-catenin expression in oral cancer with no gene mutation: Correlation with expression of cyclin D1 and epidermal growth factor receptor, Ki-67 labeling index, and clinicopathological features. Hum Pathol 36:234–41.

Oka H, Shiozaki H, Kobayashi K, Inoue M, Tahara H, Kobayashi T, Takatsuka Y, Matsuyoshi N, Hirano S, Takeichi M, et al. (1993) Expression of E-cadherin cell adhesion molecules in human breast cancer tissues and its relationship to metastasis. Cancer Res 53:1696–701.

Onder TT, Gupta PB, Mani SA, Yang J, Lander ES, Weinberg RA. (2008) Loss of E-cadherin promotes metastasis via multiple downstream transcriptional pathways. Cancer Res 68: 3645–54.

Orsulic S, Huber O, Aberle H, Arnold S, Kemler R. (1999) E-cadherin binding prevents beta-catenin nuclear localization and beta-catenin/LEF-1-mediated transactivation. J Cell Sci 112 (Pt 8):1237–1245.

Ozdamar B, Bose R, Barrios-Rodiles M, Wang HR, Zhang Y, Wrana JL. (2005) Regulation of the polarity protein Par6 by TGFbeta receptors controls epithelial cell plasticity. Science 307: 1603–9.

Palacios F, Tushir JS, Fujita Y, D'Souza-Schorey C. (2005) Lysosomal targeting of E-cadherin: A unique mechanism for the down-regulation of cell-cell adhesion during epithelial to mesenchymal transitions. Mol Cell Biol 25:389–402.

Park D, Karesen R, Axcrona U, Noren T, Sauer T. (2007) Expression pattern of adhesion molecules (E-cadherin, alpha-, beta-, gamma-catenin and claudin-7), their influence on survival in primary breast carcinoma, and their corresponding axillary lymph node metastasis. Apmis 115: 52–65.

Park SM, Gaur AB, Lengyel E, Peter ME. (2008) The miR-200 family determines the epithelial phenotype of cancer cells by targeting the E-cadherin repressors ZEB1 and ZEB2. Genes Dev 22:894–907.

Pedersen KB, Nesland JM, Fodstad O, Maelandsmo GM. (2002) Expression of S100A4, E-cadherin, al-pha-and beta-catenin in breast cancer biopsies. Br J Cancer 87:1281–6.

Peinado H, Olmeda D, Cano A. (2007) Snail, Zeb and bHLH factors in tumour progression: An alliance against the epithelial phenotype? Nat Rev Cancer 7:415–28.

Perez-Moreno MA, Locascio A, Rodrigo I, Dhondt G, Portillo F, Nieto MA, Cano A. (2001) A new role for E12/E47 in the repression of E-cadherin expression and epithelial-mesenchymal transitions. J Biol Chem 276:27424–31.

Perez-Moreno M, Jamora C, Fuchs E. (2003) Sticky business: Orchestrating cellular signals at adherens junctions. Cell 112:535–48.

Perl AK, Wilgenbus P, Dahl U, Semb H, Christofori G. (1998) A causal role for E-cadherin in the transition from adenoma to carcinoma. Nature 392:190–3.

Perrais M, Chen X, Perez-Moreno M, Gumbiner BM. (2007) E-cadherin homophilic ligation inhibits cell growth and epidermal growth factor receptor signaling independently of other cell interactions. Mol Biol Cell 18:2013–25.

Pizarro A, Benito N, Navarro P, Palacios J, Cano A, Quintanilla M, Contreras F, Gamallo C. (1994) E-cadherin expression in basal cell carcinoma. Br J Cancer 69:157–62.

Pizarro A, Gamallo C, Benito N, Palacios J, Quintanilla M, Cano A, Contreras F. (1995) Differential patterns of placental and epithelial cadherin expression in basal cell carcinoma and in the epidermis overlying tumours. Br J Cancer 72:327–32.

Qian X, Karpova T, Sheppard AM, McNally J, Lowy DR. (2004) E-cadherin-mediated adhesion inhibits ligand-dependent activation of diverse receptor tyrosine kinases. Embo J 23: 1739–48.

Rakha EA, Abd El Rehim D, Pinder SE, Lewis SA, Ellis IO. (2005) E-cadherin expression in invasive non-lobular carcinoma of the breast and its prognostic significance. Histopathology 46:685–93.

Ramasami S, Kerr KM, Chapman AD, King G, Cockburn JS, Jeffrey RR. (2000) Expression of CD44v6 but not E-cadherin or beta-catenin influences prognosis in primary pulmonary adenocarcinoma. J Pathol 192:427–32.

Reshetnikova G, Troyanovsky S, Rimm DL. (2007) Definition of a direct extracellular interaction between Met and E-cadherin. Cell Biol Int 31:366–73.

Reynolds AB. (2007) p120-catenin: Past and present. Biochim Biophys Acta 1773:2–7.

Ribeiro-Filho LA, Franks J, Sasaki M, Shiina H, Li LC, Nojima D, Arap S, Carroll P, Enokida H, Nakagawa M, Yonezawa S, Dahiya R. (2002) CpG hypermethylation of promoter region and inactivation of E-cadherin gene in human bladder cancer. Mol Carcinog 34:187–98.

Richmond PJ, Karayiannakis AJ, Nagafuchi A, Kaisary AV, Pignatelli M. (1997) Aberrant E-cadherin and alpha-catenin expression in prostate cancer: Correlation with patient survival. Cancer Res 57:3189–93.

Rieger-Christ KM, Pezza JA, Dugan JM, Braasch JW, Hughes KS, Summerhayes IC. (2001) Disparate E-cadherin mutations in LCIS and associated invasive breast carcinomas. Mol Pathol 54:91–7.

Risinger JI, Berchuck A, Kohler MF, Boyd J. (1994) Mutations of the E-cadherin gene in human gynecologic cancers. Nat Genet 7:98–102.

Rocha AS, Soares P, Seruca R, Máximo V, Matias-Guiu X, Cameselle-Teijeiro J, Sobrinho-Simões M. (2001) Abnormalities of the E-cadherin/catenin adhesion complex in classical papillary thyroid carcinoma and in its diffuse sclerosing variant. J Pathol 194:358–66.

Rocha AS, Soares P, Fonseca E, Cameselle-Teijeiro J, Oliveira MC, Sobrinho-Simoes M. (2003) E-cadherin loss rather than beta-catenin alterations is a common feature of poorly differentiated thyroid carcinomas. Histopathology 42:580–7.

Roura S, Miravet S, Piedra J, Garcia de Herreros A, Dunach M. (1999) Regulation of E-cadherin/catenin association by tyrosine phosphorylation. J Biol Chem 274:36734–40.

Rubin MA, Mucci NR, Figurski J, Fecko A, Pienta KJ, Day ML. (2001) E-cadherin expression in prostate cancer: A broad survey using high-density tissue microarray technology. Hum Pathol 32:690–7.

Sahai E, Marshall CJ. (2002) ROCK and Dia have opposing effects on adherens junctions downstream of Rho. Nat Cell Biol 4:408–15.

Saito Y, Takazawa H, Uzawa K, Tanzawa H, Sato K. (1998) Reduced expression of E-cadherin in oral squamous cell carcinoma: Relationship with DNA methylation of 5' CpG island. Int J Oncol 12:293–8.

Sakaki T, Wato M, Tamura I, Nakajima M, Morita S, Kakudo K, Shirasu R, Tanaka A, Sakaki T. (1999) Correlation of E-cadherin and alpha-catenin expression with differentiation of oral squamous cell carcinoma. J Osaka Dent Univ 33:75–81.

Saldanha G, Ghura V, Potter L, Fletcher A. (2004) Nuclear beta-catenin in basal cell carcinoma correlates with increased proliferation. Br J Dermatol 151:157–64.

Salon C, Moro D, Lantuejoul S, Brichon Py P, Drabkin H, Brambilla C, Brambilla E. (2004) E-cadherin-beta-catenin adhesion complex in neuroendocrine tumors of the lung: A suggested role upon local invasion and metastasis. Hum Pathol 35:1148–55.

Salon C, Lantuejoul S, Eymin B, Gazzeri S, Brambilla C, Brambilla E. (2005) The E-cadherin-beta-catenin complex and its implication in lung cancer progression and prognosis. Future Oncol 1:649–60.

Savagner P, Yamada KM, Thiery JP. (1997) The zinc-finger protein slug causes desmosome dissociation, an initial and necessary step for growth factor-induced epithelial-mesenchymal transition. J Cell Biol 137:1403–19.

Schipper JH, Frixen UH, Behrens J, Unger A, Jahnke K, Birchmeier W. (1991) E-cadherin expression in squamous cell carcinomas of head and neck: Inverse correlation with tumor dedifferentiation and lymph node metastasis. Cancer Res 51:6328–37.

Sehgal RN, Gumbiner BM, Reichardt LF. (1997) Antagonism of cell adhesion by an alpha-catenin mutant, and of the Wnt-signaling pathway by alpha-catenin in Xenopus embryos. J Cell Biol 139:1033–46.

Setoyama T, Natsugoe S, Okumura H, Matsumoto M, Uchikado Y, Yokomakura N, Ishigami S, Aikou T. (2007) alpha-catenin is a significant prognostic factor than E-cadherin in esophageal squamous cell carcinoma. J Surg Oncol 95:148–55.

Shen Y, Hirsch DS, Sasiela CA, Wu WJ. (2008) Cdc42 regulates E-cadherin ubiquitination and degradation through an epidermal growth factor receptor to Src-mediated pathway. J Biol Chem 283:5127–37.

Shun CT, Wu MS, Lin JT, Wang HP, Houng RL, Lee WJ, Wang TH, Chuang SM. (1998) An immunohistochemical study of E-cadherin expression with correlations to clinicopathological features in gastric cancer. Hepatogastroenterology 45:944–9.

Si HX, Tsao SW, Lam KY, Srivastava G, Liu Y, Wong YC, Shen ZY, Cheung AL. (2001) E-cadherin expression is commonly downregulated by CpG island hypermethylation in esophageal carcinoma cells. Cancer Lett 173:71–8.

Simcha I, Shtutman M, Salomon D, Zhurinsky J, Sadot E, Geiger B, Ben-Ze'ev A. (1998) Differential nuclear translocation and transactivation potential of beta-catenin and plakoglobin. J Cell Biol 141:1433–48.

Stefanou D, Goussia AC, Arkoumani E, Agnantis NJ. (2003) Expression of vascular endothelial growth factor and the adhesion molecule E-cadherin in non-small cell lung cancer. Anticancer Res 23:4715–20.

Suyama K, Shapiro I, Guttman M, Hazan RB. (2002) A signaling pathway leading to metastasis is controlled by N-cadherin and the FGF receptor. Cancer Cell 2:301–14.

Tada H, Hatoko M, Muramatsu T, Shirai T. (1996) Expression of E-cadherin in skin carcinomas. J Dermatol 23:104–10.

Takahashi K, Suzuki K. (1996) Density-dependent inhibition of growth involves prevention of EGF receptor activation by E-cadherin-mediated cell-cell adhesion. Exp Cell Res 226:214–22.

Tamura S, Shiozaki H, Miyata M, Kadowaki T, Inoue M, Matsui S, Iwazawa T, Takayama T, Takeichi M, Monden M. (1996) Decreased E-cadherin expression is associated with haematogenous recurrence and poor prognosis in patients with squamous cell carcinoma of the oesophagus. Br J Surg 83:1608–14.

Tamura G, Yin J, Wang S, Fleisher AS, Zou T, Abraham JM, Kong D, Smolinski KN, Wilson KT, James SP, Silverberg SG, Nishizuka S, Terashima M, Motoyama T, Meltzer SJ. (2000) E-Cadherin gene promoter hypermethylation in primary human gastric carcinomas. J Natl Cancer Inst 92:569–73.

Theisen CS, Wahl JK, 3rd, Johnson KR, Wheelock MJ. (2007) NHERF links the N-cadherin/catenin complex to the platelet-derived growth factor receptor to modulate the actin cytoskeleton and regulate cell motility. Mol Biol Cell 18:1220–32.

Thiery JP, Sleeman JP. (2006) Complex networks orchestrate epithelial-mesenchymal transitions. Nat Rev Mol Cell Biol 7:131–42.

Torres M, Stoykova A, Huber O, Chowdhury K, Bonaldo P, Mansouri A, Butz S, Kemler R, Gruss P. (1997) An alpha-E-catenin gene trap mutation defines its function in preimplantation development. Proc Natl Acad Sci U S A 94:901–6.

Toyoshima M, Tanaka N, Aoki J, Tanaka Y, Murata K, Kyuuma M, Kobayashi H, Ishii N, Yaegashi N, Sugamura K. (2007) Inhibition of tumor growth and metastasis by depletion of vesicular sorting protein Hrs: Its regulatory role on E-cadherin and beta-catenin. Cancer Res 67: 5162–71.

Toyoyama H, Nuruki K, Ogawa H, Yanagi M, Matsumoto H, Nishijima H, Shimotakahara T, Aikou T, Ozawa M. (1999) The reduced expression of e-cadherin, alpha-catenin and gamma-catenin but not beta-catenin in human lung cancer. Oncol Rep 6:81–5.

Umbas R, Schalken JA, Aalders TW, Carter BS, Karthaus HF, Schaafsma HE, Debruyne FM, Isaacs WB. (1992) Expression of the cellular adhesion molecule E-cadherin is reduced or absent in high-grade prostate cancer. Cancer Res 52:5104–9.

Umbas R, Isaacs WB, Bringuier PP, Schaafsma HE, Karthaus HF, Oosterhof GO, Debruyne FM, Schalken JA. (1994) Decreased E-cadherin expression is associated with poor prognosis in patients with prostate cancer. Cancer Res 54:3929–33.

van Oort IM, Tomita K, van Bokhoven A, Bussemakers MJ, Kiemeney LA, Karthaus HF, Witjes JA, Schalken JA. (2007) The prognostic value of E-cadherin and the cadherin-associated molecules alpha-, beta-, gamma-catenin and p120ctn in prostate cancer specific survival: A long-term follow-up study. Prostate 67:1432–8.

Vasioukhin V, Bauer C, Yin M, Fuchs E. (2000) Directed actin polymerization is the driving force for epithelial cell-cell adhesion. Cell 100:209–19.

Vasioukhin V, Bauer C, Degenstein L, Wise B, Fuchs E. (2001) Hyperproliferation and defects in epithelial polarity upon conditional ablation of alpha-catenin in skin. Cell 104:605–17.

Vleminckx K, Vakaet L, Jr, Mareel M, Fiers W, van Roy F. (1991) Genetic manipulation of E-cadherin expression by epithelial tumor cells reveals an invasion suppressor role. Cell 66: 107–19.

Voeller HJ, Truica CI, Gelmann EP. (1998) Beta-catenin mutations in human prostate cancer. Cancer Res 58:2520–23.

von Wasielewski R, Rhein A, Werner M, Scheumann GF, Dralle H, Pötter E, Brabant G, Georgii A. (1997) Immunohistochemical detection of E-cadherin in differentiated thyroid carcinomas correlates with clinical outcome. Cancer Res 57:2501–7.

Vos CB, Cleton-Jansen AM, Berx G, de Leeuw WJ, ter Haar NT, van Roy F, Cornelisse CJ, Peterse JL, van de Vijver MJ. (1997) E-cadherin inactivation in lobular carcinoma in situ of the breast: An early event in tumorigenesis. Br J Cancer 76:1131–3.

Watabe M, Nagafuchi A, Tsukita S, Takeichi M. (1994) Induction of polarized cell-cell association and retardation of growth by activation of the E-cadherin-catenin adhesion system in a dispersed carcinoma line. J Cell Biol 127:247–56.

Wehbi NK, Dugger AL, Bonner RB, Pitha JV, Hurst RE, Hemstreet GP, 3rd. (2002) Pan-cadherin as a high level phenotypic biomarker for prostate cancer. J Urol 167:2215–21.

Wheelock MJ, Shintani Y, Maeda M, Fukumoto Y, Johnson KR. (2008) Cadherin switching. J Cell Sci 121:727–35.

Wiseman SM, Masoudi H, Niblock P, Turbin D, Rajput A, Hay J, Filipenko D, Huntsman D, Gilks B. (2006) Derangement of the E-cadherin/catenin complex is involved in transformation of differentiated to anaplastic thyroid carcinoma. Am J Surg 191:581–7.

Wong SC, Lo SF, Lee KC, Yam JW, Chan JK, Wendy Hsiao WL. (2002) Expression of frizzled-related protein and Wnt-signalling molecules in invasive human breast tumours. J Pathol 196:145–53.

Wood LD, Parsons DW, Jones S, Lin J, Sjöblom T, Leary RJ, Shen D, Boca SM, Barber T, Ptak J, Silliman N, Szabo S, Dezso Z, Ustyanksky V, Nikolskaya T, Nikolsky Y, Karchin R, Wilson PA, Kaminker JS, Zhang Z, Croshaw R, Willis J, Dawson D, Shipitsin M, Willson JK, Sukumar S, Polyak K, Park BH, Pethiyagoda CL, Pant PV, Ballinger DG, Sparks AB, Hartigan J, Smith DR, Suh E, Papadopoulos N, Buckhaults P, Markowitz SD, Parmigiani G, Kinzler KW, Velculescu VE, Vogelstein B. (2007) The genomic landscapes of human breast and colorectal cancers. Science 318 (5853): 1108–13.

Wu TT, Hsu YS, Wang JS, Lee YH, Huang JK. (2003) The role of p53, bcl-2 and E-cadherin expression in predicting biochemical relapse for organ confined prostate cancer in Taiwan. J Urol 170:78–81.

Yamazaki F, Aragane Y, Kawada A, Tezuka T. (2001) Immunohistochemical detection for nuclear beta-catenin in sporadic basal cell carcinoma. Br J Dermatol 145:771–7.

Yang J, Mani SA, Donaher JL, Ramaswamy S, Itzykson RA, Come C, Savagner P, Gitelman I, Richardson A, Weinberg RA. (2004) Twist, a master regulator of morphogenesis, plays an essential role in tumor metastasis. Cell 117:927–39.

Yang JY, Zong CS, Xia W, Wei Y, Ali-Seyed M, Li Z, Broglio K, Berry DA, Hung MC. (2006) MDM2 promotes cell motility and invasiveness by regulating E-cadherin degradation. Mol Cell Biol 26:7269–82.

Yoshiura K, Kanai Y, Ochiai A, Shimoyama Y, Sugimura T, Hirohashi S. (1995) Silencing of the E-cadherin invasion-suppressor gene by CpG methylation in human carcinomas. Proc Natl Acad Sci U S A 92:7416–19.

Young P, Boussadia O, Halfter H, Grose R, Berger P, Leone DP, Robenek H, Charnay P, Kemler R, Suter U. (2003) E-cadherin controls adherens junctions in the epidermis and the renewal of hair follicles. Embo J 22:5723–33.

Zechner D, Fujita Y, Hülsken J, Müller T, Walther I, Taketo MM, Crenshaw EB 3rd, Birchmeier W, Birchmeier C. (2003) Beta-catenin signals regulate cell growth and the balance between progenitor cell expansion and differentiation in the nervous system. Dev Biol 258:406–18.

Zeng G, Apte U, Micsenyi A, Bell A, Monga SP. (2006) Tyrosine residues 654 and 670 in beta-catenin are crucial in regulation of Met-beta-catenin interactions. Exp Cell Res 312:3620–30.

Zhong C, Kinch MS, Burridge K. (1997) Rho-stimulated contractility contributes to the fibroblastic phenotype of Ras-transformed epithelial cells. Mol Biol Cell 8:2329–44.

Zhou YN, Xu CP, Han B, Li M, Qiao L, Fang DC, Yang JM. (2002) Expression of E-cadherin and beta-catenin in gastric carcinoma and its correlation with the clinicopathological features and patient survival. World J Gastroenterol 8:987–93.

Zhou YN, Xu CP, Chen Y, Han B, Yang SM, Fang DC. (2005) Alpha-catenin expression is decreased in patients with gastric carcinoma. World J Gastroenterol 11:3468–72.

Chapter 4
Rho GTPases in Regulation of Cancer Cell Motility, Invasion, and Microenvironment

Donita C. Brady, Jamie K. Alan, and Adrienne D. Cox

Cast of Characters

Unlike Ras proteins that are oncogenically mutated in 30% of human cancers, known naturally occurring mutations in Rho GTPases are limited to RhoH (a.k.a. ARHH), which undergoes translocations and hypermutations, especially in hematopoietic cancers. Despite this lack of common activating mutations, a large body of evidence points to misregulation of Rho protein function as a widespread occurence in epithelial-mesenchymal transition (EMT) to promote cancer cell motility and invasiveness. Deregulated Rho protein signaling occurs through aberrant expression of the GTPases themselves, altered expression or function of their regulators, or changes in activity of their upstream and downstream signaling components. Here we discuss how Rho GTPases are aberrantly regulated in cancer, and how their activity contributes to the alterations in cell-cell adhesion, cell-matrix adhesion, cell migration, and the tumor microenviroment that promote tumor cell motility, invasion, and metastasis.

Introduction

Epithelial–mesenchymal transitions (EMT) that promote cancer cell motility and invasiveness require dynamic epigenetic and morphogenetic changes. The acquisition of a motile and invasive program by cancer cells involves the activation of signaling pathways and induction of transcriptional profiles that promote the loss of cell–cell adhesions, loss of cell polarity, cytoskeletal reorganization, and proteolytic degradation and remodeling of the extracellular matrix (ECM) (Berx et al. 2007; Guarino et al. 2007). In addition to these morphological changes, cancer cells exhibit excessive cell proliferation and inhibition of normal apoptosis programs that promote cell survival (Hanahan and Weinberg 2000).

A.D. Cox (✉)
Departments of Radiation Oncology and Pharmacology, Lineberger Comprehensive Cancer Center, University of North Carolina at Chapel Hill, Campus Box 7512, Chapel Hill, NC, USA
e-mail: adrienne_cox@med.unc.edu

A. Thomas-Tikhonenko (ed.), *Cancer Genome and Tumor Microenvironment*, 67
DOI 10.1007/978-1-4419-0711-0_4, © Springer Science+Business Media, LLC 2010

It is well appreciated that aberrant activation of Ras small GTPases contributes to multiple human diseases (Schubbert et al. 2007). However, Ras isoforms were originally characterized as viral oncogenes and subsequently discovered to be mutated in 30% of human cancers (Shih et al. 1978; Chien et al. 1979; Der et al. 1982; Bos 1989). These oncogenic mutations render Ras proteins GTPase deficient, resulting in constitutive activation and thus leading to excessive activation of their downstream signaling pathways that promote many of the steps involved in cancer (Wennerberg et al. 2005).

Rho GTPases are instrumental in regulating many of the normal cellular processes that are misregulated during cancer progression, suggesting that, like members of the Ras superfamily, Rho GTPases may also be mutationally activated in human cancers. However, unlike Ras proteins that are oncogenically mutated in 30% of human cancers, no naturally occurring mutations in Rho GTPases have been found, with the exception of one Rho protein to be discussed later (Ellenbroek and Collard 2007). The absence of mutationally activated Rho GTPases in human cancers suggests that GTP/GDP cycling of these proteins may be required. Nevertheless, many of the morphological changes that contribute to tumor cell invasion and migration can be attributed to misregulation of Rho GTPase-driven cell motility (Ridley 2004; Ellenbroek and Collard 2007). Therefore, this chapter will focus on alterations of Rho GTPases in cancer at the level of expression or activation of the small GTPases and the underlying cellular mechanisms by which epigenetic changes in Rho GTPases contribute to cancer cell migration and invasion. More importantly, it will specifically focus on how misregulation of Rho GTPase signaling contributes to cancer cell motility in the context of tumor microenvironment. To that end, it is essential to first understand Rho GTPase regulation and function during normal cell conditions.

Overview of Rho GTPases: Regulation and Function

Small GTPases of the Ras superfamily function as molecular switches to elicit a diverse range of cellular processes through numerous signaling pathways (Mitin et al. 2005; Wennerberg et al. 2005). These cellular processes are initiated by the release of a myriad of extracellular stimuli, such as hormones, growth factors, and other signaling molecules, which bind to and activate cell surface receptors capable of transducing signals to promote multiple biological activities. Extensive research over the past several decades has implicated the Ras superfamily of small GTPases as central signaling nodes in regulating such processes as gene transcription, vesicle trafficking, cytoskeleton reorganization, cell survival, and cell cycle progression (Mitin et al. 2005).

The Ras superfamily of small GTPases includes over 150 GTP-binding proteins, based on their sequence identity and GTP-binding motifs. The Ras superfamily of small GTPases can be divided into five subfamilies: Ras, Ran, Rab, Arf, and Rho, based on sequence and functional similarities (Wennerberg et al. 2005). Most small GTPases share this biochemical mechanism, allowing them to function as molecular switches cycling between GTP- and GDP-bound states, a feature that is important for their regulation and function (Vetter and Wittinghofer 2001). When in the GTP-bound state, small GTPases are in an active conformation that allows them to interact with their downstream effectors, which mediate their diverse biological activities in response to extracellular stimuli. In addition to conformational changes and protein regulators of GTP/GDP cycling, small GTPase function is also regulated by posttranslational modification by prenyl and/or palmitoyl lipid moieties. C-terminal modification of small GTPases by prenylation and/or palmitoylation helps them associate with cellular membranes where they can both be activated and be associated with downstream effectors (Takai et al. 2001; Wennerberg et al. 2005). This chapter will focus on the Rho subfamily of GTPases that, like Ras subfamily members, respond to various extracellular stimuli to promote multiple biological activities, but are best known for regulating the actin cytoskeleton (Hall 1998; Etienne-Manneville and Hall 2002).

Rho Subfamily of Small GTPases

Rho GTPases are a subfamily of Ras-related small GTPases whose GTPase domains share 30% sequence identity with members of the Ras subfamily and 40–95% sequence identity within the Rho subfamily (Wennerberg and Der 2004). The evolutionarily conserved inclusion of the Rho insert domain distinguishes the Rho family of small GTPases from the other members of the Ras superfamily (Valencia et al. 1991). Like Ras, classic Rho GTPases contain a GTPase domain and short N- and C-terminal extensions. However, many of the less studied Rho GTPases can be classified as atypical members of the family based on their divergent structure, function, and modes of regulation (Aspenstrom et al. 2007).

The Rho GTPase family is comprised of 23 members that can be divided into 6 major branches based on sequence homology and function: RhoA related (RhoA, RhoB, RhoC), Rac related (Rac1, Rac2, Rac3, RhoG), Cdc42 related (Cdc42, TC10, TCL, Wrch-1, Wrch-2/Chp), Rnd (Rnd1, Rnd2, Rnd3/RhoE), RhoBTB (RhoBTB1, RhoBTB2, RhoBTB3), and Miro (Miro1, Miro2). RhoD, Rif, and RhoH/TTF are also Rho GTPases but are not usually stratified into one of the six subfamilies because their primary sequences are divergent. The inclusion of the Miro subfamily is controversial in the GTPase field due to their divergence in structure, and they are sometimes considered instead to be a distinct subfamily within the Ras superfamily. Alternative splicing of Rac1 and Cdc42 encodes Rac1b and the brain isoform of Cdc42, respectively, bringing the family to 25 distinct proteins (Wennerberg and Der 2004). The Rho family GTPases that have the more divergent structure and function, including the Rnd and RhoBTB subfamilies, RhoH, Wrch-1, and Wrch-2/Chp, are sometimes grouped together as "atypical" Rho GTPases (Aspenstrom et al. 2007).

It is well appreciated that Rho GTPases orchestrate diverse cellular processes in a variety of mammalian cell types as well as in yeast, flies, and worms (Boureux et al. 2007). Many of the biological functions associated with Rho GTPase activation, from cytoskeletal rearrangement to gene transcription, have been elucidated through studying the three classical family members: RhoA, Rac1, and Cdc42. More thorough investigation of other family members of Rho GTPases, such as Wrch-1, Rnd3, and RhoBTB, has the potential to uncover and understand additional important signaling pathways and biological functions.

Regulators of Rho GTPase GTP/GDP Cycling

Like other members of the Ras superfamily, Rho GTPases function as molecular switches, cycling between an active, GTP-bound state and an inactive, GDP-bound state. When GTP-bound, Rho GTPases elicit various biological functions through interaction with their downstream effectors. Their slow intrinsic GTPase activity turns Rho family proteins off to their GDP-bound state, thus terminating their signaling capabilities. However, members of the Rnd subfamily and RhoH are chronically GTP-bound in their wild-type forms (Foster et al. 1996; Li et al. 2002; Wennerberg and Der 2004). Since GTP-bound Rho GTPases mediate diverse cellular functions, tight regulation of their GTP/GDP cycling is necessary for normal cellular homeostasis.

Three classes of regulatory proteins facilitate GTP/GDP cycling of Rho GTPases: guanine nucleotide exchange factors (GEFs), GTPase-activating proteins (GAPs), and guanine nucleotide dissociation inhibitors (GDIs) (Wennerberg and Der 2004). GEFs accelerate the release of GDP and subsequent binding of GTP to GTPases by inducing specific conformational changes within their switch regions. These changes allow for high-affinity interaction of Rho GTPases with their effectors, leading to downstream signaling (Schmidt and Hall 2002). To date there are two distinct groups of Rho GEFs. The largest group of Rho GEFs comprises the Dbl family, characterized by tandem Dbl homology (DH) and Pleckstrin homology (PH) domains that are important for their exchange activity. The central dogma of Dbl family activation of Rho GTPases is that the PH domain interacts with phospholipids, which promotes the proper localization and subsequent activation of the catalytic DH domain through allosteric mechanisms. There are 69 human Dbl family Rho GEFs that contain the tandem DH/PH cassette; these have divergent domain architecture in regions outside of this cassette that reflect the diversity of signals and cellular functions mediated by activated Rho GTPases (Rossman et al. 2005). The second group of Rho GEFs consists of 11 proteins that form the Dock family (Cote and Vuori 2007). Members of the Dock family of GEFS do not contain the catalytic DH domain but are comprised of two regions of high sequence conservation, Dock homology region-1 and -2 (DHR-1 and DHR-2). The DHR-2 domain alone or in combination with its partner protein Elmo catalyzes nucleotide exchange, while the DHR-1 domain is structurally similar to C2 domains known to interact with phospholipids (Meller et al. 2005). The vast number of Rho GEFs highlights the diversity of signaling inputs capable of activating Rho GTPases to elicit their biological activities.

As stated previously, the GTPase activity of GTP-binding proteins is intrinsically slow and thus mechanisms to accelerate their GTPase activity are necessary to terminate their signaling outputs. GAPs increase the slow intrinsic GTP hydrolysis of GTPases and thus promote the formation of the GDP-bound, inactive state (Vetter and Wittinghofer 2001). GAPs for Rho GTPases contain a major structural element, the "arginine finger," which promotes their shared mechanism of action (Moon and Zheng 2003). When GAPs interact with a GTP-bound GTPase, this "arginine finger" present in the GAP is inserted into the active site of the GTPase to facilitate the transition from the GTP-bound state to a nucleotide-free state and subsequent reloading with GDP (Lamarche and Hall 1994; Vetter and Wittinghofer 2001). The human genome contains 160 potential GAPs for the Ras superfamily of GTPases, with approximately 70 of these identified proteins being GAPs for the Rho subfamily alone (Bernards 2003). Like the numerous GEFs, the existence of such a copious number of GAPs for the proportionately small number of Rho GTPases points out the importance of regulating their activation and inactivation in response to diverse extracellular stimuli.

The third class of regulatory proteins is that of the GDIs, which were first characterized as inhibitors of nucleotide exchange, thus blocking effector and GAP binding of GTP-bound Rho GTPases (Fukumoto et al. 1990; Chuang et al. 1993; DerMardirossian and Bokoch 2005). In addition, Rho GDIs recognize prenyl groups, which enables them to regulate the membrane association and dissociation of prenylated Rho family members, effectively blocking their activity (Michaelson et al. 2001). There is distinct binding specificity for different Rho GTPases to the three known human Rho GDIs (RhoGDIα/GDI1, Ly/D4GDIβ/GDI2, and RhoGDIγ/GDI3). Rho GDI-mediated masking of the prenyl group on Rho GTPases functions to sequester Rho proteins to the cytosol, preventing membrane association and downstream biological consequences (Hoffman et al. 2000; Dovas and Couchman 2005).

Although these three distinct classes of regulators for Rho GTPases have proven to be fundamental in regulating their GTP/GDP cycling, several Rho GTPases are not regulated in this manner. These proteins fall into the atypical subgroup of Rho GTPases that includes the Rnd and RhoBTB subfamilies, RhoH, Wrch-1, and Chp. Evidence for the existence of GEFs and GAPs for atypical Rho GTPases is lacking, although for at least some of these proteins, GAPs are likely because mutations analogous to those that cause constitutive activation of their classical relatives do confer additional activity, indicating that their activity is normally restrained by one or more GAPs in vivo. In contrast to classic Rho GTPases that are regulated by GEFs, GAPs, and GDIs, the atypical Rho GTPases are often regulated by their level of expression or additional domains involved in protein–protein interactions (Aspenstrom et al. 2007). RhoH, Rnd proteins, and RhoBTB proteins harbor "activating" amino acid substitutions at positions important for GTP hydrolysis, rendering these proteins GTPase deficient (Li et al. 2002; Chardin 2006; Aspenstrom et al. 2007). However, Wrch-1 and Chp, members of the Cdc42 subfamily of GTPases, do not contain activating mutations that render them GTPase deficient. Although Wrch-1 possesses a rapid rate of nucleotide exchange, it was shown to be predominantly in the GDP-bound conformation in vivo (Jordan et al. 1999; Saras et al. 2004; Shutes et al. 2004). Whether Chp, like Wrch-1, has an enhanced nucleotide exchange rate remains to be investigated, since detailed biochemical analysis has not yet been done.

Rho GTPases as Master Regulators of Actin Cytoskeletal Dynamics

The founding members of the Rho subfamily of GTPases, RhoA, Rac1, and Cdc42, are activated in response to extracellular stimuli and subsequently induce dynamic rearrangement of the actin cytoskeleton to regulate cell morphology and polarity (Hall 1998). Specifically, constitutive activation of RhoA leads to the formation of contractile actin–myosin filaments (stress fibers) and focal adhesions (Ridley and Hall 1992). However, membrane ruffling and lamellipodia formation at the plasma membrane are characteristics of Rac1 activation (Ridley et al. 1992). Cdc42 activation induces filopodia, which are specific actin filament protrusions at the plasma membrane (Kozma et al. 1995; Nobes et al. 1995). These effects on the actin cytoskeleton are mediated by diverse signaling pathways upstream and downstream of each Rho family GTPase to promote cell polarity, cell motility, and cell morphology (Nobes and Hall 1995).

The ability of Rho GTPases to function as master regulators of cell morphology via manipulation of the actin cytoskeleton to drive diverse cellular functions requires coordinated actin polymerization and contraction (Bishop and Hall 2000; Ridley 2001). Therefore, it is not surprising that extensive research has been conducted to investigate the actin polymerization machinery and contractile machinery regulated by Rho proteins. Simplistically, activated RhoA, Rac1, and Cdc42 drive actin polymerization and contraction through distinct downstream effectors. The best characterized downstream effectors of RhoA responsible for stress fiber formation are the serine–threonine kinases, ROCKI and ROCKII (Maekawa et al. 1999; Riento and Ridley 2003). One major pathway downstream of RhoA-mediated activation of ROCK leads to direct phosphorylation of myosin light chain (MLC) phosphatase, which indirectly leads to an increase in MLC phosphorylation (Kimura et al. 1996; Kawano et al. 1999). Upon phosphorylation of MLC, the ATPase activity of myosin II is stimulated and promotes the assembly of stress fibers (Amano et al. 1996; Bresnick 1999). The other target of ROCK serine/threonine kinases downstream of RhoA is LIM kinase (LIMK) that, when activated by phosphorylation, inhibits the actin severing protein, cofilin, thereby promoting the stabilization of actin filaments (Bamburg et al. 1999; Maekawa et al. 1999). Additionally, RhoA stimulates actin polymerization through its effector proteins, mDia1 and mDia2, through an indirect interaction with G-actin-binding protein, profilin (Watanabe et al. 1997; Nakano et al. 1999; Hotulainen and Lappalainen 2006; Gupton et al. 2007).

In contrast, Rac1 and Cdc42 coordinately regulate actin polymerization to promote lamellae, lamellipodia, and filopodia by regulating the Arp2/3 complex through distinct effectors or through the common downstream target, p21-activated kinase (PAK) (Cotteret and Chernoff 2002). One major downstream effector that allows Cdc42 to promote actin polymerization and subsequent filopodia formation is the scaffolding protein neuronal Wiskott–Aldrich syndrome protein (N-WASP) (Rohatgi et al. 1999). Rac1 regulates actin polymerization by activating WASP family verprolin-homologous protein (WAVE), resulting in altered actin nucleation activity of the Arp2/3 complex to promote lamellipodia formation (Miki et al. 2000). Like the ROCK serine/threonine kinases, activation of PAK kinase activity downstream of Rac1 or Cdc42 induces phosphorylation of LIMK, promoting actin filament stabilization (Edwards et al. 1999). In addition, active Rac- and Cdc42-stimulated PAK activation increases MLC kinase (MLCK) phosphorylation to decrease actomyosin contraction (Sanders et al. 1999). Coordinated spatiotemporal activation of these major pathways downstream of Rho GTPases is required for cell motility, which is driven by cycles of actin polymerization, cell adhesion, and actomyosin contraction. Therefore, misregulation of Rho GTPases during tumor progression can contribute to cancer cell motility by modulating actin dynamics and cell adhesion, which are necessary for invasion and metastasis (Price and Collard 2001; Ridley 2001; Ridley 2004; Olson and Sahai 2008).

Aberrations of Rho Activity in Cancer

It is clear that misregulation of Rho protein signaling occurs in cancer and contributes to aberrant growth, dedifferentiation, invasion, and metastasis. However, no activating mutations of Rho GTPases have been isolated from human cancers analogous to those identified in Ras subfamily members. Therefore, deregulation of Rho protein signaling must occur through altered expression of the GTPases themselves or of their activation that can in turn be achieved through alterations in Rho GTPase regulators or in their upstream and downstream signaling components. Extensive studies have elucidated several alterations in Rho GTPase signaling components that contribute to cancer initiation and progression.

Alteration of Rho GTPases in Cancer

RhoH is the only Rho GTPase whose sequence has been found to be genetically altered in human cancers. The RhoH gene has been found to be rearranged in non-Hodgkin's lymphomas and multiple myeloma, along with mutations in the 5′UTR in diffuse large cell lymphomas (Preudhomme et al. 2000; Pasqualucci et al. 2001). The common rearrangement found in these hematopoietic cancers is caused by a t(3;4)(q27;p11–13) chromosomal translocation resulting in a gene fusion with the BCL3/LAZ3 oncogene (Dallery-Prudhomme et al. 1997). However, it is unknown whether or how these RhoH translocations and hypermutations contribute to the pathology of these cancers. Although other Rho GTPases have not been found to

be genetically altered in cancer, the expression and activation of several of the Rho
GTPases have been reported to be misregulated in human cancers. Altered expression of RhoA, RhoB, RhoC, Rac1, Rac1b, Rac2, Rac3, RhoG, Cdc42, RhoH/TTF,
and Rnd3/RhoE have been reported in various human cancers, including breast,
colon, lung, pancreatic and gastric carcinomas, as well as melanoma and lymphomas
(Ellenbroek and Collard 2007).

Specifically, upregulation of RhoC is associated with aggressive cancers such
as pancreatic ductal adenocarcinoma, metastatic gastric carcinoma and melanoma,
inflammatory breast cancer, and non-small cell lung cancer (NSCLC) (Suwa et al.
1998; van Golen et al. 2002; Shikada et al. 2003; Liu et al. 2004). Expression of the
Rac1 splice variant Rac1b, that is known to be constitutively active due to accelerated GDP/GTP exchange, is elevated in colorectal and breast tumors (Jordan et al.
1999; Schnelzer et al. 2000). The selective advantage for Rac1b overexpression in
these cancer types may involve Rac1b-induced cell survival due to its activation
of NFκB (Matos and Jordan 2005; Radisky et al. 2005). Interestingly, Rac1b is
also thought to contribute to EMT by upregulating the transcription factor Snail
(Radisky et al. 2005). Other specific contributions of these individual GTPases to
tumorigenesis, tumor progression, and maintenance require further investigations.

Alteration in Regulators of Rho GTPases in Cancer

Misregulated expression of Rho GTPase regulators resulting in deregulated signaling downstream of Rho proteins is also associated with various human cancers.
Several Rho family GEFs, positive regulators of Rho family activation, are found
either overexpressed or truncated in human tumors, leading to constitutive activation of Rho GTPase-mediated signaling pathways and tumorigenesis. In leukemia,
chromosomal translocations result in BCR-ABL and MLL-LARG chimeras that
contribute to tumorigenesis (Kourlas et al. 2000; Kin et al. 2001). The chromosomal translocation resulting in the MLL-LARG fusion protein promotes constitutive RhoA activation that potentially contributes to the development of leukemia
(Reuther et al. 2001), while the contribution of the BCR-ABL fusion protein to cancer is related to BCR-mediated activation of Abl kinase activity (Arlinghaus 2002).
Not all Rho GEFs are involved in human cancers through chromosomal translocations. The Rac-specific GEF Tiam1 is the best characterized GEF in terms of
involvement in cancer initiation and progression. Tiam1 ablation in mice prevents
Ras-induced skin tumor formation, suggesting that Rac activation is involved in
cancer initiation (Malliri et al. 2002). In addition, overexpression of Tiam1 correlates positively with increased invasiveness of both breast and prostate cancer
(Adam et al. 2001; Minard et al. 2005; Engers et al. 2006). However, whether
Tiam1-mediated Rac activation is essential for many of these tumor types remains
to be elucidated. In addition, the Rho family GEF β-Pix is overexpressed in breast
cancer (Ahn et al. 2003), while Vav1 overexpression is associated with both pancreatic adenocarcinoma and neuroblastoma (Hornstein et al. 2003; Fernandez-Zapico
et al. 2005).

Upregulation of the positive regulators of Rho family signaling are not the only alterations that occur in Rho protein regulators during cancer initiation and progression. Genomic deletion and promoter methylation results in downregulation of the RhoGAPs, DLC-1 and DLC-2, in breast cancer and in hepatocellular carcinoma (Ching et al. 2003; Wong et al. 2003; Yuan et al. 2003a; Yuan et al. 2003b; Yuan et al. 2004). A recent study shows that DLC-1 loss promotes growth and invasion of NSCLC through RhoGAP-dependent and -independent mechanisms, suggesting that increased RhoA activation contributes to this tumor type (Healy et al. 2007). Overexpression and downregulation of each of the RhoGDIs has been reported in human cancers of different origins, but the role and mechanism by which this may contribute to tumor progression remains to be determined (Dovas and Couchman 2005; Zhang and Zhang 2006). Together, these reports of alterations in Rho GTPases themselves and of their positive and negative regulators in human cancers illustrate the importance of validating these proteins as drug targets for cancer treatment and of discovering pharmacologic inhibitors of the validated proteins to combat cancer development and progression.

Alteration of Rho GTPase Downstream Effectors in Cancer

Another mechanism by which Rho GTPase signaling deregulation can contribute to cancer is through alteration in their downstream effectors. Many of the PAK serine/threonine kinase isoforms are overexpressed in different tumor types and may contribute to tumor initiation and progression (Kumar and Vadlamudi 2002). PAK-1 upregulation in breast cancer cell lines promotes anchorage-independent growth and abnormal mitotic spindle organization (Vadlamudi et al. 2000). In addition, overexpression of ROCKI and ROCKII in bladder and testicular cancer may contribute to the invasiveness of these cancer cells by modulating actin dynamics to promote cell motility (Kamai et al. 2003; Kamai et al. 2004). Further investigation into small molecule inhibitors of the PAK kinase and ROCK kinase and their ability to block cancer progression will be an interesting endeavor. More importantly, determining whether other Rho GTPase downstream effectors are misregulated in cancer remains to be elucidated.

Rho GTPase Contributions to Tumor Cell Motility, Invasion, and Metastasis

The central role of Rho GTPases in regulating cytoskeletal architecture is key to their ability to promote cancer progression. As stated previously, the ability of cancer cells to detach from ECM and each other and acquire motile and invasive properties is dependent on the activation of signaling pathways associated with the developmental process of EMT (Guarino et al. 2007). Extensive research has uncovered an integral role for members of the Rho GTPase family in many of the steps that lead to cancer cell dissemination into secondary sites. In normal cells Rho GTPase signaling is tightly regulated so that normal cell–cell contact and cell–matrix contact is maintained. However, genetic or epigenetic changes in Rho GTPases or their regulators leads to the breakdown of cell–cell adhesion that subsequently promotes altered cell–matrix adhesion, invasion, and metastasis. This section focuses on mechanisms by which misregulation of Rho GTPases can contribute to tumor cell motility, invasion, and metastasis.

Altered Cell–Cell Adhesion

Cell junctions and the cytoskeletal network, important structural components of epithelial cells, contribute to the formation and maintenance of normal cell morphology and promote regulated cell growth and survival. Normal epithelial cell morphology is maintained by two types of intercellular adhesive junctions: adherens junctions and tight junctions that together form the apical junctional complex. Adherens junctions are adhesive structures formed through calcium-dependent interactions between cadherin molecules on adjacent epithelial cells. Cadherin molecules, such as E-cadherin, in turn form membrane anchor sites for the actin cytoskeleton through interactions with catenins, such as β-catenin and α-catenin. The association of adherens junctions with the cytoskeleton provides strength and stability to cell–cell contacts (Yap et al. 1997). Interestingly, the formation of adherens junctions is a prerequisite to the formation of other cellular junctions such as tight junctions and gap junctions (Gumbiner et al. 1988). Therefore, it is not surprising that the breakdown of adherens junctions is one of the first steps to promote cancer cell progression and is a prerequisite for cancer cells to acquire motile and invasive properties.

It is well appreciated that downregulation of E-cadherin-mediated cell–cell adhesion promotes EMT and is associated with cancer progression (Birchmeier and Behrens 1994; Bracke et al. 1996). The cycle of Rho GTPase activation and inactivation regulates both assembly and disassembly of adherens junctions, suggesting that the alterations in Rho GTPase signaling discussed above could promote cancer progression by downregulating E-cadherin-mediated cell–cell adhesion (Evers et al. 2000; Lozano et al. 2003; Malliri and Collard 2003). In some cases hyperactivation of Rac1 and RhoA disrupts the assembly of adherens junctions, yet other reports suggest that normal activity of Rac1 and RhoA is required for adherens junctions formation and maintenance (Braga et al. 1997; Braga et al. 1999; Braga et al. 2000; Sahai and Marshall 2002). These apparently contradictory findings suggest that tight regulation of Rho GTPase activity is necessary for junction stability. Activation of Rac1 downstream of Tiam1 expression disrupts adherens junction engagement in breast cancer cells (Adam et al. 2001). The mechanism by which Rac1 may contribute to the disassembly of cadherin-based adhesion in this system is by increasing the turnover of cadherins and catenins through regulation of endocytosis (Quinlan 1999; Akhtar and Hotchin 2001). In contrast, Tiam1 has been shown in various other systems to enhance E-cadherin-mediated cell–cell adhesions, thus suppressing invasion of these epithelial cells. Specifically, Tiam1 overexpression blocks hepatocyte growth factor (HGF)-mediated MDCK cell scattering (Hordijk et al. 1997). Tiam1-mediated Rac1 activation reverts the Ras-induced fibroblastoid phenotype of MDCK cells by restoring their E-cadherin adhesions (Sander et al. 1998). While Rac1 may inhibit cancer cell invasion by strengthening cell–cell contacts, in colon cancer cell lines the constitutively active Rac1 splice variant Rac1b promotes disruption of adherens junctions by downregulating E-cadherin expression downstream of Wnt signaling (Esufali et al. 2007). Together, these data suggest that proper titration of Rac1 activation is necessary for both the stabilization and disassembly of adherens junctions, and that cell context is a critical determinant of the role of Rac GTPase activity in the disruption of cadherin-based cell adhesion associated with cancer progression (Sander et al. 1998; Braga et al. 1999).

In contrast to the complex and context-dependent role for Rac1 in adherens junction regulation, RhoA signaling is clearly linked to the disassembly of adherens junctions. RhoA signaling is essential for the EMT program elicited by activation of both HGF and TGF-β that involves the disruption of cadherin engagement (Takaishi et al. 1994; Bhowmick et al. 2001). A very recent report has established that EphA2 receptor-mediated dissolution of adherens junctions in human cancer cell lines occurs via a RhoA-dependent mechanism and suggests that RhoA activation is necessary for malignant progression (Fang et al. 2008). RhoA stimulates contractile forces that promote adherens junctions dissolution. RhoA-mediated actin filament contraction was shown to be essential for the Ras-mediated fibroblastic morphology of MCF10A mammary epithelial cells and MDCK kidney epithelial cells (Zhong et al. 1997; Zondag et al. 2000). The proposed mechanism by which both RhoA and RhoC contribute to the loss of adherens junctions to promote the motile and invasive phenotype is through activation of the best characterized Rho effector, ROCK. ROCK activation promotes actin filament contraction that can strip from the cell surface cadherin molecules that are linked to the actin cytoskeletal network. Overexpression of ROCK in HCT116 colon cancer cells is sufficient to induce disassembly of adherens junctions (Sahai and Marshall 2002).

Recent investigation of the crosstalk between Rac and Rho signaling has uncovered distinct mechanisms to spatially and temporally regulate the activity of these small GTPases to modulate adherens junction engagement in normal and cancer cells. As stated above, in general, Rac activation promotes junction assembly whereas Rho activation disrupts junction assembly. One study showed that p120-catenin and p190RhoGAP regulate cell–cell adhesion by coordinating the antagonism between Rho and Rac (Wildenberg et al. 2006). The data indicate that, upon receptor activation, Rac stimulates adherens junction complex formation, which then recruits p190RhoGAP to cadherin-based junctions via a direct interaction with p120-catenin. The controlled recruitment of p190RhoGAP in turn results in localized inhibition of RhoA (Wildenberg et al. 2006). In the context of a cancer cell, these data suggest that adherens junction dissolution may be promoted by aberrant overactivation of RhoA or RhoC that overcomes the normal Rac-mediated downregulation of Rho. The degree to which this finding is generalizable and whether other Rho GTPases also contribute to the disruption of cell junctions associated with the EMT program necessary for tumor progression remains to be elucidated.

Altered Cell–Matrix Adhesion

In addition to breakdown of cell junctions, activation of signaling pathways capable of increasing cell motility and remodeling the ECM is required for cancer cells to invade. Degradation and remodeling of ECM are critical to the ability of cancer cells to become locally invasive. It is well established that Rho GTPases play a role in the induction of matrix metalloproteinase (MMP) expression. Supporting data for this contention has been elucidated in both normal and cancer cells. One recent study highlighted the finding that activation of Vav1 and Vav2 is required for Rac-mediated upregulation of MMP2 to promote CXCR4 chemokine receptor-mediated melanoma invasion (Bartolome et al. 2006). Rac1 activation in HT1080 fibrosarcoma cells grown in three-dimensional (3D) culture promotes MMP2-dependent degradation of ECM and subsequent migration through collagen barrier (Matsumoto et al. 2001). A study of lung cancer cell metastasis in an orthotopic mouse model has shown that expression of RhoC induces MMP2 and enhances metastatic potential, whereas dominant negative RhoC inhibits these processes (Ikoma et al. 2004). Similarly, RhoA activation downstream of LPA in invasive osteosarcoma cells promotes the induction of MMP2 and requires ROCK activity (Matsumoto et al. 2001). These are only a few examples that highlight the importance of investing future research efforts aimed at determining the involvement of Rho GTPases in MMP production during tumor progression to promote cancer cell invasion and metastasis.

Whether inhibitors of MMPs will prove to be successful anti-metastasis therapy remains to be seen. One study has shown that, in the presence of MMP inhibitors, cancer cells transition to an amoeboid type migration and are still capable of invading into 3D matrices (Wolf et al. 2003). Specifically, HT-1080 fibrosarcoma and MDA-MB-231 cancer cells treated with protease inhibitors adapted to a flexible spherical type of migration that allows these cancer cells to squeeze through small pores in 3D matrices and dissemination to distant sites when injected into mouse dermis. Therefore, inhibiting MMPs secreted from cancer cells themselves or their supporting stroma may not be fruitful to block cancer cell invasion.

In addition to MMP formation, Rho GTPases are essential for integrin-mediated motility of cancer cells (Wu et al. 2007). In addition, it is well appreciated that the formation and remodeling of focal contacts is a dynamic process regulated by Rho GTPases and that increased turnover of focal contacts in cancer cells promotes migration. The engagement of focal complexes via integrin binding to components of ECM and the subsequent activation of Rho GTPases involved in cancer cell motility will be discussed in the following section.

Altered Cell Migration

The migration of normal cells and cancer cells is driven by coordinated cycles of protrusion, adhesion, and contraction. Spatial and temporal regulation of Rho GTPase activation is intimately involved in the formation of actin-based protrusions and contractions along with integrin-mediated adhesions (Ridley 2001). The central dogma in the field of Rho GTPase-regulated migration is that temporally regulated activation of Cdc42 initiates the polarity of cell migration, while Rac-mediated lamellipodia extension and integrin adhesion complex formation promotes the leading edge protrusions in motile cells necessary for forward movement. RhoA activation stimulates cell body contraction and also promotes tail detachment (Schmitz et al. 2000; Ridley 2001). In addition to their regulation of actin cytoskeletal dynamics to drive cell motility, Rho GTPases are instrumental in modulating migration-inhibitory cell–cell interactions and migration-promoting cell–ECM interactions, as discussed above.

As stated above, activation of Cdc42 is essential for regulation of microtubule dynamics at the leading edge of polarized cells, in order to establish the polarized cell morphology with a front and a rear. During both single cell and coordinated cell migration, inhibition of Cdc42 activation disrupts the orientation of the microtubule organizing center (MTOC), leading to misdirected cell protrusion formation and subsequent random cell migration (Allen et al. 1998; Etienne-Manneville and Hall 2001; Etienne-Manneville and Hall 2003). Specifically, Cdc42 activation downstream of integrin-mediated cell adhesion in cell protrusion at the leading edge of migration cells stimulates MTOC orientation and cell polarization in both astrocytes and fibroblasts (Etienne-Manneville 2004). This suggests that Cdc42 activation is essential for coordinating external cues that govern the direction of cell migration. Cdc42-mediated filopodia extension through its effectors WASP and N-WASP and subsequent regulation of the Arp2/3 complex is thought to be an integral mediator of extracellular environment sensing in many cell types.

The next step essential for cell migration is coordination of lamellipodia extension and focal complex formation by activated Rac (Small et al. 2002). Active Rac promotes actin polymerization at the leading edge of cells through various downstream targets, with its major target being the Arp2/3 complex capable of promoting de novo actin nucleation of actin polymerization and the formation of new filament branches (Bailly et al. 2001; Condeelis 2001). The trigger to activate Rac at the leading edge of migrating cells remains to be elucidated, but the formation of integrin–ECM interactions could be one potential mechanism.

It is well appreciated that focal complexes enriched in integrins are localized in the lamellipodia of migrating cells and important for linking the Rac-mediated lamellipodia extension to the ECM. Both Rac and Cdc42 activation are required for focal complex assembly and both Rac and Cdc42 are activated in response to cell adhesion to ECM (Nobes and Hall 1995; Price et al. 1998; Rottner et al. 1999). These data suggest a potential mechanism by which Rac and Cdc42 activation is maintained at the leading edge of migrating cells when new interactions between integrins and ECM are engaged. Activation of Rac and Cdc42 subsequently promotes a positive feedback loop in which lamellipodia formation and cell polarity are initiated and are capable of driving cell migration in the absence of growth factor signaling. Not surprisingly, ECM composition varies during cell migration and as a result the speed of cell migration is altered. This alteration is thought to be dependent on changes in the relative activation of Rac, Rho, and Cdc42 in response to different ECM components (Ridley 2000). Although focal complex formation is necessary for cell migration, their turnover is equally important because a high level of integrin-mediated adhesion inhibits cell migration. Therefore, Rac-mediated activation of Pak or Rac antagonism of Rho activity each represents a major mechanism by which focal complex disassembly and turnover are modulated (Sander et al. 1999; Zhao et al. 2000).

The final steps involved in the cyclical process (cell body contraction and tail detachment) of cell migration are regulated by Rho activation. Cell body contraction is regulated by actomyosin contractility downstream of Rho activation of its major effector, the serine–threonine kinase ROCK. In many cell types, inhibition of Rho activity has a negative effect on cell body contraction that subsequently blocks cell migration (Allen et al. 1997, 1998; Totsukawa et al. 2000). Interestingly, the cell body contraction mediated by active Rho is associated with amoeboid cell migration upon protease inhibition (Friedl and Wolf 2003). Like the activation of Rac and Cdc42, activation of Rho must be regulated in both a spatially and a temporally controlled manner. Rho activity can block cell migration by strengthening stress fiber and focal contact formation (Cox and Huttenlocher 1998; Cox et al. 2001). Inhibition of Rho can promote cell migration by blocking cell body contraction and by weakening focal complex formation, which then promotes tail detachment in some cell types (Zhao et al. 2000; Cox et al. 2001), which is often the rate-limiting step of migration (Palecek et al. 1998).

The mechanisms described above by which Rho GTPases are integral to cell migration are not unique to normal cells. There are numerous examples of the dependence of cancer cell migration, invasion, and metastasis on aberrant regulation of Rho GTPases. For example, aberrant activation of RhoC and ROCK promotes tumor cell dissemination in mouse models in vivo (Itoh et al. 1999; Clark et al. 2000; Somlyo et al. 2000; Murata et al. 2001). In addition, RhoC overexpression has been shown to be important in both colon carcinoma and melanoma metastasis (Clark et al. 2000; Bellovin et al. 2006). Another study has determined that RhoC is required for tumor progression and metastasis in mice but is not essential for the initiation of these tumors (Hakem et al. 2005). SiRNA-mediated degradation of either RhoA or RhoC is known to inhibit the invasion of the highly invasive breast cancer cell line MDA-MB-231 in vitro and in vivo (Pille et al. 2005). A recent report showed a role for RhoA, RhoC, and Rac1 in the regulation of tumor cell morphology, invasion, and tumor cell diapedesis of PC-3 prostate cancer cells (Sequeira et al. 2008).

In contrast to the more extensive investigations of the role of Rho subfamily proteins in both normal and cancer cell migration, invasion, and metastasis, the contribution of Rac and Cdc42 subfamily members has been well studied primarily in cell migration. Two intriguing studies suggest that Cdc42 activation of its effectors PDK1 and MRCK (myotonic dystrophy kinase-related Cdc42-binding protein kinase) is important for directed migration of cancer cells in 3D matrix (Gaggioli et al. 2007; Pinner and Sahai 2008). Investigation into effective inhibitors of the RhoA and RhoC pathways to block cancer progression and into the involvement of Rac and Cdc42 subfamily members in invasion and metastasis may be essential to guide development of optimal treatments for primary tumors before they undergo EMT.

Dynamic Interplay Between Rho GTPases and the Tumor Microenvironment

It is becoming widely accepted in the cancer biology field that tumor growth and metastasis are not driven solely by genetic or epigenetic changes in the cancer cells themselves but can be supported by the tumor microenvironment. Recent advances in experimental models have highlighted the importance of tumor–stromal interactions that promote cancer initiation and progression. Tumor-associated stroma includes a heterogeneous population of cells that can consist of myofibroblasts, fibroblasts, adipocytes, blood and lymph vessels, and hematopoietic cells, depending on the tumor origin. In addition, tumor-associated stroma consists of ECM components such as collagen that influence tumor cell growth and survival, along with promoting tumor cell migration and invasion. Tumor progression occurs when stromal cells and cancer cells secrete enzymes and growth factors capable of remodeling ECM, stimulating migration, and promoting proliferation and survival. By producing growth factors and cytokines, tumor cells recruit vasculature and stroma that when active can stimulate the proliferative and invasive properties of the tumor cells (Liotta and Kohn 2001). As discussed above, Rho GTPases are essential modulators of tumor cell migration and invasion through various downstream signaling pathways. Therefore, it is not surprising that recent studies investigating the dynamic interplay between tumor cells and their associated stroma has highlighted the importance of Rho GTPases as major players in mediating tumor cell migration and invasion in response to stromal cells and ECM components, as described below.

Rho GTPase Involvement in ECM Contraction as a Driving Force Behind Cancer Initiation and Invasion

The role of ECM in tumor initiation and invasion has been most thoroughly investigated in human breast cancer. Pivotal work by Bissell, Keely, and Weaver has highlighted the importance of tumor–ECM interactions as driving forces behind breast cancer progression. Specifically, the use of 3D cell culture systems and mouse models has demonstrated that the tissue microenvironment regulates mammary gland development and that alterations in tissue homeostasis contribute to the loss of architecture observed in breast cancer. One critical factor that influences mammary gland function and morphology is the response of tensional forces within the gland to stresses and stiffness in the local environment (Paszek and Weaver 2004; Paszek et al. 2005). Increased tension within the mammary gland is associated with perturbations of differentiation and with breast cancer initiation and progression. To date there are only a few studies that have investigated a role for Rho GTPases in this process.

Keely and colleagues recently highlighted the importance of collagen density as a mediator of tumor initiation and invasion (Provenzano et al. 2006; Provenzano et al. 2008). These studies used a transgenic mouse mammary tumor model in which stromal collagen was elevated in the mammary tissue. The use of multiphoton laser scanning microscopy allowed these researchers to visualize tumors and the interface between these tumors and their associated stroma. By comparing tumor properties in otherwise syngeneic mice with or without elevated stromal collagen, this study provided the first causal evidence that an increase in stromal collagen density is sufficient to promote both tumor formation and the invasiveness and metastatic capacity of these tumors (Provenzano et al. 2008). These researchers hypothesized that the increased breast density associated with a stiffer ECM results in altered tensional homeostasis in breast epithelial cells as discussed above. These changes in ECM have been shown previously to alter the focal adhesion and Rho GTPase signaling that results in increased proliferation and the acquisition of an invasive phenotype (Wozniak et al. 2003; Paszek et al. 2005; Wozniak and Keely 2005). In addition, it has been suggested that Rho GTPase-mediated cancer cell contractility promotes ECM reorganization aligning a path for local invasion.

Two independent studies have investigated the role of Rho-mediated contractility in breast epithelial cells in response to increases in the stiffness of ECM. Previous experiments had shown that growing breast epithelial cells in detached, floating 3D collagen gels maintains differentiated structures that produce milk proteins, in contrast to their counterparts grown in attached, 3D collagen gels (Lee et al. 1984). Wozniak et al. reported that growth in the detached but not the attached gels downregulated RhoA activity (Wozniak et al. 2003). This suggested to the authors that the levels of Rho activation must be tightly regulated in order to maintain proper mammary gland differentiation, and they demonstrated that the mechanism by which breast epithelial cells sense the rigidity of the extracellular environment is through the Rho effector ROCK (Wozniak et al. 2003), which promotes cellular contraction of the surrounding ECM. Therefore, these data suggest that an increase in ECM stiffness by enhanced collagen density surrounding the mammary gland promotes high levels of Rho activity, which subsequently drives cell proliferation, dedifferentiation, and migration as a mechanism to promote cancer initiation and progression.

In a subsequent study, Paszek et al. set out to determine whether increased tissue stiffness associated with the breast tumor microenvironment could modulate mechanotransduction pathways downstream of integrin engagement (Paszek et al. 2005). This study also determined that matrix stiffness perturbs epithelial morphogenesis and promotes cell growth by a mechanism involving stimulation of integrin clustering that enhanced tumor cell ERK activation and RhoA-mediated contractility (Paszek et al. 2005). These two independent examples provide evidence that increased ECM stiffness promotes excessive cell growth, survival, migration, and invasion through the activation of mechanoresponsive signaling pathways like the Rho–ROCK signaling cascade in breast cancer. The involvement of tumor–ECM interactions in other cancer types remains to be elucidated, along with the involvement of other Rho GTPases.

Rho GTPase Involvement in Fibroblast-Led Invasion of Cancer Cells

ECM is not the only stromal component known to promote tumor cell invasion. Countless examples exist in the literature in which tumor cell interactions with the associated stromal cells help to maintain the transformed phenotype. As stated above, tumor-associated stroma includes endothelial cells, fibroblasts, myofibroblasts, and hematopoietic cells (Liotta and Kohn 2001; Weinberg 2008). Endothelial cells are recruited to a developing tumor by tumor-secreted cytokines to support the malignancy with nutrients and oxygen. The vast numbers of fibroblasts found in carcinomas are known to be important in maintaining and supporting normal epithelial tissues. Myofibroblasts are normally involved in tissue reconstruction as components of wound healing, and their recruitment to the sites of tumors suggesting that the surrounding tissue responds to tumor formation with normal wound-healing responses. Unfortunately, the tumor hijacks the wound-healing capabilities of myofibroblasts to sustain its growth (Orimo and Weinberg 2006; Orimo and Weinberg 2007). In addition, an influx of macrophages is also associated with tumor mass, consistent with research suggesting that chronic inflammation promotes cancer initiation and progression (Pollard 2004). Although many studies have highlighted an importance for tumor-associated stromal cells in cancer initiation and progression, the signaling pathways activated in cancer cells in response to stromal interactions are only now beginning to be elucidated.

One elegant study employed the use of organotypic culture systems coupled with confocal, transmission electron, or reflectance microscopy to investigate the process by which squamous cell carcinoma (SCC) cells could undergo collective invasion without first undergoing EMT (Gaggioli et al. 2007). To determine the mechanism by which SCC cells invade through ECM, Gaggioli et al. grew SCC cell lines on top of a dense matrix composed of collagen and laminins. Interestingly, the ability of SCC cells having epithelial cell characteristics to invade through ECM was dependent on co-culture with stromal fibroblasts, while SCC cells having mesenchymal characteristics invaded whether stromal fibroblasts were present or absent. These data suggest that stromal fibroblasts are essential for cancer cells that retain epithelial characteristics to invade through ECM. When closely examined with the use of multiphoton confocal time lapse imaging, it was noted that fluorescently labeled fibroblasts were always the leading cell type in the invading chain of cells. Surprisingly, ECM degradation and reorganization mediated by the leading fibroblasts was capable of promoting the invasion of SCC cells, suggesting that the fibroblasts were generating tracks within the ECM for SCC cells to follow. Inhibition of either Rho (with C3 toxin) or ROCK1/2 (with the pharmacological inhibitors Y27632 or H1152) in the leading stromal fibroblasts was sufficient to block the invasion of SCC cells, by modulating the ability of the leading fibroblasts to degrade and remodel the ECM. Loss of RhoA expression (siRNA) or function (C3) in fibroblasts but not SCC cells blocked collective invasion. Interestingly, inhibition of Cdc42-mediated activation of its effector MRCK in SCC cells was also necessary for their ability to follow tracks formed by the fibroblasts (Gaggioli et al. 2007). This study was the first of its kind to elucidate a mechanism by which Rho GTPases are involved in tumor–stromal cell interface to influence invasion. Another recent study showed that tumor cells follow macrophages to promote their intravasation, but the involvement of Rho GTPases in this process was not investigated.

Conclusions

The use of sophisticated imaging technology and co-culture systems or mouse models may continue to promote promising research efforts aimed at investigating the role of the tumor microenvironment in tumor formation and progression. In addition, the involvement of Rho GTPase signaling pathways can be elucidated. It will be interesting to unravel the specific genetic changes in different tumor types and in their surrounding stroma that alter Rho family GTPase function to promote these processes.

References

Adam L, Vadlamudi RK, McCrea P, Kumar R (2001) Tiam1 overexpression potentiates heregulin-induced lymphoid enhancer factor-1/beta-catenin nuclear signaling in breast cancer cells by modulating the intercellular stability. J Biol Chem 276:28443–28450.

Ahn SJ, Chung KW, Lee RA, Park IA, Lee SH, Park DE, Noh DY (2003) Overexpression of betaPix-a in human breast cancer tissues. Cancer Lett 193:99–107.

Akhtar N and Hotchin NA (2001) RAC1 regulates adherens junctions through endocytosis of E-cadherin. Mol Biol Cell 12:847–862.

Allen WE, Jones GE, Pollard JW, Ridley AJ (1997) Rho, Rac and Cdc42 regulate actin organization and cell adhesion in macrophages. J Cell Sci 110 (Pt 6):707–720.

Allen WE, Zicha D, Ridley AJ, Jones GE (1998) A role for Cdc42 in macrophage chemotaxis. J Cell Biol 141:1147–1157.

Amano M, Ito M, Kimura K, Fukata Y, Chihara K, Nakano T, Matsuura Y, Kaibuchi K (1996) Phosphorylation and activation of myosin by Rho-associated kinase (Rho-kinase). J Biol Chem 271:20246–20249.

Arlinghaus RB (2002) Bcr: A negative regulator of the Bcr-Abl oncoprotein in leukemia. Oncogene 21:8560–8567.

Aspenstrom P, Ruusala A, Pacholsky D (2007) Taking Rho GTPases to the next level: The cellular functions of atypical Rho GTPases. Exp Cell Res 313:3673–3679.

Bailly M, Ichetovkin I, Grant W, Zebda N, Machesky LM, Segall JE, Condeelis J (2001) The F-actin side binding activity of the Arp2/3 complex is essential for actin nucleation and lamellipod extension. Curr Biol 11:620–625.

Bamburg JR, McGough A, Ono S (1999) Putting a new twist on actin: ADF/cofilins modulate actin dynamics. Trends Cell Biol 9:364–370.

Bartolome RA, Molina-Ortiz I, Samaniego R, Sanchez-Mateos P, Bustelo XR, Teixido J (2006) Activation of Vav/Rho GTPase signaling by CXCL12 controls membrane-type matrix metalloproteinase-dependent melanoma cell invasion. Cancer Res 66:248–258.

Bellovin DI, Simpson KJ, Danilov T, Maynard E, Rimm DL, Oettgen P, Mercurio AM (2006) Reciprocal regulation of RhoA and RhoC characterizes the EMT and identifies RhoC as a prognostic marker of colon carcinoma. Oncogene 25:6959–6967.

Bernards A (2003) GAPs galore! A survey of putative Ras superfamily GTPase activating proteins in man and Drosophila. Biochim Biophys Acta 1603:47–82.

Berx G, Raspe E, Christofori G, Thiery JP, Sleeman JP (2007) Pre-EMTing metastasis? Recapitulation of morphogenetic processes in cancer. Clin Exp Metastasis 24:587–597.

Bhowmick NA, Ghiassi M, Bakin A, Aakre M, Lundquist CA, Engel ME, Arteaga CL, Moses HL (2001) Transforming growth factor-beta1 mediates epithelial to mesenchymal transdifferentiation through a RhoA-dependent mechanism. Mol Biol Cell 12:27–36.

Birchmeier W and Behrens J (1994) Cadherin expression in carcinomas: Role in the formation of cell junctions and the prevention of invasiveness. Biochim Biophys Acta 1198:11–26.

Bishop AL and Hall A (2000) Rho GTPases and their effector proteins. Biochem J 348 Pt 2: 241–255.

Bos JL (1989) ras oncogenes in human cancer: A review. Cancer Res 49:4682–4689.

Boureux A, Vignal E, Faure S, Fort P (2007) Evolution of the Rho family of ras-like GTPases in eukaryotes. Mol Biol Evol 24:203–216.

Bracke ME, Van Roy FM, Mareel MM (1996) The E-cadherin/catenin complex in invasion and metastasis. Curr Top Microbiol Immunol 213 (Pt 1):123–161.

Braga VM, Betson M, Li X, Lamarche-Vane N (2000) Activation of the small GTPase Rac is sufficient to disrupt cadherin-dependent cell-cell adhesion in normal human keratinocytes. Mol Biol Cell 11:3703–3721.

Braga VM, Del Maschio A, Machesky L, Dejana E (1999) Regulation of cadherin function by Rho and Rac: Modulation by junction maturation and cellular context. Mol Biol Cell 10: 9–22.

Braga VM, Machesky LM, Hall A, Hotchin NA (1997) The small GTPases Rho and Rac are required for the establishment of cadherin-dependent cell-cell contacts. J Cell Biol 137: 1421–1431.

Bresnick AR (1999) Molecular mechanisms of nonmuscle myosin-II regulation. Curr Opin Cell Biol 11:26–33.

Chardin P (2006) Function and regulation of Rnd proteins. Nat Rev Mol Cell Biol 7:54–62.

Chien UH, Lai M, Shih TY, Verma IM, Scolnick EM, Roy-Burman P, Davidson N (1979) Heteroduplex analysis of the sequence relationships between the genomes of Kirsten and Harvey sarcoma viruses, their respective parental murine leukemia viruses, and the rat endogenous 30S RNA. J Virol 31:752–760.

Ching YP, Wong CM, Chan SF, Leung TH, Ng DC, Jin DY, Ng IO (2003) Deleted in liver cancer (DLC) 2 encodes a RhoGAP protein with growth suppressor function and is underexpressed in hepatocellular carcinoma. J Biol Chem 278:10824–10830.

Chuang TH, Bohl BP, Bokoch GM (1993) Biologically active lipids are regulators of Rac.GDI complexation. J Biol Chem 268:26206–26211.

Clark EA, Golub TR, Lander ES, Hynes RO (2000) Genomic analysis of metastasis reveals an essential role for RhoC. Nature 406:532–535.

Condeelis J (2001) How is actin polymerization nucleated in vivo? Trends Cell Biol 11:288–293.

Cote JF and Vuori K (2007) GEF what? Dock180 and related proteins help Rac to polarize cells in new ways. Trends Cell Biol 17:383–393.

Cotteret S and Chernoff J (2002) The evolutionary history of effectors downstream of Cdc42 and Rac. Genome Biol 3:REVIEWS0002–8.

Cox EA and Huttenlocher A (1998) Regulation of integrin-mediated adhesion during cell migration. Microsc Res Tech 43:412–419.

Cox EA, Sastry SK, Huttenlocher A (2001) Integrin-mediated adhesion regulates cell polarity and membrane protrusion through the Rho family of GTPases. Mol Biol Cell 12:265–277.

Dallery-Prudhomme E, Roumier C, Denis C, Preudhomme C, Kerckaert JP, Galiegue-Zouitina S (1997) Genomic structure and assignment of the RhoH/TTF small GTPase gene (ARHH) to 4p13 by in situ hybridization. Genomics 43:89–94.

Der CJ, Krontiris TG, Cooper GM (1982) Transforming genes of human bladder and lung carcinoma cell lines are homologous to the ras genes of Harvey and Kirsten sarcoma viruses. Proc Natl Acad Sci U S A 79:3637–3640.

DerMardirossian C and Bokoch GM (2005) GDIs: Central regulatory molecules in Rho GTPase activation. Trends Cell Biol 15:356–363.

Dovas A and Couchman JR (2005) RhoGDI: Multiple functions in the regulation of Rho family GTPase activities. Biochem J 390:1–9.

Edwards DC, Sanders LC, Bokoch GM, Gill GN (1999) Activation of LIM-kinase by Pak1 couples Rac/Cdc42 GTPase signalling to actin cytoskeletal dynamics. Nat Cell Biol 1:253–259.

Ellenbroek SI and Collard JG (2007) Rho GTPases: Functions and association with cancer. Clin Exp Metastasis 24:657–672.

Engers R, Mueller M, Walter A, Collard JG, Willers R, Gabbert HE (2006) Prognostic relevance of Tiam1 protein expression in prostate carcinomas. Br J Cancer 95:1081–1086.

Esufali S, Charames GS, Pethe VV, Buongiorno P, Bapat B (2007) Activation of tumor-specific splice variant Rac1b by dishevelled promotes canonical Wnt signaling and decreased adhesion of colorectal cancer cells. Cancer Res 67:2469–2479.

Etienne-Manneville S (2004) Cdc42 – The centre of polarity. J Cell Sci 117:1291–1300.

Etienne-Manneville S and Hall A (2001) Integrin-mediated activation of Cdc42 controls cell polarity in migrating astrocytes through PKCzeta. Cell 106:489–498.

Etienne-Manneville S and Hall A (2002) Rho GTPases in cell biology. Nature 420:629–635.

Etienne-Manneville S and Hall A (2003) Cdc42 regulates GSK-3beta and adenomatous polyposis coli to control cell polarity. Nature 421:753–756.

Evers EE, Zondag GC, Malliri A, Price LS, ten Klooster JP, van der Kammen RA, Collard JG (2000) Rho family proteins in cell adhesion and cell migration. Eur J Cancer 36:1269–1274.

Fang WB, Ireton RC, Zhuang G, Takahashi T, Reynolds A, Chen J (2008) Overexpression of EPHA2 receptor destabilizes adherens junctions via a RhoA-dependent mechanism. J Cell Sci 121:358–368.

Fernandez-Zapico ME, Gonzalez-Paz NC, Weiss E, Savoy DN, Molina JR, Fonseca R, Smyrk TC, Chari ST, Urrutia R, Billadeau DD (2005) Ectopic expression of VAV1 reveals an unexpected role in pancreatic cancer tumorigenesis. Cancer Cell 7:39–49.

Foster R, Hu KQ, Lu Y, Nolan KM, Thissen J, Settleman J (1996) Identification of a novel human Rho protein with unusual properties: GTPase deficiency and in vivo farnesylation. Mol Cell Biol 16:2689–2699.

Friedl P, Wolf K (2003) Tumour-cell invasion and migration: Diversity and escape mechanisms. Nat Rev Cancer 3:362–374.

Fukumoto Y, Kaibuchi K, Hori Y, Fujioka H, Araki S, Ueda T, Kikuchi A, Takai Y (1990) Molecular cloning and characterization of a novel type of regulatory protein (GDI) for the rho proteins, ras p21-like small GTP-binding proteins. Oncogene 5:1321–1328.

Gaggioli C, Hooper S, Hidalgo-Carcedo C, Grosse R, Marshall JF, Harrington K, Sahai E (2007) Fibroblast-led collective invasion of carcinoma cells with differing roles for RhoGTPases in leading and following cells. Nat Cell Biol 9:1392–1400.

Guarino M, Rubino B, Ballabio G (2007) The role of epithelial-mesenchymal transition in cancer pathology. Pathology 39:305–318.

Gumbiner B, Stevenson B, Grimaldi A (1988) The role of the cell adhesion molecule uvomorulin in the formation and maintenance of the epithelial junctional complex. J Cell Biol 107:1575–1587.

Gupton SL, Eisenmann K, Alberts AS, Waterman-Storer CM (2007) mDia2 regulates actin and focal adhesion dynamics and organization in the lamella for efficient epithelial cell migration. J Cell Sci 120:3475–3487.

Hakem A, Sanchez-Sweatman O, You-Ten A, Duncan G, Wakeham A, Khokha R, Mak TW (2005) RhoC is dispensable for embryogenesis and tumor initiation but essential for metastasis. Genes Dev 19:1974–1979.

Hall A (1998) Rho GTPases and the actin cytoskeleton. Science 279:509–514.

Hanahan D and Weinberg RA (2000) The hallmarks of cancer. Cell 100:57–70.

Healy KD, Hodgson L, Kim TY, Shutes A, Maddileti S, Juliano RL, Hahn KM, Harden TK, Bang YJ, Der CJ (2007) DLC-1 suppresses non-small cell lung cancer growth and invasion by RhoGAP-dependent and independent mechanisms. Mol Carcinog 47:326–337.

Hoffman GR, Nassar N, Cerione RA (2000) Structure of the Rho family GTP-binding protein Cdc42 in complex with the multifunctional regulator RhoGDI. Cell 100:345–356.

Hordijk PL, ten Klooster JP, van der Kammen RA, Michiels F, Oomen LC, Collard JG (1997) Inhibition of invasion of epithelial cells by Tiam1-Rac signaling. Science 278:1464–1466.

Hornstein I, Pikarsky E, Groysman M, Amir G, Peylan-Ramu N, Katzav S (2003) The haematopoietic specific signal transducer Vav1 is expressed in a subset of human neuroblastomas. J Pathol 199:526–533.

Hotulainen P and Lappalainen P (2006) Stress fibers are generated by two distinct actin assembly mechanisms in motile cells. J Cell Biol 173:383–394.

Ikoma T, Takahashi T, Nagano S, Li YM, Ohno Y, Ando K, Fujiwara T, Fujiwara H, Kosai K (2004) A definitive role of RhoC in metastasis of orthotopic lung cancer in mice. Clin Cancer Res 10:1192–1200.

Itoh K, Yoshioka K, Akedo H, Uehata M, Ishizaki T, Narumiya S (1999) An essential part for Rho-associated kinase in the transcellular invasion of tumor cells. Nat Med 5:221–225.

Jordan P, Brazao R, Boavida MG, Gespach C, Chastre E (1999) Cloning of a novel human Rac1b splice variant with increased expression in colorectal tumors. Oncogene 18:6835–6839.

Kamai T, Tsujii T, Arai K, Takagi K, Asami H, Ito Y, Oshima H (2003) Significant association of Rho/ROCK pathway with invasion and metastasis of bladder cancer. Clin Cancer Res 9: 2632–2641.

Kamai T, Yamanishi T, Shirataki H, Takagi K, Asami H, Ito Y, Yoshida K (2004) Overexpression of RhoA, Rac1, and Cdc42 GTPases is associated with progression in testicular cancer. Clin Cancer Res 10:4799–4805.

Kawano Y, Fukata Y, Oshiro N, Amano M, Nakamura T, Ito M, Matsumura F, Inagaki M, Kaibuchi K (1999) Phosphorylation of myosin-binding subunit (MBS) of myosin phosphatase by Rho-kinase in vivo. J Cell Biol 147:1023–1038.

Kimura K, Ito M, Amano M, Chihara K, Fukata Y, Nakafuku M, Yamamori B, Feng J, Nakano T, Okawa K, Iwamatsu A, Kaibuchi K (1996) Regulation of myosin phosphatase by Rho and Rho-associated kinase (Rho-kinase). Science 273:245–248.

Kin Y, Li G, Shibuya M, Maru Y (2001) The Dbl homology domain of BCR is not a simple spacer in P210BCR-ABL of the Philadelphia chromosome. J Biol Chem 276:39462–39468.

Kourlas PJ, Strout MP, Becknell B, Veronese ML, Croce CM, Theil KS, Krahe R, Ruutu T, Knuutila S, Bloomfield CD, Caligiuri MA (2000) Identification of a gene at 11q23 encoding a guanine nucleotide exchange factor: Evidence for its fusion with MLL in acute myeloid leukemia. Proc Natl Acad Sci U S A 97:2145–2150.

Kozma R, Ahmed S, Best A, Lim L (1995) The Ras-related protein Cdc42Hs and bradykinin promote formation of peripheral actin microspikes and filopodia in Swiss 3T3 fibroblasts. Mol Cell Biol 15:1942–1952.

Kumar R and Vadlamudi RK (2002) Emerging functions of p21-activated kinases in human cancer cells. J Cell Physiol 193:133–144.

Lamarche N and Hall A (1994) GAPs for rho-related GTPases. Trends Genet 10:436–440.

Lee EY, Parry G, Bissell MJ (1984) Modulation of secreted proteins of mouse mammary epithelial cells by the collagenous substrata. J Cell Biol 98:146–155.

Li X, Bu X, Lu B, Avraham H, Flavell RA, Lim B (2002) The hematopoiesis-specific GTP-binding protein RhoH is GTPase deficient and modulates activities of other Rho GTPases by an inhibitory function. Mol Cell Biol 22:1158–1171.

Liotta LA and Kohn EC (2001) The microenvironment of the tumour-host interface. Nature 411:375–379.

Liu N, Bi F, Pan YL, Xue Y, Han ZY, Liu CJ, Fan DM (2004) [Expression of RhoC in gastric cancer cell lines and construction and identification of RhoC-specific siRNA expression vector]. Xi Bao Yu Fen Zi Mian Yi Xue Za Zhi 20:148–151.

Lozano E, Betson M, Braga VM (2003) Tumor progression: Small GTPases and loss of cell-cell adhesion. Bioessays 25:452–463.

Maekawa M, Ishizaki T, Boku S, Watanabe N, Fujita A, Iwamatsu A, Obinata T, Ohashi K, Mizuno K, Narumiya S (1999) Signaling from Rho to the actin cytoskeleton through protein kinases ROCK and LIM-kinase. Science 285:895–898.

Malliri A and Collard JG (2003) Role of Rho-family proteins in cell adhesion and cancer. Curr Opin Cell Biol 15:583–589.

Malliri A, van der Kammen RA, Clark K, van der Valk M, Michiels F, Collard JG (2002) Mice deficient in the Rac activator Tiam1 are resistant to Ras-induced skin tumours. Nature 417:867–871.

Matos P and Jordan P (2005) Expression of Rac1b stimulates NF-kappaB-mediated cell survival and G1/S progression. Exp Cell Res 305:292–299.

Matsumoto Y, Tanaka K, Harimaya K, Nakatani F, Matsuda S, Iwamoto Y (2001) Small GTP-binding protein, Rho, both increased and decreased cellular motility, activation of matrix metalloproteinase 2 and invasion of human osteosarcoma cells. Jpn J Cancer Res 92:429–438.

Meller N, Merlot S, Guda C (2005) CZH proteins: A new family of Rho-GEFs. J Cell Sci 118:4937–4946.

Michaelson D, Silletti J, Murphy G, D'Eustachio P, Rush M, Philips MR (2001) Differential localization of Rho GTPases in live cells: Regulation by hypervariable regions and RhoGDI binding. J Cell Biol 152:111–126.

Miki H, Yamaguchi H, Suetsugu S, Takenawa T (2000) IRSp53 is an essential intermediate between Rac and WAVE in the regulation of membrane ruffling. Nature 408:732–735.

Minard ME, Herynk MH, Collard JG, Gallick GE (2005) The guanine nucleotide exchange factor Tiam1 increases colon carcinoma growth at metastatic sites in an orthotopic nude mouse model. Oncogene 24:2568–2573.

Mitin N, Rossman KL, Der CJ (2005) Signaling interplay in Ras superfamily function. Curr Biol 15:R563–574.

Moon SY and Zheng Y (2003) Rho GTPase-activating proteins in cell regulation. Trends Cell Biol 13:13–22.

Murata T, Arii S, Nakamura T, Mori A, Kaido T, Furuyama H, Furumoto K, Nakao T, Isobe N, Imamura M (2001) Inhibitory effect of Y-27632, a ROCK inhibitor, on progression of rat liver fibrosis in association with inactivation of hepatic stellate cells. J Hepatol 35:474–481.

Nakano K, Takaishi K, Kodama A, Mammoto A, Shiozaki H, Monden M, Takai Y (1999) Distinct actions and cooperative roles of ROCK and mDia in Rho small G protein-induced reorganization of the actin cytoskeleton in Madin-Darby canine kidney cells. Mol Biol Cell 10:2481–2491.

Nobes CD and Hall A (1995) Rho, rac, and cdc42 GTPases regulate the assembly of multi-molecular focal complexes associated with actin stress fibers, lamellipodia, and filopodia. Cell 81:53–62.

Nobes CD, Hawkins P, Stephens L, Hall A (1995) Activation of the small GTP-binding proteins rho and rac by growth factor receptors. J Cell Sci 108 (Pt 1):225–233.

Olson MF and Sahai E (2008)The actin cytoskeleton in cancer cell motility. Clin Exp Metastasis 26:273–287.

Orimo A and Weinberg RA (2006) Stromal fibroblasts in cancer: A novel tumor-promoting cell type. Cell Cycle 5:1597–1601.

Orimo A and Weinberg RA (2007) Heterogeneity of stromal fibroblasts in tumors. Cancer Biol Ther 6:618–619.

Palecek SP, Huttenlocher A, Horwitz AF, Lauffenburger DA (1998) Physical and biochemical regulation of integrin release during rear detachment of migrating cells. J Cell Sci 111 (Pt 7):929–940.

Pasqualucci L, Neumeister P, Goossens T, Nanjangud G, Chaganti RS, Kuppers R, Dalla-Favera R (2001) Hypermutation of multiple proto-oncogenes in B-cell diffuse large-cell lymphomas. Nature 412:341–346.

Paszek MJ and Weaver VM (2004) The tension mounts: Mechanics meets morphogenesis and malignancy. J Mammary Gland Biol Neoplasia 9:325–342.

Paszek MJ, Zahir N, Johnson KR, Lakins JN, Rozenberg GI, Gefen A, Reinhart-King CA, Margulies SS, Dembo M, Boettiger D, Hammer DA, Weaver VM (2005) Tensional homeostasis and the malignant phenotype. Cancer Cell 8:241–254.

Pille JY, Denoyelle C, Varet J, Bertrand JR, Soria J, Opolon P, Lu H, Pritchard LL, Vannier JP, Malvy C, Soria C, Li H (2005) Anti-RhoA and anti-RhoC siRNAs inhibit the proliferation and invasiveness of MDA-MB-231 breast cancer cells in vitro and in vivo. Mol Ther 11: 267–274.

Pinner S, Sahai E (2008) PDK1 regulates cancer cell motility by antagonising inhibition of ROCK1 by RhoE. Nat Cell Biol 10:127–137.

Pollard JW (2004) Tumour-educated macrophages promote tumour progression and metastasis. Nat Rev Cancer 4:71–78.

Preudhomme C, Roumier C, Hildebrand MP, Dallery-Prudhomme E, Lantoine D, Lai JL, Daudignon A, Adenis C, Bauters F, Fenaux P, Kerckaert JP, Galiegue-Zouitina S (2000) Nonrandom 4p13 rearrangements of the RhoH/TTF gene, encoding a GTP-binding protein, in non-Hodgkin's lymphoma and multiple myeloma. Oncogene 19:2023–2032.

Price LS and Collard JG (2001) Regulation of the cytoskeleton by Rho-family GTPases: Implications for tumour cell invasion. Semin Cancer Biol 11:167–173.

Price LS, Leng J, Schwartz MA, Bokoch GM (1998) Activation of Rac and Cdc42 by integrins mediates cell spreading. Mol Biol Cell 9:1863–1871.

Provenzano PP, Eliceiri KW, Campbell JM, Inman DR, White JG, Keely PJ (2006) Collagen reorganization at the tumor-stromal interface facilitates local invasion. BMC Med 4:38.

Provenzano PP, Inman DR, Eliceiri KW, Knittel JG, Yan L, Rueden CT, White JG, Keely PJ (2008) Collagen density promotes mammary tumor initiation and progression. BMC Med 6:11.

Quinlan MP (1999) Rac regulates the stability of the adherens junction and its components, thus affecting epithelial cell differentiation and transformation. Oncogene 18:6434–6442.

Radisky DC, Levy DD, Littlepage LE, Liu H, Nelson CM, Fata JE, Leake D, Godden EL, Albertson DG, Nieto MA, Werb Z, Bissell MJ (2005) Rac1b and reactive oxygen species mediate MMP-3-induced EMT and genomic instability. Nature 436:123–127.

Reuther GW, Lambert QT, Booden MA, Wennerberg K, Becknell B, Marcucci G, Sondek J, Caligiuri MA, Der CJ (2001) Leukemia-associated Rho guanine nucleotide exchange factor, a Dbl family protein found mutated in leukemia, causes transformation by activation of RhoA. J Biol Chem 276:27145–27151.

Ridley A (2000) Rho GTPases. Integrating integrin signaling. J Cell Biol 150:F107–109.

Ridley AJ (2001) Rho GTPases and cell migration. J Cell Sci 114:2713–2722.

Ridley AJ (2004) Rho proteins and cancer. Breast Cancer Res Treat 84:13–19.

Ridley AJ and Hall A (1992) The small GTP-binding protein rho regulates the assembly of focal adhesions and actin stress fibers in response to growth factors. Cell 70:389–399.

Ridley AJ, Paterson HF, Johnston CL, Diekmann D, Hall A (1992) The small GTP-binding protein rac regulates growth factor-induced membrane ruffling. Cell 70:401–410.

Riento K and Ridley AJ (2003) Rocks: Multifunctional kinases in cell behaviour. Nat Rev Mol Cell Biol 4:446–456.

Rohatgi R, Ma L, Miki H, Lopez M, Kirchhausen T, Takenawa T, Kirschner MW (1999) The interaction between N-WASP and the Arp2/3 complex links Cdc42-dependent signals to actin assembly. Cell 97:221–231.

Rossman KL, Der CJ, Sondek J (2005) GEF means go: Turning on RHO GTPases with guanine nucleotide-exchange factors. Nat Rev Mol Cell Biol 6:167–180.

Rottner K, Hall A, Small JV (1999) Interplay between Rac and Rho in the control of substrate contact dynamics. Curr Biol 9:640–648.

Sahai E, Marshall CJ (2002) ROCK and Dia have opposing effects on adherens junctions downstream of Rho. Nat Cell Biol 4:408–415.

Sander EE, ten Klooster JP, van Delft S, van der Kammen RA, Collard JG (1999) Rac downregulates Rho activity: Reciprocal balance between both GTPases determines cellular morphology and migratory behavior. J Cell Biol 147:1009–1022.

Sander EE, van Delft S, ten Klooster JP, Reid T, van der Kammen RA, Michiels F, Collard JG (1998) Matrix-dependent Tiam1/Rac signaling in epithelial cells promotes either cell-cell adhesion or cell migration and is regulated by phosphatidylinositol 3-kinase. J Cell Biol 143:1385–1398.

Sanders LC, Matsumura F, Bokoch GM, de Lanerolle P (1999) Inhibition of myosin light chain kinase by p21-activated kinase. Science 283:2083–2085.

Saras J, Wollberg P, Aspenstrom P (2004) Wrch1 is a GTPase-deficient Cdc42-like protein with unusual binding characteristics and cellular effects. Exp Cell Res 299:356–369.

Schmidt A and Hall A (2002) Guanine nucleotide exchange factors for Rho GTPases: Turning on the switch. Genes Dev 16:1587–1609.

Schmitz AA, Govek EE, Bottner B, Van Aelst L (2000) Rho GTPases: Signaling, migration, and invasion. Exp Cell Res 261:1–12.

Schnelzer A, Prechtel D, Knaus U, Dehne K, Gerhard M, Graeff H, Harbeck N, Schmitt M, Lengyel E (2000) Rac1 in human breast cancer: Overexpression, mutation analysis, and characterization of a new isoform, Rac1b. Oncogene 19:3013–3020.

Schubbert S, Shannon K, Bollag G (2007) Hyperactive Ras in developmental disorders and cancer. Nat Rev Cancer 7:295–308.

Sequeira L, Dubyk CW, Riesenberger TA, Cooper CR, van Golen KL (2008) Rho GTPases in PC-3 prostate cancer cell morphology, invasion and tumor cell diapedesis. Clin Exp Metastasis 25:569–579.

Shih TY, Williams DR, Weeks MO, Maryak JM, Vass WC, Scolnick EM (1978) Comparison of the genomic organization of Kirsten and Harvey sarcoma viruses. J Virol 27:45–55.

Shikada Y, Yoshino I, Okamoto T, Fukuyama S, Kameyama T, Maehara Y (2003) Higher expression of RhoC is related to invasiveness in non-small cell lung carcinoma. Clin Cancer Res 9:5282–5286.

Shutes A, Berzat AC, Cox AD, Der CJ (2004) Atypical mechanism of regulation of the Wrch-1 Rho family small GTPase. Curr Biol 14:2052–2056.

Small JV, Stradal T, Vignal E, Rottner K (2002) The lamellipodium: Where motility begins. Trends Cell Biol 12:112–120.

Somlyo AV, Bradshaw D, Ramos S, Murphy C, Myers CE, Somlyo AP (2000) Rho-kinase inhibitor retards migration and in vivo dissemination of human prostate cancer cells. Biochem Biophys Res Commun 269:652–659.

Suwa H, Ohshio G, Imamura T, Watanabe G, Arii S, Imamura M, Narumiya S, Hiai H, Fukumoto M (1998) Overexpression of the rhoC gene correlates with progression of ductal adenocarcinoma of the pancreas. Br J Cancer 77:147–152.

Takai Y, Sasaki T, Matozaki T (2001) Small GTP-binding proteins. Physiol Rev 81:153–208.

Takaishi K, Sasaki T, Kato M, Yamochi W, Kuroda S, Nakamura T, Takeichi M, Takai Y (1994) Involvement of Rho p21 small GTP-binding protein and its regulator in the HGF-induced cell motility. Oncogene 9:273–279.

Totsukawa G, Yamakita Y, Yamashiro S, Hartshorne DJ, Sasaki Y, Matsumura F (2000) Distinct roles of ROCK (Rho-kinase) and MLCK in spatial regulation of MLC phosphorylation for assembly of stress fibers and focal adhesions in 3T3 fibroblasts. J Cell Biol 150:797–806.

Vadlamudi RK, Adam L, Wang RA, Mandal M, Nguyen D, Sahin A, Chernoff J, Hung MC, Kumar R (2000) Regulatable expression of p21-activated kinase-1 promotes anchorage-independent growth and abnormal organization of mitotic spindles in human epithelial breast cancer cells. J Biol Chem 275:36238–36244.

Valencia A, Chardin P, Wittinghofer A, Sander C (1991) The ras protein family: Evolutionary tree and role of conserved amino acids. Biochemistry 30:4637–4648.

van Golen KL, Bao L, DiVito MM, Wu Z, Prendergast GC, Merajver SD (2002) Reversion of RhoC GTPase-induced inflammatory breast cancer phenotype by treatment with a farnesyl transferase inhibitor. Mol Cancer Ther 1:575–583.

Vetter IR and Wittinghofer A (2001) The guanine nucleotide-binding switch in three dimensions. Science 294:1299–1304.

Watanabe N, Madaule P, Reid T, Ishizaki T, Watanabe G, Kakizuka A, Saito Y, Nakao K, Jockusch BM, Narumiya S (1997) p140mDia, a mammalian homolog of Drosophila diaphanous, is a target protein for Rho small GTPase and is a ligand for profilin. Embo J 16:3044–3056.

Weinberg RA (2008) Coevolution in the tumor microenvironment. Nat Genet 40:494–495.

Wennerberg K and Der CJ (2004) Rho-family GTPases: It's not only Rac and Rho (and I like it). J Cell Sci 117:1301–1312.

Wennerberg K, Rossman KL, Der CJ (2005) The Ras superfamily at a glance. J Cell Sci 118:843–846.

Wildenberg GA, Dohn MR, Carnahan RH, Davis MA, Lobdell NA, Settleman J, Reynolds AB (2006) p120-catenin and p190RhoGAP regulate cell-cell adhesion by coordinating antagonism between Rac and Rho. Cell 127:1027–1039.

Wolf K, Mazo I, Leung H, Engelke K, von Andrian UH, Deryugina EI, Strongin AY, Brocker EB, Friedl P (2003) Compensation mechanism in tumor cell migration: Mesenchymal-amoeboid transition after blocking of pericellular proteolysis. J Cell Biol 160:267–277.

Wong CM, Lee JM, Ching YP, Jin DY, Ng IO (2003) Genetic and epigenetic alterations of DLC-1 gene in hepatocellular carcinoma. Cancer Res 63:7646–7651.

Wozniak MA, Desai R, Solski PA, Der CJ, Keely PJ (2003) ROCK-generated contractility regulates breast epithelial cell differentiation in response to the physical properties of a three-dimensional collagen matrix. J Cell Biol 163:583–595.

Wozniak MA and Keely PJ (2005) Use of three-dimensional collagen gels to study mechanotransduction in T47D breast epithelial cells. Biol Proced Online 7:144–161.

Wu M, Wu ZF, Merajver SD (2007) Rho proteins and cell-matrix interactions in cancer. Cells Tissues Organs 185:100–103.

Yap AS, Brieher WM, Gumbiner BM (1997) Molecular and functional analysis of cadherin-based adherens junctions. Annu Rev Cell Dev Biol 13:119–146.

Yuan BZ, Durkin ME, Popescu NC (2003a) Promoter hypermethylation of DLC-1, a candidate tumor suppressor gene, in several common human cancers. Cancer Genet Cytogenet 140:113–117.

Yuan BZ, Jefferson AM, Baldwin KT, Thorgeirsson SS, Popescu NC, Reynolds SH (2004) DLC-1 operates as a tumor suppressor gene in human non-small cell lung carcinomas. Oncogene 23:1405–1411.

Yuan BZ, Zhou X, Durkin ME, Zimonjic DB, Gumundsdottir K, Eyfjord JE, Thorgeirsson SS, Popescu NC (2003b) DLC-1 gene inhibits human breast cancer cell growth and in vivo tumorigenicity. Oncogene 22:445–450.

Zhang Y and Zhang B (2006) D4-GDI, a Rho GTPase regulator, promotes breast cancer cell invasiveness. Cancer Res 66:5592–5598.

Zhao ZS, Manser E, Loo TH, Lim L (2000) Coupling of PAK-interacting exchange factor PIX to GIT1 promotes focal complex disassembly. Mol Cell Biol 20:6354–6363.

Zhong C, Kinch MS, Burridge K (1997) Rho-stimulated contractility contributes to the fibroblastic phenotype of Ras-transformed epithelial cells. Mol Biol Cell 8:2329–2344.

Zondag GC, Evers EE, ten Klooster JP, Janssen L, van der Kammen RA, Collard JG (2000) Oncogenic Ras downregulates Rac activity, which leads to increased Rho activity and epithelial-mesenchymal transition. J Cell Biol 149:775–782.

Chapter 5
Merlin/NF2 Tumor Suppressor and Ezrin–Radixin–Moesin (ERM) Proteins in Cancer Development and Progression

L. Ren and C. Khanna

Cast of characters

The first evidence that mutations in the *NF2* (a.k.a. merlin) gene cause neurofibromatosis II was obtained over 15 years ago (Rouleau et al. 1993; Trofatter et al. 1993). The hallmark of this disorder is the occurrence of schwannomas and other central nervous system tumors, such as meningiomas. Both somatic and germline mutations were discovered in NF2 patients and in NF2-related tumors. Loss of the wild-type allele was demonstrated in 75% of all neoplasms, suggesting that NF2 is indeed a classical tumor suppressor. Curiously, no consistent or recurrent mutations have been identified in the genes encoding closely related ERM (ezrin–radixin–moesin) protein genes. There is a single known case of anaplastic large-cell lymphoma, where a fusion protein of truncated moesin and anaplastic lymphoma kinase was identified (Tort et al. 2001). However, ERM proteins are important regulators of the Rho GTPases (see Chapter 4), firmly implicating them in the control of cancer cell motility, invasion and metastasis.

Introduction: Discovery, Functional Relationship, and Structural Organization

ERM proteins

Homology

Ezrin, radixin, and moesin are widely expressed proteins known as ERMs that link the actin cytoskeleton to membrane and membrane-associated proteins. Ezrin, the prototype ERM protein, is a 585-amino-acid polypeptide first identified in microvillar structures and shown to be present in actin-containing surface structures

C. Khanna (✉)
Head, Tumor and Metastasis Biology Section, Pediatric Oncology Branch, National Cancer Institute, 37 Convent Drive, Suite 2144, Bethesda, MD, USA
e-mail: khannac@mail.nih.gov

A. Thomas-Tikhonenko (ed.), *Cancer Genome and Tumor Microenvironment*,
DOI 10.1007/978-1-4419-0711-0_5, © Springer Science+Business Media, LLC 2010

(Bretscher 1983; Gould et al. 1986; Pakkanen et al. 1987; Turunen et al. 1989). Radixin, a 583-amino-acid protein with 77% identity to ezrin, was initially isolated from hepatic adherent junctions and was subsequently shown to localize to microvilli in hepatocytes and other cell types and to the cleavage furrow (Tsukita et al. 1989; Funayama et al. 1991; Sato et al. 1991). Moesin, which was originally identified by its ability to bind heparin, was found to be mainly expressed in endothelial cells and lymphocytes. The cDNA sequence of moesin encodes a protein of 577 amino acids with 74% identity to ezrin (Sato et al. 1992). The genes encoding ERM proteins reside on different human chromosomes: radixin is on chromosome 11 with 11 exons (Wilgenbus et al. 1993); ezrin is on chromosome 6 with 13 exons (Turunen et al. 1989; Majander-Nordenswan et al. 1998); and moesin is on the X chromosome with 12 exons (Wilgenbus et al. 1993). Homologues of ERM proteins have been identified in *Drosophila* and *C. elegans*, although the number of family members is limited to only one in flies and two nearly identical genes in nematodes. While this may suggest a single basic function for ERM proteins, recent genetic studies in mice do not point to complete functional redundancy but rather to overlapping and distinct functions for ERM proteins (Doi et al. 1999; Kikuchi et al. 2002; Saotome et al. 2004).

Structure and Domain Organization

ERM proteins share homology in sequence structure and function. They are composed of three domains, an N-terminal globular domain (N-terminal ERM association domain, N-ERMAD); an extended alpha-helical domain; and a charged C-terminal domain (C-terminal ERM association domain, C-ERMAD). The N-terminal domain of ERM proteins, called the FERM (*f*our-point-one protein, *e*zrin, *r*adixin, *m*oesin) domain, is highly conserved and is also found in merlin, band 4.1 proteins, and members of the band 4.1 superfamily. The crystal structures of ERM proteins have revealed the FERM domain to be composed of three modules that together form a compact clover-shaped structure. Although no sequence conservation is evident, all three subdomains (F1, F2, and F3) have structural homology to ubiquitin, acyl-CoA-binding protein, and the pleckstrin-homology (PH) domain. In contrast to the globular FERM domain, the carboxy-terminal domain adopts an extended structure and is composed of one β-strand and six helical regions that bind to and cover an extensive area on the FERM domain surface, potentially masking recognition sites of other proteins. There are possibly very different conformations for the C-terminal domain depending on whether it is free or bound to F-actin. Ezrin and radixin also contain a polyproline region between the helical and C-terminal domains. ERM proteins can undergo intramolecular and/or intermolecular head-to-tail interactions: both monomers and oligomers exist in cells, but it is not clear whether all forms are biologically active (Fig. 5.1).

Tissue Localization and Functional Relationship

Although ezrin, radixin, and moesin are coexpressed in most cultured cells, they exhibit somewhat distinctive tissue-specific expression patterns. For example, ezrin

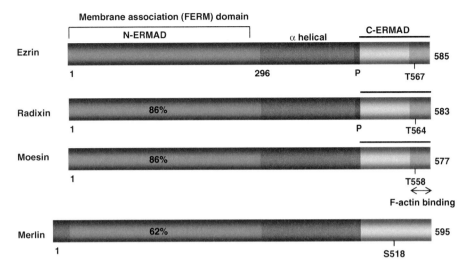

Fig. 5.1 ERM family members (ezrin, radixin, and moesin) and merlin/NF2. ERM proteins consist of three domains: a globular N-terminal, membrane-binding domain (FERM domain or N-ERMAD), followed by an extended α-helical domain, and a positively charged C-terminal, actin-binding domain(C-ERMAD). The percentage sequence identity with ezrin in N-terminal domain is indicated at amino acid sequence level

is highly concentrated in intestine, stomach, lung, and kidney. Moesin is predominantly expressed in lung and spleen, and radixin is primarily found in the liver and intestine. Ezrin is expressed in epithelial and mesothelial cells, while moesin is expressed in lymphoid and endothelial cells. The brush border of intestinal epithelial cells expresses only ezrin, and hepatocytes express only radixin.

The functional redundancy that exists between ERM proteins is supported by the phenotype of moesin, radixin, and ezrin gene knockout mice. *Moesin–/–* mice do not carry any observable phenotype in any of the tissue examined (Doi et al. 1999). Interestingly, the expression and subcellular distribution of ezrin and radixin in the tissues from the moesin –/– mice are not changed. Similarly, *Rdx* (encoding radixin)–/– animals are viable and only exhibit deafness and hepatic abnormalities (Kikuchi et al. 2002). Deafness in these mice results from defective stereocilia in the inner and outer hair cells, which exclusively express radixin (Kitajiri et al. 2004). The ezrin knockout mouse is viable at birth, suggesting the ability of radixin and moesin to compensate for ezrin during development. Interestingly the fatal phenotype of this mouse is characterized by intestinal villous malformations seen at day 13 postpartum. Of note, normal intestinal epithelial cells nearly exclusively express ezrin (Saotome et al. 2004). Genetic studies using *Drosophila* and *C. elegans* extend further to support the functional redundancy of ERM proteins (Polesello and Payre 2004). In *Drosophila*, only a single ERM protein/orthologue (Dmoesin) is present. The functional loss of Dmoesin, in *Drosophila*, leads to a wide range of developmental and morphogenic defects which can be largely attributed to abnormal epithelial morphogenesis (Jankovics et al. 2002; Polesello et al. 2002; Hipfner et al. 2004; Pilot et al. 2006).

Merlin

Structure

The *NF2* tumor suppressor gene encodes the merlin protein (moesin, ezrin, radixin-like protein). Also known as schwannomin (Rouleau et al. 1993), merlin is an ERM-related protein with tumor suppressor functions. These tumor suppressor functions are surprising since no other ERM family members or related proteins that are associated with the cytoskeleton have been shown to negatively regulate cell proliferation or growth. In this way, merlin may be a novel type of tumor suppressor. More importantly, the high degree of structural similarity between merlin and ERM proteins indicates that these proteins might share regulatory mechanisms and possibly also cellular functions. Human *NF2* gene is located on chromosome 22 with 17 exons (Rouleau et al. 1993). Alternative splicing of exon 16 gives rise to two isoforms of merlin protein, which differ in the last 11 amino acids of the C terminus. Isoform I has 595 residues and isoform II has 590 residues (Haase et al. 1994; Pykett et al. 1994). Merlin protein is enriched in mouse lung, intestine, spleen, kidney, spinal cord, and brain (Claudio et al. 1995) and especially enriched during fetal development in extra-embryonic tissues, heart, and the nervous and skeletal systems (Huynh et al. 1996). In cultured mammalian cells, merlin is concentrated in cell protrusions and cell–cell boundaries. Some merlin exhibits diffuse localization throughout the membrane and cytoplasm, and occasionally has a punctate distribution that has been attributed to localization in intracellular vesicles or membrane lipid rafts (McCartney and Fehon 1996; Stickney et al. 2004). A nuclear localization of merlin has also been reported (Kressel and Schmucker 2002; Muranen et al. 2005).

Structural similarities between merlin and ERM proteins exist (Fig. 5.1). ERM proteins and merlin can be divided into three apparent functional domains: the amino-terminal FERM domain, an extended coil–coil region, and a short carboxy-terminal domain. Furthermore, the merlin FERM domain forms a three-dimensional structure that is similar to that of ERM proteins (discussed above). Despite these similarities, there are clear structural differences between merlin and ERM proteins. One obvious difference is that merlin lacks the carboxy-terminal, actin-binding domain that is found in ERM proteins. Several studies have shown that merlin can instead interact with F-actin through actin-binding sites within the FERM domain (Xu and Gutmann 1998; Brault et al. 2001; James et al. 2001) or indirectly through βII-spectrin (Scoles et al. 1998). Although the FERM domains are quite similar, the regions in the merlin FERM domain that are conserved between human and *Drosophila* are distinct from ERM proteins. Crystallographic analysis of merlin FERM domain has shown that most divergent residues are found clustered on the globular surface, which indicates that they might serve as sites for distinct effector binding or regulatory interactions. In addition, a seven-amino-acid stretch known as the "blue box," which is unique to merlin homologues, probably forms an essential part of the interface between the FERM domain and the tail domain in the folded conformation (LaJeunesse et al. 1998).

Conformational Regulation

ERM proteins

ERM proteins are conformationally regulated. ERM proteins exist in proposed dormant forms in which the C-terminal tail binds to and masks the N-terminal FERM domain. The activation of ERM proteins is mediated by both exposure to PIP2 and phosphorylation of the C-terminal threonine (T567 in ezrin, T564 in radixin, T558 in moesin). It is likely that phosphorylation of other residues in ERM proteins is needed to maintain an open activated conformation for ezrin and to direct ezrin-specific effects in cells (Wu et al. 2000). Recent studies of ezrin using atomic force microscopy (AFM) demonstrated that the ezrin activation induced by T567 phosphorylation is a two-step process (Liu et al. 2007). In the resting stage, ezrin is initially folded, with an association of C-ERMAD with the α-helical region followed by a second association of N-FERM/C-ERMAD, which forms a completely closed ezrin molecule. During the process of ezrin activation, modification of the N terminus following PIP2 binding disrupts the N-FERM/C-ERMAD contact to allow Thr567 to be exposed for subsequent phosphorylation (Hamada et al. 2000). This phosphorylation subsequently releases the extreme carboxyl-terminal region from the F-actin binding (Fievet et al. 2004).

Several protein kinases have been found to phosphorylate the C-terminal threonine residue of the ERM proteins. Examples include PKCα (Ng et al. 2001), PKCθ (Pietromonaco et al. 1998), PKCι (Wald et al. 2008), Rho kinases/ROCK (Matsui et al. 1998), G protein-coupled receptor kinase 2 (GRK2) (Cant and Pitcher 2005), myotonic dystrophy kinase-related Cdc42-binding kinase (MRCK) (Nakamura et al. 2000), and the Ste20-related kinase Nck-interacting kinase (NIK) (Baumgartner et al. 2006).

The deactivation of ERM proteins is also important for physiological functions including the dynamics of actin-rich membrane projections. This process might be triggered by ERM protein dephosphorylation. Moesin T558 dephosphorylation has been suggested to be a crucial step for lymphocyte adhesion and transendothelial migration. The disassembly of microvilli on lymphocyte cell surfaces caused by dephosphorylation of moesin facilitates the cell–cell (lymphocyte–endothelium) contact. Protein phosphatase 2C is involved in the dephosphorylation of moesin through the activation of Rac1 small GTPase (Nijhara et al. 2004). In vivo, dephosphorylation of ERM proteins correlates with microvilli breakdown induced by anoxia and apoptosis (Chen and Mandel 1997; Kondo et al. 1997) (Fig. 5.2).

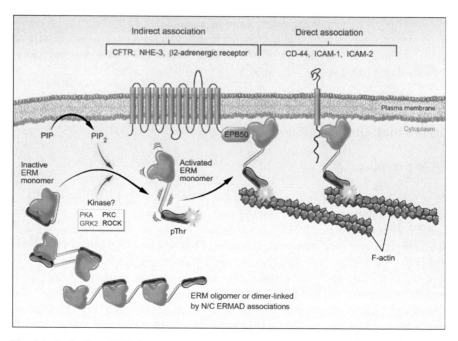

Fig. 5.2 Activation of ERM proteins. ERM proteins exist as monomers, dimers, and oligomers with a closed conformation. The activation of ERM proteins is mediated by both exposure to PIP2 and phosphorylation of the C-terminal threonine. The C-terminal residue of activated ERM proteins binds to F-actin filaments. The N-terminal domains of activated ERM proteins are associated directly with the adhesion molecules such as CD44 and ICAM-1, -2, and -3 or indirectly with other transmembrane proteins such as NHE3 through EPB50

Beyond the putative C-terminal threonine-activating residues, ERM proteins also have tyrosine phosphorylation sites (Y145, Y353, Y477 on ezrin). Although not completely understood, tyrosine phosphorylation may contribute to the regulation of changes in the actin cytoskeleton. Ezrin tyrosine phosphorylation seems to be key in the control of cell shape and signaling of epithelial cells, following EGF, PDGF, and HGF stimulation (Bretscher 1989; Fazioli et al. 1993; Chen et al. 1994; Crepaldi et al. 1997; Gautreau et al. 2002).

Merlin

Although there is considerable evidence that the open conformation of ERM proteins represents the "active" state of the molecule, the case for merlin is less clear. Merlin isoform I is also capable of inter-and intramolecular interactions. Merlin isoform II does not show intramolecular interactions and therefore exists in a constitutively "open" confirmation owing to its exposed ligand-binding sites (Sherman et al. 1997; Gonzalez-Agosti et al. 1999; Gronholm et al. 1999). Available data suggest that the phosphorylation of the merlin C-terminal serine residue (S518) is not analogous to ezrin T567 phosphorylation. Phosphorylation of merlin S518 weakens merlin self-association and inactivates merlin's growth-suppressing function. Studies in mammalian cells have shown that the S518D mutation, which mimics the phosphorylated state, blocks intermolecular interactions between the C/N termini of merlin (Shaw et al. 1998b; Shaw et al. 2001). Conversely, a S518A mutation, which blocks phosphorylation at this site, promotes this intermolecular interaction. Nonphosphorylated merlin has been shown to mediate contact inhibition of growth through its interaction with CD44 by integrating signals from the extracellular matrix (Morrison et al. 2001). However, studies in *Drosophila* indicate that merlin mutations that remove the carboxy-terminal tail and therefore eliminate the possibility of head-to-tail folding result in a constitutively active form of the protein that provides full genetic rescue of a null merlin mutation (LaJeunesse et al. 1998). These data indicate that, like ERM proteins, the unfolded form of merlin is active in vivo. While the lack of S518 phosphorylation correlates well with the growth-suppressing function of merlin, it has not been definitely shown that active merlin is necessarily closed. Further work, including in vivo functional analysis in transgenic mice, will be required to clarify this issue.

The best studied stimulus for merlin S518 phosphorylation is activation of the small GTPase Rac1 (Shaw et al. 2001). Rac-induced phosphorylation of merlin S518 appears to be mediated by the major Rac effector p21-activated kinase (Pak) (Kissil et al. 2002; Xiao et al. 2002). Phospholipids probably also have a role in merlin regulation (Gonzalez-Agosti et al. 1999). S518 can be phosphorylated in a Pak-independent manner by cAMP-dependent protein kinase A (PKA) (Alfthan et al. 2004). Merlin dephosphorylation is accomplished by myosin phosphatase MYPT-1-PPIδ (Jin et al. 2006). Intriguingly, the merlin C-term domain has a stronger affinity for ezrin N-term domain than for merlin N-term domain, and ezrin–merlin hetero-oligomers have been detected (Gronholm et al. 1999; Nguyen et al. 2001). These observations suggest that ERM proteins might control the activation of merlin or, reciprocally, that merlin might be a regulator of ERM activation. The biological significance of merlin–ERM interactions is not well understood.

Cellular Functions

ERM Proteins

Membrane and Cytoskeleton Linker

ERM proteins either directly associate with the cytoplasmic domains of adhesive type I membrane proteins, such as CD44 (Tsukita et al. 1994; Legg and Isacke 1998; Legg et al. 2002), CD43 (Serrador et al. 1998; Yonemura et al. 1998), ICAM-1, -2, and -3 (Heiska et al. 1998; Barreiro et al. 2002; Serrador et al. 2002), or indirectly associate with membrane proteins via PDZ-containing adaptors EBP50 and E3KARP (Reczek and Bretscher 1998; Donowitz et al. 2005; Fievet et al. 2007). ERM proteins not only recruit the membrane proteins to the correct localization on the cell membrane but also regulate their physiological functions (Fievet et al. 2007). ERM proteins can localize signaling molecules that regulate the activity of membrane proteins (Dransfield et al. 1997; Lamprecht et al. 1998; Sun et al. 2000; Weinman et al. 2000). ERM may also contribute to the transport/delivery of membrane proteins for their recycling and vesicular trafficking (Zhou et al. 2003; Cha et al. 2006; Stanasila et al. 2006). Regulated attachment of membrane proteins to F-actin is essential for many fundamental cellular processes, including the determination of cell shape, polarity and surface structure, cell adhesion, motility, cytokinesis, phagocytosis, and integration of membrane transport with signaling pathways.

Intracellular Signaling

ERM proteins directly and indirectly interact with cytoplasmic signaling molecules. ERM proteins seem to lie both downstream and upstream in signal transduction pathways in epithelial and mesenchymal tissues. As described earlier, ERM protein conformation (activity) is regulated by a combination of phospholipid binding and phosphorylation. Both events have been proposed to lie downstream of signals mediated by Rho (Kotani et al. 1997; Fukata et al. 1998; Matsui et al. 1998; Shaw et al. 1998a; Matsui et al. 1999). Recent evidence also places ERM proteins upstream of Rho-pathway activation through direct association with proteins that regulate Rho functions. In vitro studies indicate that ERM binding to RhoGDI, a potent sequestering factor, releases inactive Rho from the GDI, thereby allowing activation through the exchange of GDP to GTP (Takahashi et al. 1997). Additional evidence for this model is provided by the interaction of ERM proteins with hamartin, a product of tumor suppressor gene *TSC1*. The loss of the interaction between ERM proteins and hamartin suppresses the activity of Rho GTPase (Lamb et al. 2000). The possibility that ERM proteins function both upstream and downstream of Rho implies that ERMs may be involved in a feedback loop for Rho-pathway autoregulation.

In a similar fashion, ERM proteins seem to act as effectors in PKCα and PKCθ signaling events (Pietromonaco et al. 1998; Legg et al. 2002; Jensen and Larsson 2004). Both kinases have been shown to phosphorylate the conserved C-terminal threonine and thereby facilitate conformational activation of ERM proteins. In addition, PKC-mediated phosphorylation has been proposed to regulate interactions between CD44 and ezrin by altering phosphorylation of the intracellular domain of CD44 (Legg et al. 2002). Indeed, PKC may regulate the effects of CD44 on cell proliferation and migration by controlling phosphorylation of both CD44 and ERM proteins (personal communication, L. Ren and C. Khanna). Several lines of evidence link ERM functions to growth factor receptor signaling and/or transport. The ERM proteins are rapidly tyrosine phosphorylated following epidermal growth factor (EGF) or hepatocyte growth factor (HGF) stimulation (Bretscher 1989; Krieg and Hunter 1992; Berryman et al. 1993; Crepaldi et al. 1997). Ezrin directly interacts with HGF receptor (MET) and is required for HGF-induced motility (Crepaldi et al. 1997).

Nuclear Localization

To further complicate our understanding of ERM protein biology, Batchelor et al. recently found ERM proteins to localize in nucleus (Batchelor et al. 2004). The nuclear localization of endogenous ezrin and moesin is regulated by cell density and is resistant to detergent extraction, suggesting a tight association with nuclear structures. Phosphorylation in the C-terminal, actin-binding domain of ERM proteins is not a prerequisite for nuclear localization. A specific nuclear localization sequence has been identified and is conserved and functional in all ERM family members. Although the precise nuclear function of ERM proteins is not clear, these data provide further evidence that an increasing number of cytoskeletal components directly link the plasma membrane with nuclear events.

Merlin

Membrane and Cytoskeleton Linker

Merlin, like the ERM proteins, localizes to specific regions of cortical actin remodeling. In contrast to the ERMs, merlin does not have an actin-binding domain at the C terminus but instead may bind actin directly via an N-terminal domain or indirectly via the cytoskeletal proteins such as βII-spectrin, paxillin, or the ERM proteins. Merlin also binds to transmembrane adhesion molecules such as CD44. Based on this, there is increasing evidence to suggest a function of merlin in stabilizing adherence junctions (AJs).

Stabilizing AJs and Contact-Dependent Growth Inhibition

In normal cells, merlin is recruited to cadherin-containing complexes at nascent cell–cell contacts and is required for the formation of stable cadherin-containing adherent junctions (AJs) between cells. Several studies suggest that merlin contributes to the control of contact-dependent inhibition of proliferation (Morrison et al. 2001; Lallemand et al. 2003; Okada et al. 2005). In cultured primary cells, the key consequence of Merlin deficiency is a failure to undergo contact-dependent inhibition of proliferation. This may explain the enhanced tumorigenic and metastatic potential of NF2-deficient tumor cells. Merlin expression and phosphorylation are regulated by cell density, which also suggests Merlin's role on cell–cell communication (Shaw et al. 1998b). Most studies conclude that membrane association is necessary for the growth-suppressing function of merlin. Mutant versions of merlin that cannot localize to the membrane cannot inhibit cell proliferation (Surace et al. 2004). In some cells the association of merlin with the hyaluronic acid receptor CD44 has been shown to be required for contact-dependent inhibition of proliferation (Morrison et al. 2001). Interestingly, this study identified distinct compositions of CD44-containing complexes at low cell density [CD44 – hyperphosphorylated (inactive) merlin–ERM] and high cell density [CD44 – hypophosphorylated (active) merlin], indicating distinct functions for merlin-containing complexes. Recent studies provide further evidence that Merlin mediates contact inhibition by blocking recruitment of Rac to matrix adhesions. Pak reverses this inhibition by phosphorylating, and thus inactivating, merlin (Okada et al. 2005). In agreement with this hypothesis, new studies indicate that inactivation of merlin activates Ras signaling in confluent cells (Jin et al. 2006; Morrison et al. 2007). The fact that defective cell–cell communication can contribute to both tumor initiation and metastasis provides an explanation for the tumorigenic and metastatic consequences of *NF2* deficiency in humans and mice.

Signaling Pathways

The function of merlin and the ERM proteins has been linked to the Rho family of small GTPases that control actin cytoskeleton remodeling. Rac-induced phosphorylation of merlin S518 appears to be mediated by Pak. Recent evidence suggests that merlin can bind to and directly negatively regulates Pak (Kissil et al. 2002; Legg et al. 2002; Xiao et al. 2002; Gronholm et al. 2003). Overexpression of Merlin negatively regulates Rac-dependent signaling and *NF2–/–* cells display phenotypes that are observed in cells expressing constitutively activate Rac. This reciprocal (feedback) regulation is also observed in ERM proteins.

Merlin has been reported to physically interact with several proteins that have established roles in growth factor receptor signaling. Merlin can form a ternary complex with a novel protein named Magicin and Grb2, an adaptor that coordinates receptor tyrosine kinase and ras signaling. Merlin can also interact with EBP50/NHE-RF1, a PDZ-domain containing adaptor that has been implicated in the membrane distribution of receptor tyrosine kinases. It has been reported that merlin directly controls the surface availability and function of membrane receptors that regulate proliferation and differentiation by promoting the clearance of receptors from plasma membrane or sequestering them to a nonsignaling plasma membrane compartment (Maitra et al. 2006; Curto et al. 2007). The localization of merlin to vesicle structures under some conditions together with its reported localization to lipid rafts further supports a role in membrane receptor trafficking.

Physiological Function

ERM Proteins

Epithelial Cell Morphogenesis and Embryogenesis

A requirement for ERM proteins in the morphogenesis of specialized domains of the plasma membrane has been reported in several different systems. Ezrin is involved in the biogenesis of apical microvilli and in the formation of a functional epithelium (Crepaldi et al. 1997; Bonilha et al. 1999; Yonemura and Tsukita 1999; Dard et al. 2001). Moesin is important for the redistribution of adhesion molecules to the uropods of activated lymphocytes (Serrador et al. 1999). Radixin and moesin also play roles in the formation of nerve growth cones (Castelo and Jay 1999). In studies of early postnatal ezrin knockout mice, the loss of ezrin leads to substantial reductions in the apical microvilli and basal infoldings in retinal pigment epithelial cells and in the Muller cell apical microvilli. Ezrin also has a crucial role in the early embryogenesis in mouse. The constitutively active ezrin (ezrin T567D) localizes around the cell cortex and inhibits cell–cell adhesion and cell polarization at the eight-cell stage. In reverse, the inactive ezrin (ezrin T567A) is mainly cytoplasmic and does not perturb compaction at eight-cell stage. However, at the 16-cell stage, ezrin T567A relocalizes at the basolateral cortex, leading to a strong decrease in the surface of adherence junctions, and finally, embryos abort development.

Angiogenesis

Under normal conditions in postnatal mammals, endothelial cells (ECs) lining blood vessel walls are quiescent. Physiological and pathological stimuli can induce ECs to enter the cell cycle for the purpose of vascular repair or the formation of new vessels, e.g., during wound healing, endometrial proliferation, or tumor growth. Ezrin may play a role in the regulation of EC proliferation following exposure to TNF-α. TNF-α-treated ECs exhibit elevation of ezrin expression and phosphorylation of ezrin through activation of Rho A. Following TNF-α exposure, phosphorylated ezrin translocates to the nucleus and represses the activity of the cyclin A promoter. Overexpression of dominant negative ezrin attenuates this TNF-α-induced downregulation of the cyclin A promoter activity and mRNA expression, and abrogates TNF-α-induced repression of EC proliferation in vitro and in vivo (Kishore et al. 2005).

T-Lymphocyte Physiology

Members of the ERM family contribute to lymphocyte transendothelial migration during homing and inflammation. Ezrin is involved in the generation of the uropod (a posterior cellular protrusion) and in the anchoring of various transmembrane proteins (ICAMs, CD44, CD43, PSGL-1, and death receptor CD95/Fas) in lymphocytes. On the endothelial side of the lymphocyte–endothelial interaction, VCAM-1 and ICAM-1, two major endothelial adhesion molecules, are anchored to the actin cytoskeleton through ezrin and moesin, where they contribute to the docking structure of endothelial cells. The polarized T cell interacts with the docking structure during homing and transendothelial migration.

ERM proteins are responsible for the relocalization of ICAM-3 on the surface of T cells, which is needed for immune synapse (IS) formation (Roumier et al. 2001; Das et al. 2002; Tomas et al. 2002). It has been demonstrated that ezrin and moesin, which are generally believed to be functionally redundant, are differentially localized, and have important and complementary functions in IS formation. Moesin appears to be important to move the surface protein CD43, a negative regulator of T-cell activation, out of the center of immunological synapse (Allenspach et al. 2001;

Delon et al. 2001). In contrast, ezrin interacts with and recruits the signaling kinase ZAP-70 to the IS (Ilani et al. 2007).

The interaction of ezrin with CD95 (APO/Fas) is an important trigger for the intracellular signaling cascade, leading to apoptosis induced by this receptor (Parlato et al. 2000; Lozupone et al. 2004).

Merlin

Morphogenesis

The generation of *NF2–/–* -mutant mouse models has contributed to our understanding of merlin function in development and tumorigenesis. Merlin is required for the normal development of several tissues. *NF2*-null embryos fail to gastrulate due to extra-embryonic defects (McClatchey et al. 1997; McClatchey and Giovannini 2005). Furthermore, expression of merlin in the mouse embryo appears to be dynamically regulated during tissue fusion. Merlin expression is low at the leading front before fusion and high across the fused tissue bridge. A targeted deletion of *NF2* in the developing nerve system causes neural tube defects by impairing tissue fusion (McLaughlin et al. 2007). This phenotype appears to be derived from the inability of these merlin-deficient cells to form apico-junction complexes, consistent with the role of merlin in controlling formation and stabilization of AJs (Lallemand et al. 2003). Furthermore, merlin heterozygous (+/–) mice develop a wide variety of malignant tumors, especially fibrosarcomas and osteosarcomas, with a high rate of metastasis. Interestingly, no increase in tumor risk is seen in human patients who are heterozygous deficient for *NF2*. This difference may be explained by the fact that *NF2* and tumor suppressor *p53* genes are linked in the mouse (McClatchey et al. 1998).

Function in Cancer Development and Progression

ERM Proteins

No consistent or recurrent mutations have been identified in the *ERM* genes in cancer conditions. A single case of anaplastic large-cell lymphoma has been described, where a fusion protein of a truncated moesin and anaplastic lymphoma kinase was identified (Tort et al. 2001). ERM proteins have been connected with epithelial–mesenchymal transition (EMT) and tumorigenesis. Coexpression of ezrin and an activated c-Src mutant-enhanced cell scattering disrupted the cell–cell contacts and prevented cell aggregation in mouse mammary cancer cells. Pretreatment with an Src inhibitor PP2 partially restored aggregation of these cells. Expression of a truncated N-terminal domain of ezrin, which has dominant negative function, blocked the cell scattering effect of the activated c-Src and promoted the formation of cohesive cell–cell contacts (Elliott et al. 2004). Repression of ezrin expression by ezrin shRNA in a human breast cancer cell line MDA-MB-231 led to the disruption of the F-actin cytoskeleton and decreased cell motility and invasiveness. Furthermore, blocking ezrin function results in an increased expression of E-cadherin and a decreased phosphorylation of β-catenin by inhibiting phosphorylation levels of c-src (Li et al. 2008).

Ezrin has been recently shown to be expressed in most human cancers and linked to progression in several cancers including, carcinomas of endometrium, breast, colon, ovary, in uveal and cutaneous melanoma, brain tumors, and most recently soft tissue sarcomas. A brief summary of the associations between ezrin and some of these human cancers is presented below.

Sarcomas

Studies of ezrin expression in cancer and corresponding normal tissues have suggested uniquely aberrant expression of ezrin in tissues of mesenchymal origin. Normal human mesenchymal tissues express very little to no ezrin, whereas mesenchymal cancers (i.e., sarcomas) are amongst the highest expressors of ezrin (Bruce et al. 2007). This may suggest a distinct role for ezrin in sarcomas. In adult soft tissue sarcomas, a direct correlation has been made between histological grade and ezrin-staining intensity using immunohistochemistry. Furthermore, multivariate analysis has suggested that high ezrin-staining intensity in primary tumors is inversely associated with metastasis-free interval. A strong correlation between ezrin expression and infiltrative growth pattern of the STS was also observed (Weng et al. 2005).

The role of ezrin in the process of tumor progression and metastasis in three pediatric tumors – rhabdomyosarcoma (RMS) (Yu et al. 2004), osteosarcoma (OS) (Khanna et al. 2004), and Ewing's sarcoma (Krishnan et al. 2006) – has also been reported. In osteosarcoma and rhabdomyosarcoma, the disruption of ezrin expression using dominant-negative mutants, antisense RNA or RNA interference (RNAi), resulted in the inhibition of metastasis. Interestingly, the inhibition or overexpression of ezrin in these cells appeared to do little to influence primary tumor growth of these cancers. Mechanistically the connection between ezrin and metastasis has been explored in osteosarcoma. Ezrin expression appears to provide an early survival advantage for cancer cells that metastasize to the lung in the mouse models. Both Akt and MAPK phosphorylation and activity were reduced when ezrin protein was suppressed. Interestingly, the active phosphorylated form of ezrin does not appear to be constitutively expressed during metastasis, rather phosphorylation of ERM proteins was found to be dynamically regulated. Metastatic OS cells express phosphorylated ERMs early after their arrival in the lung. Surprisingly a loss of phosphorylated ERM was seen within the growing metastatic lesion, followed by a re-expression of phosphorylated ERM at the invasive front of larger metastatic lesions (Ren et al. 2009). This observation indicates that the regulation of ERM activation/phosphorylation may also play an important role in tumor metastasis and progression. The connection between ezrin and metastatic progression was further supported by studies of ezrin protein expression in both pet dogs that naturally develop osteosarcoma and pediatric osteosarcoma patients where the intensity of ezrin expression was linked to poor outcome (Khanna et al. 2001, 2004). In RMS, ezrin was found to be a direct transcriptional target of Six1, a homeodomain-containing transcription factor (Yu et al. 2004). RNA interference (RNAi)-based knockdown of ezrin fully inhibited the ability of Six1 to promote metastasis in RMS cells (Yu et al. 2006).

Head and Neck Cancer

Overexpression of ERMs has been linked to tumor progression in the head and neck squamous cell carcinoma (UADT-SCC) using DNA microarrays (TMA) (Belbin et al. 2005). At the protein level, high cytoplasmic ezrin expression was significantly associated with decreased survival in patients. Strong cytoplasmic moesin expression was associated with poorer survival, albeit not significantly. In contrast, membranous ezrin expression was associated with improved overall survival (Madan et al. 2006) in these patients.

Melanoma

Ezrin is expressed in most primary melanomas of the skin and in all metastatic tumors. Ezrin expression correlates with tumor thickness and level of invasion, suggesting an association between ezrin expression and tumor progression (Ilmonen et al. 2005). In uveal melanoma, multivariate analysis has suggested that ezrin expression is an independent and significant predictor for metastasis (Makitie et al. 2001).

Serous Ovarian Carcinoma

In contrast to other cancers, low or weak ezrin expression in serous ovarian carcinoma correlated with poor patient outcome (Moilanen et al. 2003). In a recent study of 440 patients assessed by tissue microarray immunohistochemistry, ezrin-staining intensity had an inverse correlation with tumor grade. These studies suggest that ezrin may serve different functions in different cell types. Such an explanation is supported by studies showing that ezrin can mediate different intracellular signals depending on the cell type and the extracellular environment (Gautreau et al. 1999; Parlato et al. 2000).

Lung Adenocarcinoma

Radixin expression has been shown to be downregulated in lung adenocarcinoma, including an early stage bronchioloalveolar carcinoma, by differential display analysis. Similarly, the expression of moesin and ezrin is also reduced in lung adenocarcinoma. Immunohistochemistry has confirmed that lung cancer cells express very little radixin and moesin, whereas non-neoplastic alveolar and bronchiolar epithelial cells and endothelial cells express both proteins. In contrast to radixin and moesin, weak but significant staining for ezrin has been observed in the majority of cancer cells. Interestingly, a diffuse cytoplasmic staining pattern has been observed instead of the characteristic membranous staining pattern, especially in areas where tubular structures were disorganized. Moreover, ezrin expression appeared to be strongly induced in tumor cells invading the stroma in a scattered manner, which may suggest that there are cell special functions for ezrin in tumor progression (Tokunou et al. 2000).

Phagocytic Activity of Ezrin

The phagocytic-like behavior of tumor cells was first observed a century ago and confirmed more recently in murine and human tumor cells against both dead cells and inert particles (Marin-Padilla 1977; DeSimone et al. 1980). Most recently, many morphologic features associated with phagocytosis have been identified in tumors, and the phagocytic-like activity of these cells has been associated with invasiveness (Fais 2007). In studies of human malignant melanoma, this phagocytic activity was observed in tumor cells derived from metastatic lesions, whereas cells obtained from primary melanomas did not show detectable phagocytic activity (Lugini et al. 2003). The actin cytoskeleton appears to be connected to the phagocytic activity of tumor cells. Furthermore, ezrin is involved and necessary for this process. Treatment with either cytochalasin or antisense oligonucleotides against ezrin markedly inhibited the phagocytic activity of melanoma cells. Data obtained with murine professional phagocytes suggest that tumor phagocytic activity may occur through the ezrin-mediated assembly of the actin filaments on the lysosomal membranes. It is possible that many of the connections between ezrin and cancer can be explained by changes in phagocytic activity of cells that occur secondary to dysregulation of the ezrin activation/phosphorylation.

Merlin

Merlin protein levels are reduced or absent in most sporadically occurring meningiomas, schwannomas, and ependymomas, collectively these tumors are described as neurofibromatosis type 2 (NF2) tumors. Patients with NF2 may have a familial syndrome with germline heterozygosity for *NF2* or may have sporadic NF2, where both copies of the gene are germline wild type. Missense mutations occur in the *NF2* gene at an extremely low frequency in humans. Nearly all the mutations are nonsense, frameshift, or splice site mutations that all lead to the production of N-terminally truncated merlin. Strikingly, truncated merlin species are rarely detected in primary tumor samples, suggesting that mutant merlin proteins are unstable and actively degraded. Correlation between *NF2* gene mutation frequency and *NF2*-associated tumor types provides only a partial picture of merlin involvement in these tumors. This suggested that post-translational regulation of merlin expression and *merlin* gene mutations might be involved in the loss of merlin expression. The cell surface, calcium-dependent protease, calpain, can specifically cleave merlin. Interestingly, the calpain system is activated in central nervous system tumors with low or absent merlin expression. A recent report also supports this hypothesis that merlin is phosphorylated by Akt on residues Thr230 and ser315, which abolishes merlin N/C-terminal interactions and binding to other proteins. Subsequently, Akt-mediated phosphorylation leads to merlin degradation by ubiquitin (Tang et al. 2007).

Conclusions

Merlin and ERM are proteins that function as linkers between cell membrane and the actin cytoskeleton. Through this linker function and through other less well-described functions, these proteins regulate cell morphology, cell adhesion, motility, cytokinesis, phagocytosis, and integration of membrane transport with signaling pathways. Not surprisingly, connection to these cellular processes has been part of the recently described roles these proteins play in tumor biology. Although related by structure, merlin and the other ERM proteins influence tumor cell biology in distinct directions. On the one hand, merlin acts as a suppressor of cell growth through its role in contact inhibition, whereas ezrin has been associated with promoting cancer progression. The importance of conformational regulation of these proteins has been increasingly understood. Transits through conformational forms of these proteins differentially influence the transduction of growth signals in both physiology and cancer. Indeed, the Rho pathway (discussed in the previous chapter) is one of the signaling pathways linked to ERM and merlin proteins. Further studies should provide important insights into the activities of merlin and ERM proteins as linker proteins and in their regulation of signaling in cancer.

References

Alfthan K, Heiska L, Gronholm M, Renkema GH, Carpen O (2004) Cyclic AMP-dependent protein kinase phosphorylates merlin at serine 518 independently of p21-activated kinase and promotes merlin–ezrin heterodimerization. J Biol Chem 279:18559–18566.

Allenspach EJ, Cullinan P, Tong J, Tang Q, Tesciuba AG, Cannon JL, Takahashi SM, Morgan R, Burkhardt JK, Sperling AI (2001) ERM-dependent movement of CD43 defines a novel protein complex distal to the immunological synapse. Immunity 15:739–750.

Barreiro O, Yanez-Mo M, Serrador JM, Montoya MC, Vicente-Manzanares M, Tejedor R, Furthmayr H, Sanchez-Madrid F (2002) Dynamic interaction of VCAM-1 and ICAM-1 with moesin and ezrin in a novel endothelial docking structure for adherent leukocytes. J Cell Biol 157:1233–1245.

Batchelor CL, Woodward AM, Crouch DH (2004) Nuclear ERM (ezrin, radixin, moesin) proteins: Regulation by cell density and nuclear import. Exp Cell Res 296:208–222.

Baumgartner M et al. (2006) The Nck-interacting kinase phosphorylates ERM proteins for formation of lamellipodium by growth factors. Proc Natl Acad Sci U S A 103:13391–13396.

Belbin TJ, Singh B, Smith RV, Socci ND, Wreesmann VB, Sanchez-Carbayo M, Masterson J, Patel S, Cordon-Cardo C, Prystowsky MB, Childs G (2005) Molecular profiling of tumor progression in head and neck cancer. Arch Otolaryngol Head Neck Surg 131:10–18.

Berryman M, Franck Z, Bretscher A (1993) Ezrin is concentrated in the apical microvilli of a wide variety of epithelial cells whereas moesin is found primarily in endothelial cells. J Cell Sci 105 (Pt 4):1025–1043.

Bonilha VL, Finnemann SC, Rodriguez-Boulan E (1999) Ezrin promotes morphogenesis of apical microvilli and basal infoldings in retinal pigment epithelium. J Cell Boil 147:1533–1548.

Brault E, Gautreau A, Lamarine M, Callebaut I, Thomas G, Goutebroze L (2001) Normal membrane localization and actin association of the NF2 tumor suppressor protein are dependent on folding of its N-terminal domain. J Cell Sci 114:1901–1912.

Bretscher A (1983) Purification of an 80,000-dalton protein that is a component of the isolated microvillus cytoskeleton, and its localization in nonmuscle cells. J Cell Biol 97:425–432.

Bretscher A (1989) Rapid phosphorylation and reorganization of ezrin and spectrin accompany morphological changes induced in A-431 cells by epidermal growth factor. J Cell Biol 108: 921–930.

Bruce B, Khanna G, Ren L, Landberg G, Jirström K, Powell C, Borczuk A, Keller ET, Wojno KJ, Meltzer P, Baird K, McClatchey A, Bretscher A, Hewitt SM, Khanna C (2007) Expression of the cytoskeleton linker protein ezrin in human cancers. Clin Exp Metastasis 24:69–78.

Cant SH and Pitcher JA (2005) G protein-coupled receptor kinase 2-mediated phosphorylation of ezrin is required for G protein-coupled receptor-dependent reorganization of the actin cytoskeleton. Mol Biol Cell 16:3088–3099.

Castelo L, Jay DG (1999) Radixin is involved in lamellipodial stability during nerve growth cone motility. Mol Biol Cell 10:1511–1520.

Cha B, Tse M, Yun C, Kovbasnjuk O, Mohan S, Hubbard A, Arpin M, Donowitz M (2006) The NHE3 juxtamembrane cytoplasmic domain directly binds ezrin: Dual role in NHE3 trafficking and mobility in the brush border. Mol Biol Cell 17:2661–2673.

Chen J and Mandel LJ (1997) Unopposed phosphatase action initiates ezrin dysfunction: A potential mechanism for anoxic injury. Am J Physiol 273:C710–716.

Chen J, Doctor RB, Mandel LJ (1994) Cytoskeletal dissociation of ezrin during renal anoxia: Role in microvillar injury. Am J Physiol 267:C784–795.

Claudio JO, Lutchman M, Rouleau GA (1995) Widespread but cell type-specific expression of the mouse neurofibromatosis type 2 gene. Neuroreport 6:1942–1946.

Crepaldi T, Gautreau A, Comoglio PM, Louvard D, Arpin M (1997) Ezrin is an effector of hepatocyte growth factor-mediated migration and morphogenesis in epithelial cells. J Cell Biol 138:423–434.

Curto M, Cole BK, Lallemand D, Liu CH, McClatchey AI (2007) Contact-dependent inhibition of EGFR signaling by Nf2/Merlin. J Cell Biol 177:893–903.

Das V, Nal B, Roumier A, Meas-Yedid V, Zimmer C, Olivo-Marin JC, Roux P, Ferrier P, Dautry-Varsat A, Alcover A (2002) Membrane–cytoskeleton interactions during the formation of the immunological synapse and subsequent T-cell activation. Immunol Rev 189:123–135.

Delon J, Kaibuchi K, Germain RN (2001) Exclusion of CD43 from the immunological synapse is mediated by phosphorylation-regulated relocation of the cytoskeletal adaptor moesin. Immunity 15:691–701.

DeSimone PA, East R, Powell RD, Jr. (1980) Phagocytic tumor cell activity in oat cell carcinoma of the lung. Hum Pathol 11:535–539.

Doi Y, Itoh M, Yonemura S, Ishihara S, Takano H, Noda T, Tsukita S (1999) Normal development of mice and unimpaired cell adhesion/cell motility/actin-based cytoskeleton without compensatory up-regulation of ezrin or radixin in moesin gene knockout. J Biol Chem 274:2315–2321.

Donowitz M, Cha B, Zachos NC, Brett CL, Sharma A, Tse CM, Li X (2005) NHERF family and NHE3 regulation. J Physiol 567:3–11.

Dransfield DT, Bradford AJ, Smith J, Martin M, Roy C, Mangeat PH, Goldenring JR. (1997) Ezrin is a cyclic AMP-dependent protein kinase anchoring protein. Embo J 16:35–43.

Elliott BE, Qiao H, Louvard D, Arpin M (2004) Co-operative effect of c-Src and ezrin in deregulation of cell–cell contacts and scattering of mammary carcinoma cells. J Cell Biochem 92:16–28.

Fais S (2007) Cannibalism: A way to feed on metastatic tumors. Cancer Lett 258:155–164.

Fazioli F, Wong WT, Ullrich SJ, Sakaguchi K, Appella E, Di Fiore PP (1993) The ezrin-like family of tyrosine kinase substrates: Receptor-specific pattern of tyrosine phosphorylation and relationship to malignant transformation. Oncogene 8:1335–1345.

Fievet BT, Gautreau A, Roy C, Del Maestro L, Mangeat P, Louvard D, Arpin M (2004) Phosphoinositide binding and phosphorylation act sequentially in the activation mechanism of ezrin. J Cell Biol 164:653–659.

Fievet B, Louvard D, Arpin M (2007) ERM proteins in epithelial cell organization and functions. Biochim Biophys Acta 1773:653–660.

Fukata Y, Kimura K, Oshiro N, Saya H, Matsuura Y, Kaibuchi K (1998) Association of the myosin-binding subunit of myosin phosphatase and moesin: Dual regulation of moesin phosphorylation by Rho-associated kinase and myosin phosphatase. J Cell Biol 141:409–418.

Funayama N, Nagafuchi A, Sato N, Tsukita S (1991) Radixin is a novel member of the band 4.1 family. J Cell Biol 115:1039–1048.

Gautreau A, Poullet P, Louvard D, Arpin M (1999) Ezrin, a plasma membrane–microfilament linker, signals cell survival through the phosphatidylinositol 3-kinase/Akt pathway. Proc Natl Acad Sci U S A 96:7300–7305.

Gautreau A, Louvard D, Arpin M (2002) ERM proteins and NF2 tumor suppressor: The Yin and Yang of cortical actin organization and cell growth signaling. Curr Opin Cell Biol 14: 104–109.

Gonzalez-Agosti C, Wiederhold T, Herndon ME, Gusella J, Ramesh V (1999) Interdomain interaction of merlin isoforms and its influence on intermolecular binding to NHE-RF. J Biol Chem 274:34438–34442.

Gould KL, Cooper JA, Bretscher A, Hunter T (1986) The protein-tyrosine kinase substrate, p81, is homologous to a chicken microvillar core protein. J Cell Biol 102:660–669.

Gronholm M, Sainio M, Zhao F, Heiska L, Vaheri A, Carpen O (1999) Homotypic and heterotypic interaction of the neurofibromatosis 2 tumor suppressor protein merlin and the ERM protein ezrin. J Cell Sci 112 (Pt 6):895–904.

Gronholm M, Vossebein L, Carlson CR, Kuja-Panula J, Teesalu T, Alfthan K, Vaheri A, Rauvala H, Herberg FW, Taskén K, Carpén O (2003) Merlin links to the cAMP neuronal signaling pathway by anchoring the RIbeta subunit of protein kinase A. J Biol Chem 278:41167–41172.

Haase VH, Trofatter JA, MacCollin M, Tarttelin E, Gusella JF, Ramesh V (1994) The murine NF2 homologue encodes a highly conserved merlin protein with alternative forms. Hum Mol Genet 3:407–411.

Hamada K, Shimizu T, Matsui T, Tsukita S, Hakoshima T (2000) Structural basis of the membrane-targeting and unmasking mechanisms of the radixin FERM domain. Embo J 19:4449–4462.

Heiska L, Alfthan K, Gronholm M, Vilja P, Vaheri A, Carpen O (1998) Association of ezrin with intercellular adhesion molecule-1 and -2 (ICAM-1 and ICAM-2). Regulation by phosphatidylinositol 4, 5-bisphosphate. J Biol Chem 273:21893–21900.

Hipfner DR, Keller N, Cohen SM (2004) Slik Sterile-20 kinase regulates Moesin activity to promote epithelial integrity during tissue growth. Genes Dev 18:2243–2248.

Huynh DP, Tran TM, Nechiporuk T, Pulst SM (1996) Expression of neurofibromatosis 2 transcript and gene product during mouse fetal development. Cell Growth Differ 7:1551–1561.

Ilani T, Khanna C, Zhou M, Veenstra TD, Bretscher A (2007) Immune synapse formation requires ZAP-70 recruitment by ezrin and CD43 removal by moesin. J Cell Biol 179:733–746.

Ilmonen S, Vaheri A, Asko-Seljavaara S, Carpen O (2005) Ezrin in primary cutaneous melanoma. Mod Pathol 18:503–510.

James MF, Manchanda N, Gonzalez-Agosti C, Hartwig JH, Ramesh V (2001) The neurofibromatosis 2 protein product merlin selectively binds F-actin but not G-actin, and stabilizes the filaments through a lateral association. Biochem J 356:377–386.

Jankovics F, Sinka R, Lukacsovich T, Erdelyi M (2002) MOESIN crosslinks actin and cell membrane in Drosophila oocytes and is required for OSKAR anchoring. Curr Biol 12: 2060–2065.

Jensen PV and Larsson LI (2004) Actin microdomains on endothelial cells: Association with CD44, ERM proteins, and signaling molecules during quiescence and wound healing. Histochem Cell Biol 121:361–369.

Jin H, Sperka T, Herrlich P, Morrison H (2006) Tumorigenic transformation by CPI-17 through inhibition of a merlin phosphatase. Nature 442:576–579.

Khanna C, Khan J, Nguyen P, Prehn J, Caylor J, Yeung C, Trepel J, Meltzer P, Helman L (2001) Metastasis-associated differences in gene expression in a murine model of osteosarcoma. Cancer Res 61:3750–3759.

Khanna C, Wan X, Bose S, Cassaday R, Olomu O, Mendoza A, Yeung C, Gorlick R, Hewitt SM, Helman LJ (2004) The membrane–cytoskeleton linker ezrin is necessary for osteosarcoma metastasis. Nat Med 10:182–186.

Kikuchi S, Hata M, Fukumoto K, Yamane Y, Matsui T, Tamura A, Yonemura S, Yamagishi H, Keppler D, Tsukita S, Tsukita S (2002) Radixin deficiency causes conjugated hyperbilirubine-mia with loss of Mrp2 from bile canalicular membranes. Nat Genet 31:320–325.

Kishore R, Qin G, Luedemann C, Bord E, Hanley A, Silver M, Gavin M, Yoon YS, Goukassian D, Losordo DW (2005) The cytoskeletal protein ezrin regulates EC proliferation and angiogenesis via TNF-alpha-induced transcriptional repression of cyclin A. J Clin Invest 115(7):1785–1796.

Kissil JL, Johnson KC, Eckman MS, Jacks T (2002) Merlin phosphorylation by p21-activated kinase 2 and effects of phosphorylation on merlin localization. J Biol Chem 277: 10394–10399.

Kitajiri S, Fukumoto K, Hata M, Sasaki H, Katsuno T, Nakagawa T, Ito J, Tsukita S, Tsukita S (2004) Radixin deficiency causes deafness associated with progressive degeneration of cochlear stereocilia. J Cell Biol 166:559–570.

Kondo T, Takeuchi K, Doi Y, Yonemura S, Nagata S, Tsukita S (1997) ERM (ezrin/radixin/moesin)-based molecular mechanism of microvillar breakdown at an early stage of apoptosis. J Cell Biol 139:749–758.

Kotani H, Takaishi K, Sasaki T, Takai Y (1997) Rho regulates association of both the ERM family and vinculin with the plasma membrane in MDCK cells. Oncogene 14:1705–1713.

Kressel M and Schmucker B (2002) Nucleocytoplasmic transfer of the NF2 tumor suppressor protein merlin is regulated by exon 2 and a CRM1-dependent nuclear export signal in exon 15. Hum Mol Genet 11:2269–2278.

Krieg J and Hunter T (1992) Identification of the two major epidermal growth factor-induced tyrosine phosphorylation sites in the microvillar core protein ezrin. J Biol Chem 267: 19258–19265.

Krishnan K, Bruce B, Hewitt S, Thomas D, Khanna C, Helman LJ (2006) Ezrin mediates growth and survival in Ewing's sarcoma through the AKT/mTOR, but not the MAPK, signaling pathway. Clin Exp Metastasis 23:227–236.

LaJeunesse DR, McCartney BM, Fehon RG (1998) Structural analysis of Drosophila merlin reveals functional domains important for growth control and subcellular localization. J Cell Biol 141:1589–1599.

Lallemand D, Curto M, Saotome I, Giovannini M, McClatchey AI (2003) NF2 deficiency pro-motes tumorigenesis and metastasis by destabilizing adherens junctions. Genes Dev 17: 1090–1100.

Lamb RF, Roy C, Diefenbach TJ, Vinters HV, Johnson MW, Jay DG, Hall A (2000) The TSC1 tumour suppressor hamartin regulates cell adhesion through ERM proteins and the GTPase Rho. Nat Cell Biol 2:281–287.

Lamprecht G, Weinman EJ, Yun CH (1998) The role of NHERF and E3KARP in the cAMP-mediated inhibition of NHE3. J Biol Chem 273:29972–29978.

Legg JW and Isacke CM (1998) Identification and functional analysis of the ezrin-binding site in the hyaluronan receptor, CD44. Curr Biol 8:705–708.

Legg JW, Lewis CA, Parsons M, Ng T, Isacke CM (2002) A novel PKC-regulated mechanism controls CD44 ezrin association and directional cell motility. Nat Cell Biol 4:399–407.

Li Q, Wu M, Wang H, Xu G, Zhu T, Zhang Y, Liu P, Song A, Gang C, Han Z, Zhou J, Meng L, Lu Y, Wang S, Ma D (2008) Ezrin silencing by small hairpin RNA reverses metastatic behaviors of human breast cancer cells. Cancer Lett 261:55–63.

Liu D, Ge L, Wang F, Takahashi H, Wang D, Guo Z, Yoshimura SH, Ward T, Ding X, Takeyasu K, Yao X (2007) Single-molecule detection of phosphorylation-induced plasticity changes during erzin activation. FEBS Lett 581:3563–3571.

Lozupone F, Lugini L, Matarrese P, Luciani F, Federici C, Iessi E, Margutti P, Stassi G, Malorni W, Fais S (2004) Identification and relevance of the CD95-binding domain in the N-terminal region of ezrin. J Biol Chem 279:9199–9207.

Lugini L, Lozupone F, Matarrese P, Funaro C, Luciani F, Malorni W, Rivoltini L, Castelli C, Tinari A, Piris A, Parmiani G, Fais S (2003) Potent phagocytic activity discriminates metastatic and primary human malignant melanomas: A key role of ezrin. Lab Invest 83:1555–1567.

Madan R, Brandwein-Gensler M, Schlecht NF, Elias K, Gorbovitsky E, Belbin TJ, Mahmood R, Breining D, Qian H, Childs G, Locker J, Smith R, Haigentz M Jr, Gunn-Moore F, Prystowsky MB (2006) Differential tissue and subcellular expression of ERM proteins in normal and malignant tissues: Cytoplasmic ezrin expression has prognostic significance for head and neck squamous cell carcinoma. Head Neck 28:1018–1027.

Maitra S, Kulikauskas RM, Gavilan H, Fehon RG (2006) The tumor suppressors Merlin and Expanded function cooperatively to modulate receptor endocytosis and signaling. Curr Biol 16:702–709.

Majander-Nordenswan P et al. (1998) Genomic structure of the human ezrin gene. Hum Genet 103:662–665.

Makitie T, Carpen O, Vaheri A, Kivela T (2001) Ezrin as a prognostic indicator and its relationship to tumor characteristics in uveal malignant melanoma. Invest Ophthalmol Vis Sci 42: 2442–2449.

Marin-Padilla M (1977) Erythrophagocytosis by epithelial cells of a breast carcinoma. Cancer 39:1085–1089.

Matsui T, Maeda M, Doi Y, Yonemura S, Amano M, Kaibuchi K, Tsukita S, Tsukita S (1998) Rho-kinase phosphorylates COOH-terminal threonines of ezrin/radixin/moesin (ERM) proteins and regulates their head-to-tail association. J Cell Biol 140:647–657.

Matsui T, Yonemura S, Tsukita S (1999) Activation of ERM proteins in vivo by Rho involves phosphatidyl-inositol 4-phosphate 5-kinase and not ROCK kinases. Curr Biol 9:1259–1262.

McCartney BM and Fehon RG (1996) Distinct cellular and subcellular patterns of expression imply distinct functions for the Drosophila homologues of moesin and the neurofibromatosis 2 tumor suppressor, merlin. J Cell Biol 133:843–852.

McClatchey AI and Giovannini M (2005) Membrane organization and tumorigenesis–the NF2 tumor suppressor, Merlin. Genes Dev 19:2265–2277.

McClatchey AI, Saotome I, Ramesh V, Gusella JF, Jacks T (1997) The Nf2 tumor suppressor gene product is essential for extraembryonic development immediately prior to gastrulation. Genes Dev 11:1253–1265.

McClatchey AI, Saotome I, Mercer K, Crowley D, Gusella JF, Bronson RT, Jacks T (1998) Mice heterozygous for a mutation at the Nf2 tumor suppressor locus develop a range of highly metastatic tumors. Genes Dev 12:1121–1133.

McLaughlin ME, Kruger GM, Slocum KL, Crowley D, Michaud NA, Huang J, Magendantz M, Jacks T (2007) The Nf2 tumor suppressor regulates cell–cell adhesion during tissue fusion. Proc Natl Acad Sci U S A 104:3261–3266.

Moilanen J, Lassus H, Leminen A, Vaheri A, Butzow R, Carpen O (2003) Ezrin immunoreactivity in relation to survival in serous ovarian carcinoma patients. Gynecol Oncol 90:273–281.

Morrison H, Sherman LS, Legg J, Banine F, Isacke C, Haipek CA, Gutmann DH, Ponta H, Herrlich P (2001) The NF2 tumor suppressor gene product, merlin, mediates contact inhibition of growth through interactions with CD44. Genes Dev 15:968–980.

Morrison H, Sperka T, Manent J, Giovannini M, Ponta H, Herrlich P (2007) Merlin/neurofibromatosis type 2 suppresses growth by inhibiting the activation of Ras and Rac. Cancer Res 67:520–527.

Muranen T, Gronholm M, Renkema GH, Carpen O (2005) Cell cycle-dependent nucleocytoplasmic shuttling of the neurofibromatosis 2 tumour suppressor merlin. Oncogene 24:1150–1158.

Nakamura N, Oshiro N, Fukata Y, Amano M, Fukata M, Kuroda S, Matsuura Y, Leung T, Lim L, Kaibuchi K (2000) Phosphorylation of ERM proteins at filopodia induced by Cdc42. Genes Cells 5:571–581.

Ng T, Parsons M, Hughes WE, Monypenny J, Zicha D, Gautreau A, Arpin M, Gschmeissner S, Verveer PJ, Bastiaens PI, Parker PJ. (2001) Ezrin is a downstream effector of trafficking PKC–integrin complexes involved in the control of cell motility. Embo J 20:2723–2741.

Nguyen R, Reczek D, Bretscher A (2001) Hierarchy of merlin and ezrin N- and C-terminal domain interactions in homo- and heterotypic associations and their relationship to binding of scaffolding proteins EBP50 and E3KARP. J Biol Chem 276:7621–7629.

Nijhara R, van Hennik PB, Gignac ML, Kruhlak MJ, Hordijk PL, Delon J, Shaw S (2004) Rac1 mediates collapse of microvilli on chemokine-activated T lymphocytes. J Immunol 173: 4985–4993.

Okada T, Lopez-Lago M, Giancotti FG (2005) Merlin/NF-2 mediates contact inhibition of growth by suppressing recruitment of Rac to the plasma membrane. J Cell Biol 171:361–371.

Pakkanen R, Hedman K, Turunen O, Wahlstrom T, Vaheri A (1987) Microvillus-specific Mr 75,000 plasma membrane protein of human choriocarcinoma cells. J Histochem Cytochem 35: 809–816.

Parlato S, Giammarioli AM, Logozzi M, Lozupone F, Matarrese P, Luciani F, Falchi M, Malorni W, Fais S (2000) CD95 (APO-1/Fas) linkage to the actin cytoskeleton through ezrin in human T lymphocytes: A novel regulatory mechanism of the CD95 apoptotic pathway. Embo J 19: 5123–5134.

Pietromonaco SF, Simons PC, Altman A, Elias L (1998) Protein kinase C-theta phosphorylation of moesin in the actin-binding sequence. J Biol Chem 273:7594–7603.

Pilot F, Philippe JM, Lemmers C, Lecuit T (2006) Spatial control of actin organization at adherens junctions by a synaptotagmin-like protein Btsz. Nature 442:580–584.

Polesello C and Payre F (2004) Small is beautiful: What flies tell us about ERM protein function in development. Trends Cell Biol 14:294–302.

Polesello C, Delon I, Valenti P, Ferrer P, Payre F (2002) Dmoesin controls actin-based cell shape and polarity during Drosophila melanogaster oogenesis. Nat Cell Biol 4:782–789.

Pykett MJ, Murphy M, Harnish PR, George DL (1994) The neurofibromatosis 2 (NF2) tumor suppressor gene encodes multiple alternatively spliced transcripts. Hum Mol Genet 3: 559–564.

Reczek D and Bretscher A (1998) The carboxyl-terminal region of EBP50 binds to a site in the amino-terminal domain of ezrin that is masked in the dormant molecule. J Biol Chem 273:18452–18458.

Ren L, Hong SH, Cassavaugh J, Osborne T, Chou A, Kim SY, Gorlick R, Hewitt SM, Khanna C (2009) The actin-cytoskeleton linker protein ezrin is regulated during osteosarcoma metastasis by PKC. Oncogene 28:792–802.

Rouleau GA, Merel P, Lutchman M, Sanson M, Zucman J, Marineau C, Hoang-Xuan K, Demczuk S, Desmaze C, Plougastel B, Kinzler KW, Vogelstein B (1993) Alteration in a new gene encoding a putative membrane-organizing protein causes neuro-fibromatosis type 2. Nature 363:515–521.

Roumier A, Olivo-Marin JC, Arpin M, Michel F, Martin M, Mangeat P, Acuto O, Dautry-Varsat A, Alcover A (2001) The membrane–microfilament linker ezrin is involved in the formation of the immunological synapse and in T cell activation. Immunity 15:715–728.

Saotome I, Curto M, McClatchey AI (2004) Ezrin is essential for epithelial organization and villus morphogenesis in the developing intestine. Dev Cell 6:855–864.

Sato N, Yonemura S, Obinata T, Tsukita S, Tsukita S (1991) Radixin, a barbed end-capping actin-modulating protein, is concentrated at the cleavage furrow during cytokinesis. J Cell Biol 113:321–330.

Sato N, Funayama N, Nagafuchi A, Yonemura S, Tsukita S, Tsukita S (1992) A gene family consisting of ezrin, radixin and moesin. Its specific localization at actin filament/plasma membrane association sites. J Cell Sci 103 (Pt 1):131–143.

Scoles DR, Huynh DP, Morcos PA, Coulsell ER, Robinson NG, Tamanoi F, Pulst SM (1998) Neurofibromatosis 2 tumour suppressor schwannomin interacts with betaII-spectrin. Nat Genet 18:354–359.

Serrador JM, Nieto M, Sanchez-Madrid F (1999) Cytoskeletal rearrangement during migration and activation of T lymphocytes. Trends Cell Biol 9:228–233.

Serrador JM, Nieto M, Alonso-Lebrero JL, del Pozo MA, Calvo J, Furthmayr H, Schwartz-Albiez R, Lozano F, González-Amaro R, Sánchez-Mateos P, Sánchez-Madrid F (1998) CD43 interacts with moesin and ezrin and regulates its redistribution to the uropods of T lymphocytes at the cell–cell contacts. Blood 91:4632–4644.

Serrador JM, Vicente-Manzanares M, Calvo J, Barreiro O, Montoya MC, Schwartz-Albiez R, Furthmayr H, Lozano F, Sánchez-Madrid F (2002) A novel serine-rich motif in the intercellular adhesion molecule 3 is critical for its ezrin/radixin/moesin-directed subcellular targeting. J Biol Chem 277:10400–10409.

Shaw RJ, Henry M, Solomon F, Jacks T (1998a) RhoA-dependent phosphorylation and relocalization of ERM proteins into apical membrane/actin protrusions in fibroblasts. Mol Biol Cell 9:403–419.

Shaw RJ, McClatchey AI, Jacks T (1998b) Regulation of the neurofibromatosis type 2 tumor suppressor protein, merlin, by adhesion and growth arrest stimuli. J Biol Chem 273:7757–7764.

Shaw RJ, Paez JG, Curto M, Yaktine A, Pruitt WM, Saotome I, O'Bryan JP, Gupta V, Ratner N, Der CJ, Jacks T, McClatchey AI (2001) The Nf2 tumor suppressor, merlin, functions in Rac-dependent signaling. Dev Cell 1:63–72.

Sherman L, Xu HM, Geist RT, Saporito-Irwin S, Howells N, Ponta H, Herrlich P, Gutmann DH (1997) Interdomain binding mediates tumor growth suppression by the NF2 gene product. Oncogene 15:2505–2509.

Stanasila L, Abuin L, Diviani D, Cotecchia S (2006) Ezrin directly interacts with the alpha1b-adrenergic receptor and plays a role in receptor recycling. J Biol Chem 281:4354–4363.

Stickney JT, Bacon WC, Rojas M, Ratner N, Ip W (2004) Activation of the tumor suppressor merlin modulates its interaction with lipid rafts. Cancer Res 64:2717–2724.

Sun F, Hug MJ, Lewarchik CM, Yun CH, Bradbury NA, Frizzell RA (2000) E3KARP mediates the association of ezrin and protein kinase A with the cystic fibrosis transmembrane conductance regulator in airway cells. J Biol Chem 275:29539–29546.

Surace EI, Haipek CA, Gutmann DH (2004) Effect of merlin phosphorylation on neurofibromatosis 2 (NF2) gene function. Oncogene 23:580–587.

Takahashi K et al. (1997) Direct interaction of the Rho GDP dissociation inhibitor with ezrin/radixin/moesin initiates the activation of the Rho small G protein. J Biol Chem 272:23371–23375.

Tang X, Jang SW, Wang X, Liu Z, Bahr SM, Sun SY, Brat D, Gutmann DH, Ye K (2007) Akt phosphorylation regulates the tumour-suppressor merlin through ubiquitination and degradation. Nat Cell Biol 9:1199–1207.

Tokunou M, Niki T, Saitoh Y, Imamura H, Sakamoto M, Hirohashi S (2000) Altered expression of the ERM proteins in lung adenocarcinoma. Lab Invest 80:1643–1650.

Tomas EM, Chau TA, Madrenas J (2002) Clustering of a lipid-raft associated pool of ERM proteins at the immunological synapse upon T cell receptor or CD28 ligation. Immunol Lett 83: 143–147.

Tort F, Pinyol M, Pulford K, Roncador G, Hernandez L, Nayach I, Kluin-Nelemans HC, Kluin P, Touriol C, Delsol G, Mason D, Campo E (2001) Molecular characterization of a new ALK translocation involving moesin (MSN-ALK) in anaplastic large cell lymphoma. Lab Invest 81:419–426.

Trofatter JA, MacCollin MM, Rutter JL, Murrell JR, Duyao MP, Parry DM, Eldridge R, Kley N, Menon AG, Pulaski K, Haase VH, Ambrose CM, Munroe D, Bove C, Haines JL, Martuza RL, MacDonald ME, Seizinger BR, Short MP, Buckler AJ, Gusella JF (1993) A novel moesin-, erzin-, radixin-like gene is a candidate for the neurofibromatosis 2 tumor suppressor. Cell 75:826.

Tsukita S, Hieda Y, Tsukita S (1989) A new 82-kD barbed end-capping protein (radixin) local-
    ized in the cell-to-cell adherens junction: Purification and characterization. J Cell Biol 108:
    2369–2382.
Tsukita S, Oishi K, Sato N, Sagara J, Kawai A (1994) ERM family members as molecular link-
    ers between the cell surface glycoprotein CD44 and actin-based cytoskeletons. J Cell Biol
    126:391–401.
Turunen O, Winqvist R, Pakkanen R, Grzeschik KH, Wahlstrom T, Vaheri A (1989) Cytovillin,
    a microvillar Mr 75,000 protein. cDNA sequence, prokaryotic expression, and chromosomal
    localization. J Biol Chem 264:16727–16732.
Wald FA, Oriolo AS, Mashukova A, Fregien NL, Langshaw AH, Salas PJ (2008) Atypical protein
    kinase C (iota) activates ezrin in the apical domain of intestinal epithelial cells. J Cell Sci
    121:644–654.
Weinman EJ, Steplock D, Donowitz M, Shenolikar S (2000) NHERF associations with sodium-
    hydrogen exchanger isoform 3 (NHE3) and ezrin are essential for cAMP-mediated phosphory-
    lation and inhibition of NHE3. Biochemistry 39:6123–6129.
Weng WH, Ahlen J, Astrom K, Lui WO, Larsson C (2005) Prognostic impact of immunohis-
    tochemical expression of ezrin in highly malignant soft tissue sarcomas. Clin Cancer Res
    11:6198–6204.
Wilgenbus KK, Milatovich A, Francke U, Furthmayr H (1993) Molecular cloning, cDNA
    sequence, and chromosomal assignment of the human radixin gene and two dispersed
    pseudogenes. Genomics 16:199–206.
Wu YX, Uezato T, Fujita M (2000) Tyrosine phosphorylation and cellular redistribution of ezrin
    in MDCK cells treated with pervanadate. J Cell Biochem 79:311–321.
Xiao GH, Beeser A, Chernoff J, Testa JR (2002) p21-activated kinase links Rac/Cdc42 signaling
    to merlin. J Biol Chem 277:883–886.
Xu HM and Gutmann DH (1998) Merlin differentially associates with the microtubule and actin
    cytoskeleton. J Neurosci Res 51:403–415.
Yonemura S, Hirao M, Doi Y, Takahashi N, Kondo T, Tsukita S, Tsukita S (1998)
    Ezrin/radixin/moesin (ERM) proteins bind to a positively charged amino acid cluster in the
    juxta-membrane cytoplasmic domain of CD44, CD43, and ICAM-2. J Cell Biol 140:885–895.
Yonemura S, Tsukita S (1999) Direct involvement of erzin/radixin/moesin (ERM)-binding mem-
    brane proteins in the organization of microvilli in collaboration with activated ERM proteins.
    J Cell Biol 145:1497–1509.
Yu Y, Khan J, Khanna C, Helman L, Meltzer PS, Merlino G (2004) Expression profiling identifies
    the cytoskeletal organizer ezrin and the developmental homeoprotein Six-1 as key metastatic
    regulators. Nat Med 10:175–181.
Yu Y, Davicioni E, Triche TJ, Merlino G (2006) The homeoprotein six1 transcriptionally acti-
    vates multiple protumorigenic genes but requires ezrin to promote metastasis. Cancer Res 66:
    1982–1989.
Zhou R, Cao X, Watson C, Miao Y, Guo Z, Forte JG, Yao X (2003) Characterization of protein
    kinase A-mediated phosphorylation of ezrin in gastric parietal cell activation. J Biol Chem
    278:35651–35659.

Part III
Coming Up for Air:
Hypoxia and Angiogenesis

Chapter 6
von Hippel–Lindau Tumor Suppressor, Hypoxia-Inducible Factor-1, and Tumor Vascularization

Huafeng Zhang and Gregg L. Semenza

Cast of Characters

von Hippel–Lindau (VHL) disease is an autosomal dominant, familial cancer syndrome that is characterized by the development of various benign and malignant tumors. The most frequent tumors are hemangioblastoma (HB) in the central nervous system (CNS), pheochromocytoma (Pheo), and renal-cell carcinoma of the clear-cell type (RCC). VHL families have been subdivided into those with a low risk of pheochromocytoma (type 1 VHL disease) and those with a high risk of pheochromocytoma (type 2 VHL disease). VHL type 2 disease is further classified into three categories: type 2A, type 2B, and type 2C. Type 2A VHL disease has pheochromocytoma and hemangioblastoma in the CNS, but not RCC. Type 2B exhibits pheochromocytoma, RCC, and hemangioblastoma. Type 2C disease has only pheochromocytoma, without hemangioblastoma or RCC.

Individuals with VHL disease harbor a germline mutation in one allele of the *VHL* gene and somatic inactivation or silencing of the remaining wild-type allele results in tumor development (Kim and Kaelin 2004). Type 2 families almost invariably have missense *VHL* mutations, while type 1 VHL disease is linked to many different types of mutations, including nonsense mutations and deletions. In type 1, type 2A, and type 2B VHL diseases, *VHL* alleles encode proteins that are at least partially defective with respect to the regulation of hypoxia-inducible factor (HIF) 1α and 2α, whereas the products of type 2C *VHL* alleles are not defective in this regard (Clifford et al. 2001; Hoffman et al. 2001). However, the products of type 2C *VHL* alleles are defective with respect to another VHL function, i.e., down-regulation of atypical protein kinase C activity (Pal et al. 1997; Okuda et al. 1999, 2001). Increased atypical protein kinase C activity and consequent upregulation of JunB seem to promote the survival of pheochromocytoma cells (Lee et al. 2005).

G.L. Semenza (✉)
Departments of Pediatrics, Medicine, Oncology, and Radiation Oncology, The Johns Hopkins University School of Medicine, Broadway Research Building, Suite 671, Baltimore, MD, USA
e-mail: gsemenza@jhmi.edu

A. Thomas-Tikhonenko (ed.), *Cancer Genome and Tumor Microenvironment*, DOI 10.1007/978-1-4419-0711-0_6, © Springer Science+Business Media, LLC 2010

The most common sites for hemangioblastoma (HB) development are the cerebellum and spinal cord. The symptoms of this disease are largely characterized by the expansion of the tumor in the cranial space or the spinal cord. Pheochromocytoma develops in the adrenal gland or paraganglia. RCC develops in the kidney and is the tumor that most commonly metastasizes to other organs in VHL disease.

Introduction

In adult life, little angiogenesis occurs in the absence of disease (Hanahan and Folkman 1996). However, the growth of cancers is dependent on angiogenesis (Folkman 1995; Carmeliet and Jain 2000). During the earliest stages of tumor growth, tumors do not demonstrate significant angiogenesis. At sizes up to approximately 1–2 mm tumors can obtain oxygenation via passive diffusion. When tumors grow beyond a volume of several cubic millimeters, passive diffusion cannot provide enough oxygen, and the availability of O_2 and nutrients is limited by competition among actively proliferating cells, and diffusion of metabolites is also inhibited by high interstitial pressure (Stohrer et al. 2000). Thus, tumors are required to establish their own vascular supply, which is also referred as tumor neovascularization. New vessels are required not only to provide oxygen, but also to provide nutrients and dispose of cellular metabolic waste. Thus, a major event in tumor development is the angiogenic switch, an alteration in the balance between pro- and anti-angiogenic factors that leads to tumor vascularization, following which the tumor assumes a more aggressive form characterized by rapid growth (Hanahan and Folkman 1996).

Angiogenesis, which refers to the budding of new capillary branches from preexisting capillaries, may be stimulated by changes within the endothelial cell microenvironment including genetic change, trauma, hypoxia, oxidative stress, and mechanical strain. Hypoxia is perhaps the best-characterized initiator of angiogenesis, and HIF-1-regulated factors are involved in different steps in angiogenesis (Semenza 2000). The rapid growth of solid tumors creates an hypoxic microenvironment. Hypoxia-induced and HIF-1-mediated angiogenic growth factor production plays a major role in tumor vascularization. HIF-1 gain-of-function in human cancer cells resulted in increased vascularization of tumor xenografts (Ravi et al. 2000). The following chapter will describe molecular events underlying hypoxic responses and angiogenesis in RCC.

Renal-Cell Carcinoma

RCC is a highly vascular tumor which originates from the proximal tubule cells of nephrons, accounts for approximately 2.6% of all cancers in the United States, and is the sixth leading cause of cancer deaths in developed nations. A quarter of the patients present with advanced disease, including locally invasive or metastatic

RCC. A third of the patients who undergo resection of localized disease will have a recurrence. Although with the emergence of nephron-sparing surgery and other non-surgical techniques, such as radiofrequency ablation, early stage RCC is becoming a curable condition, the median survival for patients with metastatic disease is only 13 months. Each year in the United States, there are approximately 36,000 new cases of RCC and 13,000 related deaths (Cohen and McGovern 2005). Though there are different pathologic subtypes, the majority (~75%) of RCC cases are referred to as "conventional" or "clear-cell" type (ccRCC) (Cohen and McGovern 2005). More than 95% of clear-cell kidney cancers occur sporadically within the population, while the remainder occur as part of relatively rare, inherited genetic syndromes (Choyke et al. 2003; Cohen and McGovern 2005), which arise from one inherited mutated *VHL* allele and the inactivation or silencing of the remaining normal (wild-type) *VHL* allele. Thus, the primary genetic defect of clear-cell kidney cancer (in both sporadic and hereditary forms) involves inactivation of the *VHL* gene pathway. Remarkably, in sporadic clear-cell renal carcinomas, somatic *VHL* gene defects are detected in 60–90% of patients with this cancer and up to 20% exhibit decreased VHL expression due to hypermethylation (Gallou et al. 1999; Brauch et al. 2000; Ma et al. 2001; Kondo et al. 2002). However, *VHL* mutations are not observed in non-clear-cell (papillary or chromophobe) histologies. In this chapter, the term RCC will be used to refer to the clear-cell type renal-cell carcinoma.

The defining feature of RCC is the histologic appearance of large cells with abundant cytoplasm packed with glycogen and neutral lipids that do not stain with hematoxylin/eosin. The accumulation of immense quantities of glycogen probably results from the high level of glucose metabolism observed in RCC; moreover, the neutral lipid may be contributed by the expression of adipose differentiation-related peptide (ADRP). ADRP is a HIF-1 target gene that encodes a cell surface lipid transport molecule, which may promote the cytoplasmic neutral lipid accumulation (Yao et al. 2005). Additional tumor-specific metabolic characteristics, such as the elevated lactate levels within RCC, may relate to the high rates of glucose metabolism and the impaired oxidative phosphorylation process for generating ATP.

VHL Gene

The *VHL* tumor-suppressor gene, which is located on chromosome 3p25–26, was identified in 1993 (Latif et al. 1993). The gene consists of 3 exons and encodes a short protein (pVHL) with 213 amino acids. pVHL is a potent tumor suppressor, as demonstrated by the introduction of a wild-type *VHL* cDNA into VHL-null RCC cells, which represses the growth of tumor xenografts in immunocompromised mice (Iliopoulos et al. 1995). There are two start codons in the first exon of the *VHL* gene. Thus, an alternate N-terminal truncated version is produced by utilization of an in-frame internal ATG translation start site located 54 codons downstream of the 5′-most ATG, producing a 19-kDa product in addition to the 30-kDa 213-amino acid pVHL product (Blankenship et al. 1999). This second gene product retains the tumor-suppressor function of the full-length protein, but its specific role is not clear. The relative levels of the two pVHL proteins appears to be of little consequence with respect to the promotion of cancer, as few disease-causing mutations have been localized in this N-terminal 54-amino acid region. Instead, the tumor-suppressor activity of pVHL is relegated to the central and C-terminal portions of the protein (Gao et al. 1995). This gene is evolutionarily conserved in organisms ranging from *Caenorhabditis elegans* to humans. $Vhl^{-/-}$ mouse embryos are not viable due to defective placental vasculogenesis, and conditional, systemic inactivation of *Vhl* in adult mice is also lethal (Gnarra et al. 1997; Ma et al. 2003).

In 1971, Knudson hypothesized that germ line inactivation of one tumor-suppressor allele in a hereditary cancer syndrome, followed by somatic inactivation in the remaining allele, led to cancer, whereas somatic inactivation of both tumor-suppressor alleles led to the sporadic cases (Knudson 1971). Individuals carrying one wild-type *VHL* allele and one mutated *VHL* allele in their germ line develop VHL syndrome, which is associated with an increased risk of a variety of tumors, including central nervous system (especially cerebellum and spinal cord) hemangioblastomas, pheochromocytomas, as well as RCC. Whereas individuals with sporadic RCC usually have unilateral kidney involvement, patients with VHL syndrome often have bilateral multifocal disease of early onset.

VHL Protein

pVHL functions in the proteolysis of HIF-1α and HIF-2α by the ubiquitin proteasome system (Fig. 6.1). The ubiquitin proteasome system is highly regulated and involves several steps: initiation by a ubiquitin-activating enzyme (E1), transfer of activated ubiquitin to a ubiquitin-conjugating enzyme (E2), and conjugation of ubiquitin to target proteins by an E3 ubiquitin–ligase complex. The E3 ligase complex contains an adaptor molecule, such as pVHL, that determines the substrate specificity. Successive transfers of activated ubiquitin to lysine-48 of the previously conjugated ubiquitin molecule lead to the formation of polyubiquitin chains, which serve as recognition markers for degradation by the 26S proteasome. pVHL functions as the substrate recognition component of an E3 ubiquitin–ligase complex that contains elongin B, elongin C, Ring box protein 1 (Rbx1), and Cul2 (Pause et al. 1997). X-ray crystallographic analysis of pVHL has revealed two major protein domains: an α domain and a β domain. The surface of the α domain (residues 155–192) is primarily responsible for the interaction between pVHL and Elongin C. The surface of the β domain consists of a seven-stranded β sandwich (residues 63–154) and α helix (residues 193–204) and is primarily responsible for binding target proteins for ubiquitination (Stebbins, Kaelin and Pavletich 1999).

Known and putative substrates of the pVHL E3 ubiquitin–ligase complex include atypical protein kinase C; hyperphosphorylated large subunit of RNA polymerase II; VHL deubiquitinating enzymes (VDU)-1 and -2; and HIF-1α and HIF-2α. The substrates that have been most extensively studied are HIF-1α and HIF-2α, both

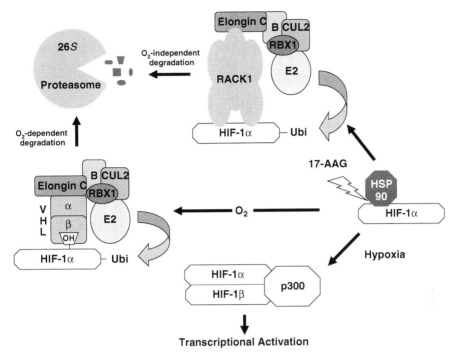

Fig. 6.1 HIF-1α protein degradation pathways. Two pathways regulate HIF-1α protein stability. Under normoxic condition, HIF-1α is hydroxylated at proline residue(s) 402 and/or 564. Hydroxylated HIF-1α is recognized by pVHL, recruited to the E3 ubiquitin–ligase complex containing Elongin C, Elongin B, Cullin 2, and RBX1, polyubiquitinated, and targeted for proteasomal degradation. RACK1 competes with heat shock protein 90 (HSP90) for binding to HIF-1α. RACK1 also binds to Elongin C and thereby (as in the case of pVHL) recruits an ubiquitin–ligase complex. Inhibitors of HSP90, such as 17-AAG, dissociate HSP90 from HIF-1α and thus promote RACK1 binding. Under hypoxic conditions, HIF-α is not hydroxylated, not ubiquitinated, and accumulates at high levels to form transcriptionally active HIF-1, leading to the transcription of downstream target genes

of which are induced in response to hypoxia. In the presence of O_2, one (or both) of two prolyl residues in the HIF-α oxygen degradation domain (Pro-402 and Pro-564 in human HIF-1α) is hydroxylated by members of the EglN family of prolyl hydroxylases. Hydroxylated HIF-α is recognized by pVHL, recruited to the E3 ubiquitin–ligase complex, polyubiquitinated, and targeted for proteasomal degradation (Maxwell et al. 1999; Bruick and McKnight 2001; Ivan et al. 2001; Jaakkola et al. 2001; Yu et al. 2001). Under hypoxic conditions, HIF-α is not hydroxylated, can not bind to pVHL, and accumulates in the cell. When *VHL* is lost or mutated, as in RCC, the pVHL target proteins, HIF-1α and HIF-2α are not degraded and accumulate at high levels to form transcriptionally active HIF-1, leading to the transcription of downstream target genes (Iliopoulos et al. 1996; Kaelin 2004).

Hypoxia-inducible genes regulated by HIF-1 encode proteins involved in angiogenesis (e.g., vascular endothelial growth factor, VEGF), cell proliferation (e.g., transforming growth factor α, TGF-α) and migration (e.g., C-MET), glucose uptake (e.g., the GLUT1 glucose transporter), and acid–base balance (e.g., carbonic anhydrase IX, CA9). Overproduction of such hypoxia-inducible mRNAs is a hallmark of pVHL-defective tumors. When VHL protein is lost, these proteins are overexpressed, creating a microenvironment favorable for cell proliferation, migration, and invasion. Thus, cells deficient in *VHL* behave as if they are hypoxic, even in conditions of normoxia. The hypervascularity of these tumors can be explained by a pVHL-dependent defect in ubiquitin-mediated degradation of HIF-α proteins, leading to increased HIF-1 transcriptional activity with consequent upregulation of VEGF and other angiogenic growth factors that promote tumor progression (Semenza 2003).

HIF-1

HIF-1, which functions as a global regulator of oxygen homeostasis in all metazoan species, is a heterodimeric transcription factor that consists of an oxygen-regulated subunit, which is designated HIF-1α, and a constitutively expressed subunit, which is designated as HIF-1β (Semenza and Wang 1992; Wang et al. 1995). Both HIF-1 subunits are members of the basic helix-loop-helix (bHLH) PER-ARNT-SIM (PAS)-domain family of transcription factors (Wang et al. 1995). The HLH and PAS domains mediate heterodimer formation between the HIF-1α and HIF-1β subunits, which is necessary for DNA binding by the basic domains (Jiang et al. 1996). Exposure of cells to graded hypoxia revealed that HIF-1α protein expression induced by hypoxia was half-maximal at $1.5 - 2\%$ O_2 and maximal at 0.5% O_2. A second oxygen-regulated protein, which is designated HIF-2α (also known as endothelial PAS domain protein 1, EPAS1) can also dimerize with HIF-1β. The specific cellular biological processes or tissue-specific contexts that dictate the utilization of HIF-1α vs HIF-2α remain incompletely understood. HIF-1α and HIF-2α regulate distinct, but overlapping, batteries of target genes (Tian et al.1997; Elvidge et al. 2006). Another related protein, HIF-3α (also known as inhibitory PAS domain protein, IPAS), is expressed in certain cell types in the eye and brain and functions as an inhibitor that is involved in the negative regulation of transcriptional responses to hypoxia (Makino et al. 2001), but its role in cancer pathophysiology has not been established.

VHL protein binds the transcriptional factors HIF-1α and HIF-2α directly and destabilizes them (Maxwell et al. 1999). Under normoxic conditions, HIF-1α (as well as HIF-2α and HIF-3α) is subjected to O_2-dependent ubiquitination that is initiated by the binding of the pVHL and its recruitment of an E3 ubiquitin–ligase complex that contains Elongin C, Elongin B, Cullin 2, and RBX1 (Pause et al. 1997; Ohh et al. 2000). The binding of pVHL is dependent on the hydroxylation of proline residue(s) 402 and/or 564 of HIF-1α within the so-called oxygen-dependent degradation domain (Bruick and McKnight 2001; Ivan et al. 2001; Jaakkola et al. 2001;

Yu et al. 2001). The HIF-1α prolyl hydroxylases are dioxygenases that utilize O_2 and α-ketoglutarate as substrates. A family of three human HIF-1α prolyl hydroxylases (HPHs), alternatively designated prolyl hydroxylase domain-containing proteins (PHDs), was identified and shown to be encoded by the *EGLN2, EGLN1*, and *EGLN3* genes, respectively (Epstein et al. 2001). Under hypoxic conditions, the hydroxylase activity is inhibited and HIF-1α and HIF-2α accumulate in the cell as a result of decreased hydroxylation, ubiquitination, and degradation. In the absence of VHL, which occurs in the majority of clear-cell type renal-cell carcinoma, HIF-1α and HIF-2α are hydroxylated but pVHL-dependent ubiquitylation does not occur, which thus results in the accumulation of high levels of HIF-1α and HIF-2α protein even under non-hypoxic conditions (Kaelin 2004).

Besides the O_2-dependent degradation of HIF-1α mediated by PHD/VHL/ Elongin-C/B/Cul2 E3 ubiquitin ligase and proteasome, the receptor for activated C kinase 1 (RACK1), which was originally identified as an anchoring protein for activated protein kinase C, promotes the O_2/PHD/VHL independent but proteasome-dependent degradation of HIF-1α (Fig. 6.1). Inhibitors of heat shock protein 90 (HSP90) dissociate HSP90 from HIF-1α and induce O_2/PHD/VHL-independent degradation of HIF-1α. RACK1 competes with HSP90 for binding to the PAS-A domain of HIF-1α. RACK1 also binds to Elongin C via an amino acid sequence with striking similarity to the region of pVHL that interacts with Elongin C. Thus, RACK1 recruits an ubiquitin–ligase complex similar to that which is recruited by pVHL, establishing a parallel but O_2-independent pathway for the proteasomal degradation of HIF-1α (Liu et al. 2007).

In addition to prolyl hydroxylation, HIF-1α is also subjected to O_2-dependent hydroxylation of asparagine residue 803 in the carboxyl-terminal transactivation domain by factor inhibiting HIF-1 (FIH-1), which is another dioxygenase that utilizes O_2 and α-ketoglutarate (also known as 2-oxoglutarate) (Lando et al. 2002). The prolyl and asparaginyl hydroxylation reactions require O_2, Fe (II), and α-ketoglutarate and generate succinate and CO_2 as side-products. Hydroxylation of asparagine-803 prevents the interaction of HIF-1α with the co-activators p300 and CBP. Thus, both the half-life and transcriptional activity of HIF-1α are regulated by O_2-dependent hydroxylation events that provide a direct mechanism by which changes in O_2 concentration can be linked to changes in the gene expression mediated by HIF-1.

In addition to VHL loss of function, many other genetic alterations that inactivate tumor suppressors or activate oncoproteins have been shown to increase HIF-1 activity in cancer cells through a variety of molecular mechanisms (Semenza 2003). Immunohistochemical analysis of human tumor biopsies has revealed overexpression of HIF-1α in the majority of common cancers (Zhong et al. 1999; Talks et al. 2000). High HIF-1α levels in tumors reflect the frequent presence of intratumoral hypoxia and the fact that many common genetic alterations in cancer cells upregulate HIF-1α expression. In general, these changes serve to increase the basal levels of HIF-1α in cancer cells, which serves to amplify the physiological response of cancer cells to hypoxia.

Target Genes Transcriptionally Regulated by HIF-1

A recent study of global gene expression using DNA microarrays indicates that more than 2% of all human genes are directly or indirectly regulated by HIF-1 in arterial endothelial cells (Manalo et al. 2005). HIF-1 binding sites, designated as hypoxia response elements, all contain the core consensus nucleotide sequence 5'-RCGTG-3', and can be located in the 5'-flanking region of the gene, introns, or 3'-flanking region. One major function of HIF-1 is to increase O_2 delivery to cells subjected to reduced O_2 availability (hypoxia). When the entire organism is hypoxic, HIF-1 activates transcription of the gene encoding erythropoietin EPO, the glycoprotein hormone that controls the production of red blood cells and thereby determines blood O_2-carrying capacity. When hypoxia results from inadequate perfusion of a specific tissue (ischemia), vascular endothelial growth factor (VEGF) and other angiogenic cytokines are produced to stimulate new blood vessel formation and/or the remodeling of existing blood vessels to increase blood flow. HIF-1 also promotes cell survival under conditions of O_2 deprivation. HIF-1 activates the transcription of genes encoding glucose transporters and glycolytic enzymes, such as the glucose transporter (GLUT1), enzymes of glucose metabolism, such as hexokinase and lactate dehydrogenase A, and the lactate transporter MCT-4, and thereby increases the capacity for anaerobic ATP synthesis. In addition, HIF-1 controls the expression of survival factors that can block hypoxia-induced apoptosis, including insulin-like growth factor 2 (IGF-2) and adrenomedullin (Semenza 2003).

HIF-1α expression levels are correlated with an increased risk of mortality in several types of carcinoma. The basis for this association is that many genes that are regulated by HIF-1 play critical roles in many key aspects of cancer biology, especially angiogenesis, metabolic reprogramming, invasion/metastasis, and drug resistance (Semenza 2003).

Angiogenesis/Hypoxia

HIF-1α is necessary and sufficient for the hypoxia-induced expression of multiple angiogenic growth factors including angiopoietin 1, angiopoietin 2, placental growth factor, platelet-derived growth factor B, stromal-derived factor 1, and VEGF (Kelly et al. 2003). These factors promote the proliferation, migration, and maturation of endothelial cells and pericytes during angiogenesis, which is necessary to establish and maintain blood supply to the growing tumor mass (Fig. 6.2). Collectively, these results implicate dysregulation of HIF target genes playing a causal role in the pathogenesis of different tumors, especially the VHL-defective RCC.

Consistent with a major role for hypoxia in the overall process, many genes involved in different steps of angiogenesis are independently regulated by hypoxia/HIF-1. Those genes include vascular endothelial growth factor (VEGF), angiopoietin 1 and angiopoietin 2, platelet-derived growth factor B (PDGFB), placental growth factor (PLGF) and stromal-derived factor 1, and genes involved

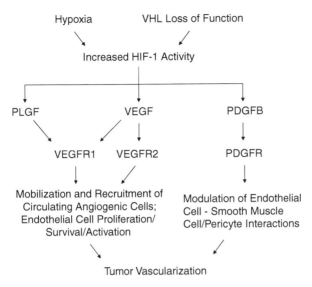

Fig. 6.2 Tumor angiogenesis regulated by VHL and HIF-1. Hypoxia or VHL loss-of-function stabilizes HIF-1α protein, leading to increased HIF-1 transcriptional activity. HIF-1 activates the transcription of genes encoding pro-angiogenic factors including vascular endothelial growth factor (VEGF), placental growth factor (PLGF), platelet-derived growth factor B (PDGFB). PLGF and VEGF bind to the receptor tyrosine kinases, VEGFR1 and/or VEGFR2, which mediate mobilization and recruitment of circulating angiogenic cells as well as endothelial cell proliferation, survival and activation. PDGFB interacts with its receptor PDGFR, modulating the interaction of endothelial cells with smooth muscle cells/pericytes

in matrix metabolism, including matrix metalloproteinases, plasminogen activator receptors and inhibitors, and procollagen prolyl hydroxylases, and lysyl oxidase (Kelly et al. 2003, Semenza 2003; Alvarez et al. 2006).

Under hypoxic conditions HIF-1 activates the transcription of genes encoding pro-angiogenic factors, most notably VEGF (Wang et al. 1995). VEGF is dramatically overexpressed throughout RCC tissue and may be the most important tumor angiogenic factor. VEGF is a pleiotropic growth factor that mediates multiple functions including regulation of vessel permeability, endothelial cell activation, survival, proliferation, invasion and migration. In order to exert biological effects, VEGF binds to the receptor tyrosine kinases, VEGFR1 and VEGFR2, which are expressed on the surface of endothelial cells. VEGFR2 mediates the majority of VEGF downstream angiogenic effects, leading to the most robust upregulation of angiogenesis, while VEGFR1 is critical in developmental angiogenesis. VEGF can also bind to neuropilin 1 and 2, which function as co-receptors to activate endothelial cells and promote angiogenesis.

Another angiogenic factor that is regulated by hypoxia/HIF-1 is PDGF-B (Alvarez et al. 2006). Mature PDGF proteins are the dimers PDGF-AA, PDGF-AB, and PDGF-BB, which interact with two cognate receptors, PDGFRα and PDGFRß, the activation of which is critical for pericyte proliferation and survival (Alvarez et al. 2006). Pericytes are an important supporting cell in blood vessels that maintain endothelial cell viability. Although the cell biology of angiogenesis has been recognized to be far more complicated than originally anticipated, the VEGF and PDGF systems are still thought to occupy a central role in tumor angiogenesis.

Angiopoietins, which are also HIF-1 target genes, appear to modulate angiogenesis in concert with VEGF. Angiopoietin 1 binds to a tyrosine kinase receptor, Tie-2, to promote endothelial cell pericyte interaction. Angiopoietin 2 binds to the same Tie-2 receptor, but blocks endothelial cell interaction with pericytes, which is required for endothelial cell sprouting. Several matrix metalloproteases (MMPs) are also regulated by HIF-1. The best-characterized proteases regulating tumor angiogenesis are MMP-2 and MMP-9, which are encoded by HIF-1 target genes, as is the membrane-type MMP, MT1-MMP.

Anti-angiogenic Therapy

Prior to the development of anti-angiogenic therapy, treatment for renal cancer was limited to the immunotherapeutic agents IFN-α and interleukin-2, which have had only modest success. Given the paucity of angiogenesis in adults, the growing vessels in tumors present a therapeutic target with fewer potential side effects than traditional chemotherapies. Besides, endothelial cells have a stable genome and may not develop drug resistance as rapidly as tumor cells.

Avastin (Bevacizumab), a humanized VEGF-neutralizing antibody, is the first Food and Drug Administration (FDA) approved drug for anti-angiogenic therapy in metastatic RCC (Yang et al. 2003). Other strategies have targeted the VEGFR family. Recently, the FDA approved two new agents for the treatment of advanced kidney cancer, Sutent (Sunitinib) and Nexavar (Sorafenib). Both agents are small molecule tyrosine kinase inhibitors that can selectively inhibit both VEGFRs and PDGFRs (Motzer et al. 2006a,b; Escudier et al. 2007).

As aforementioned, hypoxia/HIF-1 is a potent initiator of tumor angiogenesis, and inhibitors designed specific for HIF-1 may be useful in combination with anti-angiogenic therapy. A large number of novel compounds have been shown to inhibit HIF-1. 2-Methoxyestradiol, which inhibits HIF-1α protein accumulation, is already in clinical trials (Mabjeesh et al. 2003). Other HIF-1 inhibitors, such as PX-478, YC-1, and chetomin, also have shown anti-cancer activity in tumor xenograft models (Kung et al. 2004; Macpherson and Figg 2004; Welsh et al. 2004). Importantly, as mentioned above, small molecule inhibitors of HSP90 promote degradation of HIF-1α proteins (Fig. 6.1) in a pVHL-independent manner (Liu et al. 2007). The HSP90 inhibitors 17-AAG (17-allylamino-17-geldanamycin) and 17-DMAG (17-N-allylamino-17-demethoxygeldanamycin), which inhibit HIF-1 activity, are currently in clinical trials in patients with RCC (Isaacs et al. 2003). Inhibitors of the mTOR (mammalian target of rapamycin) pathway reduce HIF-1α protein levels and thereby inhibit HIF-1 transcriptional activity (Hudson et al. 2002). Clinical trials have shown that the novel mTOR inhibitor CCI779 (temsirolimus, Torisel) has promising activity in patients with advanced RCC (Atkins et al. 2004).

Conclusions

Advanced renal cancers are notoriously resistant to chemotherapy and radiotherapy, and novel therapeutic approaches are desperately needed. Multi-drug regimens that include angiogenesis inhibitors, e.g., targeting of both mTOR and VEGF/PDGF pathways simultaneously, will need to be studied. The identification of drug combinations that are safe and effective remains a major challenge.

References

Alvarez R.H., Kantarjian H.M., Cortes J.E. (2006) Biology of platelet-derived growth factor and its involvement in disease. Mayo Clin Proc 81:1241–1257.

Atkins M.B., Hidalgo M., Stadler W.M., Logan T.F., Dutcher J.P., Hudes G.R., Park Y., Liou S.H., Marshall B., Boni J.P., Dukart G., Sherman M.L. (2004) Randomized phase II study of multiple dose levels of CCI-779, a novel mammalian target of rapamycin kinase inhibitor, in patients with advanced refractory renal cell carcinoma. J Clin Oncol 22:909–918.

Blankenship C., Naglich J.G., Whaley J.M., Seizinger B., Kley N. (1999) Alternate choice of initiation codon produces a biologically active product of the von Hippel Lindau gene with tumor suppressor activity. Oncogene 18:1529–1535.

Brauch H., Weirich G., Brieger J., Glavac D., Rodl H., Eichinger M., Feurer M., Weidt E., Puranakanitstha C., Neuhaus C., Pomer S., Brenner W., Schirmacher P., Storkel S., Rotter M., Masera A., Gugeler N., Decker H.J. (2000) VHL alterations in human clear cell renal cell carcinoma: association with advanced tumor stage and a novel hot spot mutation. Cancer Res 60:1942–1948.

Bruick R.K. and McKnight S.L. (2001) A conserved family of prolyl-4-hydroxylases that modify HIF. Science 294: 1337–1340.

Carmeliet P. and Jain R.K. (2000) Angiogenesis in cancer and other diseases. Nature 407: 249–257.

Choyke P.L, Glenn G.M., Walther M.M., Zbar B., Linehan W.M. (2003) Hereditary renal cancers. Radiology 226:33–46.

Clifford S., Cockman M., Smallwood A.C., Mole D.R., Woodward E.R., Maxwell P.H., Ratcliffe P.J., Maher E.R. (2001) Contrasting effects on HIF-1α regulation by disease-causing pVHL mutations correlate with patterns of tumourigenesis in von Hippel-Lindau disease. Hum Mol Genet 10: 1029–1038.

Cohen H.T. and McGovern F.J. (2005) Renal-cell carcinoma. N Engl J Med 353:2477–2490.

Elvidge G.P., Glenny L., Appelhoff R.J., Ratcliffe P.J., Ragoussis J., Gleadle J.M. (2006) Concordant regulation of gene expression by hypoxia and 2-oxoglutarate-dependent dioxygenase inhibition: the role of HIF-1α, HIF-2α, and other pathways. J Biol Chem 281: 15215–15226.

Epstein A.C., Gleadle J.M., McNeill L.A., Hewitson K.S., O'Rourke J., Mole D.R., Mukherji M., Metzen E., Wilson M.I., Dhanda A., Tian Y.M., Masson N., Hamilton D.L., Jaakkola P., Barstead R., Hodgkin J., Maxwell P.H., Pugh C.W., Schofield C.J., Ratcliffe P.J. (2001) C. elegans EGL-9 and mammalian homologs define a family of dioxygenases that regulate HIF by prolyl hydroxylation. Cell 107:43–54.

Escudier B., Eisen T., Stadler W.M., Szczylik C., Oudard S., Siebels M., Negrier S., Chevreau C., Solska E., Desai A.A., Rolland F., Demkow T., Hutson T.E., Gore M., Freeman S., Schwartz B., Shan M., Simantov R., Bukowski R.M. (2007) TARGET Study Group. Sorafenib in advanced clear-cell renal-cell carcinoma. N Engl J Med 356:125–134.

Folkman J. (1995) Angiogenesis in cancer, vascular, rheumatoid and other disease. Nat Med 1: 27–31.

Gallou C., Joly D., Mejean A., Staroz F., Martin N., Tarlet G., Orfanelli M.T., Bouvier R., Droz D., Chretien Y., Marechal J.M., Richard S., Junien C., Beroud C. (1999) Mutations of the VHL gene in sporadic renal cell carcinoma: definition of a risk factor for VHL patients to develop an RCC. Hum Mutat 13: 464–475.

Gao J., Naglich J.G., Laidlaw J., Whaley J.M., Seizinger B.R., Kley N. (1995) Cloning and characterization of a mouse gene with homology to the human von Hippel–Lindau disease tumor suppressor gene: implications for the potential organization of the human von Hippel–Lindau disease gene. Cancer Res 55:743–747.

Gnarra J., Ward J., Porter F., Wagner J.R., Devor D.E., Grinberg A., Emmert-Buck M.R., Westphal H., Klausner R.D., Linehan W.M. (1997) Defective placental vasculogenesis causes embryonic lethality in VHL-deficient mice. Proc Natl Acad Sci U S A 94:9102–9107.

Hanahan D. and Folkman J. (1996) Patterns and emerging mechanisms of the angiogenic switch during tumorigenesis. Cell 86:353 – 647.

Hoffman M., Ohh M., Yang H., Klco J., Ivan M., Kaelin W. J. (2001) von Hippel-Lindau protein mutants linked to type 2C VHL disease preserve the ability to downregulate HIF. Hum Mol Genet 10:1019–1027.

Hudson C.C., Liu M., Chiang G.G., Otterness D.M., Loomis D.C., Kaper F., Giaccia A.J., Abraham R.T. (2002) Regulation of hypoxia-inducible factor 1α expression and function by the mammalian target of rapamycin. Mol Cell Biol 22:7004–7014.

Iliopoulos O., Kibel A., Gray S., Kaelin W.G. (1995) Tumour suppression by the human von Hippel–Lindau gene product. Nat Med 1:822–826.

Iliopoulos O., Levy A.P., Jiang C., Kaelin W.G. (1996) Goldberg MA. Negative regulation of hypoxia-inducible genes by the von Hippel-Lindau protein. Proc Natl Acad Sci U S A 93:10595–10599.

Isaacs J.S., Xu W., Neckers L. (2003) Heat shock protein 90 as a molecular target for cancer therapeutics, Cancer Cell 3:213–217.

Ivan M., Kondo K., Yang H., Kim W., Valiando J., Ohh M., Salic A., Asara J.M., Lane W.S., Kaelin W.G. (2001) HIFα targeted for VHL-mediated destruction by proline hydroxylation: implications for O2 sensing. Science 292:464–468.

Jaakkola P., Mole D.R., Tian Y.M., Wilson M.I., Gielbert J., Gaskell S.J., Kriegsheim A.v. , Hebestreit H.F., Mukherji M., Schofield C.J., Maxwell P.H., Pugh C.W., Ratcliffe P.J. (2001) Targeting of HIF-α to the von Hippel–Lindau ubiquitylation complex by O2-regulated prolyl hydroxylation. Science 292:468–472.

Jiang B.H., Rue E., Wang G.L., Semenza G.L. (1996) Dimerization, DNA binding, and transactivation properties of hypoxia-inducible factor 1. J Biol Chem 271:17771–17778.

Kaelin W.G. (2004) The von Hippel-Lindau tumor suppressor gene and kidney cancer. Clin Cancer Res 10:6290–6295S

Kelly B.D., Hackett S.F., Hirota K., Oshima Y., Cai Z., Berg-Dixon S., Rowan A., Yan Z., Campochiaro P.A., Semenza G.L. (2003) Cell type-specific regulation of angiogenic growth factor gene expression and induction of angiogenesis in nonischemic tissue by a constitutively active form of hypoxia-inducible factor 1. Circ Res. 93:1074–1081.

Kim W.Y. and Kaelin W.G. (2004) Role of VHL gene mutation in human cancer. J Clin Oncol 22:4991–5004.

Knudson A.G. (1971) Mutation and cancer: statistical study of retinoblastoma. Proc Natl Acad Sci U S A 68:820–823.

Kondo K., Yao M., Yoshida M., Kishida T., Shuin T., Miura T., Moriyama M., Kobayashi K., Sakai N., Kaneko S., Kawakami S., Baba M., Nakaigawa N., Nagashima Y., Nakatani Y., Hosaka M. (2002) Comprehensive mutational analysis of the VHL gene in sporadic renal cell carcinoma: relationship to clinicopathological parameters. Genes Chromosomes Cancer 34:58–68.

Kung A.L., Zabludoff S.D., France D.S., Freedman S.J., Tanner E.A., Vieira A., Cornell-Kennon S., Lee J., Wang B., Wang J., Memmert K., Naegeli H.U., Petersen F., Eck M.J., Bair K.W., Wood A.W., Livingston D.M. (2004) Small molecule blockade of transcriptional coactivation of the hypoxia-inducible factor pathway, Cancer Cell 6:33–34.

Lando D., Peet D.J., Gorman J.J., Whelan D.A., Whitelaw M.L., Bruick R.K. (2002) FIH-1 is an asparaginyl hydroxylase enzyme that regulates the transcriptional activity of hypoxia-inducible factor. Genes Dev 16:1466–1471.

Latif F., Tory K., Gnarra J., Yao M., Duh F.M., Orcutt M.L., Stackhouse T., Kuzmin I., Modi W., Geil L. (1993) Identification of the von Hippel–Lindau disease tumor suppressor gene. Science 260:1317–1320.

Lee S., Nakamura E., Yang H., Wei W., Linggi M.S., Sajan M.P., Farese R.V., Freeman R.S., Carter B.D., Kaelin W.G., Schlisio S. (2005) Neuronal apoptosis linked to EglN3 prolyl hydroxy-lase and familial pheochromocytoma genes: developmental culling and cancer. Cancer Cell 8: 155–167.

Liu Y.V., Baek J.H., Zhang H., Diez R., Cole R.N., Semenza G.L. (2007) RACK1 competes with HSP90 for binding to HIF-1α and is required for O2-independent and HSP90 inhibitor-induced degradation of HIF-1α. Mol Cell 25:207–217.

Ma X., Yang K., Lindblad P., Egevad L., Hemminki K. (2001) VHL gene alterations in renal cell carcinoma patients: novel hotspot or founder mutations and linkage disequilibrium. Oncogene 20:5393–5400.

Ma W., Tessarollo L., Hong S.B., Baba M., Southon E., Back T.C., Spence S., Lobe C.G., Sharma N., Maher G.W., Pack S., Vortmeyer A.O., Guo C., Zbar B., Schmidt L.S. (2003) Hepatic vascular tumors, angiectasis in multiple organs, and impaired spermatogenesis in mice with conditional inactivation of the VHL gene. Cancer Res 63:5320–5328.

Mabjeesh N.J., Escuin D., LaVallee T.M., Pribluda V.S., Swartz G.M., Johnson M.S., Willard M.T., Zhong H., Simons J.W., Giannakakou P. (2003) 2ME2 inhibits tumor growth and angiogenesis by disrupting microtubules and dysregulating HIF. Cancer Cell 3:363–375.

Macpherson G.R. and Figg W.D. (2004) Small molecule-mediated anti-cancer therapy via hypoxia-inducible factor-1 blockade. Cancer Biol Ther 3:503–504.

Makino Y., Cao R., Svensson K., Bertilsson G., Asman M., Tanaka H., Cao Y., Berkenstam A., Poellinger L. (2001) Inhibitory PAS domain protein is a negative regulator of hypoxia-inducible gene expression. Nature 414:550–554.

Manalo D.J., Rowan A., Lavoie T., Natarajan L., Kelly B.D., Ye S.Q., Garcia J.G., Semenza G.L. (2005) Transcriptional regulation of vascular endothelial cell responses to hypoxia by HIF-1. Blood 105:659–669.

Maxwell P.H., Wiesener M.S., Chang G.W., Clifford S.C., Vaux E.C., Cockman M.E., Wykoff C.C., Pugh C.W., Maher E.R., Ratcliffe P.J. (1999) The tumour suppressor protein VHL targets hypoxia-inducible factors for oxygen-dependent proteolysis. Nature 399:271–275.

Motzer R.J., Michaelson M.D., Redman B.G., Hudes G.R., Wilding G., Figlin R.A., Ginsberg M.S., Kim S.T., Baum C.M., DePrimo S.E., Li J.Z., Bello C.L., Theuer C.P., George D.J., Rini B.I. (2006a) Activity of SU11248, a multitargeted inhibitor of vascular endothelial growth factor receptor and platelet-derived growth factor receptor, in patients with metastatic renal cell carcinoma. J Clin Oncol 24:16–24.

Motzer R.J., Rini B.I., Bukowski R.M., Curti B.D., George D.J., Hudes G.R., Redman B.G., Margolin K.A., Merchan J.R., Wilding G., Ginsberg M.S., Bacik J., Kim S.T., Baum C.M., Michaelson M.D. (2006b) Sunitinib in patients with metastatic renal cell carcinoma. JAMA 295:2516–2524.

Ohh M., Park C.W., Ivan M., Hoffman M.A., Kim T.Y., Huang L.E., Pavletich N., Chau V., Kaelin W.G. (2000) Ubiquitination of hypoxia-inducible factor requires direct binding to the beta-domain of the von Hippel-Lindau protein. Nat Cell Biol 2:423–427.

Okuda H., Hirai S., Takaki Y., Kamada M., Baba M., Sakai N., Kishida T., Kaneko S., Yao M., Ohno S., Shuin T. (1999) Direct interaction of the ß-domain of VHL tumor suppressor pro-tein with the regulatory domain of atypical PKC isotypes. Biochem Biophys Res Commun 263:491–497.

Okuda H., Saitoh K., Hirai S., Iwai K., Takaki Y., Baba M., Minato N., Ohno S., Shuin T. (2001) The von Hippel-Lindau tumor suppressor protein mediates ubiquitination of activated atypical protein kinase C. J Biol Chem 276:43611–43617.

Pal S., Claffey K., Dvorak H., Mukhopadhyay D. (1997) The von Hippel-Lindau gene product inhibits vascular permeability factor/vascular endothelial growth factor expression in renal cell carcinoma by blocking protein kinase C pathways. J Biol Chem 272:27509–27512.

Pause A., Lee S., Worrell R.A., Chen D.Y., Burgess W.H., Linehan W.M., Klausner R.D. (1997) The von Hippel-Lindau tumor-suppressor gene product forms a stable complex with human CUL-2, a member of the Cdc53 family of proteins. Proc Natl Acad Sci U S A 94: 2156–2161.

Ravi R., Mookerjee B., Bhujwalla Z.M., Sutter C.H., Artemov D., Zeng Q., Dillehay L.E., Madan A., Semenza G.L., Bedi A. (2000) Regulation of tumor angiogenesis by p53-induced degradation of hypoxia-inducible factor 1α. Genes Dev 14:34–44.

Semenza G.L. (2000) HIF-1: using two hands to flip the angiogenic switch, Cancer Metastasis Rev 19:59–65.

Semenza G.L. (2003) Targeting HIF-1 for cancer therapy. Nat Rev Cancer 3:721–732.

Semenza G.L. and Wang G.L. (1992) A nuclear factor induced by hypoxia via de novo protein synthesis binds to the human erythropoietin gene enhancer at a site required for transcriptional activation. Mol Cell Biol 12:5447–5454.

Stebbins C.E., Kaelin W.G., Pavletich N.P. (1999) Structure of the VHL-ElonginC-ElonginB complex: implications for VHL tumor suppressor function. Science 284:455–461.

Stohrer M., Boucher Y., Stangassinger M. and Jain R.K. (2000) Oncotic pressure in solid tumors is elevated, Cancer Res 60:4215–4255.

Talks K.L., Turley H., Gatter K.C., Maxwell P.H., Pugh C.W., Ratcliffe P.J., Harris A.L. (2000) The expression and distribution of the hypoxia-inducible factors HIF-1α and HIF-2α in normal human tissues, cancers, and tumor-associated macrophages, Am J Pathol 157:411–421.

Tian H., McKnight S.L., Russell D.W. (1997) Endothelial PAS domain protein 1 (EPAS1), a transcription factor selectively expressed in endothelial cells. Genes Dev 11:72–82.

Wang G.L., Jiang B.H., Rue E.A., Semenza G.L. (1995) Hypoxia-inducible factor 1 is a basic-helix-loop-helix-PAS heterodimer regulated by cellular O2 tension. Proc Natl Acad Sci U S A 92:5510–5514.

Welsh S., Williams R., Kirkpatrick L., Paine-Murrieta G., Powis G. (2004) Antitumor activity and pharmacodynamic properties of PX-478, an inhibitor of hypoxia-inducible factor-1α. Mol Cancer Ther 3:233–244.

Yang J.C., Haworth L., Sherry R.M., Hwu P., Schwartzentruber D.J., Topalian S.L., Steinberg S.M., Chen H.X., Rosenberg S.A. (2003) A randomized trial of bevacizumab, an anti-vascular endothelial growth factor antibody, for metastatic renal cancer. N Engl J Med 349:427–434.

Yao M., Tabuchi H., Nagashima Y., Baba M., Nakaigawa N., Ishiguro H., Hamada K., Inayama Y., Kishida T., Hattori K., Yamada-Okabe H., Kubota Y. (2005) Gene expression analysis of renal carcinoma: adipose differentiation-related protein as a potential diagnostic and prognostic biomarker for clear-cell renal carcinoma. J Pathol 205:377–387.

Yu F., White S.B., Zhao Q., Lee F.S. (2001) HIF-1α binding to VHL is regulated by stimulus-sensitive proline hydroxylation. Proc. Natl Acad. Sci. USA 98:9630–9635.

Zhong H., De Marzo A.M., Laughner E., Lim M., Hilton D.A., Zagzag D., Buechler P., Isaacs W.B., Semenza G.L., Simons J.W. (1999) Overexpression of hypoxia-inducible factor 1α in common human cancers and their metastases. Cancer Res 59:5830–5835.

Chapter 7
RAS Oncogenes and Tumor–Vascular Interface

Janusz Rak

Cast of Characters

The discovery of *ras* oncogenes is amongst the most breathtaking events in the quest to understand the molecular nature of human cancers. After several years, during which various laboratories were zooming in on viral oncogenes (Malumbres and Barbacid, 2003), in 1981, the laboratory led by Robert Weinberg succeeded in transferring DNA sequences from human cancer cells to immortalized murine fibroblasts (NIH-3T3), causing their overt malignant transformation (Malumbres and Barbacid, 2003; Karnoub and Weinberg, 2008). Frantic efforts during the subsequent 2–3 years led to the identification of the responsible mutant genes present in either bladder (*T24, EJ*) or lung cancer (*LX-1*) cell lines. An almost serendipitous comparison of their sequences to that of the viral gene present in the rat sarcoma (*v-ras*) led to the realization that these oncogenic DNAs were similar and correspond to genes presently known as H-*ras* and K-*ras*, respectively (Karnoub and Weinberg, 2008). This emerging family was later extended by the discovery of an additional member present in neuroblastoma cells (N-*ras*) and currently includes several, more distantly related entities with different functions (Karnoub and Weinberg, 2008). It became apparent early on that oncogenic mutations of *ras* genes are not a result of tissue culture artifacts but rather are present in naturally occurring human lung cancers and, as subsequent decades of studies revealed conclusively, in a wide spectrum of human malignancies (Karnoub and Weinberg, 2008). This did not dissipate the mystery of these fascinating genes. Indeed, while *ras* genes share considerable sequence homology, biochemical similarity, and analogous manner of oncogenic activation, they likely have different roles in normal cells and tissues. Their oncogenic mutation, usually within codons 12, 13, or 61, results in a similarly reduced GTPase activity and altered patterns of molecular interactions, but they occur with different frequencies in different human cancers: K-*ras* being mutated most frequently, especially in pancreatic, colorectal, and lung cancers, while H-*ras* and

J. Rak (✉)
Montreal Children's Hospital Research Institute, Montreal, QC, H3Z 3Z2, Canada
e-mail: janusz.rak@mcgill.ca

A. Thomas-Tikhonenko (ed.), *Cancer Genome and Tumor Microenvironment*,
DOI 10.1007/978-1-4419-0711-0_7, © Springer Science+Business Media, LLC 2010

133

N-*ras* are mutated in urinary tract and hematopoietic malignancies, respectively (Karnoub and Weinberg, 2008). The specific means by which *ras* mutations trigger malignant growth are still being studied, and one of many such mechanisms is described in this chapter.

Introduction

The Link Between Oncogenes and Tumor Angiogenesis

In spite of the steady progress in the management of human malignancies, many remain resistant to presently available therapies and are ultimately incurable. Therefore, the advent of new therapeutic paradigms, such as biologically based anticancer therapies and the resulting derivation of, now several hundreds of, targeted agents, inspired great hopes and considerable expectations. Indeed, targeted drugs were conceived as means to obliterate two major components of the circuitry driving cancer progression, namely the various predefined intrinsic oncogenic pathways (signal transduction inhibitors) and the host components essential for aggressive tumor growth and metastasis (antiangiogenics) (Folkman and Kalluri, 2003; Perez-Atayde et al., 1997).

While long studied as separate entities, tumor angiogenesis (Folkman, 1971; Folkman and Kalluri, 2003) and molecular oncogenesis (Bishop, 1995; Malumbres and Barbacid, 2003) have begun to intersect in the late 1980s and the early 1990s. The turning point in this regard has been the discovery made by the group led by Noel Bouck of the tumor suppressor (p53)-driven mechanism that controls the production of thrombospondin-1 (TSP-1), one of the most potent and well-studied endogenous, matricellular inhibitors of angiogenesis (Rastinejad et al., 1989; Dameron et al., 1994; Bouck et al., 1996). Shortly thereafter, this finding was complemented by the realization that dominant-acting oncogenes may also directly control the angiogenic process in cancer (Thomson and Mackie, 1989). It was also originally found that this may occur by deregulation of an antithetical mechanism, namely the increase in expression of proangiogenic molecules, such as vascular endothelial growth factor (VEGF) in cells harboring oncogenic *ras* (Rak et al., 1995, 2000; Grugel et al., 1995; Rak and Kerbel, 2003). Indeed, several oncogenes and tumor suppressors are now known to control both positive and negative influences that modulate vascular processes in the growing tumors (Rak et al., 2000b; Rak and Kerbel, 2003; Dews et al., 2006; Janz et al., 2000; Weinstat-Saslow et al., 1994; Zabrenetzky et al., 1994; Teodoro et al., 20069, 2007; Bouck et al., 1996), thereby firmly placing the angiogenic phenotype amongst the inherent hallmarks of cancer (Hanahan and Weinberg, 2000).

It is important to point out that these findings did not negate the traditional views of tumor angiogenesis as a microenvironmentally driven and somewhat 'unspecific' response of the vasculature to the very anomaly of tumorigenesis. In fact, it is now understood that oncogenic alterations may either drive constitutive changes in the cancer cell angiome that mimic microenvironmental stresses (Rak et al., 1995,

2000; Janz et al., 2000; Berra et al., 2000; Bouck et al., 1996) or sensitize such cells to the effects of hypoxia, inflammation, procoagulant mediators, cell–cell contact, growth factors, and other influences commonly present in the growing tumor (Mazure et al., 1996, 1997; Laderoute et al., 2000; Giaccia, 2003). Still, it was realized that some of the oncogene-directed anticancer agents may exert their effects in vivo, at least in part, via reversal/downmodulation of the angiogenic switch driven by their respective molecular targets (Rak et al., 1995). Finally, this linkage suggested the possibility that the inherently pleiotropic effects of oncogenic lesions may reset wider molecular networks not only within cancer cells themselves but also outside of them, in the adjacent host cell compartments, such as tumor-associated stroma, and even at distant sites, thereby conditioning the host to the development of the systemic malignancy (Rak and Kerbel, 2003). In this chapter we will discuss the scope of these oncogene-dependent vascular alterations, especially as they relate to mutant *ras*.

Tumor–Vascular Interface and Cancer Progression

One of the most striking features in the progression of human malignancies is the associated emergence of new and abnormal points of direct contact between the cellular compartments, from which the disease originates (e.g., epithelia), and the various facets of the host vascular system. Thus, most of the normal epithelial tissues (e.g., in the gut, skin, and exocrine glands) are separated from the vasculature by connective tissue layers and basement membranes. These barriers are compromised during the course of the malignant process, resulting in the reciprocal structural interdigitations and functional interactions of vascular (cells, blood, and lymph) and parenchymal components (cancer cells). Several increasingly well-described processes exemplify this transition, including blood vessel co-option by cancer cells, vascular invasion, onset of capillary hyperpermeability and interstitial leakage of plasma macromolecules into the proximity of cancer cells, angiogenesis, lymphangiogenesis, onset of coagulation, and distant metastasis (Fig. 7.1) (Folkman and Kalluri, 2003; Holash et al., 1999; Dvorak and Rickles, 2006; Carmeliet, 2005).

The sum of these dynamic contacts and interactions could be described as *tumor–vascular interface* (Fig. 7.1) and represents both the outcome and the causal element in the pathogenesis of the malignant process. This role includes several 'outside-in' effects, such as supply of oxygen, growth factors, metabolites to the growing tumor cell masses, paracrine and adhesive tumor–vascular interactions, remodeling of the extracellular matrix (ECM), recruitment/retention of the host immune, inflammatory and bone marrow-derived progenitor cells, delivery of drugs, hormones, and regulatory peptides, and several other effects. However, this interface also mediates several 'inside-out' processes responsible for the systemic manifestations of the malignant disease, notably extravasation of metastatic cancer cells, emission of angiogenesis-regulating, proinflammatory, hormonal, and metabolic (e.g., cachexia-inducing) signals, shedding/uptake of tumor-related microvesicles

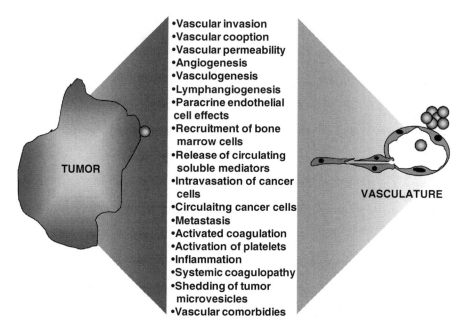

Tumor-vascular interface

(points of contact between cancer cells and the structures, cells
and molecules of the vascular system)

TUMOR

- •Vascular invasion
- •Vascular cooption
- •Vascular permeability
- •Angiogenesis
- •Vasculogenesis
- •Lymphangiogenesis
- •Paracrine endothelial
  cell effects
- •Recruitment of bone
  marrow cells
- •Release of circulating
  soluble mediators
- •Intravasation of cancer
  cells
- •Circulaitng cancer cells
- •Metastasis
- •Activated coagulation
- •Activation of platelets
- •Inflammation
- •Systemic coagulopathy
- •Shedding of tumor
  microvesicles
- •Vascular comorbidies

VASCULATURE

Fig. 7.1 Constituents of the tumor–vascular interface. Multiple biological processes and variables are engaged during tumor progression. Many of them are affected by events controlled by the oncogenic RAS pathway

containing biologically active molecules (Folkman and Kalluri, 2003; Rak et al., 2006) as well as systemic changes in the status of the coagulation system (Rickles, 2006; Dvorak and Rickles, 2006). While the entire tumor–vascular interface likely responds to the succession of oncogenic alterations in cancer cells (or cancer stem cells) (Rak et al., 1995, 2006; Rak and Klement, 2000; Rak and Kerbel, 2003), the best described vascular consequence of oncogenic mutations is the onset of tumor angiogenesis (Folkman, 1985)

Tumor Angiogenesis

It is now well established that tumors cannot grow beyond a few millimeters in diameter, or metastasize, without generating or gaining access to vascular (and lymphatic) networks (Folkman, 1990; Alitalo and Carmeliet, 2002). Tumor cells may actively 'seek' blood vessel proximity through processes of vascular invasion (Folkman, 1985) or co-option (Holash et al., 1999), provoke the assembly of endothelial progenitor cells into new vascular structures (vasculogenesis), or else, at least in some cases, transdifferentiate into endothelial-like cells (vasculogenic mimicry) (Hendrix et al., 2003). Blood vessels could also form through the partition of larger vessels by the invaginating external tissue pillars (intussusception) (Burri, 1991) or through the formation of intraluminal endothelial septa (splitting) (Carmeliet and Jain, 2000; Carmeliet, 2000). Perhaps, the largest proportion of the tumor microcirculation, however, originates by a directional branching and extension (sprouting) of the preexisting vascular channels (*angiogenesis*) (Carmeliet and Jain, 2000; Carmeliet, 2000).

Deployment of vascular sprouts is well described (Paku and Paweletz, 1991; Paweletz and Knierim, 1989; Dvorak et al., 1991; Carmeliet and Jain, 2000; Gerhardt et al., 2003) and usually entails the initial circumferential enlargement of the affected capillary of venule, resulting in the formation of a thin-walled mother vessel (Pettersson et al., 2000). This is followed by focal dissolution of the plasma membrane, detachment of pericytes, and activation of endothelial cell migration and proliferation capacities, all of which result in the extension of a cellular cohort composed of functionally and molecularly distinct endothelial cell subsets of *stalk* and *tip cells*. These cells are programmed for growth/migration and for recognition of the angiogenic gradient (e.g., immobilized VEGF), respectively, and establish the rudiment and topology of the newly formed capillary (Gerhardt et al., 2003). Under the normal circumstances, vascular sprouts eventually anastomose with each other to permit the blood flow to occur. They also mature by attracting pericytes and smooth muscle cells, and by developing the basement membrane (Carmeliet and Jain, 2000; Carmeliet, 2000). These processes are largely triggered by a host of external proangiogenic stimuli and their gradients, but they are 'supervised' by endogenous programs of participating cells, notably endothelial cells and pericytes and increasingly recognized bone marrow-derived cells. These include circulating endothelial progenitor cells (Rafii et al., 2002; Asahara et al., 1997; Bertolini et al., 2006; Shaked et al., 2006), hematopoietic progenitors (Rafii et al., 2002), various populations of macrophages (Carmeliet et al., 2001), and other bone marrow-derived accessory, regulatory, or vasculogenic cells with functions that may depend on the stage and the nature of the angiogenic process (Shojaei et al., 2008).

Tumor-associated blood vessels are structurally (Ocak et al., 2007), functionally (Dvorak et al., 1991; Jain, 2001), and molecularly (Neri and Bicknell, 2005; St. Croix et al., 2000; Seaman et al., 2007) different than their quiescent counterparts, or the vasculature generated during developmental and reparative processes. This is believed to be the basis of their selective responses to presently available antiangiogenics and relative tolerability of these agents to normal tissues (Rak and Kerbel, 1996; Verheul and Pinedo, 2007). However, it is increasingly clear that, contrary to prior predictions (Folkman, 1971), tumor-associated endothelial cells not only are distinct from their tumor-unrelated counterparts but also differ in a tumor-specific fashion, notably with respect to their molecular characteristics often referred to as tumor endothelial markers (TEMs) (Nanda and St Croix, 2004; St.Croix et al., 2000; Seaman et al., 2007). While increasing numbers of such endothelial signatures are being revealed by gene and protein expression profiling techniques (Seaman et al.,

2007; Carver and Schnitzer, 2003; Ho et al., 2003; Neri and Bicknell, 2005), the exact reasons why such profound *reprogramming of endothelial cells* seems to occurs in the context of cancer are presently unknown.

Nonetheless, the dynamics of tumor neovascularization is controlled by the detection systems deployed by endothelial (and other) cells to translate the tumor-derived cues into formation of new vascular sprouts. This apparatus includes several key entities, such as three VEGF receptor tyrosine kinases (VEGFR-1, -2, and -3), along with their soluble isoforms, e.g., sVEGFR-1/Flt-1, and non-kinase receptors, e.g., neuropilins 1 and 2, all of which interact with various members of the VEGF family (Ferrara and Gerber, 2001; Yancopoulos et al., 2000). Another essential regulatory system consists of angiopoietins (especially Ang-1 and Ang-2) and their Tie-2/Tek receptors, as well as the related orphan Tie-1 receptor (Jones et al., 2001; Yancopoulos et al., 2000). In addition, vascular responses are influenced by the Notch/Dll4 pathway (Noguera-Troise et al., 2006; Leong and Karsan, 2006; Ridgway et al., 2006), integrins, vascular endothelial cadherin (VE-cadherin), and several other adhesion molecules (Liebner et al., 2006). Important roles are also ascribed to platelet-derived growth factors and their receptors (PDGFRs) that control pericyte and tip cell behavior (Nystrom et al., 2006; Lundkvist et al., 2007; Hellstrom et al., 2007; Bergers et al., 2003; Carmeliet and Jain, 2000; Carmeliet, 2000). More recently, it was uncovered that ephrinB2/EphB4 pathway is involved in arteriovenous determination of endothelial cell identity (Wang et al., 1998), while several other pathways provide cues for cellular guidance and patterning (e.g., Slit/Robo or UNC5B) (Klagsbrun and Eichmann, 2005; Carmeliet and Tessier-Lavigne, 2005). The specific roles of these vascular effectors in the angiogenic responses observed in different tumor settings is only beginning to emerge and the details of the related studies exceed the scope of this review (for reference, see Carmeliet, 2005).

Angiogenic Factors and Their Interactions

Traditionally, the onset of angiogenesis is described as a consequence of the change in balance between various pro- and antiangiogenic factors produced in a given context (Folkman and Kalluri, 2003; Hanahan and Folkman, 1996; Bouck et al., 1996; Bergers and Benjamin, 2003). However, the increasingly well-understood finesse of the endothelial/vascular homeostatic apparatus suggests that it may be more accurate to describe this regulation as a multidimensional signaling network, where the impact of a particular effector molecule may be modulated by the status of many others, and the output may not necessarily translate into 'more angiogenesis,' and hence 'more tumor growth.' For instance, while upregulation of VEGF by cancer cells (Ferrara and Kerbel, 2005) and stimulation of VEGFR-2/KDR/Flk-1 are amongst the most consistent correlates and driving forces involved in tumor progression, several other events take place to shape and modulate this reaction.

In this regard, it should be kept in mind that VEGF is produced in multiple molecular splice isoforms ranging from more abundant, such as VEGF121, VEGF165, and VEGF189, to less common, including VEGFs 145, 162, 183, and 206 (Poltorak et al., 1997; Lange et al., 2003; Jingjing et al., 2001). Importantly, these isoforms differ in their ability to bind to the extracellular heparinoids and the plasma membrane in the following increasing order: VEGF121<VEGF165<VEGF189 (Neufeld et al., 1999). These properties profoundly affect the spatial distribution of the respective ligands, formation of their gradients, and consequently impact the organization of the vascular growth. For instance, VEGF121 does not bind heparin, is highly soluble, and therefore inefficient at forming well-defined gradients. In contrast, heparin-binding and partially soluble VEGF165 readily forms gradients recognized by sprouting tip cells (Gerhardt et al., 2003). As somewhat different compositions of VEGF isoforms may be produced in different tumors, these properties may impact the nature of their respective vascular networks (Yu et al., 2002b; Grunstein et al., 2000).

In addition to the ligands encoded by the *VEGF* gene and described collectively as VEGF-A, VEGF receptors are also stimulated by other VEGR-related proteins. Thus, VEGF-A interacts mainly with VEGFR-1/Flt-1 and VEGFR-2/Flk-1. The related molecules VEGF-B and placenta growth factor (PlGF) are ligands for VEGFR-1, while VEGF-C and VEGF-D (lymphangiogenic factors) activate mainly VEGFR-3 on lymphatic endothelial cells. VEGF-E interacts selectively with VEGFR-2 (Carmeliet, 2005; Alitalo et al., 2005; Ferrara and Kerbel, 2005). It is also worth mentioning that the proangiogenic actions of VEGF-A may be opposed by the naturally produced, soluble ectodomain of VEGFR-1 (sFlt-1) (Shibuya, 2006; Levine et al., 2004) or the recently described antiangiogenic VEGF165b isoform (Woolard et al., 2004). In addition, numerous endogenous angiogenesis inhibitors, such as thrombospondins 1 and 2 (TSP-1 and -2), angiostatin, endostatin, tumstatin, castatin, arresten, interferons (IFNs), antiangiogenic antithrombin (aaAT), platelet factor 4 (PF4), brain-derived inhibitors (GD-AIF and BAI1), pigment epithelium-derived factor (PEDF), and several other entities, act at various stages of the angiogenic cascade (mostly downstream of the VEGF/VEGFR pathway) to control the activity and survival of endothelial cells (Folkman and Kalluri, 2003).

As mentioned earlier, VEGF-stimulated angiogenesis begins by the formation of mother vessels (Pettersson et al., 2000), the induction of vascular permeability (Dvorak, 2002; Paul et al., 2001), and triggering the production of two important endothelial cell-derived ligands: angiopoietin 2 (Ang-2) and delta-like 4 (Dll4) (Hanahan, 1997; Yancopoulos et al., 2000; Noguera-Troise et al., 2006; Noguera-Troise et al., 2006). The former is now understood to antagonize the stabilizing effects of Ang-1, which are mediated via the Tie-2 receptor expressed by endothelial cells (Yancopoulos et al., 2000; Jones and Dumont, 2000; Hanahan, 1997). As a result, pericytes separate from the endothelial tube and thereby enable endothelial cell sprouting (Yancopoulos et al., 2000; Hanahan, 1997). During the latter process, the ratio of tip cells to stalk cells (and ultimately the branching pattern) is maintained by the interaction between Dll4, a membrane-bound ligand, and its endothelial Notch receptor (Thurston et al., 2007).

In the absence of VEGF, vascular density in tumors may decrease (at least in some settings – see below), often below the functional threshold required for cancer cell viability (Grunstein et al., 1999; Grunstein et al., 2000; Kim et al., 1993; Noguera-Troise et al., 2006). In contrast, inhibition of Dll4 leads to the formation of hyperdense, but nonproductive, vascular networks (i.e., more angiogenesis is accompanied by less blood flow). Importantly, both of these diametrically different scenarios are associated with impaired tumor growth (Noguera-Troise et al., 2006; Noguera-Troise et al., 2006; Thurston et al., 2007; Patel et al., 2005; Ferrara and Kerbel, 2005). Similarly paradoxical could be the effects of Ang-1, which is generally considered to be a proangiogenic factor. For instance, the expression of Ang-1 in tumor cells stimulates the formation of more stable vessels, amidst mitigated tumor growth (Ahmad et al., 2001). Thus, the capacity of specific mediators to produce more sprouts, or more vascular branches in various experimental settings, may not accurately reflect their mode of action in vivo, their net impact on vascular growth, remodeling, or perfusion. Cancer cells constitute the important source of signals that control the repertoire of tumor-associated vascular effectors. In the remaining sections of this chapter, we will illustrate how Ras oncoproteins regulate these processes and their consequences (Rak and Kerbel, 2003; Kranenburg et al., 2004).

RAS Oncogenes in Cancer Progression and Angiogenesis

Ras GTPases are central to how a cell responds to changes in the microenvironment (Malumbres and Barbacid, 2003; Khosravi-Far et al., 1998; Rajalingam et al., 2007). Discovered as retroviral oncogenes nearly 50 years ago, the corresponding *ras* genes are mutated in approximately 20% of all human cancers (Malumbres and Barbacid, 2003; Rajalingam et al., 2007), but most frequently in pancreatic (59–90%), colorectal (20–50%), lung (20%), and hematopoietic (11%) malignancies (Rajalingam et al., 2007; Malumbres and Barbacid, 2003; Hasegawa et al., 1995; Downward, 2003; Fearon and Vogelstein, 1990). Still, the activation of the RAS pathway is even more widespread (Guha, 1998). In addition to the three major *ras* genes (H-*ras*, K-*ras*, and N-*ras*) and four related proteins (HRAS, KRASA, KRASB, NRAS), the *ras* superfamily also includes numerous related (RAS-like) entities, usually assigned to distinct subfamilies, such as RAS, RHO, RAB, ARF, α, and several others (MRAS, RRAS, ERAS) on the basis of a similar structure and the basic mode of activation (Rajalingam et al., 2007). However, the cellular functions of these proteins are vastly different (Rajalingam et al., 2007).

RAS proteins are recruited to the inner leaflet of the plasma membrane, mostly as a result of the posttranslational prenylation of their C-termini, notably by protein farnesyl transferases (PFT) and the related enzymes (Gibbs et al., 1994; Grimbacher et al., 1998; Prendergast and Oliff, 2000). This facilitates their interactions with receptor tyrosine kinases and participation in other events that may lead to RAS activation (Rajalingam et al., 2007). The latter can also occur or persist in other than plasma membrane cellular compartments, such as endoplasmic reticulum and Golgi (Cox, 2003; Di Guglielmo et al., 1994; Rajalingam et al., 2007). Activation of RAS consists of binding to the GTP and is catalyzed by guanosine exchange factors (GEFs), e.g., SOS, RAS-GRF, or RAS-GRP (Rajalingam et al., 2007). Conversely, inactivation of RAS entails replacement of GTP with GDP, which is mediated mainly by factors with RAS-GTPase activity (e.g., p120GAP, neurofibromin, GAP1IP4BP, GAP1m) (Rajalingam et al., 2007). Mutations in codons 12, 13, or 61, as it occurs in cancer cells, render RAS proteins resistant to these latter influences and thereby constitutively active (Malumbres and Barbacid, 2003; Khosravi-Far et al., 1998; Rajalingam et al., 2007). KRAS is the most commonly mutated isoform in human cancer and one that is essential for survival during murine embryogenesis (Rajalingam et al., 2007). However, all RAS isoforms possess potent transforming capacities in experimental assays (Rajalingam et al., 2007).

In the activated GTP-bound state, RAS assumes the conformation, which exposes the switch regions I and II to interactions with proteins that contain ras-binding domains (RBDs) and thereby can act as RAS effectors, whereby they effectively transmit the related cellular signals (Rajalingam et al., 2007). The growing number of such molecules currently includes RAF, p110/catalytic subunit of PI3K, PKCζ, PLCϵ, GAP, RalGDS, RIN1, TIAM1, AF6, and Nore1 (Rajalingam et al., 2007) and signifies the diversity of intracellular signals that branch out of the activated RAS 'node' of this network (Khosravi-Far et al., 1998).

The aforementioned RAS effectors interact with several downstream signaling cascades that are crucial for various aspects of cellular function and participate in malignant transformation (Downward, 2003). The best characterized of those are the RAF/MEK/MAPK and the PI3K/Akt modules that control several major aspects of the cancer cell phenotype, such as growth factor-independent mitogenesis, survival, and angiogenesis (Hanahan and Weinberg, 2000). However, the impact of mutant *ras* on the signaling circuitry is much wider and involves changes in cell shape and motility (via RHO, Rac, Cdc42) (Bar-Sagi and Hall, 2000), resistance to anoikis (via PI3K) (Downward, 2003; Rosen et al., 2000), hypoxia response pathways (HIF1) (Berra et al., 2000; Feldkamp et al., 1999; Sodhi et al., 2001), oxidative and prostaglandin pathways (Khosravi-Far et al., 1998; Sheng et al., 1998c), regulation of gene transcription (SP1, AP1, NF(B)) (Zuber et al., 2000; Irani et al., 1997), RNA stability (White et al., 1997), protein translation (eIF4E) (Kevil et al., 1996), and very likely also changes in the regulatory microRNA species, similarly to other oncoproteins that may lie downstream of RAS (Dews et al., 2006).

The consequences of these events depend on the cellular context, the expression and compartmentalization of the respective molecules, temporal characteristics of RAS activation (e.g., chronic versus intermittent), and interactions with other signaling pathways (Rajalingam et al., 2007). For instance, expression of the mutant *ras* transgenes in mice leads to the formation of hyperplastic or cancerous outgrowths (Tuveson et al., 2004; Guerra et al., 2003; Ding et al., 2001). However, overexpression of *ras* in cultured primary cells precipitates cell senescence and death, while similar exposure of immortalized, but nontumorigenic (quail-normal) cell lines results in a robust cellular transformation. This is due to the influence of the presence or the absence of tumor suppressors (e.g., p53 and p16) on RAS-mediated signaling (Serrano et al., 1995, 1997; McCormick, 2003; Weinberg, 1996). The latter process entails a profound change in the cellular gene expression patterns (Agudo-Ibanez et al., 2007; Zuber et al., 2000), including deregulation of genes that control the capacity of cell to interact with the vascular system.

RAS-Dependent Multicellular Angiogenic Phenotype

In 1995 we reported that the expression of mutant H-*ras* in immortalized, but nontumorigenic intestinal epithelial cells, IEC-18, leads to their acquisition of the overtly tumorigenic and angiogenic capacity, along with the exuberant production of VEGF-A (Rak et al., 1995). In addition, removal of a single, naturally occurring mutant K-*ras* allele from two human colorectal cancer cell lines (HCT116 and DLD1) resulted not only in the reversal of their cellular transformation and tumorigenic phenotype (Shirasawa et al., 1993), but also in their reduced production of VEGF (Rak et al., 1995), and their ability to stimulate angiogenesis in vivo (Okada et al., 1998). These findings reveal only a small fragment of what could be referred to a *RAS-dependent angiome*, which involves a number of gene products with a direct or an indirect ability to impact tumor–vascular interface (Rak et al., 2006) (Fig. 7.2; Table 7.1).

In general terms, RAS-dependent transformation shifts the expression of angiogenesis-related genes toward a more stimulatory profile (Rak et al., 2000a). This involves upregulation of mediators that directly promote endothelial sprouting, survival and angiogenic expansion (e.g., VEGF, FGF, IL-8; Gro-1) (Rak et al., 1995; Iberg et al., 1989; Sparmann and Bar-Sagi, 2004; Yang et al., 2006), reduction in levels of angiogenic inhibitors (TSP-1, PEDF) (Zabrenetzky et al., 1994; Watnick et al., 2003; Rak et al., 2000a; Viloria-Petit et al., 2003), and changes in factors involved in vascular remodeling (e.g., Ang-1) (Viloria-Petit et al., 2003; Larcher et al., 2003).

Although cells expressing mutant *ras* are often constitutively and robustly proangiogenic, as detected by the ability of their conditioned media (CM) to stimulate endothelial cells, it is unlikely that in natural settings this phenotype is sufficient to act as a cell-autonomous trigger of the angiogenic switch (Rak et al., 2000b). This is for a number of reasons. First, regardless of the degree of the preceding genetic instability, oncogenic *ras* mutations would be expected to occur relatively rarely, a circumstance that would lead to the emergence of individual mutant cells in the midst of the overwhelming majority of their counterparts expressing wild-type *ras*, along with normal host cells (Kalas et al., 2005b). The latter cells could be expected to be non- or even antiangiogenic, as they would produce little or no VEGF. The presence of such cells may 'dilute' the impact of this factor produced by the cellular minority expressing mutant *ras*. Second, in the absence of *ras* mutations, the cellular majority would produce considerable levels of TSP-1 and other inhibitors, the compound effect of which would likely eclipse TSP-1 downregulation in *ras*-expressing single cells. In other words, it is difficult to foresee a mechanism by

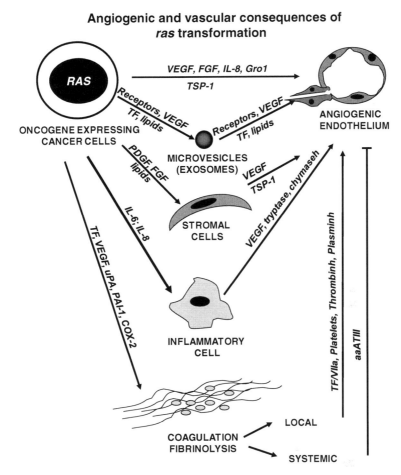

Fig. 7.2 Angiogenic and vascular consequences of *ras* transformation. The expression of mutant *ras* or the activation of the RAS pathway in cancer cells triggers several processes that impact tumor angiogenesis in a direct or an indirect manner (see text). These events include production of angiogenic growth factors (VEGF), microvesicles (MVs), factors stimulating stromal cells (FGF), proinflammatory cytokines (IL-6) or chemokines (IL-8), and activation of the coagulation system, all of which can potentially impact tumor neovascularization

which the angiogenic switch in a single *ras*-mutated cell would, in itself, produce the impact required for reaching the proangiogenic threshold (Rak et al., 2000b; Kalas et al., 2005b).

For these reasons it was proposed that the angiogenic switching should, perhaps, be viewed as a multicellular event, where a number of cells would need to participate in mounting the stimulatory signal (a *proangiogenic unit*). This could be accomplished by a selective amplification and survival of *ras*-expressing cells to such a degree as to achieve their sheer number sufficient to produce angiogenic activity able to impact the vasculature (Rak et al., 1999). Alternatively, small numbers of

Table 7.1 Vascular mediators regulated by oncogenic *ras*

Mediator	Function	References
VEGF	Stimulator of angiogenesis, vasculogenesis, and vascular permeability	Rak et al., 1995; Grugel et al., 1995
FGF	Stimulator of angiogenesis	Iberg et al., 1989
TGF-α	Stimulator of angiogenesis	Filmus et al., 1993
IL-8	Stimulator of angiogenesis and inflammation	Sparmann and Bar-Sagi, 2004
IL-6	Proinflammatory cytokine involved in tumor angiogenesis	Ancrile et al., 2007
Gro-1	Proangiogenic chemokine	Yang et al., 2006
uPA	Proangiogenic protease	Testa et al., 1989
MMP-2	Proangiogenic protease	Kranenburg et al., 2004; Gum et al., 1996; Meade-Tollin et al., 1998
MMP-9	Proangiogenic protease	Kranenburg et al., 2004; Gum et al., 1996; Meade-Tollin et al., 1998
COX-2	Procoagulant and proangiogenic via prostaglandin synthesis	Sheng et al., 1998; Subbaramaiah et al., 1996
TSP-1	Antiangiogenic	Volpert et al., 1997; Zabrenetzky et al., 1994; Rak et al., 2000a; Watnick et al., 2003
PEDF	Antiangiogenic	Dawson et al., 1999; Viloria-Petit et al., 2003
Ang-1	Angiogenesis modulator involved in endothelial cell survival and vascular stabilization	Viloria-Petit et al., 2003; Larcher et al., 2003
PlGF	Pathological angiogenesis	Larcher et al., 2003
SDF-1	Proangiogenic factor involved in the recruitment of bone marrow cells	Moskovits et al., 2006
TF	Procoagulant, signaling, and proangiogenic receptor for clotting factor VII	Yu et al., 2005

ras-expressing cells could change the angiogenic properties or their cellular surroundings. Indeed, such a property was recently uncovered and found to depend on the *ras*-regulated release of small molecular mediators that are able to trigger downregulation of TSP-1 in adjacent normal fibroblasts (Kalas et al., 2005b). Notably, stromal fibroblasts are frequently activated in the presence of tumor cells and this leads to production of angiogenic factors (Hlatky et al., 1994; Dong et al., 2004; Viloria-Petit et al., 2003), or decrease in the production of angiogenic inhibitors (Mettouchi et al., 1994). Another plausible mechanism of multicellular proangiogenic conversion is via intercellular exchange of microvesicles, microparticles, or exosomes. In this regard, cancer cells harboring mutant oncogenes were found to exhibit increased vesiculation and to emit exosomes carrying active mediators of angiogenesis (Gesierich et al., 2006; Baj-Krzyworzeka et al., 2006; Yu et al., 2005), as well as oncoproteins (Al-Nedawi et al., 2008). Uptake of this material by adjacent cells can reprogram their gene expression profiles, rendering them more proangiogenic (Al-Nedawi et al., 2008). These observations suggest that oncogenic *ras* may exert pleiotropic effects, not only on cells that contain the respective mutation but also on their wider surroundings, a process that may likely produce a coordinated proangiogenic, multicellular change (*angiogenic field effect*) (Kalas et al., 2005b; Rak et al., 2000b).

In addition to the aforementioned changes in direct-acting angiogenic effectors, RAS-transformed cells also acquire the ability to mobilize the proangiogenic potential of the coagulation and inflammatory systems (Rak et al., 2006; Yu et al., 2005; Ancrile et al., 2008; Sparmann and Bar-Sagi, 2004). For instance, recent studies suggested that activated oncogenes in general (Shchors et al., 2006; Coussens et al., 1999) and RAS in particular play direct roles in the recruitment of inflammatory cells to the tumor site and thereby induce inflammatory neoangiogenesis (Sparmann and Bar-Sagi, 2004; Ancrile et al., 2007). In this regard, Sparmann and Bar-Sagi first documented a *ras*-dependent upregulation of interleukin-8 (IL-8) by cancer cells, an effect that led not only to direct stimulation of angiogenesis but also to recruitment of inflammatory cells into the tumor (Sparmann and Bar-Sagi, 2004). In another study, *ras*-driven production of IL-6 was shown to trigger the inflammatory infiltration and the accompanying angiogenesis, both of which were essential for the aggressive tumor growth (Ancrile et al., 2007). As tumor cells in this case did not express IL-6 receptors, this effect was strictly paracrine in nature (Ancrile et al., 2007). As mentioned earlier, several populations of bone marrow-derived cells participate in the angiogenic process, including inflammatory macrophages, granulocytes, mast cells, hematopoietic cells, and endothelial-like progenitors, the recruitment and retention of which is driven by a network of growth factors, cytokines, and chemokines generated within the tumor microenvironment, including VEGF, Bv8, SDF-1, IL-8, IL-6, and probably many others (Asahara et al., 1997; Bertolini et al., 2006; Shaked et al., 2006; Shojaei et al., 2008) (Table 7.1).

Systemic Vascular Consequences of the Oncogenic Transformation

In addition to the relatively well-studied local control of angiogenesis, oncogenic transformation may also impact vascular homeostasis at the wider and more systemic level. This is implicit in the context of the aforementioned and still poorly understood processes whereby bone marrow-derived progenitor, accessory, and regulatory cells are recruited to the sites of neovascularization. These processes are thought to be driven by the release of several soluble mediators (Bv8, SDF1, PlGF, or VEGF) into the circulation (Shojaei et al., 2008; Asahara et al., 1999; Grunewald et al., 2006; Li et al., 2006). Interestingly, the expression of at least some of these entities (VEGF, SDF-1) is controlled by oncogenic pathways, including RAS (Rak et al., 2000b; Moskovits et al., 2006).

Exuberant expression of VEGF, but also the presence of inflammatory cytokines, is implicated in tumor-related hepatotoxicity, paraneoplastic syndrome, and cachexia (Wong et al., 2001; Ravasco et al., 2007). Indeed, the combined effects of the expanding tumor burden, the activation of RAS, and severe hypoxia could potentially explain the high systemic levels of VEGF and other cytokines in colorectal cancer patients and the related morbidity (Ravasco et al., 2007). The nature of these events remains unclear, but it is possible that stimulation of endothelial cell mitogenesis, vascular permeability and organ damage in distant organ sites (Wong et al., 2001), as well as prothrombotic effects of certain RAS targets, could be a part of the related pathomechanism (Rak et al., 2006; Yu et al., 2005; Contrino et al., 1996; Mechtcheriakova et al., 2001).

Coagulation system and the ECM are also rich sources of systemically acting regulators of angiogenesis (Folkman and Kalluri, 2003). This includes the well-studied angiogenesis inhibitors such as platelet factor 4 (PF4), antithrombin fragment (aaAT), and angiostatin (O'Reilly et al., 1994; Bouck et al., 1996; Folkman and Kalluri, 2003), all derivatives of hemostatic proteins (Browder et al., 2000). Moreover, endostatin, tumstatin, arresten, and several other proteins and peptides (O'Reilly et al., 1997; Folkman and Kalluri, 2003; Kalluri, 2003) are produced by proteolytic cleavage of tumor-associated ECM components (e.g., collagens XVIII and IV) (Kalluri, 2003). As this occurs in a tumor cell-regulated manner (O'Reilly et al., 1994; Gimbrone et al., 1972; Folkman and Kalluri, 2003), it is possible that the synthesis, the posttranslational modification, and/or the proteolytic generation of these entities could be influenced by oncogenic events.

Indeed, the loss of p53 expression in several types of cancer cells was recently shown to downregulate the levels of collagen prolyl hydroxylase (αIIPH), which is required for the formation of mature fibers of collagens 4 and 18 (Teodoro et al., 2007; Teodoro et al., 2006). Hence, the loss of p53 denies the substrate to proteolytic enzymes that generate antiangiogenic fragments of these molecules (e.g., tumstatin and endostatin), relieves systemic angiogenesis inhibition, and potentially promotes tumor growth and dissemination (Teodoro et al., 2006). Interestingly, enzymes that participate in the production of the circulating, antiangiogenic ECM fragments include matrix metalloproteinase 2 (MMP-2), which is itself a target of p53 (Teodoro et al., 2006), as well as RAS (Kim et al., 2007; Gum et al., 1996; Kranenburg et al., 2004). RAS regulates several proteolytic activities, including MMP-2, MMP-9, and urokinase plasminogen activator (uPA) (Testa et al., 1989; Kranenburg et al., 2004), which possess well-documented angiogenesis-regulating activities (Bergers et al., 2000; Pepper, 2001). Taken together, these observations suggest that oncogenic *ras* mutations can change the state of the angiogenic network not only locally but also systemically.

RAS, Coagulopathy, and Tumor Angiogenesis

It has recently come to light that oncogenic transformation may profoundly influence the local and systemic activation of the coagulation system in cancer patients. The latter condition was recognized over 140 years ago (Trousseau, 1865), is found in up to 90% cases of metastatic malignancy, and is commonly referred to as cancer coagulopathy or Trousseau's syndrome (Rak et al., 2006; Varki, 2007). While cancer coagulopathy was originally viewed as an 'unspecific' consequence of vascular invasion, blood vessel leakiness, flow stasis, inflammation, and iatrogenic manipulations related to anticancer therapy (Rickles, 2006; Levine et al., 1988), it is increasingly clear that it also involves changes linked to oncogenic transformation (Rak et al., 2006).

This possibility is illustrated by the consequences of the exuberant production of VEGF in *ras*-driven malignancies, namely by an increase in vascular permeability. This condition promotes abnormal contacts between coagulation proenzymes of blood plasma (factors VII, X, and prothrombin) and their activators present in the extravascular tumor microenvironment (Dvorak and Rickles, 2006). Tissue factor (TF) is amongst the most important mediators in this regard, especially since this molecule is ubiquitously expressed in human and experimental tumors (Contrino et al., 1996), where it acts as cell-associated (transmembrane) receptor for the coagulation factor VII (FVII) (Mackman, 2008). As a result of this interaction, FVII becomes activated to FVIIa and, in turn, activates factor X (FX) to FXa (Mackman, 2008). Generation of FXa activity triggers conversion of prothrombin to thrombin (FIIa), which catalyses the formation of the fibrin clot and the activation of platelets along with triggering promitotic, migratory, and proangiogenic cellular effects (Nierodzik and Karpatkin, 2006). The latter are mediated by G protein-coupled, protease-activated receptors (PARs) with which coagulation factors interact, especially PAR-1 (Xa, IIa) and PAR-2 (TF/VIIa complex) (Mackman, 2008). TF may also signal more directly through its short cytoplasmic tail (Morrissey, 2004; Mackman, 2008; Coughlin, 2005).

Thus, VEGF-mediated vascular permeability and constant vascular remodeling promote activation of the coagulation system in cancer and precipitate the related cellular and clotting effects. One consequence of this protracted process is the development of the systemic hypercoagulable state in cancer patients, a source of a considerable morbidity (thrombosis) and a contributing factor in disease progression, metastasis, and patient mortality (Dvorak and Rickles, 2006; Rickles, 2006; Dvorak and Rickles, 2006; Buller et al., 2007).

Some of the causes of cancer coagulopathy could be viewed as especially cancer-specific. For instance, TF expression/activity is elevated up to 1000-fold in cancer cells relative to their normal counterparts (Ruf, 2007; Rickles, 2006) and sometimes higher in cells that are more metastatic (Mueller et al., 1992) or express stem cell markers (CD133) (Milsom et al., 2007a). Moreover, in colorectal cancer cells, TF expression is directly linked to the status of mutant K-*ras* and is further increased upon disruption of *p53* (Yu et al., 2005). Similarly, oncogenic *EGFR, HER-2, PML-RARα*, and loss of *PTEN* precipitate increases in TF expression and activity, especially when combined with microenvironmental stresses, such as hypoxia and cellular compaction (Yu et al., 2004; Rong et al., 2005; Milsom et al., 2007b; Milsom.C and Rak, 2005). Cancer cells expressing some of these oncogenic changes not only produce TF locally but also shed TF-containing (procoagulant) microvesicles into the systemic circulation (Yu and Rak, 2004; Yu et al., 2005).

This may signify the oncogene-driven nature of the hypercoagulable state that is often associated with malignancy. Indeed, in one study the expression of oncogenic *c-Met* in mice led to a fulminant thrombohemorrhagic syndrome mediated in this case not by TF but by the oncogene-dependent upregulation of cyclooxygenase 2 (COX-2) and plasminogen activator inhibitor 1 (PAI-1) (Boccaccio et al., 2005). Spectacular procoagulant events in these mice were driven by the activation of the prostaglandin synthesis and the inhibition of clot resolution (fibrinolysis) (Boccaccio et al., 2005). As mentioned earlier, oncogene-dependent procoagulant changes can potentially facilitate metastasis (Palumbo et al., 2007), impact primary tumor growth and angiogenesis (Yu et al., 2005), and alter vascular morphology (Milsom et al., 2007b). These properties point to the involvement of the coagulation system in the formation of the tumor–vascular interface and to the potential utility of anticoagulants in the treatment of oncogene (*ras*)-driven cancers (Rak et al., 2006).

Mechanisms of RAS-Dependent Regulation of Vascular Effectors

The large number of molecular regulators affected by the expression of mutant *ras* (Table 7.1) or by the activation of the RAS pathway makes the comprehensive analysis of the related regulatory cascades extremely challenging. Because some of the key processes in this regard have recently been reviewed, we would like to limit our comments to only those paradigmatic events that can best illustrate the related complexities and point to questions that might be answerable versus those that may be too complex or context dependent to be generalized. In this regard, the regulation of VEGF expression by mutant *ras* has attracted much experimental attention, largely due to the prevalence and the perceived critical role of this factor in a large number of human malignancies (Rak and Kerbel, 2003).

The impact of RAS on VEGF regulation was reported to occur at a number of levels, including gene transcription, mRNA stability, and protein translation (Kranenburg et al., 2004; Rak and Kerbel, 2003). The related transcriptional mechanisms that have been implicated include several regulatory sites (SP1, AP1, and HIF) identified within the *VEGF* gene promoter (Grugel et al., 1995; Sodhi et al., 2001; Gille et al., 1997; Tischer et al., 1991) and often controlled downstream of the two main RAS effector pathways: Raf/MEK/MAPK and PI3K/Akt (Sodhi et al., 2001; Rak et al., 2000a; Grugel et al., 1995; Berra et al., 2000; Milanini et al., 1998).

Of special interest in this regard is the role of the hypoxia-inducible factor alpha (HIF-α), which represents one of the key regulators of VEGF expression under physiological conditions. Normally, HIF-α is constitutively synthesized and degraded by the von Hippel–Lindau (VHL) protein-directed ubiquitination pathway, which is controlled by the oxygen-sensitive system of prolyl and aspargyl hydroxylases (Semenza, 2003; Harris, 2002; Pugh and Ratcliffe, 2003). Under anoxic conditions, prolyl hydroxylases fail to mark HIF-α for degradation, leading to the accumulation of HIF-α in the cell and increase in the expression of HIF-α-responsive genes (Semenza, 2003; Harris, 2002). During this process, HIF-α translocates to the nucleus, dimerizes with its partner HIF-β/ARNT, and acts on the hypoxia-responsive elements (HREs) of the *VEGF* promoter (and other genes), leading to an increase in the production and angiogenic activity of the respective protein product (Semenza, 2003; Harris, 2002). RAS transformation can trigger or synergize with this HIF-α activity. For instance, while RAS-expressing cells produce elevated amounts of VEGF (Rak et al., 1995), this production can be further increased under hypoxic conditions due to the synergistic impact of both stimuli on PI3K-dependent signaling (Mazure et al., 1996, 1997). Another mechanism of this cross talk is exemplified by the phosphorylation of HIF-α by the activated MAPK module downstream of activated RAS (Berra et al., 2000).

Several additional mechanisms of RAS-dependent VEGF regulation have also been identified (Fig. 7.3). For instance, RAS could influence VEGF mRNA stability through Rac/JNK pathway (White et al., 1997; Kranenburg et al., 2004) or enhance VEGF translation by activating cap protein eIF-4E (Kevil et al., 1996; Polunovsky et al., 2000). RAS can cooperate with other oncoproteins (e.g., c-Myc, SRC), which are implicated in VEGF regulation. In addition, VEGF and other angiogenesis effectors could be influenced by some of the less studied pathways that can be activated downstream of RAS, including generation of reactive oxygen species (ROI), activation of NF-κB, lipooxygenase, cyclooxygenase, prostaglandins and their receptors, phospholipids, autocrine cytokine and growth factor pathways, and microRNA (Irani et al., 1997; Jiang et al., 1997; Sheng et al., 1998; Timoshenko

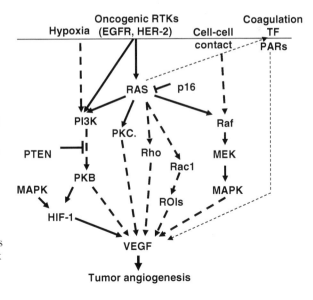

Fig. 7.3 The complexity of RAS-dependent regulation of VEGF. Some pathways emanating from the activated or mutant RAS have been depicted to illustrate the multifactorial and context-dependent nature of this regulation. For more detailed description of these events, see text and references (Kranenburg et al., 2004; Rak and Kerbel, 2001; Rak et al., 2000b)

et al., 2007; Kalas et al., 2005b; Dlugosz et al., 1997; Chen et al., 1997; Ancrile
et al., 2007; Dews et al., 2006).

While activation of the aforementioned pathways could clearly be a part of
the signaling circuitry that drives VEGF expression downstream of mutant *ras*,
several influences may alter and modulate these events (Fig. 7.3). For instance,
ras-dependent transformation in general (Serrano et al., 1997) and VEGF expression in particular are influenced by the status of tumor suppressor genes, e.g., *p53*,
p130, and *p16* (Teodoro et al., 2006; Harada et al., 1999; Claudio et al., 2001).
Activation of the RAS pathway facilitates VEGF upregulation due to extracellular cues such as hypoxia (Mazure et al., 1996) and cell–cell contact (Rak et al.,
2000a). Moreover, activated RAS pathway may set in motion a number of indirect
autocrine and paracrine influences, e.g., by triggering the expression of TF, PAR-1
receptor, and the related sensitization of cells to signals generated by the coagulation proteases, which results in the deregulation of VEGF and angiogenesis (Yu
et al., 2005; Abe et al., 1999; Cohen et al., 1996; Ancrile et al., 2007). Similarly,
RAS-dependent upregulation of TGF-α, IL-6, and IL-1 may trigger autocrine signals in cancer cells expressing the respective receptors (Lu et al., 1992; Dlugosz
et al., 1997) and lead to further VEGF upregulation (Cohen et al., 1996; Rak et al.,
1996; Gille et al., 1997). It is noteworthy that the capacity of specific cell types
to mobilize these complex direct and indirect responses depends on a number of
associated circumstances in addition to the presence or the absence of the activated
RAS. For instance, we observed that the enforced expression of comparable levels
of oncogenic H-*ras* in fibroblasts and intestinal epithelial cells led in both cases to
a marked VEGF upregulation, but via completely different signaling pathways, i.e.,
MEK/MAPK and PI3K/Akt, respectively (Rak et al., 2000a,b). Thus, while several studies successfully mapped the signaling cascades operative downstream of
various oncogenes and responsible for deregulation of specific vascular regulators
(Kranenburg et al., 2004; Berra et al., 2000; Watnick et al., 2003), a more complete
understanding of these events in vivo remains to be a formidable challenge.

Redundancy of RAS-Regulated Angiogenic Pathways

Several studies, including our own (Okada et al., 1998; Viloria-Petit et al., 2003;
Yu et al., 2005), attempted to establish the relative roles of various RAS-regulated
vascular effectors in tumor angiogenesis (Inoue et al., 2002; Casanovas et al., 2005;
Shi and Ferrara, 1999; Detmar, 1996; Watnick et al., 2003). This was motivated, at
least in part, by hopes of finding ways to obliterate oncogene-driven tumor growth
though disruption of angiogenesis, the regulatory apparatus of which was felt to
be more accessible to therapeutic intervention than the mutant *ras* itself (Rak and
Kerbel, 2003). Notable in this regard were the efforts to establish the requirement
for VEGF during RAS-driven tumor angiogenesis (Rak et al., 1995, 2000; Watnick
et al., 2003; Chin et al., 1999; Grunstein et al., 1999, 2000; Shi and Ferrara, 1999;
Okada et al., 1998; Viloria-Petit et al., 2003; Inoue et al., 2002; Casanovas et al.,
2005; Kim et al., 1993).

It was originally felt that the indispensable role of VEGF (VEGF-A) and VEGF receptors during development of the vascular system, vasculogenesis, and angiogenesis in mice (Carmeliet et al., 1996; Ferrara et al., 1996; Fong et al., 1995; Shalaby et al., 1995; Shibuya, 2006) would likely mandate a similar role of this pathway during tumor-related neovascularization (Rak et al., 1995). Indeed, initial studies suggested that pharmacological blockade of the VEGF activity in experimental tumor models (Kim et al., 1993; Warren et al., 1995), genetic inactivation of VEGF receptors (Millauer et al., 1994, 1996), or disruption of the *VEGF* gene in cancer cells (Inoue et al., 2002; Shi and Ferrara, 1999; Grunstein et al., 1999, 2000) may result in the inhibition of tumor growth and blood vessel formation.

However, our concurrent studies with *VEGF–/–* tumorigenic but 'oncogene-less' embryonic stem (ES) cell-derived teratomas and their related, isogenic *VEGF–/–* fibrosarcomas harboring mutant *ras* or *neu* oncogenes led to a fundamentally different conclusion (Viloria-Petit et al., 2003). Thus, deletion of the *VEGF* gene and/or antibody-mediated inhibition of the VEGFR-2 in vivo produced a complete growth arrest only in the former (ES stem cell-driven) but not in the latter (*ras*-driven) tumors (Viloria-Petit et al., 2003). Interestingly, both *ras*- and *neu*-dependent and VEGF-deficient fibrosarcomas were highly vascular and almost as aggressive as their counterparts producing elevated amounts of VEGF. This was ascribed to several alternative proangiogenic mechanisms that these cells were able to mobilize due to the pleiotropic nature of the oncogenic transformation. These changes included downregulation of several angiogenesis inhibitors (TSP-1, PEDF) and release of factors impacting the angiogenic properties of tumor stroma (Viloria-Petit et al., 2003; Kalas et al., 2005b). The latter effect resulted in the production of VEGF by tumor-associated host stromal cells (Viloria-Petit et al., 2003) in vivo and in the suppression of TSP-1 synthesis by fibroblasts exposed to small molecule mediators released by *ras*-expressing fibrosarcoma cells (Kalas et al., 2005a,b). Indeed, subsequent analyses revealed that the disruption of VEGF release or therapeutic blockade of VEGF receptors can be circumvented by tumors through the onset of endogenous expression of alternative angiogenic factors (e.g., FGF) or by the involvement of tumor stroma in angiogenesis stimulation (Dong et al., 2004; Casanovas et al., 2005).

The existence of such redundancy was in agreement with the prior predictions based on the analysis of changes in the angiogenic profile of human breast cancers over the course of their natural history (Relf et al., 1997). This is also consistent with the emerging clinical experience with agents blocking VEGF/VEGFR-2-driven angiogenesis, especially with Avastin/bevacizumab and kinase inhibitors (Hurwitz et al., 2005; Ince et al., 2005; Ferrara, 2005; Kerbel and Folkman, 2002). Overall, these studies suggest that in patients with advanced and metastatic cancers, VEGF inhibitors (Avastin) may often exhibit clinically encouraging but hardly curative effects (Hurwitz et al., 2003), greater in some contexts than in others (Jubb et al., 2006). Thus, the appropriate stratification, disease- and case-specific approaches, and multipronged antiangiogenic protocols may be required to achieve the optimal effects in patient populations where the disease may involve high degree of oncogenic transformation and redundant changes in cellular/tissue angiome.

RAS and the Responses of Cancer Cells to Vascular Proximity

Diffusion of essential metabolites, growth factors, and oxygen between blood and tumor parenchyma can occur only at relatively short distances. Over time this may lead to selection within the cancer cell population of two fundamentally different sets of biological properties, namely the ability to trigger the increasingly robust angiogenic response and/or to survive under conditions of declining tumor perfusion (Rak and Kerbel, 1996; Rak et al., 1996). Oncogenic events, including *ras*, play causative roles in both of these processes (Rak and Yu, 2004).

In colorectal adenoma, oncogenic *ras* mutations occur with greater frequency in the context of a polypoid, three-dimensional tumor growth pattern relative to tumors that grow superficially (Hasegawa et al., 1995; Yamagata et al., 1995; Minamoto et al., 1994), i.e., in proximity to the intestinal vasculature (Rak et al., 2000b). In these disease settings, *ras* mutations predominate at the stage of intermediate adenoma when the lesions assume a more three-dimensional configuration (Fearon and Vogelstein, 1990), and when the angiogenic switch is found to occur in vivo (Staton et al., 2007), coupled with an increased production of VEGF (Rak et al., 1995). While this may be interpreted simply as a reflection of the impact mutant *ras* has on the angiogenic phenotype, the related cellular transformation also has other effects.

Mutant *ras* profoundly alters several intrinsic cellular properties, such as growth factor dependence, survival, and metabolic requirements (Dong et al., 2004; Malumbres and Barbacid, 2003; Downward, 2003; Dang and Semenza, 1999). In experiments involving mixed tumors containing both high and low RAS-expressing cell subsets, the former, but not the latter cells, were able to survive in hypoxic regions, distant from the perfused capillary networks (Rak et al., 1996). Moreover, the expression of mutant *ras* was found to be essential for sustained tumor growth (tumor maintenance) in several experimental settings (Shirasawa et al., 1993; Chin et al., 1999), while VEGF expression alone was not (Chin et al., 1999). Conversely, injection of human colorectal cancer cells (Hkh-2), in which mutant K-*ras* was genetically disrupted (Shirasawa et al., 1993), into immunodeficient mice led to a prolonged tumor latency (Yu et al., 2005). However, when the tumors eventually emerged, they contained de novo mutations within the previously intact K-*ras* allele and expressed RAS-regulated genes (Yu et al., 2005). Similarly, when cancer cells were exposed to hypoxia and glucose deprivation in vitro or to antiangiogenic therapy in vivo, K-*ras* mutations occurred spontaneously and with increased frequency (Yu et al., 2005; Shahrzad et al., 2005, 2008). Collectively, these observations suggest that activation of the oncogenic RAS in cancer cells not only provokes the aforementioned proangiogenic switching, but also changes the relationship between cancer cells and tumor-associated perfused vasculature. As in the case of other genetic alterations (Yu et al., 2002a), mutant *ras* appears to control metabolic and survival pathways and thereby may confer the increased capacity to withstand ischemic conditions on certain types of cancer cells (Rak and Yu, 2004).

Conclusions

Oncogenic *ras* plays a significant role in conditioning host tissues to accommodate malignant growth. RAS proteins not only drive cell-autonomous processes of mitogenesis and survival but also profoundly impact the tumor vascular interface and related events involved in disease progression.

Of interest in this regard is the potential linkage between *ras* mutations and the relative ability of cancer cell subsets to initiate growth or repopulate the tumor mass, i.e., act as tumor-initiating cells (TICs) or cancer stem cells (CSCs) (Reya et al., 2001). It is intriguing that experimental expression of mutant *ras* in various types of cells greatly enhances their clonogenic and tumor-initiating (stem cell) potential (Shih and Weinberg, 1982; Filmus et al., 1993; Rak et al., 1995) and affects the expression of genes that are often viewed as stem cell markers, e.g., CD44 (Jamal et al., 1994).

It is noteworthy that in order to initiate tumor growth or metastasis, TICs must rely on a permissive extracellular microenvironment, which is therefore often referred to as a tumor stem cell niche (Reya et al., 2001). Recent studies suggest that vascular elements significantly contribute to this protective milieu (Kaplan et al., 2005; Calabrese et al., 2007; Bao et al., 2006; Milsom et al., 2007a). This is consistent with the observation that vascular defects, aging, and comorbidities modulate tumor growth in the experimental (Pili et al., 1994; Klement et al., 2007) and clinical (Balducci and Ershler, 2005) settings. Moreover, TICs are often localized in the physical proximity of tumor blood vessels (Calabrese et al., 2007) or are found to be particularly efficient in producing TF (Milsom et al., 2007a), VEGF, or vascular growth (Bao et al., 2006). It is unclear to what extent RAS controls these properties of TICs and whether it contributes to the formation of their niches.

The effects of the RAS activation are context dependent and differ not only in various disease settings but also as a function of tumor microenvironment and cancer cell heterogeneity (e.g., in TICs versus their progeny). While targeting RAS proteins for therapeutic purposes has thus far been challenging, a better understanding of the context in which oncogenic RAS is expressed and how it controls tumor–vascular interface may unveil some hitherto unappreciated opportunities.

Acknowledgments I am indebted to my collaborators Drs Nigel Mackman, George Broze, Mark Anderson, Abhijit Guha, Jeffrey Weitz, and Petr Klement and above all to my family for continuous support and understanding, with special thanks to Danuta and Anna Rak. This work was supported by funds from the Canadian Cancer Society, Canadian Institutes of Health Research, and Cancer Research Society. Infrastructure funding was provided by Fonds de la recherche en sante du Quebec (FRSQ). The author holds the Jack Cole Chair in Pediatric Oncology at McGill University.

References

Abe K, Shoji M, Chen J, Bierhaus A, Danave I, Micko C, Casper K, Dillehay DL, Nawroth PP, Rickles FR (1999) Regulation of vascular endothelial growth factor production and angiogenesis by the cytoplasmic tail of tissue factor. Proc Natl Acad Sci U S A 96:8663–8668.

Agudo-Ibanez L, Nunez F, Calvo F, Berenjeno IM, Bustelo XR, Crespo P (2007) Transcriptomal profiling of site-specific Ras signals. Cell Signal 19:2264–2276.

Ahmad SA, Liu W, Jung YD, Fan F, Wilson M, Reinmuth N, Shaheen RM, Bucana CD, Ellis LM (2001) The effects of angiopoietin-1 and -2 on tumor growth and angiogenesis in human colon cancer. Cancer Res 61:1255–1259.

Al-Nedawi K, Meehan B, Micelef J, May L, Guha A, Rak J (2008) Intercellular transfer of the oncogenic EGFRvIII *via* tumor cell derived microvesicles. Nature Cell Biology 10(5):619–24.

Alitalo K and Carmeliet P (2002) Molecular mechanisms of lymphangiogenesis in health and disease. Cancer Cell 1:219–227.

Alitalo K, Tammela T, Petrova TV (2005) Lymphangiogenesis in development and human disease. Nature 438:946–953.

Ancrile B, Lim KH, Counter CM (2007) Oncogenic Ras-induced secretion of IL6 is required for tumorigenesis. Genes Dev 21:1714–1719.

Ancrile BB, O'Hayer KM, Counter CM (2008) Oncogenic ras-induced expression of cytokines: A new target of anti-cancer therapeutics. Mol Interv 8:22–27.

Asahara T, Murohara T, Sullivan A, Silver M, van der Zee R, Li T, Witzenbichler B, Schatteman G, Isner JM (1997) Isolation of putative progenitor endothelial cells for angiogenesis. Science 275:964–967.

Asahara T, Takahashi T, Masuda H, Kalka C, Chen D, Iwaguro H, Inai Y, Silver M, Isner JM (1999) VEGF contributes to postnatal neovascularization by mobilizing bone marrow-derived endothelial progenitor cells. EMBO J 18:3964–3972.

Baj-Krzyworzeka M, Szatanek R, Weglarczyk K, Baran J, Urbanowicz B, Branski P, Ratajczak MZ, Zembala M (2006) Tumour-derived microvesicles carry several surface determinants and mRNA of tumour cells and transfer some of these determinants to monocytes. Cancer Immunol Immunother 55:808–818.

Balducci L and Ershler WB (2005) Cancer and ageing: A nexus at several levels. Nat Rev Cancer 5:655–662.

Bao S, Wu Q, Sathornsumetee S, Hao Y, Li Z, Hjelmeland AB, Shi Q, McLendon RE, Bigner DD, Rich JN (2006) Stem Cell-like Glioma Cells Promote Tumor Angiogenesis through Vascular Endothelial Growth Factor. Cancer Res 66:7843–7848.

Bar-Sagi D and Hall A (2000) Ras and Rho GTPases: A family reunion. Cell 103:227–238.

Bergers G and Benjamin LE (2003) Tumorigenesis and the angiogenic switch. Nat Rev Cancer 3:401–410.

Bergers G, Brekken R, McMahon G, Vu TH, Itoh T, Tamaki K, Tanzawa K, Thorpe P, Itohara S, Werb Z, Hanahan D (2000) Matrix metalloproteinase-9 triggers the angiogenic switch during carcinogenesis. Nat Cell Biol 2:737–744.

Bergers G, Song S, Meyer-Morse N, Bergsland E, Hanahan D (2003) Benefits of targeting both pericytes and endothelial cells in the tumor vasculature with kinase inhibitors. J Clin Invest 111:1287–1295.

Berra E, Pages G, Pouyssegur J (2000) MAP kinases and hypoxia in the control of VEGF expression. Cancer Metastasis Rev 19:139–145.

Bertolini F, Shaked Y, Mancuso P, Kerbel RS (2006) The multifaceted circulating endothelial cell in cancer: Towards marker and target identification. Nat Rev Cancer 6:835–845.

Bishop JM (1995) Cancer: The rise of the genetic paradigm. Genes Dev 9:1309–1315.

Boccaccio C, Sabatino G, Medico E, Girolami F, Follenzi A, Reato G, Sottile A, Naldini L, Comoglio PM (2005) The MET oncogene drives a genetic programme linking cancer to haemostasis. Nature 434:396–400.

Bouck N, Stellmach V, Hsu SC (1996) How tumors become angiogenic. Adv Cancer Res 69: 135–174.

Browder T, Folkman J, Pirie-Shepherd S (2000) The hemostatic system as a regulator of angiogenesis. J Biol Chem 275:1521–1524.

Buller HR, van Doormaal FF, van Sluis GL, Kamphuisen PW (2007) Cancer and thrombosis: From molecular mechanisms to clinical presentations. J Thromb Haemost 5(Suppl 1):246–254.

Burri PH (1991) Intussusceptive microvascular growth, a new mechanism of capillary network expansion. Angiogenesis, International Symposium, St Gallen, March 13–15, 1991 Abstract:88.

Calabrese C, Poppleton H, Kocak M, Hogg TL, Fuller C, Hamner B, Oh EY, Gaber MW, Finklestein D, Allen M, Frank A, Bayazitov IT, Zakharenko SS, Gajjar A, Davidoff A, Gilbertson RJ (2007) A perivascular niche for brain tumor stem cells. Cancer Cell 11: 69–82.

Carmeliet P (2000) Mechanisms of angiogenesis and arteriogenesis. Nat Med 6:389–395.

Carmeliet P (2005) Angiogenesis in life, disease and medicine. Nature 438:932–936.

Carmeliet P and Jain RK (2000) Angiogenesis in cancer and other diseases. Nature 407:249–257.

Carmeliet P and Tessier-Lavigne M (2005) Common mechanisms of nerve and blood vessel wiring. Nature 436:193–200.

Carmeliet P, Ferreira V, Breier G, Pollefeyt S, Kieckens L, Gertsenstein M, Fahrig M, Vandenhoeck A, Harpal K, Eberhardt C, Declercq C, Pawling J, Moons L, Collen D, Risau W, Nagy A (1996) Abnormal blood vessel development and lethality in embryos lacking a single VEGF allele. Nature 380:435–439.

Carmeliet P, Moons L, Luttun A, Vincenti V, Compernolle V, De Mol M, Wu Y, Bono F, Devy L, Beck H, Scholz D, Acker T, DiPalma T, Dewerchin M, Noel A, Stalmans I, Barra A, Blacher S, Vandendriessche T, Ponten A, Eriksson U, Plate KH, Foidart JM, Schaper W, Charnock-Jones DS, Hicklin DJ, Herbert JM, Collen D, Persico MG (2001) Synergism between vascular endothelial growth factor and placental growth factor contributes to angiogenesis and plasma extravasation in pathological conditions. Nat Med 7:575–583.

Carver LA and Schnitzer JE (2003) Caveolae: Mining little caves for new cancer targets. Nat Rev Cancer 3:571–581.

Casanovas O, Hicklin DJ, Bergers G, Hanahan D (2005) Drug resistance by evasion of antiangiogenic targeting of VEGF signaling in late-stage pancreatic islet tumors. Cancer Cell 8:299–309.

Chen BK, Liu YW, Yamamoto S, Chang WC (1997) Overexpression of Ha-ras enhances the transcription of human arachidonate 12-lipoxygenase promoter in A431 cells. Biochim Biophys Acta 1344:270–277.

Chin L, Tam A, Pomerantz J, Wong M, Holash J, Bardeesy N, Shen Q, O'Hagan R, Pantginis J, Zhou H, Horner JW, Cordon-Cardo C, Yancopoulos GD, DePinho RA (1999) Essential role for oncogenic Ras in tumour maintenance. Nature 400:468–472.

Claudio PP, Stiegler P, Howard CM, Bellan C, Minimo C, Tosi GM, Rak J, Kovatich A, De Fazio P, Micheli P, Caputi M, Leoncini L, Kerbel R, Giordano GG, Giordano A (2001) RB2/p130 gene-enhanced expression down-regulates vascular endothelial growth factor expression and inhibits angiogenesis in vivo. Cancer Res 61:462–468.

Cohen T, Nahari D, Cerem LW, Neufeld G, Levi B-Z (1996) Interleukin 6 induces the expression of vascular endothelial growth factor. J Biol Chem 271:736–741.

Contrino J, Hair G, Kreutzer DL, Rickles FR (1996) In situ detection of tissue factor in vascular endothelial cells: Correlation with the malignant phenotype of human breast disease. Nat Med 2:209–215.

Coughlin SR (2005) Protease-activated receptors in hemostasis, thrombosis and vascular biology. J Thromb Haemost 3:1800–1814.

Coussens LM, Raymond WW, Bergers G, Laig-Webster M, Behrendtsen O, Werb Z, Caughey GH, Hanahan D (1999) Inflammatory mast cells up-regulate angiogenesis during squamous epithelial carcinogenesis. Genes Dev 13:1382–1397.

Cox AD (2003) Farnesyltransferase inhibitors as anticancer agents. In: Rak, J (ed) Oncogene-Directed Therapies. Humana Press, Totowa, pp. 353–362.

Dameron KM, Volpert OV, Tainsky MA, Bouck N (1994) Control of angiogenesis in fibroblasts by p53 regulation of thrombospondin-1. Science 265:1582–1584.

Dang CV and Semenza GL (1999) Oncogenic alterations of metabolism. Trends Biochem Sci 24:68–72.

Dawson DW, Volpert OV, Gillis P, Crawford SE, Xu H, Benedict W, Bouck NP (1999) Pigment epithelium-derived factor: A potent inhibitor of angiogenesis. Science 285:245–248.

Detmar M (1996) Molecular regulation of angiogenesis in the skin. J Invest Dermatol 106: 207–208.

Dews M, Homayouni A, Yu D, Murphy D, Sevignani C, Wentzel E, Furth EE, Lee WM, Enders GH, Mendell JT, Thomas-Tikhonenko A (2006) Augmentation of tumor angiogenesis by a Myc-activated microRNA cluster. Nat Genet 38:1060–1065.

Di Guglielmo GM, Baass PC, Ou WJ, Posner BI, Bergeron JJ (1994) Compartmentalization of SHC, GRB2 and mSOS, and hyperphosphorylation of Raf-1 by EGF but not insulin in liver parenchyma. EMBO J 13:4269–4277.

Ding H, Roncari L, Shannon P, Wu X, Lau N, Karaskova J, Gutmann DH, Squire JA, Nagy A, Guha A (2001) Astrocyte-specific expression of activated p21-ras results in malignant astrocytoma formation in a transgenic mouse model of human gliomas. Cancer Res 61:3826–3836.

Dlugosz AA, Hansen L, Cheng C, Alexander N, Denning MF, Threadgill DW, Magnuson T, Coffey RJ, Jr., Yuspa SH (1997) Targeted disruption of the epidermal growth factor receptor impairs growth of squamous papillomas expressing the v-ras(Ha) oncogene but does not block in vitro keratinocyte responses to oncogenic ras. Cancer Res 57:3180–3188.

Dong J, Grunstein J, Tejada M, Peale F, Frantz G, Liang WC, Bai W, Yu L, Kowalski J, Liang X, Fuh G, Gerber HP, Ferrara N (2004) VEGF-null cells require PDGFR alpha signaling-mediated stromal fibroblast recruitment for tumorigenesis. EMBO J 23:2800–2810.

Downward J (2003) Targeting RAS signalling pathways in cancer therapy. Nat Rev Cancer 3: 11–22.

Dvorak FH and Rickles FR (2006) Malignancy and Hemostasis. In: Coleman RB, Marder VJ, Clowes AW, George JN Goldhaber SZ (eds) Hemostasis and Thrombosis: Basic Principles and Clinical Practice, Fifth edn. Lippincott Company Williams & Wilkins, Philadelphia, pp 851–873.

Dvorak HF (2002) Vascular permeability factor/vascular endothelial growth factor: A critical cytokine in tumor angiogenesis and a potential target for diagnosis and therapy. J Clin Oncol 20:4368–4380.

Dvorak HF, Nagy JA, Dvorak AM (1991) Structure of solid tumors and their vasculature: Implications for therapy with monoclonal antibodies. Cancer Cells 3:77–85.

Fearon ER and Vogelstein B (1990) A genetic model for colorectal tumorigenesis. Cell 61: 759–767.

Feldkamp MM, Lau N, Rak J, Kerbel RS, Guha A (1999) Normoxic and hypoxic regulation of vascular endothelial growth factor (VEGF) by astrocytoma cells is mediated by Ras. Int J Cancer 81:118–124.

Ferrara N (2005) VEGF as a therapeutic target in cancer. Oncology 69 Suppl 3:11–16.

Ferrara N and Gerber HP (2001) The role of vascular endothelial growth factor in angiogenesis. Acta Haematol 106:148–156.

Ferrara N and Kerbel RS (2005) Angiogenesis as a therapeutic target. Nature 438:967–974.

Ferrara N, Carver-Moore K, Chen H, Dowd M, Lu L, O'Shea KS, Powell-Braxton L, Hillan KJ, Moore MW (1996) Heterozygous embryonic lethality induced by targeted inactivation of the VEGF gene. Nature 380:439–442.

Filmus J, Shi W, Spencer T (1993) Role of transforming growth factor alpha (TGF-α) in the transformation of *ras*-transfected rat intestinal epithelial cells. Oncogene 8:1017–1022.

Folkman J (1971) Tumor angiogenesis: Therapeutic implications. N Engl J Med 285: 1182–1186.

Folkman J (1985) Tumor angiogenesis. Adv Cancer Res 43:175–203.

Folkman J (1990) What is the evidence that tumors are angiogenesis-dependent? J Natl Canc Inst 82:4–6.

Folkman J and Kalluri R (2003) Tumor Angiogenesis. In: Kufe DW, Pollock RE, Weichselbaum RR, Bast Jr., RC, Gansler TS, Holland JF, Frei, E, III (eds) Cancer Medicine, 6 edn. BC Decker Inc., Hamilton, London, pp 161–194.

Fong GH, Rossant J, Gertsenstein M, Breitman ML (1995) Role of the Flt-1 receptor tyrosine kinase in regulating the assembly of vascular endothelium. Nature 376:66–70.

Gerhardt H, Golding M, Fruttiger M, Ruhrberg C, Lundkvist A, Abramsson A, Jeltsch M, Mitchell C, Alitalo K, Shima D, Betsholtz C (2003) VEGF guides angiogenic sprouting utilizing endothelial tip cell filopodia. J Cell Biol 161:1163–1177.

Gesierich S, Berezovskiy I, Ryschich E, Zoller M (2006) Systemic induction of the angiogenesis switch by the tetraspanin D6.1A/CO-029. Cancer Res 66:7083–7094.

Giaccia A (2003) Genetic basis of altered responsiveness of cancer cells to their microenvironment. In: Rak, J (ed) Oncogene-Directed Therapies. Humana Press, Totowa, pp 113–132.

Gibbs JB, Oliff A, Kohl NE (1994) Farnesyltransferase inhibitors: ras research yields a potential cancer therapeutic. Cell 77:175–178.

Gille J, Swerlick RA, Caughman SW (1997) Transforming growth factor-alpha-induced transcriptional activation of the vascular permeability factor (VPF/VEGF) gene requires AP-2-dependent DNA binding and transactivation. EMBO J 16:750–759.

Gimbrone M, Leapman S, Cotran R, Folkman J (1972) Tumor dormancy in vivo by prevention of neovascularization. J Exp Med 136:261–276.

Grimbacher B, Huber M, von Kempis J, Kalden P, Uhl M, Kohler G, Blum HE, Peter HH (1998) Successful treatment of gastrointestinal vasculitis due to systemic lupus erythematosus with intravenous pulse cyclophosphamide: A clinical case report and review of the literature. Br J Rheumatol 37:1023–1028.

Grugel S, Finkenzeller G, Weindel K, Barleon B, Marme D (1995) Both v-Ha-ras and v-raf stimulate expression of the vascular endothelial growth factor in NIH 3T3 cells. J Biol Chem 270:25915–25919.

Grunewald M, Avraham I, Dor Y, Bachar-Lustig E, Itin A, Jung S, Chimenti S, Landsman L, Abramovitch R, Keshet E (2006) VEGF-induced adult neovascularization: Recruitment, retention, and role of accessory cells. Cell 124:175–189.

Grunstein J, Roberts WG, Mathieu-Costello O, Hanahan D, Johnson RS (1999) Tumor-derived expression of vascular endothelial growth factor is a critical factor in tumor expansion and vascular function. Cancer Res 59:1592–1598.

Grunstein J, Masbad JJ, Hickey R, Giordano F, Johnson RS (2000) Isoforms of vascular endothelial growth factor act in a coordinate fashion To recruit and expand tumor vasculature. Mol Cell Biol 20:7282–7291.

Guerra C, Mijimolle N, Dhawahir A, Dubus P, Barradas M, Serrano M, Campuzano V, Barbacid M (2003) Tumor induction by an endogenous K-ras oncogene is highly dependent on cellular context. Cancer Cell 4:111–120.

Guha A (1998) Ras activation in astrocytomas and neurofibromas. Can J Neurol Sci 25:267–281.

Gum R, Lengyel E, Juarez J, Chen JH, Sato H, Seiki M, Boyd D (1996) Stimulation of 92-kDa gelatinase B promoter activity by ras is mitogen-activated protein kinase kinase 1-independent and requires multiple transcription factor binding sites including closely spaced PEA3/ets and AP-1 sequences. J Biol Chem 271:10672–10680.

Hanahan D (1997) Signaling vascular morphogenesis and maintenance. Science 277:48–50.

Hanahan D and Folkman J (1996) Patterns and emerging mechanisms of the angiogenic switch during tumorigenesis. Cell 86:353–364.

Hanahan D and Weinberg RA (2000) The hallmarks of cancer. Cell 100:57–70.

Harada H, Nakagawa K, Iwata S, Saito M, Kumon Y, Sakaki S, Sato K, Hamada K (1999) Restoration of wild-type *p16* down-regulates vascular endothelial growth factor expression and inhibits angiogenesis in human gliomas. Cancer Res 59:3783–3789.

Harris AL (2002) Hypoxia–a key regulatory factor in tumour growth. Nat Rev Cancer 2:38–47.

Hasegawa H, Ueda M, Watanabe M, Teramoto T, Mukai M, Kitajima M (1995) K-*ras* gene mutations in early colorectal cancer . . . flat elevated vs polyp-forming cancer . . . . Oncogene 10:1413–1416.

Hellstrom M, Phng LK, Hofmann JJ, Wallgard E, Coultas L, Lindblom P, Alva J, Nilsson AK, Karlsson L, Gaiano N, Yoon K, Rossant J, Iruela-Arispe ML, Kalen M, Gerhardt H, Betsholtz C

(2007) Dll4 signalling through Notch1 regulates formation of tip cells during angiogenesis. Nature 445:776–780.

Hendrix MJ, Seftor EA, Hess AR, Seftor RE (2003) Vasculogenic mimicry and tumour-cell plasticity: Lessons from melanoma. Nat Rev Cancer 3:411–421.

Hlatky L, Tsionou C, Hahnfeldt P, Coleman CN (1994) Mammary fibroblasts may influence breast tumor angiogenesis via hypoxia-induced vascular endothelial growth factor up-regulation and protein expression. Cancer Res 54:6083–6086.

Ho M, Yang E, Matcuk G, Deng D, Sampas N, Tsalenko A, Tabibiazar R, Zhang Y, Chen M, Talbi S, Ho YD, Wang J, Tsao PS, Ben Dor A, Yakhini Z, Bruhn L, Quertermous T (2003) Identification of endothelial cell genes by combined database mining and microarray analysis. Physiol Genomics 13:249–262.

Holash J, Maisonpierre PC, Compton D, Boland P, Alexander CR, Zagzag D, Yancopoulos GD, Wiegand SJ (1999) Vessel cooption, regression, and growth in tumors mediated by angiopoietins and VEGF. Science 284:1994–1998.

Hurwitz HI, Fehrenbacher L, Hainsworth JD, Heim W, Berlin J, Holmgren E, Hambleton J, Novotny WF, Kabbinavar F (2005) Bevacizumab in combination with fluorouracil and leucovorin: An active regimen for first-line metastatic colorectal cancer. J Clin Oncol. 23(15):3502–3508

Iberg N, Rogelj S, Fanning P, Klagsbrun M (1989) Purification of 18- and 22-kDa forms of basic fibroblast growth factor from rat cells transformed by the ras oncogene. J Biol Chem 264:19951–19955.

Ince WL, Jubb AM, Holden SN, Holmgren EB, Tobin P, Sridhar M, Hurwitz HI, Kabbinavar F, Novotny WF, Hillan KJ, Koeppen H (2005) Association of k-ras, b-raf, and p53 status with the treatment effect of bevacizumab. J Natl Cancer Inst 97:981–989.

Inoue M, Hager JH, Ferrara N, Gerber HP, Hanahan D (2002) VEGF-A has a critical, nonredundant role in angiogenic switching and pancreatic beta cell carcinogenesis. Cancer Cell 1: 193–202.

Irani K, Xia Y, Zweier JL, Sollott SJ, Der CJ, Fearon ER, Sundaresan M, Finkel T, Goldschmidt-Clermont PJ (1997) Mitogenic signaling mediated by oxidants in Ras-transformed fibroblasts. Science 275:1649–1652.

Jain RK (2001) Normalizing tumor vasculature with anti-angiogenic therapy: A new paradigm for combination therapy. Nature Med 7:987–989.

Jamal H, Cano-gauci DF, Buick RN, Filmus J (1994) Activated *ras* and *src* induce CD44 overexpression in rat intestinal epithelial cells. Oncogene 9:417–423.

Janz A, Sevignani C, Kenyon K, Ngo CV, Thomas-Tikhonenko A (2000) Activation of the myc oncoprotein leads to increased turnover of thrombospondin-1 mRNA. Nucleic Acids Res 28:2268–2275.

Jiang BH, Agani F, Passaniti A, Semenza GL (1997) V-SRC induces expression of hypoxia-inducible factor 1 (HIF-1) and transcription of genes encoding vascular endothelial growth factor and enolase 1: Involvement of HIF-1 in tumor progression. Cancer Res 57: 5328–5335.

Jingjing L, Srinivasan B, Roque RS (2001) Ectodomain shedding of VEGF183, a novel isoform of vascular endothelial growth factor, promotes its mitogenic activity in vitro. Angiogenesis 4:103–112.

Jones N and Dumont DJ (2000) Tek/Tie2 signaling: New and old partners. Cancer Metastasis Rev 19:13–17.

Jones N, Iljin K, Dumont DJ, Alitalo K (2001) Tie receptors: New modulators of angiogenic and lymphangiogenic responses. Nat Rev Mol Cell Biol 2:257–267.

Jubb AM, Oates AJ, Holden S, Koeppen H (2006) Predicting benefit from anti-angiogenic agents in malignancy. Nat Rev Cancer 6:626–635.

Kalas W, Klement P, Rak J (2005a) Downregulation of the angiogenesis inhibitor thrombospondin 1 in fibroblasts exposed to platelets and their related phospholipids. Biochem Biophys Res Commun 334:549–554.

Kalas W, Yu JL, Milsom C, Rosenfeld J, Benezra R, Bornstein P, Rak J (2005b) Oncogenes and Angiogenesis: Down-regulation of Thrombospondin-1 in Normal Fibroblasts Exposed to Factors from Cancer Cells Harboring Mutant Ras. Cancer Res 65:8878–8886.

Kalluri R (2003) Basement membranes: Structure assembly and role in tumor angiogenesis. Nature Reviews Cancer 3:422–433.

Kaplan RN, Riba RD, Zacharoulis S, Bramley AH, Vincent L, Costa C, MacDonald DD, Jin DK, Shido K, Kerns SA, Zhu Z, Hicklin D, Wu Y, Port JL, Altorki N, Port ER, Ruggero D, Shmelkov SV, Jensen KK, Rafii S, Lyden D (2005) VEGFR1-positive haematopoietic bone marrow progenitors initiate the pre-metastatic niche. Nature 438:820–827.

Karnoub AE and Weinberg RA (2008) Ras oncogenes: Split personalities. Nat Rev Mol Cell Biol 9:517–531.

Kerbel RS and Folkman J (2002) Clinical translation of angiogenesis inhibitors. Nature Reviews Cancer 2:727–739.

Kevil CG, De Benedetti A, Payne DK, Coe LL, Laroux FS, Alexander JS (1996) Translational regulation of vascular permeability factor by eukaryotic initiation factor 4E: Implications for tumor angiogenesis. Int J Cancer 65:785–790.

Khosravi-Far R, Campbell S, Rossman KL, Der CJ (1998) Increasing complexity of Ras signal transduction: Involvement of Rho family proteins. Adv Cancer Res 72:57–107:57–107.

Kim IY, Jeong SJ, Kim ES, Kim SH, Moon A (2007) Type I collagen-induced pro-MMP-2 activation is differentially regulated by H-Ras and N-Ras in human breast epithelial cells. J Biochem Mol Biol 40:825–831.

Kim KJ, Li B, Winer J, Armanini M, Gillett N, Phillips HS, Ferrara N (1993) Inhibition of vascular endothelial growth factor-induced angiogenesis suppresses tumour growth in vivo. Nature 362:841–844.

Klagsbrun M and Eichmann A (2005) A role for axon guidance receptors and ligands in blood vessel development and tumor angiogenesis. Cytokine Growth Factor Rev 16:535–548.

Klement H, St CB, Milsom C, May L, Guo Q, Yu JL, Klement P, Rak J (2007) Atherosclerosis and Vascular Aging as Modifiers of Tumor Progression, Angiogenesis, and Responsiveness to Therapy. Am J Pathol 171:1342–1351.

Kranenburg O, Gebbink MF, Voest EE (2004) Stimulation of angiogenesis by Ras proteins. Biochim Biophys Acta 1654:23–37.

Laderoute KR, Alarcon RM, Brody MD, Calaoagan JM, Chen EY, Knapp AM, Yun Z, Denko NC, Giaccia AJ (2000) Opposing effects of hypoxia on expression of the angiogenic inhibitor thrombospondin 1 and the angiogenic inducer vascular endothelial growth factor. Clin Cancer Res 6:2941–2950.

Lange T, Guttmann-Raviv N, Baruch L, Machluf M, Neufeld G (2003) VEGF162, a new heparin-binding vascular endothelial growth factor splice form that is expressed in transformed human cells. J Biol Chem 278:17164–17169.

Larcher F, Franco M, Bolontrade M, Rodriguez-Puebla M, Casanova L, Navarro M, Yancopoulos G, Jorcano JL, Conti CJ (2003) Modulation of the angiogenesis response through Ha-ras control, placenta growth factor, and angiopoietin expression in mouse skin carcinogenesis. Mol Carcinog 37:83–90.

Leong KG and Karsan A (2006) Recent insights into the role of Notch signaling in tumorigenesis. Blood 107:2223–2233.

Levine MN, Gent M, Hirsh J, Arnold A, Goodyear MD, Hryniuk W, De Pauw S (1988) The thrombogenic effect of anticancer drug therapy in women with stage II breast cancer. N Engl J Med 318:404–407.

Levine RJ, Maynard SE, Qian C, Lim KH, England LJ, Yu KF, Schisterman EF, Thadhani R, Sachs BP, Epstein FH, Sibai BM, Sukhatme VP, Karumanchi SA (2004) Circulating angiogenic factors and the risk of preeclampsia. N Engl J Med 350:672–683.

Li B, Sharpe EE, Maupin AB, Teleron AA, Pyle AL, Carmeliet P, Young PP (2006) VEGF and PlGF promote adult vasculogenesis by enhancing EPC recruitment and vessel formation at the site of tumor neovascularization. FASEB J 20:1495–1497.

Liebner S, Cavallaro U, Dejana E (2006) The multiple languages of endothelial cell-to-cell communication. Arterioscler Thromb Vasc Biol 26:1431–1438.

Lu C, Vickers MF, Kerbel RS (1992) Interleukin-6: A fibroblast-derived growth inhibitor of human melanoma cells from early but not advanced stages of tumor progression. Proc Natl Acad Sci (USA) 89:9215–9219.

Lundkvist A, Lee S, Iruela-Arispe L, Betsholtz C, Gerhardt H (2007) Growth factor gradients in vascular patterning. Novartis Found Symp 283:194–201.

Mackman N (2008) Triggers, targets and treatments for thrombosis. Nature 451:914–918.

Malumbres M and Barbacid M (2003) RAS oncogenes: The first 30 years. Nat Rev Cancer 3: 459–465.

Mazure NM, Chen EY, Yeh P, Laderoute KR, Giaccia AJ (1996) Oncogenic transformation and hypoxia synergistically act to modulate vascular endothelial growth factor expression. Cancer Res 56:3436–3440.

Mazure NM, Chen EY, Laderoute KR, Giaccia AJ (1997) Induction of vascular endothelial growth factor by hypoxia is modulated by a phosphatidylinositol 3-kinase/Akt signaling pathway in Ha-ras- transformed cells through a hypoxia inducible factor-1 transcriptional element. Blood 90:3322–3331.

McCormick F (2003) Signal transduction networks. Ras as a paradigm. In: Rak, J (ed) Oncogene-Directed Therapies. Humana Press, Totowa, pp 35–46.

Meade-Tollin LC, Boukamp P, Fusenig NE, Bowen CP, Tsang TC, Bowden GT (1998) Differential expression of matrix metalloproteinases in activated c-ras-Ha-transfected immortalized human keratinocytes. Br J Cancer 77:724–730.

Mechtcheriakova D, Schabbauer G, Lucerna M, Clauss M, de Martin R, Binder BR, Hofer E (2001) Specificity, diversity, and convergence in VEGF and TNF-{alpha} signaling events leading to tissue factor up-regulation via EGR-1 in endothelial cells. FASEB J 15:230–242.

Mettouchi A, Cabon F, Montreau N, Vernier P, Mercier G, Blangy D, Tricoire H, Vigier P, Binetruy B (1994) SPARC and thrombospondin genes are repressed by the c-jun oncogene in rat embryo fibroblasts. EMBO J 13:5668–5678.

Milanini J, Vinals F, Pouyssegur J, Pages G (1998) p42/p44 MAP kinase module plays a key role in the transcriptional regulation of the vascular endothelial growth factor gene in fibroblasts. J Biol Chem 273:18165–18172.

Millauer B, Shawver LK, Plate KH, Risau W, Ullrich A (1994) Glioblastoma growth inhibited in vivo by a dominant-negative Flk-1 mutant. Nature 367:576–579.

Millauer B, Longhi MP, Plate KH, Shawver LK, Risau W, Ullrich A, Strawn LM (1996) Dominant-negative inhibition of Flk-1 suppresses the growth of many tumor types in vivo. Cancer Res 56:1615–1620.

Milsom C and Rak J (2005) Regulation of tissue factor and angiogenesis related genes by changes in cell shape. Biochem Biophys Res Commun 337(4):1267–75.

Milsom C, Anderson GM, Weitz JI, Rak J (2007a) Elevated tissue factor procoagulant activity in CD133-positive cancer cells. J Thromb Haemost 5:2550–2552.

Milsom C, Yu J, May L, Meehan B, Magnus N, Al-Nedawi K, Luyendyk J, Weitz J, Klement P, Broze G, Mackman N, Rak J (2007b) The role of tumor- and host-related tissue factor pools in oncogene-driven tumor progression. Thromb Res 120 Suppl 2:S82–S91.

Minamoto T, Sawaguchi K, Mai M, Yamashita N, Sugimura T, Esumi H (1994) Infrequent K-ras activation in superficial-type (flat) colorectal adenomas and adenocarcinomas. Cancer Res 54:2841–2844.

Morrissey JH (2004) Tissue factor: A key molecule in hemostatic and nonhemostatic systems. Int J Hematol 79:103–108.

Moskovits N, Kalinkovich A, Bar J, Lapidot T, Oren M (2006) p53 Attenuates cancer cell migration and invasion through repression of SDF-1/CXCL12 expression in stromal fibroblasts. Cancer Res 66:10671–10676.

Mueller BM, Reisfeld RA, Edgington TS, Ruf W (1992) Expression of tissue factor by melanoma cells promotes efficient hematogenous metastasis. Proc Natl Acad Sci U S A 89:11832–11836.

Nanda A and St Croix B (2004) Tumor endothelial markers: New targets for cancer therapy. Curr Opin Oncol 16:44–49.

Neri D and Bicknell R (2005) Tumour vascular targeting. Nat Rev Cancer 5:436–446.

Neufeld G, Cohen T, Gengrinovitch S, Poltorak Z (1999) Vascular endothelial growth factor (VEGF) and its receptors. FASEB J 13:9–22.

Nierodzik ML and Karpatkin S (2006) Thrombin induces tumor growth, metastasis, and angiogenesis: Evidence for a thrombin-regulated dormant tumor phenotype. Cancer Cell 10:355–362.

Noguera-Troise I, Daly C, Papadopoulos NJ, Coetzee S, Boland P, Gale NW, Lin HC, Yancopoulos GD, Thurston G (2006) Blockade of Dll4 inhibits tumour growth by promoting non-productive angiogenesis. Nature 444:1032–1037.

Nystrom HC, Lindblom P, Wickman A, Andersson I, Norlin J, Faldt J, Lindahl P, Skott O, Bjarnegard M, Fitzgerald SM, Caidahl K, Gan LM, Betsholtz C, Bergstrom G (2006) Platelet-derived growth factor B retention is essential for development of normal structure and function of conduit vessels and capillaries. Cardiovasc Res 71:557–565.

O'Reilly MS, Holmgren L, Shing Y, Chen c, Rosenthal RA, Moses M, Lane SW, Cao Y, Sage EH, Folkman J (1994) Angiostatin: A novel angiogenesis inhibitor that mediates the suppression of metastases by a Lewis lung carcinoma. Cell 79:315–328.

O'Reilly MS, Boehm T, Shing Y, Fukai N, Vasios G, Lane WS, Flynn E, Birkhead JR, Olsen BR, Folkman J (1997) Endostatin: An endogenous inhibitor of angiogenesis and tumor growth. Cell 88:277–285.

Ocak I, Baluk P, Barrett T, McDonald DM, Choyke P (2007) The biologic basis of in vivo angiogenesis imaging. Front Biosci 12:3601–3616.

Okada F, Rak J, St.Croix B, Lieubeau B, Kaya M, Roncari L, Sasazuki S, Kerbel RS (1998) Impact of oncogenes on tumor angiogenesis: Mutant *K-ras* upregulation of VEGF/VPF is necessary but not sufficient for tumorigenicity of human colorectal carcinoma cells. Proc Natl Acad Sci (USA) 95:3609–3614.

Paku S and Paweletz N (1991) First steps of tumor-related angiogenesis. Lab Invest 65:334–346.

Palumbo JS, Talmage KE, Massari JV, La Jeunesse CM, Flick MJ, Kombrinck KW, Hu Z, Barney KA, Degen JL (2007) Tumor cell-associated tissue factor and circulating hemostatic factors cooperate to increase metastatic potential through natural killer cell-dependent and-independent mechanisms. Blood 110:133–141.

Patel NS, Li JL, Generali D, Poulsom R, Cranston DW, Harris AL (2005) Up-regulation of delta-like 4 ligand in human tumor vasculature and the role of basal expression in endothelial cell function. Cancer Res 65:8690–8697.

Paul R, Zhang ZG, Eliceiri BP, Jiang Q, Boccia AD, Zhang RI., Chopp M Cheresh DA (2001). Src deficiency or blockade of Src activity in mice provides cerebral protection following stroke. Nature Medicine 7(2), 222–227. 1–2

Paweletz N and Knierim M (1989) Tumor related angiogenesis. In: CRC critical reviews in oncology/hematology. Academic Press, Orlando, pp 197–242.

Pepper MS (2001) Role of the matrix metalloproteinase and plasminogen activator-plasmin systems in angiogenesis. Arterioscler Thromb Vasc Biol 21:1104–1117.

Perez-Atayde AR, Sallan SE, Tedrow U, Connors S, Allred E, Folkman J (1997) Spectrum of tumor angiogenesis in the bone marrow of children with acute lymphoblastic leukemia. Am J Pathol 150:815–820.

Pettersson A, Nagy JA, Brown LF, Sundberg C, Morgan E, Jungles S, Carter R, Krieger JE, Manseau EJ, Harvey VS, Eckelhoefer IA, Feng D, Dvorak AM, Mulligan RC, Dvorak HF (2000) Heterogeneity of the angiogenic response induced in different normal adult tissues by vascular permeability factor/vascular endothelial growth factor. Lab Invest 80:99–115.

Pili R, Guo Y, Chang J, Nakanishi H, Martin GR, Passaniti A (1994) Altered angiogenesis underlying age-dependent changes in tumor growth. J Natl Cancer Inst 86:1303–1314.

Poltorak Z, Cohen T, Sivan R, Kandelis Y, Spira G, Vlodavsky I, Keshet E, Neufeld G (1997) VEGF145, a secreted vascular endothelial growth factor isoform that binds to extracellular matrix. J Biol Chem 272:7151–7158.

Polunovsky VA, Gingras AC, Sonenberg N, Peterson M, Tan A, Rubins JB, Manivel JC, Bitterman PB (2000) Translational control of the antiapoptotic function of Ras. J Biol Chem 275: 24776–24780.

Prendergast GC and Oliff A (2000) Farnesyltransferase inhibitors: Antineoplastic properties, mechanisms of action, and clinical prospects. Semin Cancer Biol 10:443–452.

Pugh CW and Ratcliffe PJ (2003) The von Hippel-Lindau tumor suppressor, hypoxia-inducible factor-1 (HIF-1) degradation, and cancer pathogenesis. Semin Cancer Biol 13:83–89.

Rafii S, Lyden D, Benezra R, Hattori K, Heissig B (2002) Vascular and haematopoietic stem cells: Novel targets for anti-angiogenesis therapy? Nat Rev Cancer 2:826–835.

Rajalingam K, Schreck R, Rapp UR, Albert S (2007) Ras oncogenes and their downstream targets. Biochim Biophys Acta 1773:1177–1195.

Rak J and Kerbel RS (1996) Treating cancer by inhibiting angiogenesis: New hopes and potential pitfalls. Cancer Metastasis Rev 15:231–236.

Rak J and Kerbel RS (2001) Ras regulation of vascular endothelial growth factor and angiogenesis. Methods Enzymol 333:267–83.:267–283.

Rak J and Kerbel RS (2003) Oncogenes and tumor angiogenesis. In: Rak, J (ed) Oncogene-Directed Therapies. Humana Press, Totowa, pp 171–218.

Rak J and Klement G (2000) Impact of oncogenes and tumor suppressor genes on deregulation of hemostasis and angiogenesis in cancer. Cancer Metastasis Rev 19:93–96.

Rak J and Yu JL (2004) Oncogenes and tumor angiogenesis: The question of vascular "supply" and vascular "demand". Semin Cancer Biol 14:93–104.

Rak J, Mitsuhashi Y, Bayko L, Filmus J, Sasazuki T, Kerbel RS (1995) Mutant *ras* oncogenes upregulate VEGF/VPF expression: Implications for induction and inhibition of tumor angiogenesis. Cancer Res 55:4575–4580.

Rak J, Filmus J, Kerbel RS (1996) Reciprocal paracrine interactions between tumor cells and endothelial cells. The "angiogenesis progression" hypothesis. Eur J Cancer 32A:2438–2450.

Rak J, Mitsuhashi Y, Sheehan C, Krestow JK, Florenes VA, Filmus J, Kerbel RS (1999) Collateral expression of proangiogenic and tumorigenic properties in intestinal epithelial cell variants selected for resistance to anoikis. Neoplasia 1:23–30.

Rak J, Mitsuhashi Y, Sheehan C, Tamir A, Viloria-Petit A, Filmus J, Mansour SJ, Ahn NG, Kerbel RS (2000a) Oncogenes and tumor angiogenesis: Differential modes of vascular endothelial growth factor up-regulation in ras-transformed epithelial cells and fibroblasts. Cancer Res 60:490–498.

Rak J, Yu JL, Klement G, Kerbel RS (2000b) Oncogenes and angiogenesis: Signaling three-dimensional tumor growth. J Investig Dermatol Symp Proc 5:24–33.

Rak J, Yu JL, Luyendyk J, Mackman N (2006) Oncogenes, trousseau syndrome, and cancer-related changes in the coagulome of mice and humans. Cancer Res 66:10643–10646.

Rastinejad F, Polverini PJ, Bouck N (1989) Regulation of the activity of a new inhibitor by angiogenesis by a cancer suppressor gene. Cell 56:345–355.

Ravasco P, Monteiro-Grillo I, Camilo M (2007) How relevant are cytokines in colorectal cancer wasting? Cancer J 13:392–398.

Relf M, LeJeune S, Scott PA, Fox S, Smith K, Leek R, Moghaddam A, Whitehouse R, Bicknell R, Harris AL (1997) Expression of the angiogenic factors vascular endothelial cell growth factor, acidic and basic fibroblast growth factor, tumor growth factor beta-1, platelet-derived endothelial cell growth factor, placenta growth factor, and pleiotrophin in human primary breast cancer and its relation to angiogenesis. Cancer Res 57:963–969.

Reya T, Morrison SJ, Clarke MF, Weissman IL (2001) Stem cells, cancer, and cancer stem cells. Nature 414:105–111.

Rickles FR (2006) Mechanisms of cancer-induced thrombosis in cancer. Pathophysiol Haemost Thromb 35:103–110.

Ridgway J, Zhang G, Wu Y, Stawicki S, Liang WC, Chanthery Y, Kowalski J, Watts RJ, Callahan C, Kasman I, Singh M, Chien M, Tan C, Hongo JA, de SF, Plowman G, Yan M (2006) Inhibition of Dll4 signalling inhibits tumour growth by deregulating angiogenesis. Nature 444:1083–1087.

Rong Y, Post DE, Pieper RO, Durden DL, Van Meir EG, Brat DJ (2005) PTEN and hypoxia regulate tissue factor expression and plasma coagulation by glioblastoma. Cancer Res 65: 1406–1413.

Rosen K, Rak J, Leung T, Dean NM, Kerbel RS, Filmus J (2000) Activated Ras prevents down-regulation of Bcl-X(L) triggered by detachment from the extracellular matrix. A mechanism of Ras-induced resistance to anoikis in intestinal epithelial cells. J Cell Biol 149:447–456.

Ruf W (2007) Redundant signaling of tissue factor and thrombin in cancer progression? J Thromb Haemost 5:1584–1587.

Seaman S, Stevens J, Yang MY, Logsdon D, Graff-Cherry C, St CB (2007) Genes that distinguish physiological and pathological angiogenesis. Cancer Cell 11:539–554.

Semenza GL (2003) Targeting HIF-1 for cancer therapy. Nat Rev Cancer 3:721–732.

Serrano M, Gomez-Lahoz E, DePinho RA, Beach D, Bar-Sagi D (1995) Inhibition of ras-induced proliferation and cellular transformation by p16INK4. Science 267:249–252.

Serrano M, Lin AW, McCurrach ME, Beach D, Lowe SW (1997) Oncogenic ras provokes premature cell senescence associated with accumulation of p53 and p16INK4a. Cell 88:593–602.

Shahrzad S, Quayle L, Stone C, Plumb C, Shirasawa S, Rak JW, Coomber BL (2005) Ischemia-induced K-ras mutations in human colorectal cancer cells: Role of microenvironmental regulation of MSH2 expression. Cancer Res 65:8134–8141.

Shahrzad S, Shirasawa S, Sasazuki T, Rak JW, Coomber BL (2008) Low-dose metronomic cyclophosphamide treatment mediates ischemia-dependent K-ras mutation in colorectal carcinoma xenografts. Oncogene 27:3729–3738.

Shaked Y, Ciarrocchi A, Franco M, Lee CR, Man S, Cheung AM, Hicklin DJ, Chaplin D, Foster FS, Benezra R, Kerbel RS (2006) Therapy-induced acute recruitment of circulating endothelial progenitor cells to tumors. Science 313:1785–1787.

Shalaby F, Rossant J, Yamaguchi TP, Gertsenstein M, Wu XF, Breitman ML, Schuh AC (1995) Failure of blood-island formation and vasculogenesis in Flk-1-deficient mice. Nature 376: 62–66.

Shchors K, Shchors E, Rostker F, Lawlor ER, Brown-Swigart L, Evan GI (2006) The Myc-dependent angiogenic switch in tumors is mediated by interleukin 1beta. Genes Dev 20: 2527–2538.

Sheng H, Williams CS, Shao J, Liang P, DuBois RN, Beauchamp RD (1998) Induction of cyclooxygenase-2 by activated Ha-ras oncogene in Rat-1 fibroblasts and the role of mitogen-activated protein kinase pathway. J Biol Chem 273:22120–22127.

Shi YP and Ferrara N (1999) Oncogenic ras fails to restore an in vivo tumorigenic phenotype in embryonic stem cells lacking vascular endothelial growth factor (VEGF). Biochem Biophys Res Commun 254:480–483.

Shibuya M (2006) Differential roles of vascular endothelial growth factor receptor-1 and receptor-2 in angiogenesis. J Biochem Mol Biol 39:469–478.

Shih C and Weinberg RA (1982) Isolation of a transforming sequence from a human bladder carcinoma cell line. Cell 29:161–169.

Shirasawa S, Furuse M, Yokoyama N, Sasazuki T (1993) Altered growth of human colon cancer cell lines disrupted at activated Ki-ras. Science 260:85–88.

Shojaei F, Singh M, Thompson JD, Ferrara N (2008) Role of Bv8 in neutrophil-dependent angiogenesis in a transgenic model of cancer progression. Proc Natl Acad Sci U S A 105:2640–2645.

Sodhi A, Montaner S, Miyazaki H, Gutkind JS (2001) MAPK and Akt act cooperatively but independently on hypoxia inducible factor-1alpha in rasV12 upregulation of VEGF. Biochem Biophys Res Commun 287:292–300.

Sparmann A and Bar-Sagi D (2004) Ras-induced interleukin-8 expression plays a critical role in tumor growth and angiogenesis. Cancer Cell 6:447–458.

St.Croix B, Rago C, Velculescu V, Traverso G, Romans KE, Montgomery E, Lal A, Riggins GJ, Lengauer C, Vogelstein B, Kinzler KW (2000) Genes expressed in human tumor endothelium. Science 289:1197–1202.

Staton CA, Chetwood AS, Cameron IC, Cross SS, Brown NJ, Reed MW (2007) The angiogenic switch occurs at the adenoma stage of the adenoma-carcinoma sequence in colorectal cancer. Gut 56:1426–1432.

Subbaramaiah K, Telang N, Ramonetti JT, Araki R, DeVito B, Weksler BB, Dannenberg AJ (1996) Transcription of cyclooxygenase-2 is enhanced in transformed mammary epithelial cells. Cancer Res 56:4424–4429.

Teodoro JG, Parker AE, Zhu X, Green MR (2006) p53-mediated inhibition of angiogenesis through up-regulation of a collagen prolyl hydroxylase. Science 313:968–971.

Teodoro JG, Evans SK, Green MR (2007) Inhibition of tumor angiogenesis by p53: A new role for the guardian of the genome. J Mol Med 85:1175–1186.

Testa JE, Medcalf RL, Cajot JF, Schleuning WD, Sordat B (1989) Urokinase-type plasminogen activator is induced by the EJ-Ha-ras oncogene in CL26 mouse colon carcinoma cells. Int J Cancer 43:816–822.

Thomson W and Mackie RM (1989) Comparison of five antimelanoma antibodies for identification of melanocytic cells on tissue sections in routine dermatopathology. J Am Acad Dermatol 21:1280–1284.

Thurston G, Noguera-Troise I, Yancopoulos GD (2007) The Delta paradox: DLL4 blockade leads to more tumour vessels but less tumour growth. Nat Rev Cancer 7:327–331.

Timoshenko AV, Rastogi S, Lala PK (2007) Migration-promoting role of VEGF-C and VEGF-C binding receptors in human breast cancer cells. Br J Cancer 97:1090–1098.

Tischer E, Mitchell R, Hartman T, Silva M, Gospodarowicz D, Fiddes JC, Abraham JA (1991) The human gene for vascular endothelial growth factor. Multiple protein forms are encoded through alternative exon splicing. J Biol Chem 266:11947–11954.

Trousseau, A (1865) Phlegmasia alba dolens. Clinique Medicale de l'Hotel -Dieu de Paris. The Sydenham Society Second edition, Paris, France, 654–712.

Tuveson DA, Shaw AT, Willis NA, Silver DP, Jackson EL, Chang S, Mercer KL, Grochow R, Hock H, Crowley D, Hingorani SR, Zaks T, King C, Jacobetz MA, Wang L, Bronson RT, Orkin SH, DePinho RA, Jacks T (2004) Endogenous oncogenic K-ras(G12D) stimulates proliferation and widespread neoplastic and developmental defects. Cancer Cell 5:375–387.

Varki A (2007) Trousseau's syndrome: Multiple definitions and multiple mechanisms. Blood 110:1723–1729.

Verheul HM and Pinedo HM (2007) Possible molecular mechanisms involved in the toxicity of angiogenesis inhibition. Nat Rev Cancer 7:475–485.

Viloria-Petit A, Miquerol L, Yu JL, Gertsenstein M, Sheehan C, May L, Henkin J, Lobe C, Nagy A, Kerbel RS, Rak J (2003) Contrasting effects of VEGF gene disruption in embryonic stem cell-derived versus oncogene-induced tumors. EMBO J 22:4091–4102.

Volpert OV, Dameron KM, Bouck N (1997) Sequential development of an angiogenic phenotype by human fibroblasts progressing to tumorigenicity. Oncogene 14:1495–1502.

Wang HU, Chen ZF, Anderson DJ (1998) Molecular distinction and angiogenic interaction between embryonic arteries and veins revealed by ephrin-B2 and its receptor Eph-B4. Cell 93:741–753.

Warren RS, Yuan H, Mati MR, Gillett NA, Ferrara N (1995) Regulation by vascular endothelial growth factor of human colon cancer tumorigenesis in a mouse model of experimental liver metastasis. J Clin Invest 95:1789–1797.

Watnick RS, Cheng Y-N, Rangarajan A, Ince TA, Weinberg RA (2003) Ras modulates Myc activity to repress thrombospondin-1 expression and increase tumor angiogenesis. Cancer Cell 3:219–231.

Weinberg RA (1996) How cancer arises. Sci Am 275:62–70.

Weinstat-Saslow DL, Zabrenetzky VS, VanHoutte K, Frazier WA, Roberts DD, Steeg PS (1994) Transfection of thrombospondin 1 complementary DNA into a human breast carcinoma cell line reduces primary tumor growth, metastatic potential, and angiogenesis. Cancer Res 54:6504–6511.

White FC, Benehacene A, Scheele JS, Kamps M (1997) VEGF mRNA is stabilized by ras and tyrosine kinase oncogenes, as well as by UV radiation–evidence for divergent stabilization pathways. Growth Factors 14:199–212.

Wong AK, Alfert M, Castrillon DH, Shen Q, Holash J, Yancopoulos GD, Chin L (2001) Excessive tumor-elaborated VEGF and its neutralization define a lethal paraneoplastic syndrome. Proc Natl Acad Sci U S A 19;98:7481–7486.

Woolard J, Wang WY, Bevan HS, Qiu Y, Morbidelli L, Pritchard-Jones RO, Cui TG, Sugiono M, Waine E, Perrin R, Foster R, Digby-Bell J, Shields JD, Whittles CE, Mushens RE, Gillatt DA, Ziche M, Harper SJ, Bates DO (2004) VEGF165b, an inhibitory vascular endothelial growth factor splice variant: Mechanism of action, in vivo effect on angiogenesis and endogenous protein expression. Cancer Res 64:7822–7835.

Yamagata S, Muto T, Uchida Y, Masaki T, Higuchi Y, Sawada T, Hirooka T (1995) Polypoid growth and K-ras codon 12 mutation in colorectal cancer. Cancer 75:953–957.

Yancopoulos GD, Davis S, Gale NW, Rudge JS, Wiegand SJ, Holash J (2000) Vascular-specific growth factors and blood vessel formation. Nature 407:242–248.

Yang G, Rosen DG, Zhang Z, Bast RC, Jr., Mills GB, Colacino JA, Mercado-Uribe I, Liu J (2006) The chemokine growth-regulated oncogene 1 (Gro-1) links RAS signaling to the senescence of stromal fibroblasts and ovarian tumorigenesis. Proc Natl Acad Sci U S A 103:16472–16477.

Yu JL and Rak JW (2004) Shedding of tissue factor (TF)-containing microparticles rather than alternatively spliced TF is the main source of TF activity released from human cancer cells. J Thromb Haemost 2:2065–2067.

Yu JL, Rak JW, Coomber BL, Hicklin DJ, Kerbel RS (2002a) Effect of p53 status on tumor response to antiangiogenic therapy. Science 295:1526–1528.

Yu J, Rak JW, Klement G, Kerbel RS (2002b) VEGF isoform expression as a determinant of blood vessel patterning in human melanoma xenografts. Cancer Res 62:1838–1846.

Yu JL, May L, Klement P, Weitz JI, Rak J (2004) Oncogenes as regulators of tissue factor expression in cancer: Implications for tumor angiogenesis and anti-cancer therapy. Semin Thromb Hemost 30:21–30.

Yu JL, May L, Lhotak V, Shahrzad S, Shirasawa S, Weitz JI, Coomber BL, Mackman N, Rak JW (2005) Oncogenic events regulate tissue factor expression in colorectal cancer cells: Implications for tumor progression and angiogenesis. Blood 105:1734–1741.

Zabrenetzky V, Harris CC, Steeg PS, Roberts DD (1994) Expression of the extracellular matrix molecule thrombospondin inversely correlates with malignant progression in melanoma, lung and breast carcinoma cell lines. Int J Cancer 59:191–195.

Zuber J, Tchernitsa OI, Hinzmann B, Schmitz AC, Grips M, Hellriegel M, Sers C, Rosenthal A, Schafer R (2000) A genome-wide survey of RAS transformation targets. Nat Genet 24:144–152.

Chapter 8
Myc and Control of Tumor Neovascularization

Prema Sundaram, Chi V. Dang, and Andrei Thomas-Tikhonenko

Cast of Characters

The hallmark of Burkitt's and some other non-Hodgkin lymphomas and leukemias is the (8;14) translocation that subjects the c-myc proto-oncogene to the control of a heavy chain gene enhancer (Dalla-Favera et al. 1982; Taub et al. 1982). Additionally, double minute chromosomes (dmin) containing amplified copies of the c-Myc gene are commonly detected in acute myeloid leukemia (AML) and myelodysplastic syndromes (MDS) (Storlazzi et al. 2004). In parallel, rearrangements and amplifications of the c-MYC locus are hallmarks of many solid neoplasms. For example, the LINE-1 element insertion leads to MYC rearrangement in the case of breast carcinoma (Morse et al. 1988) and up to 50% of breast carcinomas show a gain in copy number of the 8q24 band containing MYC (Ioannidis et al. 2003). Another Myc family member, MYCN, is amplified in neuroblastoma cell lines (Kohl et al. 1983) and primary tumors, where it correlates with advance disease stage (Brodeur et al. 1984). Yet, despite the wealth of data implicating Myc in the pathogenesis of cancer, its exact contribution to neoplastic traits is not completely understood. Much recent evidence points towards the involvement of Myc in cell-extrinsic processes, such as angiogenesis.

Introduction

Several essential intracellular processes are closely controlled by the c-myc oncogene, which encodes a basic helix-loop-helix/leucine zipper transcription factor. To accomplish its functions, c-Myc transcriptionally activates target genes by dimerizing with the Myc-associated protein X, or MAX, usually at the expense of another MAX-interacting protein MAD (Grandori et al. 2000). Once bound to gene promoters, the Myc–Max dimer further recruits a variety of transcriptional regulators

A. Thomas-Tikhonenko (✉)
University of Pennsylvania and the Children's Hospital of Philadelphia, 516H Abramson Research Center, Philadelphia, PA, USA
e-mail: andreit@mail.med.upenn.edu

A. Thomas-Tikhonenko (ed.), *Cancer Genome and Tumor Microenvironment*, DOI 10.1007/978-1-4419-0711-0_8, © Springer Science+Business Media, LLC 2010

including histone-modifying enzymes (McMahon et al. 1998). Myc can also act as a transcriptional repressor (or de-activator), and this function is thought to involve interactions with Miz1 (Peukert et al. 1997), Sp1 (Gartel et al. 2001), and other partners. Recently, a comprehensive set of c-Myc-regulated genes have been identified using high-throughput techniques (Coller et al. 2000; Dang et al. 2006; Zeller et al. 2006). While the exact molecular mechanisms controlling gene regulation by Myc are still being debated (Meyer and Penn 2008), it is clear that c-Myc has a profound influence on the expression of a multitude of genes, which are involved in parallel, complementary, conflicting, and sometimes frankly antagonistic pathways. The ensuing tug of war involves signals that, depending on the context, can promote cell proliferation, de-differentiation, and apoptosis (Dang 1999; Meyer and Penn 2008), which are frequent hallmarks of neoplastic transformation. According to a recent study, at physiological, low-threshold levels, c-Myc stimulates primarily proliferation, whereas at high levels it helps cells commit to apoptosis (Murphy et al. 2008). The role of c-myc in maintaining cell stemness is also well recognized (Laurenti et al. 2008); and more recently a non-transcriptional, direct replicative role of c-Myc has been demonstrated (Dominguez-Sola et al. 2007).

In addition to these fundamental processes that directly control cell numbers, Myc family proteins regulate target genes that are involved in cellular growth (i.e., increase in size) and metabolism (Coller et al. 2000; Neiman et al. 2001; Meyer and Penn 2008). When deregulated, Myc swiftly boosts protein synthesis independently of mitotic divisions, thereby directly increasing cellular mass. This can be observed in human Burkitt's lymphomas as well as in murine models of lymphomagenesis (Iritani and Eisenman 1999; Johnston et al. 1999; Schuhmacher et al. 1999). c-Myc has also been shown to directly activate rRNA synthesis and ribosome biogenesis in Drosophila as well as in human cells (Grandori et al. 2005; Grewal et al. 2005).

Another important approach that deregulated Myc takes to promote tumor growth is to compromise genome integrity and increase DNA amplification (Mai et al. 1996; Felsher and Bishop 1999; Li and Dang 1999). In addition to inflicting genotoxic stress, Myc directly activates some components of DNA damage response by promoting stability of p53 tumor suppressor featured in preceding chapters (Eischen et al. 1999). And just as p53 plays key roles in both cell-intrinsic and cell-extrinsic processes, Myc has important non-cell-autonomous effects, such as stimulation of angiogenesis.

Deregulated Myc, Tumor Neovascularization, and the Angiogenic Balance

The first genetic evidence that Myc contributes to neovascularization came from the laboratory of Gerard Evan and their papillomatosis model, wherein c-myc is conditionally overexpressed in the skin epidermis (Pelengaris et al. 1999). In that study, c-Myc was expressed from the involucrin promoter as a fusion with the mutated form of estrogen receptor (MycER^{TM}) requiring for nuclear localization the presence of the activating ligand, 4-hydroxytamoxifen (4OHT). Turning on Myc via topical application of 4OHT resulted in the thickening of the skin epidermis due to the rapid proliferation of suprabasal keratinocytes and eventually – papillomatosis. Furthermore, in vivo differentiation of post-mitotic keratinocytes was suspended and apoptosis was attenuated. Interestingly, this pathology was accompanied by a commensurate increase in new blood vasculature (Pelengaris et al. 1999). Continuous expression of c-myc was required to maintain both papillomatosis and the associated angiogenic phenotype. In fact, turning off c-myc by withdrawing 4OHT resulted in overt regression of blood vessels, demonstrating the independent role of c-myc in promoting neovascularization.

Another study of the angiogenic effects of Myc utilized Rat-1A fibroblasts which had been transformed by a retrovirus encoding human c-Myc (Ngo et al. 2000). When Rat-1A/Myc fibroblasts were injected into immunocompromised mice, they developed large tumors with abundant vasculature. To demonstrate that the observed angiogenesis was driven by Myc independently of tumor growth, corneal and Matrigel neovascularization assays were performed in parallel. In the first assay, conditioned media from myc-transformed and control fibroblast were introduced into polyvinyl sponges, which were then surgically inserted into virtually avascular rat corneas. Ten days after the implantation, endothelial cell proliferation and abundant neovascularization were observed. In parallel, fibroblasts expressing MycER^{TM} were incorporated into subcutaneous Matrigel plugs. Pronounced neovascularization of Matrigels was apparent in animals systemically treated with 4OHT but not in control mice.

A similar role for Myc as an inducer of vasculature formation has been successfully demonstrated in systems other than the mouse, namely in the chicken bursal lymphomagenesis model (Brandvold et al. 2000). Two ways to induce lymphomagenesis were used in this study – one involving the avian leukosis retrovirus integrating next to the c-myc proto-oncogene and another involving HB-1 retrovirus itself encoding the v-myc oncogene. An increase in microvascular density beginning very early (13 days) after the transplantation of both c-myc and v-myc-transformed bursal progenitor cells was observed. This vasculature has been found to be maintained through all stages of lymphomagenesis. Additionally, media conditioned by cultured myc-transformed bursal cells were found to stimulate proliferation of human microvascular endothelial cells in vitro.

Thus, at least in genetically simple systems, where c-Myc is the only transforming protein, it could be directly implicated in the induction of angiogenesis and vascular homeostasis. The latter, as mentioned in preceding chapters, is controlled by a complex set of regulatory factors. These factors could be divided into two categories – pro-angiogenic cytokines such as vascular endothelial growth factor A (VEGF A), B, and C, acidic and basic fibroblast growth factors (a/bFGF), angiopoietin-1 (Ang-1) [reviewed in (Adams and Alitalo 2007)], and anti-angiogenic inhibitors such as thrombospondins 1 and 2 (TSP-1/2) (Rastinejad et al. 1989; Volpert et al. 1995a,b), angiostatin (O'Reilly 1997), and endostatin (O'Reilly et al. 1997). An equilibrium that exists between these activating and inhibitory molecules is thought to maintain the angiogenic balance in normal tissues under physiological conditions. However, this balance is impaired during the course of neoplastic progression resulting in abnormal tumor neovascularization (Bouck et al. 1996). In light of the "balance hypothesis," the pro-angiogenic effects could be accomplished by either activating an activator, or inhibiting an inhibitor, or performing both tasks simultaneously. How does Myc go about it?

The Myc-VEGF Axis in Tumorigenesis

Myc as the Inducer of VEGF

Some early answers to this mechanistic question came from B-cell lymphoma research. It is well recognized that angiogenesis is an integral part of tumor expansion in B-cell malignancies (Perez-Atayde et al. 1997; Vacca et al. 1999; Saaristo et al. 2000). Also, B-cell tumors are known to be a good source of a secreted pro-angiogenic factor VEGF-A (herein referred to simply as VEGF). Other members of the VEGF family, notably C and D, are known to promote mainly lymphangiogenesis, or growth of new lymphatic vessels (Alitalo and Carmeliet 2002; Adams and Alitalo 2007).

The role of c-myc in VEGF-mediated angiogenesis and lymphangiogenesis has been investigated by several groups. Ruddell and colleagues observed that activation of c-Myc, placed under the control of a tetracycline-inducible promoter, increased VEGF expression up to 10-fold in both human B-cell line P493-6 and avian B cells (Mezquita et al. 2005). This is true not only in vitro but also in vivo, as noted in the murine model of Burkitt's lymphoma (Eµ-myc mice), where c-Myc is overexpressed specifically in the B-lymphocytes of bone marrow and lymph nodes (Ruddell et al. 2003). These pre-cancerous tissues showed an increase in the expression of endothelial markers VEGFR-2 and VEGFR-3. Moreover, blood vasculature and lymphatic vessel formation were pronounced in both tissues. Tracker-dye flow experiments also showed that the new lymphatic vessels were fully functional and hence capable of promoting tumor expansion by metastasis.

Another study that extensively analyzed the effect of c-Myc on VEGF expression was performed using c-myc-null embryonic stem (ES) cells (Baudino et al. 2002). The c-Myc-null mice die very early in embryogenesis with several developmental defects. A close examination of the $c\text{-}myc^{-/-}$ embryos revealed that they harbored defects in several processes such as vasculogenesis, angiogenesis, differentiation, and erythropoiesis. These defects were attributed to very low levels of VEGF expression in the absence of wild-type c-Myc. Northern blot and real-time PCR showed a reduction in the levels of VEGF mRNA. In situ hybridization performed in $c\text{-}myc^{-/-}$ embryos further confirmed the downregulation of VEGF expression in both the embryo proper and the yolk sac. When injected into *Scid* mice, $c\text{-}myc^{-/-}$ ES cells formed significantly smaller tumors compared to either $c\text{-}myc^{+/-}$ or $c\text{-}myc^{+/+}$ counterparts. Thus, c-Myc appears to be essential for VEGF expression in vivo.

However, c-Myc might not have any direct role in increasing VEGF transcription or VEGF mRNA levels. There was no evidence for direct binding of Myc to the

VEGF promoter region, although the latter does contain a conserved Myc-binding sequence. Measurement of VEGF mRNA levels by quantitative PCR revealed that c-Myc had no direct role in increasing VEGF transcription in human P493-6 cells (Mezquita et al. 2005). Instead, c-Myc was shown to indirectly increase VEGF protein levels by increasing the translation of VEGF mRNA. It was reported in an earlier work that c-Myc overexpression can increase the levels of the translation initiation factor eIF-4E (Rosenwald et al. 1993), which could in turn increase the translation of VEGF mRNA (Kevil et al. 1996). In this study, however, increased VEGF mRNA translation was not associated with an increase in this factor; rather there was an increase in the loading of VEGF mRNA onto polysomes. Thus, the mechanism by which c-Myc promotes VEGF translation is complex and may be dependent on the cell type.

This idea could be further supported by revisiting the $c\text{-}myc^{-/-}$ ES model (Baudino et al. 2002) where VEGF seems to be only partially responsible for the defects observed in the $c\text{-}myc^{-/-}$ embryos. Restoration of VEGF levels incompletely rescued the loss of tumorigenic potential of $c\text{-}myc^{-/-}$ ES cells, suggesting that additional pathways had been rendered non-functional due to the loss of c-Myc. Furthermore, induction of VEGF may not be the universal mechanism of promoting angiogenesis in all tissues or tumor types. For example, undifferentiated keratinocytes expressing MycER^{TM} show elevated VEGF levels (Pelengaris et al. 1999), whereas Rat-1A fibroblasts expressing MycER^{TM} show no noticeable changes in the levels of VEGF (Ngo et al. 2000).

Nevertheless, several lines of evidence, both in vitro and in vivo, show that c-Myc is the major regulator of VEGF and potentially other angiogenic factors, which cooperate to promote angiogenesis in embryonic as well as adult tissues under normal and pathological conditions. Depending on the tumor/cell type c-Myc may directly or indirectly stimulate VEGF expression either by transcriptional or post-transcriptional mechanisms. These and other findings led to the idea that induction of VEGF production by Myc might be contingent upon certain physiological or pathological conditions and molecular determinants thereof. What could these conditions be? Important clues have emerged from the analysis of Myc-induced phenotypes.

Myc, Hypoxia, and VEGF

As outlined above, c-Myc is a master regulator of cell proliferation, cell growth, and metabolism. Thus, induction of endogenous Myc in normal cells by growth factors is followed by the activation of a regulated program of cell growth that is dominated by ribosomal biogenesis, coupled with mitochondrial biogenesis that provides adequate energy for cellular entry into S phase, where the fidelity of DNA replication is paramount. When growth factor signaling ceases, Myc expression diminishes and the cell returns to a resting state. By contrast, deregulated Myc expression in cancer cells leads to a constitutive drive for cell growth and cell proliferation, which are both highly demanding of oxygen for energy production, such that decoupling of energy production from the drive for cell growth results in apoptosis. Hence, as deregulated c-Myc drives the cell into uncontrolled growth, its will create a hypoxic microenvironment wherein an expanding three-dimensional cellular mass is limited by diffusion of oxygen and nutrients to the core of hypoxic cells. In this regard, c-Myc-induced cell proliferation creates a hypoxic tumor microenvironment, which is known to promote angiogenesis (see Chapter 6.)

In order to determine if VEGF is involved in c-Myc-induced hypoxia and ensuing angiogenesis, the same involucrin-mycER^{TM} was employed (Pelengaris et al. 1999). In situ hybridization in post-mitotic keratinocytes isolated from the epidermal tumors overexpressing c-Myc revealed localization of VEGF mRNA to hypoxia-rich regions of the inner sheath cells of hair follicles (Knies-Bamforth et al. 2004). Similar results were obtained in vitro where high VEGF levels were attained only when cells were exposed to hypoxic conditions. Increased VEGF expression not only coincided with hypoxia-rich regions but also was shown to be responsible for promoting angiogenesis. In fact, inhibiting VEGF dramatically reduced angiogenesis in vivo in mouse epidermal tumors overexpressing c-Myc (Knies-Bamforth et al. 2004). As a separate observation, hypoxia increased the transcription of VEGF mRNA and at the same time contributed to the VEGF mRNA stability in rat glial tumor cells (Stein et al. 1995). How could this be explained mechanistically?

Hypoxia triggers the production of hypoxia-inducible factors 1 and 2 (HIF-1 and HIF-2; see Chapter 6), which transactivate target genes, thus helping tumor cells adapt to and survive the low-oxygen environment. Some of these genes encode transcription factors, metabolic enzymes, cytokines and, predictably, pro-angiogenic factors such as VEGF and Ang1 (Forsythe et al. 1996; Kelly et al. 2003; Manalo et al. 2005; Semenza 2008). It was shown as early as in 1996 that HIF-1 induces VEGF transcription by directly binding to the HIF Response Element (HRE) in the 5'region of the VEGF gene (Forsythe et al. 1996; Semenza 2008). Perhaps deregulated c-Myc works in concert with HIF-1 to increase VEGF protein output? Verification of this hypothesis proved difficult, primarily because interactions between c-Myc and HIF-1 appear to vary depending on the cellular context.

Several groups studying VHL-deficient renal carcinomas with stabilized HIF-1 have shown that HIF-1 inhibits c-Myc function under normal physiological conditions (Koshiji et al. 2004; Zhang et al. 2007), wherein HIF-1 might positively cooperate with deregulated c-Myc oncoprotein (Gordan et al. 2007a). Similar results have also been observed in the P493-6 Burkitt's lymphoma model with an inducible Myc, whereas hypoxia-induced HIF-1 cooperates with deregulated c-Myc and triggers the production of VEGF to promote angiogenesis (Kim et al. 2007). HIF-2, on the other hand, appears to cooperate with c-Myc by increasing its activity, if not steady-state levels (Gordan et al. 2007b; Gordan and Simon 2007).

Therefore, the propensity of HIF-1 to antagonize or cooperate with c-Myc depends on whether c-Myc is a deregulated oncoprotein or whether the interplay between Myc and HIF-1 unfolds in a physiological context. HIF-2, which is highly expressed naturally in endothelial cells is expected to collaborate with Myc, particularly under physiological conditions, when endothelial cells are recruited into a hypoxic region and need to proliferate in a Myc-dependent fashion (Manalo et al. 2005). On the other hand, non-endothelial cells are expected to trigger a different response to hypoxia under the pathological condition of ischemia. This is because they would be best served by withdrawing into a resting (G0/G1) phase until normal oxygen tension and supply of nutrients are restored following re-vascularization of an ischemic tissue. This physiological context is in marked contrast to a cluster of deregulated cancer cells which have escaped normal cues and hence adapted to proliferate under hypoxic conditions. There, deregulation of the c-myc gene alters the stoichiometric balance between Myc and HIF-1, to the effect that despite HIF-1 overexpression enough c-Myc is available to bind to Max and promote tumorigenesis (Dang et al. 2008).

Having concluded that HIF-1 cooperates with the c-Myc oncoprotein, one might ask if c-Myc has any direct effect on HIF-1 expression in tumors. This remains an open question, but there is one recent piece of evidence suggesting that c-Myc inhibits HIF-1 through a microRNA (miRNA)-based mechanism. miRNAs are short non-coding RNAs, which are cleaved out of exons or introns of PolII transcripts and are known to control a wide variety of developmental processes. Their physiological role is to repress gene expression by binding to the partially complementary 3'UTRs of target mRNAs and facilitating formation of RNA-interference silencing complexes (RISC). This usually leads to inhibition of translation, mRNA degradation (Chang and Mendell 2007), or sequestration of mRNA in P-bodies (Liu et al. 2005). Notably, c-Myc induces expression of the 6-microRNA cluster, mir-17-92 (O'Donnell, Wentzel 2005) which has been shown to inhibit HIF-1a expression in lung cancer cell lines (Taguchi, Yanagisawa 2008). This suggests that there might be a feedback loop that connects c-Myc and HIF-1; and that it could be either positive or negative depending on the cellular context (Fig. 8.1).

However, with more research underway, this relatively simple relationship between c-Myc and HIF might soon be replaced by a more intricate model taking

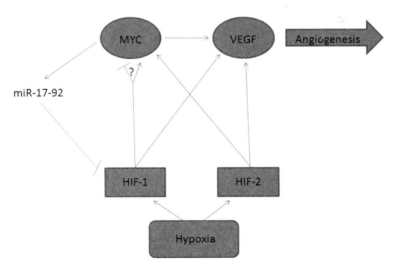

Fig. 8.1 Complex interactions between Myc, HIFs, and VEGF. Original artwork by Kathryn Simmermon, MHA/MHE

Fig. 8.2 Heterogeneity of tumor microenvironment with respect to hypoxia. Fluorescent micrograph documenting BrdU (*green*) incorporation and hypoxic areas stained (*red*) with anti-pimonidazole antibody (Hypoxyprobe™; *red*) in a section of a P493-6 human B-lymphoma xenograft (courtesy of Anne Le in C. Dang laboratory)

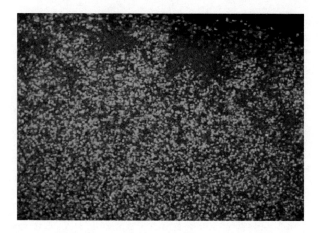

into account tumor heterogeneity. It should be noted that the tumor microenvironment is a complex jumble of areas with high- and low-proliferation rates and also of areas that are near-anoxic, hypoxic, or relatively normoxic, depending on the distance to the nearest blood vessel (Fig. 8.2). In this context, the interplay between hypoxic and non-hypoxic cells is another important arena for further studies with regard to the role of Myc and HIF in tumorigenesis.

Myc, Normoxia, Inflammation, and VEGF

c-Myc can trigger tumor angiogenesis in a hypoxia-independent manner as well. This has been demonstrated by Gerard Evan's group, which used the transgenic mouse model pIns-*MycER^{TM}; RIP7-Bcl-x_L* wherein the switchable c-MycER™ expression is under the control of the insulin promoter active exclusively in β-cells of the pancreas (Shchors et al. 2006). Two days after Myc activation in the β-cells, there was an increase in the β-cell population, as expected. However, there was also an increase in cell proliferation in the neighboring endothelial compartment which did not overexpress c-Myc. When c-Myc expression was switched off, both the β-cell compartment of the pancreas as well as the endothelial compartment showed a reduction in cell proliferation. This clearly suggested that angiogenesis is indeed c-Myc induced, with a signal from the β-cells acting in *trans* and activating the adjacent endothelial cells. However, no markers of hypoxia were detected in c-Myc expressing β-cells nor was there an increase in VEGF mRNA.

Instead, the angiogenic signal from c-Myc-expressing β-cells turned out to be interleukin-1β (IL-1β), which was induced 2 h after c-Myc activation. IL-1β in turn stimulated matrix metalloprotease (MMP) activity in β-cells which mobilized pre-existing VEGF from the extracellular matrix. MMPs, in particular MMP-9, had already been shown to be involved in the mobilization of tissue-bound VEGF (Bergers et al. 2000). Newly released VEGF was now able to instruct adjacent endothelial cells to proliferate. Interestingly, inactivation of IL-1β in the pancreatic tumor model only delayed but not completely blocked angiogenesis, suggesting that additional c-Myc-responsive pro-inflammatory stimuli might be involved in angiogenesis and tumor formation as well (Shchors et al. 2006).

Indeed, a more recent study from the same laboratory has shown that mast cells were rapidly recruited to the β-cell site upon c-Myc activation (Soucek et al. 2007). Once recruited, mast cells serve as a rich source of VEGF and various MMPs, which increase tissue angiogenesis and tumor expansion. In fact, the β-cells in mast cell-deficient mice $Kit^{W-sh/W-sh}$ lose the capacity to rapidly expand upon c-myc overexpression. Moreover, Myc activation was followed by induction of several chemokines (e.g., *Ccl2, Cxcl2, Ccl7*, and *Ccl5*) which attract not only mast cells but neutrophils and macrophages as well, thus creating a rich pro-angiogenic milieu (Soucek et al. 2007). This could be regarded as a paradox, since in other systems acute inflammation exerts anti-angiogenic effects (Hunter et al. 2001; Thomas-Tikhonenko and Hunter 2003).

Other Ways to Flip the Switch

VEGF-Independent Effects of Myc

While the connection between Myc overexpression and VEGF upregulation is well established, it is context dependent and does not occur in every cell type or organ system. Furthermore, with respect to genetically complex neoplasms, it is not entirely clear what the major genetic cues are that trigger the angiogenic switch and irrevocably alter the balance between pro- and anti-angiogenic molecules. One certainly could speculate that Myc drives tumor neovascularization when it is the only functional oncoprotein [e.g., in the papillomatosis model], but in genetically complex neoplasms activation of VEGF is attained by other oncoproteins. Indeed, both Ha- and Ki-Ras are known to activate VEGF (Grugel et al. 1995; Rak et al. 1995; Okada et al. 1998; Serban et al. 2008) and increase the activity of matrix metalloproteinases (MMP) (Arbiser et al. 1997) required for endothelial cell migration. The loss of p53 also results in upregulation of VEGF (Mukhopadhyay et al. 1995; Volpert et al. 1997) and potentially − in improved stability of hypoxia-induced factor alpha (HIF1α) (Ravi et al. 2000), the principal physiological inducer of VEGF. Thus, it was to be expected that in neoplastic cells with activated Ki-Ras and null for p53 (for example, advanced colon carcinoma cells) Myc will have little if any effect on VEGF production.

To determine if this is the case, a previously established line of p53-null murine colonocytes (Sevignani et al. 1998) was transformed by the c-Myc and Ki-Ras oncogenes. While Ki-Ras-overexpressing cells formed subcutaneous tumors within 3 weeks, no neoplasms were apparent in mice injected with Myc-overexpressing colonocytes, even after prolonged observation and in an orthotopic location (cecal wall.) While overexpression of Myc did not confer overt tumorigenicity upon p53-null colonocytes, it was possible that it would enhance the tumorigenic potential of their Ki-Ras-transformed counterparts. To this end, Ki-Ras/p53-null cells were infected with a Myc/GFP-encoding MIGR1 retrovirus. In vitro, Ras and Myc/Ras cultures grew in vitro at the same rate, but while control Ras/GFP cells formed small, indolent tumors, Ras/Myc/GFP neoplasms were on average three times larger. The same positive effect of Myc on tumor growth was observed with MycER^{TM}-overexpressing Ras-colonocytes in 4OHT-treated animals (Dews et al. 2006).

To reveal the nature of Myc effects, histological examination of size-matched tumors was performed. Most strikingly, Myc-overexpressing tumors possessed much more robust neovascularization. Especially numerous were large caliber vessels richly perfused with red blood cells. Similar differences emerged when the same sections were stained with lectin to visualize endothelial cells. While Ki-Ras tumors contained only solitary lectin-positive cells, the latter were found to surround apparent luminal structures in Myc/Ras neoplasms (Fig. 8.3). In contrast, there was no increase in the density of lymphatic vessels, as judged by LYVE-1 staining, in spite of the reported propensity of Myc to promote lymphangiogenesis (Ruddell et al. 2003).

To determine whether the effects of Myc on angiogenesis are mediated by hypoxia or VEGF production, levels of HIF1α and VEGF were assessed in Ras-alone and RasMyc tumors. Neither tumor type had detectable HIF1α levels; and

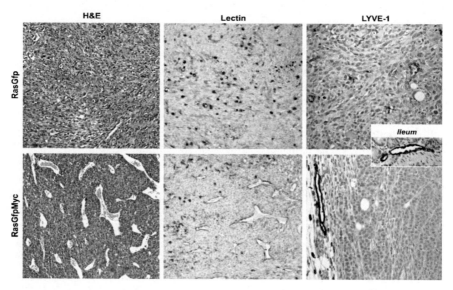

Fig. 8.3 Comparative analysis of RasGfp and RasGfpMyc tumors. Left column depicts hematoxylin+eosin staining (H&E). Perfused blood vessels contain numerous red blood cells. Middle column depicts staining of endothelial cells with lectin (*brown*). Right column depicts staining of lymphatic vessels with an antibody against LYVE-1 (*brown*). The insert depicts staining of normal ileum. From (Dews et al. 2006)

there was no upregulation, at the mRNA level, of a variety of known hypoxia-activated genes such as Glut1 or VEGF-A. To investigate possible deregulation of VEGF at the protein level, ELISA was performed on tumor cell lysates. Again, no difference in VEGF production between Ras-alone and RasMyc neoplasms was apparent (Dews et al. 2006). This suggested that Myc can induce angiogenesis in a VEGF-independent manner. How might it work?

Downregulation of Thrombospondin-1 and Related Proteins by Myc

It stood to reason that VEGF-independent pro-angiogenic effects of Myc could be explained by its propensity to downregulate endogenous anti-angiogenic factors such as thrombospondin-1. Many normal cells do maintain high levels of thrombospondin-1 (TSP-1) (Good et al. 1990) which largely accounts for their non-angiogenic phenotype. This was first shown by Noel Bouck's laboratory studying cultured fibroblasts from patients with the Li-Fraumeni syndrome (heterozygocity for p53). Following loss of the remaining allele of tp53, the levels of Tsp-1 fell dramatically, which coincided with robust angiogenicity of cultures fibroblasts (Dameron et al. 1994). Several other studies have linked downregulation of thrombospondin-1 to activating mutations in the Ras oncogene (Rak et al. 2000; Ren et al. 2006) suggesting that it is an important negative regulator of tumor neovascularization.

To a large extent, the anti-angiogenic properties of thrombospondin-1 are mediated by the so-called thrombospondin-1 type 1 repeats (TSR), a cysteine-rich amino acid sequence (Guo et al. 1997; Iruela-Arispe et al. 1999; Adams and Tucker 2000). Consistent with this notion, peptides derived from TSR have shown promise in preclinical (Bogdanov et al. 1999; Miao et al. 2001; Reiher et al. 2002) and lately clinical trials (Hoekstra et al. 2005). Interestingly, TSRs are shared by a diverse group of proteins, and some of them also possess anti-angiogenic properties, for example, SPARC (Chlenski et al. 2002), and spondin-1 (Terai et al. 2001). For other members, the anti-angiogenic connection has not been established or remains controversial. One case in point is the connective tissue growth factor (CTGF), which has been ascribed to both pro-angiogenic (Babic et al. 1999; Shimo et al. 2001a; Shimo et al. 2001b) and anti-angiogenic (Inoki et al. 2002) and anti-neoplastic (Moritani et al. 2003) properties. One possible resolution of this paradox is that while CTGF might intrinsically promote angiogenesis during embryonic development (Lau and Lam 1999; Perbal 2004), it is also known to sequester VEGF, which is required in tumor contexts for endothelial cell proliferation/survival (Brigstock 2002).

That c-Myc potently downregulates thrombospondin-1 expression was first demonstrated using transformed Rat-1A fibroblasts where c-Myc was the only functional oncoprotein (Tikhonenko et al. 1996). These cells upon c-Myc activation showed marked decrease in the TSP-1 levels, but retained unaltered levels of VEGF.

Nevertheless, the net phenotype was overtly angiogenic, both in Matrigel and cornea neovascularization assays (Ngo et al. 2000).

Subsequently, a mouse model expressing conditional Myc under the control of Tet promoter in the hematopoietic system demonstrated the cooperative role of p53 and Myc in regulating the levels of Tsp-1 (Giuriato et al. 2006). Hematopoietic tumors that have inactive Myc showed regression only in the presence of wild-type p53. Lymphomas harboring mutations in p53 showed initial regression of the tumor upon Myc inactivation but the tumorigenic phenotype relapsed later. This relapse was associated with low levels of TSP-1 in the absence of p53. However, restoration of either wild-type p53 or TSP-1 resulted in the continuous regression of tumor suggesting that c-Myc requires p53 activity to downregulate TSP-1

As Myc often works hand-in-hand with a cooperating oncogene in rodents (Land et al. 1983), it came as no surprise that Myc and Ras coordinate downregulation of TSP-1 in transformed human epithelial cells (Watnick et al. 2003). In this study, low-Ras expressing cells formed smaller tumors and were lacking in their ability to induce neo-vascularization. High-Ras expressing cells, on the other hand, were able to form large tumors when transplanted into mice, primarily by downregulating TSP-1 and thereby increasing angiogenesis. Interestingly, Ras achieves this by activating Myc via the PI3 Kinase/Rho/ROCK signaling pathway. Phosphorylated Myc, in turn, downregulates Tsp-1 thereby promoting angiogenesis and tumor formation (Watnick et al. 2003) [reviewed in (Volpert and Alani 2003)]. Given the effects on thrombospondin-1 of both p53 and Ras (through endogenous c-Myc), would deregulated Myc still downregulate thrombospondin-1 in a meaningful way in Myc/Ras/p53-null colon carcinoma cells?

To answer this question, microarray analysis was performed on mRNAs from Ras-alone vs. Ras Myc tumors. Interestingly, the list of Myc-downregulated genes prominently featured not only thrombospondin-1 but also several other members of the TSR superfamily (Adams and Tucker 2000): CTGF and its relative WISP2, spondin-1 (f-spondin), thrombospondin repeat containing [protein] 1, clusterin, SPARC (secreted acidic cysteine-rich glycoprotein), and thrombospondin type I domain containing protein 6.

A separate interesting question is how Myc achieves coordinate deregulation of many TSR family members. Early clues to underlying molecular mechanisms came from the study showing that c-Myc regulates TSP-1 levels by decreasing the stability of TSP-1 mRNA (Janz et al. 2000). This effect is now known to involve microRNAs, and more recently Myc has been shown to induce the expression of a microRNA cluster called mir-17-92 (O'Donnell et al. 2005). miR-17-92 cluster was also upregulated in MycRas overexpressing p53-null colonocytes (Dews et al. 2006). Provocatively, several members of the TSR superfamily are predicted targets of the miR-17-92 cluster [per TargetScan 5.0 algorithm (Friedman et al. 2009)], and indeed inhibition of mir-17-92 function with antisense oligoribonucleotides partly restores the levels of Tsp-1 and CTGF, suggesting that these and some other TSR family members are direct targets of mir-17-92 cluster. Most importantly, overexpression of mir-17-92 in Ras-only colonocytes increased tumor neovascularization and overall growth in a manner reminiscent of Myc activity (Dews et al. 2006).

Recently, another Myc family member N-Myc was shown to upregulate mir-17-92 (Fontana et al. 2008; Schulte et al. 2008; Chayka et al., 2009), suggesting that it may promote angiogenesis as well.

N-Myc and Angiogenesis

N-Myc is a proto-oncogene initially identified based on its homology to c-Myc and is frequently associated with human neuroblastoma (Kohl et al. 1983; Brodeur et al. 1984). In fact, N-Myc promotes angiogenesis and tumor progression by mechanisms both similar to and different from c-Myc. N-Myc induces angiogenesis in proliferating neuroblastoma cells at least in part by increasing VEGF expression (Kang et al. 2008). It has been shown that PI3K/Akt signaling is required to maintain N-Myc induction of VEGF. Inhibition of PI3K or Akt in neuroblastoma cells by using siRNAs significantly reduced the expression of both N-myc itself and independently – VEGF. Furthermore, it has been reported that N-myc inhibits activin A, a negative regulator of angiogenesis (Breit et al. 2000). This downregulation, unlike that by c-Myc, involves a direct interaction of N-Myc with the activin A promoter region. Another report suggests that N-Myc overexpression downregulates leukemia inhibitory factor (LIF) which affects proliferation of endothelial cells (Hatzi et al. 2002). The downregulation of LIF has been shown to be independent of c-myc and is involved in tumor progression and angiogenesis rather than increasing neuroblastoma cell proliferation and expansion. Although still sketchy, these studies have shed light on the molecular mechanisms by which N-Myc induces angiogenesis in N-Myc-amplified neuroblastoma cells. While it is not known whether N-Myc downregulates thrombospondin-1, there is evidence that thrombospondin-1-based peptide ABT-510 combined with valproic acid is an effective anti-angiogenesis strategy in neuroblastoma (Yang et al. 2007).

Conclusions

The effects of Myc family members on the expression of pro- and anti-angiogenic factors are manifold. As detailed above, one common theme is the context-dependent upregulation of VEGF expression and availability, by both hypoxia-dependent and hypoxia-independent pathways. This property alone is not unique to Myc (p53 and Ras do it!) and does not appear to be sufficient for angiogenesis. Myc also needs to downregulate key anti-angiogenic factors such as thrombospondin-1. This is achieved at least in part by modulating miRNA activity, and to the extent that levels of miRNA are highly amenable to biochemical manipulations, they represent attractive targets for therapeutic anti-angiogenesis.

There is overwhelming evidence that the angiogenic switch is one of the key events in tumor progression. Once it is turned on, neovascularization closely follows tumor cell mass expansion (Folkman and Hanahan 1991; Shpitz et al. 2003;

Takahashi et al. 2003). In most oncogene-driven multi-step mouse tumor models, it has been demonstrated that angiogenesis is a pre-requisite for tumor growth and metastasis (Hanahan 1985; Folkman et al. 1989; Bergers et al. 1999; Coussens et al. 1999; Bergers et al. 2000; Nyberg et al. 2008). In fact, some tumors might remain dormant due exclusively to their failure to recruit new blood vessels (Udagawa et al. 2002; Naumov et al. 2006; Naumov et al. 2008). To the extent that c-Myc family members aid and abet angiogenesis in a variety of ways and in different settings (Shchors and Evan, 2007), they should be regarded as key cell-extrinsic regulators of tumor progression.

Acknowledgments The authors wish to thank the members of their laboratories, in particular Dr Michael Dews, and also Dr. Celeste Simon (Penn), for many stimulating discussions concerning the nature of Myc-driven angiogenesis.

References

Adams, J. C. and R. P. Tucker (2000). "The thrombospondin type 1 repeat (TSR) superfamily: diverse proteins with related roles in neuronal development." *Dev Dyn* **218**(2): 280–99.

Adams, R. H. and K. Alitalo (2007). "Molecular regulation of angiogenesis and lymphangiogenesis." *Nat Rev Mol Cell Biol* **8**(6): 464–78.

Alitalo, K. and P. Carmeliet (2002). "Molecular mechanisms of lymphangiogenesis in health and disease." *Cancer Cell* **1**(3): 219–27.

Arbiser, J. L., M. A. Moses, C. A. Fernandez, N. Ghiso, Y. Cao, N. Klauber, D. Frank, M. Brownlee, E. Flynn, S. Parangi, H. R. Byers and J. Folkman (1997). "Oncogenic H-ras stimulates tumor angiogenesis by two distinct pathways." *Proc Natl Acad Sci U S A* **94**(3): 861–6.

Babic, A. M., C. C. Chen and L. F. Lau (1999). "Fisp12/mouse connective tissue growth factor mediates endothelial cell adhesion and migration through integrin alphavbeta3, promotes endothelial cell survival, and induces angiogenesis in vivo." *Mol Cell Biol* **19**(4): 2958–66.

Baudino, T. A., C. McKay, H. Pendeville-Samain, J. A. Nilsson, K. H. Maclean, E. L. White, A. C. Davis, J. N. Ihle and J. L. Cleveland (2002). "c-Myc is essential for vasculogenesis and angiogenesis during development and tumor progression." *Genes Dev* **16**(19): 2530–43.

Bergers, G., K. Javaherian, K. M. Lo, J. Folkman and D. Hanahan (1999). "Effects of angiogenesis inhibitors on multistage carcinogenesis in mice." *Science* **284**(5415): 808–12.

Bergers, G., R. Brekken, G. McMahon, T. H. Vu, T. Itoh, K. Tamaki, K. Tanzawa, P. Thorpe, S. Itohara, Z. Werb and D. Hanahan (2000). "Matrix metalloproteinase-9 triggers the angiogenic switch during carcinogenesis." *Nat Cell Biol* **2**(10): 737–44.

Bogdanov, A., Jr., E. Marecos, H. C. Cheng, L. Chandrasekaran, H. C. Krutzsch, D. D. Roberts and R. Weissleder (1999). "Treatment of experimental brain tumors with trombospondin-1 derived peptides: an in vivo imaging study." *Neoplasia* **1**(5): 438–45.

Bouck, N., V. Stellmach and S. C. Hsu (1996). "How tumors become angiogenic." *Adv Cancer Res* **69**: 135–74.

Brandvold, K. A., P. Neiman and A. Ruddell (2000). "Angiogenesis is an early event in the generation of myc-induced lymphomas." *Oncogene* **19**(23): 2780–5.

Breit, S., K. Ashman, J. Wilting, J. Rossler, E. Hatzi, T. Fotsis and L. Schweigerer (2000). "The N-myc oncogene in human neuroblastoma cells: down-regulation of an angiogenesis inhibitor identified as activin A." *Cancer Res* **60**(16): 4596–601.

Brigstock, D. R. (2002). "Regulation of angiogenesis and endothelial cell function by connective tissue growth factor (CTGF) and cysteine-rich 61 (CYR61)." *Angiogenesis* **5**(3): 153–65.

Brodeur, G. M., R. C. Seeger, M. Schwab, H. E. Varmus and J. M. Bishop (1984). "Amplification of N-myc in untreated human neuroblastomas correlates with advanced disease stage." *Science* **224**(4653): 1121–4.

Chang, T. C. and J. T. Mendell (2007). "microRNAs in vertebrate physiology and human disease." *Annu Rev Genomics Hum Genet* **8**: 215–39.

Chayka O., Corvetta, D., Dews, M., Caccamo, A. E., Piotrowska, I., Santilli, G., Gibson, S., Sebire, N. J., Himoudi, N., Hogarty, M. D., Anderson, J., Bettuzzi, S., Thomas-Tikhonenko, A., and Sala, A. (2009) "Clusterin, a haploinsufficient tumour suppressor gene in neuroblastomas." *J Natl Cancer Inst* **101**(g): 663–77.

Chlenski, A., S. Liu, S. E. Crawford, O. V. Volpert, G. H. DeVries, A. Evangelista, Q. Yang, H. R. Salwen, R. Farrer, J. Bray and S. L. Cohn (2002). "SPARC is a key Schwannian-derived inhibitor controlling neuroblastoma tumor angiogenesis." *Cancer Res* **62**(24): 7357–63.

Coller, H. A., C. Grandori, P. Tamayo, T. Colbert, E. S. Lander, R. N. Eisenman and T. R. Golub (2000). "Expression analysis with oligonucleotide microarrays reveals that MYC regulates genes involved in growth, cell cycle, signaling, and adhesion." *Proc Natl Acad Sci U S A* **97**(7): 3260–5.

Coussens, L. M., W. W. Raymond, G. Bergers, M. Laig-Webster, O. Behrendtsen, Z. Werb, G. H. Caughey and D. Hanahan (1999). "Inflammatory mast cells up-regulate angiogenesis during squamous epithelial carcinogenesis." *Genes Dev* **13**(11): 1382–97.

Dalla-Favera, R., M. Bregni, J. Erikson, D. Patterson, R. C. Gallo and C. M. Croce (1982). "Human c-myc onc gene is located on the region of chromosome 8 that is translocated in Burkitt lymphoma cells." *Proc Natl Acad Sci U S A* **79**(24): 7824–7.

Dameron, K. M., O. V. Volpert, M. A. Tainsky and N. Bouck (1994). "Control of angiogenesis in fibroblasts by p53 regulation of thrombospondin-1." *Science* **265**(5178): 1582–4.

Dang, C. V. (1999). "c-Myc target genes involved in cell growth, apoptosis, and metabolism." *Mol Cell Biol* **19**(1): 1–11.

Dang, C. V., K. A. O'Donnell, K. I. Zeller, T. Nguyen, R. C. Osthus and F. Li (2006). "The c-Myc target gene network." *Semin Cancer Biol* **16**(4): 253–64.

Dang, C. V., J. W. Kim, P. Gao and J. Yustein (2008). "The interplay between MYC and HIF in cancer." *Nat Rev Cancer* **8**(1): 51–6.

Dews, M., A. Homayouni, D. Yu, D. Murphy, C. Sevignani, E. Wentzel, E. E. Furth, W. M. Lee, G. H. Enders, J. T. Mendell and A. Thomas-Tikhonenko (2006). "Augmentation of tumor angiogenesis by a Myc-activated microRNA cluster." *Nat Genet* **38**(9): 1060–5.

Dominguez-Sola, D., C. Y. Ying, C. Grandori, L. Ruggiero, B. Chen, M. Li, D. A. Galloway, W. Gu, J. Gautier and R. Dalla-Favera (2007). "Non-transcriptional control of DNA replication by c-Myc." *Nature* **448**(7152): 445–51.

Eischen, C. M., J. D. Weber, M. F. Roussel, C. J. Sherr and J. L. Cleveland (1999). "Disruption of the ARF-Mdm2-p53 tumor suppressor pathway in Myc-induced lymphomagenesis." *Genes Dev* **13**(20): 2658–69.

Felsher, D. W. and J. M. Bishop (1999). "Transient excess of MYC activity can elicit genomic instability and tumorigenesis." *Proc Natl Acad Sci U S A* **96**(7): 3940–4.

Folkman, J. and D. Hanahan (1991). "Switch to the angiogenic phenotype during tumorigenesis." *Princess Takamatsu Symp* **22**: 339–47.

Folkman, J., K. Watson, D. Ingber and D. Hanahan (1989). "Induction of angiogenesis during the transition from hyperplasia to neoplasia." *Nature* **339**(6219): 58–61.

Fontana, L., M. E. Fiori, S. Albini, L. Cifaldi, S. Giovinazzi, M. Forloni, R. Boldrini, A. Donfrancesco, V. Federici, P. Giacomini, C. Peschle and D. Fruci (2008). "Antagomir-17-5p abolishes the growth of therapy-resistant neuroblastoma through p21 and BIM." *PLoS ONE* **3**(5): e2236.

Forsythe, J. A., B. H. Jiang, N. V. Iyer, F. Agani, S. W. Leung, R. D. Koos and G. L. Semenza (1996). "Activation of vascular endothelial growth factor gene transcription by hypoxia-inducible factor 1." *Mol Cell Biol* **16**(9): 4604–13.

Friedman, R. C., K. K. Farh, C. B. Burge and D. P. Bartel (2009). "Most mammalian mRNAs are conserved targets of microRNAs." *Genome Res* **19**(1): 92–105.

Gartel, A. L., X. Ye, E. Goufman, P. Shianov, N. Hay, F. Najmabadi and A. L. Tyner (2001). "Myc represses the p21(WAF1/CIP1) promoter and interacts with Sp1/Sp3." *Proc Natl Acad Sci U S A* **98**(8): 4510–15.

Giuriato, S., S. Ryeom, A. C. Fan, P. Bachireddy, R. C. Lynch, M. J. Rioth, J. van Riggelen, A. M. Kopelman, E. Passegue, F. Tang, J. Folkman and D. W. Felsher (2006). "Sustained regression of tumors upon MYC inactivation requires p53 or thrombospondin-1 to reverse the angiogenic switch." *Proc Natl Acad Sci U S A* **103**(44): 16266–71.

Good, D. J., P. J. Polverini, F. Rastinejad, M. M. Le Beau, R. S. Lemons, W. A. Frazier and N. P. Bouck (1990). "A tumor suppressor-dependent inhibitor of angiogenesis is immunologically and functionally indistinguishable from a fragment of thrombospondin." *Proc Natl Acad Sci U S A* **87**(17): 6624–8.

Gordan, J. D. and M. C. Simon (2007). "Hypoxia-inducible factors: central regulators of the tumor phenotype." *Curr Opin Genet Dev* **17**(1): 71–7.

Gordan, J. D., C. B. Thompson and M. C. Simon (2007a). "HIF and c-Myc: sibling rivals for control of cancer cell metabolism and proliferation." *Cancer Cell* **12**(2): 108–13.

Gordan, J. D., J. A. Bertout, C. J. Hu, J. A. Diehl and M. C. Simon (2007b). "HIF-2alpha promotes hypoxic cell proliferation by enhancing c-myc transcriptional activity." *Cancer Cell* **11**(4): 335–47.

Grandori, C., S. M. Cowley, L. P. James and R. N. Eisenman (2000). "The Myc/Max/Mad network and the transcriptional control of cell behavior." *Annu Rev Cell Dev Biol* **16**: 653–99.

Grandori, C., N. Gomez-Roman, Z. A. Felton-Edkins, C. Ngouenet, D. A. Galloway, R. N. Eisenman and R. J. White (2005). "c-Myc binds to human ribosomal DNA and stimulates transcription of rRNA genes by RNA polymerase I." *Nat Cell Biol* **7**(3): 311–8.

Grewal, S. S., L. Li, A. Orian, R. N. Eisenman and B. A. Edgar (2005). "Myc-dependent regulation of ribosomal RNA synthesis during Drosophila development." *Nat Cell Biol* **7**(3): 295–302.

Grugel, S., G. Finkenzeller, K. Weindel, B. Barleon and D. Marme (1995). "Both v-Ha-Ras and v-Raf stimulate expression of the vascular endothelial growth factor in NIH 3T3 cells." *J Biol Chem* **270**(43): 25915–9.

Guo, N. H., H. C. Krutzsch, J. K. Inman, C. S. Shannon and D. D. Roberts (1997). "Antiproliferative and antitumor activities of D-reverse peptides derived from the second type-1 repeat of thrombospondin-1." *J Pept Res* **50**(3): 210–21.

Hanahan, D. (1985). "Heritable formation of pancreatic beta-cell tumours in transgenic mice expressing recombinant insulin/simian virus 40 oncogenes." *Nature* **315**(6015): 115–22.

Hatzi, E., C. Murphy, A. Zoephel, H. Ahorn, U. Tontsch, A. M. Bamberger, K. Yamauchi-Takihara, L. Schweigerer and T. Fotsis (2002). "N-myc oncogene overexpression down-regulates leukemia inhibitory factor in neuroblastoma." *Eur J Biochem* **269**(15): 3732–41.

Hoekstra, R., F. Y. de Vos, F. A. Eskens, J. A. Gietema, A. van der Gaast, H. J. Groen, R. A. Knight, R. A. Carr, R. A. Humerickhouse, J. Verweij and E. G. de Vries (2005). "Phase I safety, pharmacokinetic, and pharmacodynamic study of the thrombospondin-1-mimetic angiogenesis inhibitor ABT-510 in patients with advanced cancer." *J Clin Oncol* **23**(22): 5188–97.

Hunter, C. A., D. Yu, M. Gee, C. V. Ngo, C. Sevignani, M. Goldschmidt, T. V. Golovkina, S. Evans, W. F. Lee and A. Thomas-Tikhonenko (2001). "Cutting edge: systemic inhibition of angiogenesis underlies resistance to tumors during acute toxoplasmosis." *J Immunol* **166**(10): 5878–81.

Inoki, I., T. Shiomi, G. Hashimoto, H. Enomoto, H. Nakamura, K. Makino, E. Ikeda, S. Takata, K. Kobayashi and Y. Okada (2002). "Connective tissue growth factor binds vascular endothelial growth factor (VEGF) and inhibits VEGF-induced angiogenesis." *FASEB J* **16**(2): 219–21.

Ioannidis, P., L. Mahaira, A. Papadopoulou, M. R. Teixeira, S. Heim, J. A. Andersen, E. Evangelou, U. Dafni, N. Pandis and T. Trangas (2003). "8q24 Copy number gains and expression of the c-myc mRNA stabilizing protein CRD-BP in primary breast carcinomas." *Int J Cancer* **104**(1): 54–9.

Iritani, B. M. and R. N. Eisenman (1999). "c-Myc enhances protein synthesis and cell size during B lymphocyte development." *Proc Natl Acad Sci U S A* **96**(23): 13180–5.

Iruela-Arispe, M. L., M. Lombardo, H. C. Krutzsch, J. Lawler and D. D. Roberts (1999). "Inhibition of angiogenesis by thrombospondin-1 is mediated by 2 independent regions within the type 1 repeats." *Circulation* **100**(13): 1423–31.

Janz, A., C. Sevignani, K. Kenyon, C. V. Ngo and A. Thomas-Tikhonenko (2000). "Activation of the myc oncoprotein leads to increased turnover of thrombospondin-1 mRNA." *Nucleic Acids Res* **28**(11): 2268–75.

Johnston, L. A., D. A. Prober, B. A. Edgar, R. N. Eisenman and P. Gallant (1999). "Drosophila myc regulates cellular growth during development." *Cell* **98**(6): 779–90.

Kang, J., P. G. Rychahou, T. A. Ishola, J. M. Mourot, B. M. Evers and D. H. Chung (2008). "N-myc is a novel regulator of PI3K-mediated VEGF expression in neuroblastoma." *Oncogene* **27**(28): 3999–4007.

Kelly, B. D., S. F. Hackett, K. Hirota, Y. Oshima, S. Cai, S. Berg-Dixon, A. Rowan, Z. Yan, P. A. Campochiaro and G. L. Semenza (2003). "Cell type-specific regulation of angiogenic growth factor gene expression and induction of angiogenesis in nonischemic tissue by a constitutively active form of hypoxia-inducible factor 1." *Circ Res* **93**(11): 1074–81.

Kevil, C. G., A. De Benedetti, D. K. Payne, L. L. Coe, F. S. Laroux and J. S. Alexander (1996). "Translational regulation of vascular permeability factor by eukaryotic initiation factor 4E: implications for tumor angiogenesis." *Int J Cancer* **65**(6): 785–90.

Kim, J. W., P. Gao, Y. C. Liu, G. L. Semenza and C. V. Dang (2007). "Hypoxia-inducible factor 1 and dysregulated c-Myc cooperatively induce vascular endothelial growth factor and metabolic switches hexokinase 2 and pyruvate dehydrogenase kinase 1." *Mol Cell Biol* **27**(21): 7381–93.

Knies-Bamforth, U. E., S. B. Fox, R. Poulsom, G. I. Evan and A. L. Harris (2004). "c-Myc interacts with hypoxia to induce angiogenesis in vivo by a vascular endothelial growth factor-dependent mechanism." *Cancer Res* **64**(18): 6563–70.

Kohl, N. E., N. Kanda, R. R. Schreck, G. Bruns, S. A. Latt, F. Gilbert and F. W. Alt (1983). "Transposition and amplification of oncogene-related sequences in human neuroblastomas." *Cell* **35**(2 Pt 1): 359–67.

Koshiji, M., Y. Kageyama, E. A. Pete, I. Horikawa, J. C. Barrett and L. E. Huang (2004). "HIF-1alpha induces cell cycle arrest by functionally counteracting Myc." *EMBO J* **23**(9): 1949–56.

Land, H., L. F. Parada and R. A. Weinberg (1983). "Tumorigenic conversion of primary embryo fibroblasts requires at least two cooperating oncogenes." *Nature* **304**(5927): 596–602.

Lau, L. F. and S. C. Lam (1999). "The CCN family of angiogenic regulators: the integrin connection." *Exp Cell Res* **248**(1): 44–57.

Laurenti, E., B. Varnum-Finney, A. Wilson, I. Ferrero, W. E. Blanco-Bose, A. Ehninger, P. S. Knoepfler, P. F. Cheng, H. R. MacDonald, R. N. Eisenman, I. D. Bernstein and A. Trumpp (2008). "Hematopoietic stem cell function and survival depend on c-Myc and N-Myc activity." *Cell Stem Cell* **3**(6): 611–24.

Li, Q. and C. V. Dang (1999). "c-Myc overexpression uncouples DNA replication from mitosis." *Mol Cell Biol* **19**(8): 5339–51.

Liu, J., M. A. Valencia-Sanchez, G. J. Hannon and R. Parker (2005). "MicroRNA-dependent localization of targeted mRNAs to mammalian P-bodies." *Nat Cell Biol* **7**(7): 719–23.

Mai, S., J. Hanley-Hyde and M. Fluri (1996). "c-Myc overexpression associated DHFR gene amplification in hamster, rat, mouse and human cell lines." *Oncogene* **12**(2): 277–88.

Manalo, D. J., A. Rowan, T. Lavoie, L. Natarajan, B. D. Kelly, S. Q. Ye, J. G. Garcia and G. L. Semenza (2005). "Transcriptional regulation of vascular endothelial cell responses to hypoxia by HIF-1." *Blood* **105**(2): 659–69.

McMahon, S. B., H. A. Van Buskirk, K. A. Dugan, T. D. Copeland and M. D. Cole (1998). "The novel ATM-related protein TRRAP is an essential cofactor for the c-Myc and E2F oncoproteins." *Cell* **94**(3): 363–74.

Meyer, N. and L. Z. Penn (2008). "Reflecting on 25 years with MYC." *Nat Rev Cancer* **8**(12): 976–90.

Mezquita, P., S. S. Parghi, K. A. Brandvold and A. Ruddell (2005). "Myc regulates VEGF production in B cells by stimulating initiation of VEGF mRNA translation." *Oncogene* **24**(5): 889–901.

Miao, W. M., W. L. Seng, M. Duquette, P. Lawler, C. Laus and J. Lawler (2001). "Thrombospondin-1 type 1 repeat recombinant proteins inhibit tumor growth through transforming growth factor-beta-dependent and -independent mechanisms." *Cancer Res* **61**(21): 7830–9.

Moritani, N. H., S. Kubota, T. Nishida, H. Kawaki, S. Kondo, T. Sugahara and M. Takigawa (2003). "Suppressive effect of overexpressed connective tissue growth factor on tumor cell growth in a human oral squamous cell carcinoma-derived cell line." *Cancer Lett* **192**(2): 205–14.

Morse, B., P. G. Rotherg, V. J. South, J. M. Spandorfer and S. M. Astrin (1988). "Insertional mutagenesis of the myc locus by a LINE-1 sequence in a human breast carcinoma." *Nature* **333**(6168): 87–90.

Mukhopadhyay, D., L. Tsiokas and V. P. Sukhatme (1995). "Wild-type p53 and v-Src exert opposing influences on human vascular endothelial growth factor gene expression." *Cancer Res* **55**(24): 6161–5.

Murphy, D. J., M. R. Junttila, L. Pouyet, A. Karnezis, K. Shchors, D. A. Bui, L. Brown-Swigart, L. Johnson and G. I. Evan (2008). "Distinct thresholds govern Myc's biological output in vivo." *Cancer Cell* **14**(6): 447–57.

Naumov, G. N., L. A. Akslen and J. Folkman (2006). "Role of angiogenesis in human tumor dormancy: animal models of the angiogenic switch." *Cell Cycle* **5**(16): 1779–87.

Naumov, G. N., J. Folkman and O. Straume (2008). "Tumor dormancy due to failure of angiogenesis: role of the microenvironment." *Clin Exp Metastasis*.

Neiman, P. E., A. Ruddell, C. Jasoni, G. Loring, S. J. Thomas, K. A. Brandvold, R. Lee, J. Burnside and J. Delrow (2001). "Analysis of gene expression during myc oncogene-induced lymphomagenesis in the bursa of Fabricius." *Proc Natl Acad Sci U S A* **98**(11): 6378–83.

Ngo, C. V., M. Gee, N. Akhtar, D. Yu, O. Volpert, R. Auerbach and A. Thomas-Tikhonenko (2000). "An in vivo function for the transforming Myc protein: elicitation of the angiogenic phenotype." *Cell Growth Differ* **11**(4): 201–10.

Nyberg, P., T. Salo and R. Kalluri (2008). "Tumor microenvironment and angiogenesis." *Front Biosci* **13**: 6537–53.

O'Donnell, K. A., E. A. Wentzel, K. I. Zeller, C. V. Dang and J. T. Mendell (2005). "c-Myc-regulated microRNAs modulate E2F1 expression." *Nature* **435**(7043): 839–43.

O'Reilly, M. S. (1997). "Angiostatin: an endogenous inhibitor of angiogenesis and of tumor growth." *EXS* **79**: 273–94.

O'Reilly, M. S., T. Boehm, Y. Shing, N. Fukai, G. Vasios, W. S. Lane, E. Flynn, J. R. Birkhead, B. R. Olsen and J. Folkman (1997). "Endostatin: an endogenous inhibitor of angiogenesis and tumor growth." *Cell* **88**(2): 277–85.

Okada, F., J. W. Rak, B. S. Croix, B. Lieubeau, M. Kaya, L. Roncari, S. Shirasawa, T. Sasazuki and R. S. Kerbel (1998). "Impact of oncogenes in tumor angiogenesis: mutant K-ras up-regulation of vascular endothelial growth factor/vascular permeability factor is necessary, but not sufficient for tumorigenicity of human colorectal carcinoma cells." *Proc Natl Acad Sci U S A* **95**(7): 3609–14.

Pelengaris, S., T. Littlewood, M. Khan, G. Elia and G. Evan (1999). "Reversible activation of c-Myc in skin: induction of a complex neoplastic phenotype by a single oncogenic lesion." *Mol Cell* **3**(5): 565–77.

Perbal, B. (2004). "CCN proteins: multifunctional signalling regulators." *Lancet* **363**(9402): 62–4.

Perez-Atayde, A. R., S. E. Sallan, U. Tedrow, S. Connors, E. Allred and J. Folkman (1997). "Spectrum of tumor angiogenesis in the bone marrow of children with acute lymphoblastic leukemia." *Am J Pathol* **150**(3): 815–21.

Peukert, K., P. Staller, A. Schneider, G. Carmichael, F. Hanel and M. Eilers (1997). "An alternative pathway for gene regulation by Myc." *EMBO J* **16**(18): 5672–86.

Rak, J., Y. Mitsuhashi, L. Bayko, J. Filmus, S. Shirasawa, T. Sasazuki and R. S. Kerbel (1995). "Mutant ras oncogenes upregulate VEGF/VPF expression: implications for induction and inhibition of tumor angiogenesis." *Cancer Res* **55**(20): 4575–80.

Rak, J., J. L. Yu, G. Klement and R. S. Kerbel (2000). "Oncogenes and angiogenesis: signaling three-dimensional tumor growth." *J Investig Dermatol Symp Proc* **5**(1): 24–33.

Rastinejad, F., P. J. Polverini and N. P. Bouck (1989). "Regulation of the activity of a new inhibitor of angiogenesis by a cancer suppressor gene." *Cell* **56**(3): 345–55.

Ravi, R., B. Mookerjee, Z. M. Bhujwalla, C. H. Sutter, D. Artemov, Q. Zeng, L. E. Dillehay, A. Madan, G. L. Semenza and A. Bedi (2000). "Regulation of tumor angiogenesis by p53-induced degradation of hypoxia-inducible factor 1alpha." *Genes Dev* **14**(1): 34–44.

Reiher, F. K., O. V. Volpert, B. Jimenez, S. E. Crawford, C. P. Dinney, J. Henkin, F. Haviv, N. P. Bouck and S. C. Campbell (2002). "Inhibition of tumor growth by systemic treatment with thrombospondin-1 peptide mimetics." *Int J Cancer* **98**(5): 682–9.

Ren, B., K. O. Yee, J. Lawler and R. Khosravi-Far (2006). "Regulation of tumor angiogenesis by thrombospondin-1." *Biochim Biophys Acta* **1765**(2): 178–88.

Rosenwald, I. B., D. B. Rhoads, L. D. Callanan, K. J. Isselbacher and E. V. Schmidt (1993). "Increased expression of eukaryotic translation initiation factors eIF-4E and eIF-2 alpha in response to growth induction by c-myc." *Proc Natl Acad Sci U S A* **90**(13): 6175–8.

Ruddell, A., P. Mezquita, K. A. Brandvold, A. Farr and B. M. Iritani (2003). "B lymphocyte-specific c-Myc expression stimulates early and functional expansion of the vasculature and lymphatics during lymphomagenesis." *Am J Pathol* **163**(6): 2233–45.

Saaristo, A., T. Karpanen and K. Alitalo (2000). "Mechanisms of angiogenesis and their use in the inhibition of tumor growth and metastasis." *Oncogene* **19**(53): 6122–9.

Schuhmacher, M., M. S. Staege, A. Pajic, A. Polack, U. H. Weidle, G. W. Bornkamm, D. Eick and F. Kohlhuber (1999). "Control of cell growth by c-Myc in the absence of cell division." *Curr Biol* **9**(21): 1255–8.

Schulte, J. H., S. Horn, T. Otto, B. Samans, L. C. Heukamp, U. C. Eilers, M. Krause, K. Astrahantseff, L. Klein-Hitpass, R. Buettner, A. Schramm, H. Christiansen, M. Eilers, A. Eggert and B. Berwanger (2008). "MYCN regulates oncogenic MicroRNAs in neuroblastoma." *Int J Cancer* **122**(3): 699–704.

Semenza, G. L. (2008). "Hypoxia-inducible factor 1 and cancer pathogenesis." *IUBMB Life* **60**(9): 591–7.

Serban, D., J. Leng and D. Cheresh (2008). "H-ras regulates angiogenesis and vascular permeability by activation of distinct downstream effectors." *Circ Res* **102**(11): 1350–8.

Sevignani, C., P. Wlodarski, J. Kirillova, W. E. Mercer, K. G. Danielson, R. V. Iozzo and B. Calabretta (1998). "Tumorigenic conversion of p53-deficient colon epithelial cells by an activated Ki-ras gene." *J Clin Invest* **101**(8): 1572–80.

Shchors K and Evan G (2007) "Tumor angiogenesis: cause or consequence of cancer?" *Cancer Res* 67:7059–7061.

Shchors, K., E. Shchors, F. Rostker, E. R. Lawlor, L. Brown-Swigart and G. I. Evan (2006). "The Myc-dependent angiogenic switch in tumors is mediated by interleukin 1beta." *Genes Dev* **20**(18): 2527–38.

Shimo, T., S. Kubota, S. Kondo, T. Nakanishi, A. Sasaki, H. Mese, T. Matsumura and M. Takigawa (2001a). "Connective tissue growth factor as a major angiogenic agent that is induced by hypoxia in a human breast cancer cell line." *Cancer Lett* **174**(1): 57–64.

Shimo, T., T. Nakanishi, T. Nishida, M. Asano, A. Sasaki, M. Kanyama, T. Kuboki, T. Matsumura and M. Takigawa (2001b). "Involvement of CTGF, a hypertrophic chondrocyte-specific gene product, in tumor angiogenesis." *Oncology* **61**(4): 315–22.

Shpitz, B., S. Gochberg, D. Neufeld, M. Grankin, G. Buklan, E. Klein and J. Bernheim (2003). "Angiogenic switch in earliest stages of human colonic tumorigenesis." *Anticancer Res* **23**(6D): 5153–7.

Soucek, L., E. R. Lawlor, D. Soto, K. Shchors, L. B. Swigart and G. I. Evan (2007). "Mast cells are required for angiogenesis and macroscopic expansion of Myc-induced pancreatic islet tumors." *Nat Med* **13**(10): 1211–18.

Stein, I., M. Neeman, D. Shweiki, A. Itin and E. Keshet (1995). "Stabilization of vascular endothelial growth factor mRNA by hypoxia and hypoglycemia and coregulation with other ischemia-induced genes." *Mol Cell Biol* **15**(10): 5363–8.

Storlazzi, C. T., T. Fioretos, K. Paulsson, B. Strombeck, C. Lassen, T. Ahlgren, G. Juliusson, F. Mitelman, M. Rocchi and B. Johansson (2004). "Identification of a commonly amplified 4.3 Mb region with overexpression of C8FW, but not MYC in MYC-containing double minutes in myeloid malignancies." *Hum Mol Genet* **13**(14): 1479–85.

Taguchi, A., K. Yanagisawa, M. Tanaka, K. Cao, Y. Matsuyama, H. Goto and T. Takahashi (2008). "Identification of hypoxia-inducible factor-1 alpha as a novel target for miR-17–92 microRNA cluster." *Cancer Res* **68**(14): 5540–5.

Takahashi, Y., L. M. Ellis and M. Mai (2003). "The angiogenic switch of human colon cancer occurs simultaneous to initiation of invasion." *Oncol Rep* **10**(1): 9–13.

Taub, R., I. Kirsch, C. Morton, G. Lenoir, D. Swan, S. Tronick, S. Aaronson and P. Leder (1982). "Translocation of the c-myc gene into the immunoglobulin heavy chain locus in human Burkitt lymphoma and murine plasmacytoma cells." *Proc Natl Acad Sci U S A* **79**(24): 7837–41.

Terai, Y., M. Abe, K. Miyamoto, M. Koike, M. Yamasaki, M. Ueda, M. Ueki and Y. Sato (2001). "Vascular smooth muscle cell growth-promoting factor/F-spondin inhibits angiogenesis via the blockade of integrin alphavbeta3 on vascular endothelial cells." *J Cell Physiol* **188**(3): 394–402.

Thomas-Tikhonenko, A. and C. A. Hunter (2003). "Infection and cancer: the common vein." *Cytokine Growth Factor Rev* **14**(1): 67–77.

Tikhonenko, A. T., D. J. Black and M. L. Linial (1996). "Viral Myc oncoproteins in infected fibroblasts down-modulate thrombospondin-1, a possible tumor suppressor gene." *J Biol Chem* **271**(48): 30741–7.

Udagawa, T., A. Fernandez, E. G. Achilles, J. Folkman and R. J. D'Amato (2002). "Persistence of microscopic human cancers in mice: alterations in the angiogenic balance accompanies loss of tumor dormancy." *FASEB J* **16**(11): 1361–70.

Vacca, A., D. Ribatti, L. Ruco, F. Giacchetta, B. Nico, F. Quondamatteo, R. Ria, M. Iurlaro and F. Dammacco (1999). "Angiogenesis extent and macrophage density increase simultaneously with pathological progression in B-cell non-Hodgkin's lymphomas." *Br J Cancer* **79**(5–6): 965–70.

Volpert, O. V. and R. M. Alani (2003). "Wiring the angiogenic switch: Ras, Myc, and Thrombospondin-1." *Cancer Cell* **3**(3): 199–200.

Volpert, O. V., V. Stellmach and N. Bouck (1995a). "The modulation of thrombospondin and other naturally occurring inhibitors of angiogenesis during tumor progression." *Breast Cancer Res Treat* **36**(2): 119–26.

Volpert, O. V., S. S. Tolsma, S. Pellerin, J. J. Feige, H. Chen, D. F. Mosher and N. Bouck (1995b). "Inhibition of angiogenesis by thrombospondin-2." *Biochem Biophys Res Commun* **217**(1): 326–32.

Volpert, O. V., K. M. Dameron and N. Bouck (1997). "Sequential development of an angiogenic phenotype by human fibroblasts progressing to tumorigenicity." *Oncogene* **14**(12): 1495–502.

Watnick, R. S., Y. N. Cheng, A. Rangarajan, T. A. Ince and R. A. Weinberg (2003). "Ras modulates Myc activity to repress thrombospondin-1 expression and increase tumor angiogenesis." *Cancer Cell* **3**(3): 219–31.

Yang, Q., Y. Tian, S. Liu, R. Zeine, A. Chlenski, H. R. Salwen, J. Henkin and S. L. Cohn (2007). "Thrombospondin-1 peptide ABT-510 combined with valproic acid is an effective antiangiogenesis strategy in neuroblastoma." *Cancer Res* **67**(4): 1716–24.

Zeller, K. I., X. Zhao, C. W. Lee, K. P. Chiu, F. Yao, J. T. Yustein, H. S. Ooi, Y. L. Orlov, A. Shahab, H. C. Yong, Y. Fu, Z. Weng, V. A. Kuznetsov, W. K. Sung, Y. Ruan, C. V. Dang and C. L. Wei (2006). "Global mapping of c-Myc binding sites and target gene networks in human B cells." *Proc Natl Acad Sci U S A* **103**(47): 17834–9.

Zhang, H., P. Gao, R. Fukuda, G. Kumar, B. Krishnamachary, K. I. Zeller, C. V. Dang and G. L. Semenza (2007). "HIF-1 inhibits mitochondrial biogenesis and cellular respiration in VHL-deficient renal cell carcinoma by repression of C-MYC activity." *Cancer Cell* **11**(5): 407–20.

Chapter 9
p53 and Angiogenesis

Jose G. Teodoro, Sara K. Evans, and Michael R. Green

Cast of Characters

The *TP53* gene is the most mutated gene in human cancer and as a consequence
has been one of the most extensively studied genes in the human genome. Over
half of all human cancers carry direct mutations of the p53 coding region. In addition to sporadic mutations in human cancer, inherited mutations in *TP53* cause a
genetic predisposition to cancer called Li–Fraumeni syndrome. Individuals with
Li–Fraumeni exhibit early onset of a wide variety of cancers including soft-tissue
sarcoma, leukemia, osteosarcoma, and tumors of the breast and brain (Li et al.,
1988). The *TP53* gene is not essential for development but seems to have evolved
a primary function to prevent neoplasia in multicellular organisms. The p53 tumor
suppressor protein has the structure of a classical transcription factor possessing
a central domain with sequence-specific DNA binding activity and an N-terminal
acidic region required for transcriptional regulation of target genes. The majority
of mutations observed in human cancer fall within the DNA binding region of p53
and hence disrupts its ability to modify gene expression (Soussi et al., 2006). The
major tumor suppressive properties of p53 are derived from increasing expression
of hundreds of target genes that inhibit cell cycle progression and promote apoptosis. In addition, p53 is also thought to regulate target genes that can affect the tumor
microenvironment to inhibit angiogenesis and metastasis.

Introduction: Hardwiring the Angiogenic Switch

Mammalian cells have intensive requirements for oxygen and nutrients and are
provided with a constant supply of both via the capillary network of the vascular
system. In general, cells cannot be located further than approximately 100 μm from

J.G. Teodoro (✉)
McGill Cancer Centre and Department of Biochemistry, McGill University, Montreal,
Quebec, Canada
e-mail: jose.teodoro@mcgill.ca

A. Thomas-Tikhonenko (ed.), *Cancer Genome and Tumor Microenvironment*,
DOI 10.1007/978-1-4419-0711-0_9, © Springer Science+Business Media, LLC 2010

a capillary, which represents the diffusion limit of oxygen through tissues. As a result, an inherent property of rapidly proliferating tissues is the formation of new blood vessels – a process termed angiogenesis. During angiogenesis, cells comprising the vasculature (endothelial cells) are stimulated to divide and migrate to regions of low oxygen (hypoxia) requiring vascularization. Part of the angiogenic response also involves the proteolytic breakdown of the extracellular matrix (ECM) to allow for expansion and growth of existing blood vessels. Widespread angiogenesis occurs during the normal physiological processes of embryogenesis and at specific periods in adulthood such as wound healing and cycling of the female reproductive system. The inappropriate induction of angiogenesis is associated with several pathologies including psoriasis, macular degeneration, inflammation, and atherosclerosis. Aberrant angiogenesis is also associated with the progression of cancer, where it plays a critical role in the growth, invasion, and metastases of solid tumors.

The process of angiogenesis is promoted by the production of growth factors that stimulate endothelial cells to divide and sprout into new blood vessels. This angiogenic potential is countered by the production of endogenous factors that actively inhibit angiogenesis. The resulting balance of pro- and anti-angiogenic factors determines whether a given tissue or tumor cell mass undergoes angiogenesis. The early stages of tumor development are thought to be characterized by an "angiogenic switch" in which the output of pro-angiogenic factors exceeds that of anti-angiogenic factors, resulting in the tumor becoming highly vascularized and aggressive. Prior to the angiogenic switch, a small occult tumor can lie dormant for many years before transitioning to become a vascularized, rapidly growing tumor.

Because new blood vessel formation is an inherent property of rapidly dividing tissues, genes that promote cell division are often hardwired to concomitantly stimulate angiogenesis. For example, some of the most potent growth-promoting genes, such as the oncogenes *ras* (Rak et al. 2000), *src* (Mukhopadhyay, Tsiokas and Sukhatme 1995a; Mukhopadhyay et al. 1995b)], *myc* (Pelengaris et al. 1999), and *fos* (Saez et al. 1995), are also powerful stimulators of angiogenesis. Conversely, the same logic applies to tumor suppressor proteins, which are capable of limiting cellular division and at the same time preventing angiogenesis. The Rb tumor suppressor, for example, is a key regulator of cell cycle progression and has been shown to inhibit angiogenesis through several mechanisms (Gabellini, Del Bufalo and Zupi 2006). As discussed in this chapter, p53 – a crucial cell cycle regulator and major tumor suppressor protein in humans – also plays an important role in inhibiting angiogenesis and is key to maintaining the angiogenic switch in an "off" state.

p53: The Guardian of the Genome

The tumor suppressor protein p53 is a key regulator of the cellular response to genotoxic damage, and thus plays a pivotal role in preventing cancer formation. Once DNA damage has been incurred, p53 can elicit several different responses to either correct the error(s) or destroy the damaged cell. First, p53 can induce G1 cell cycle arrest, which stops the cell from dividing and allows time to repair the damage before the DNA is replicated. Second, p53 can activate DNA repair proteins to drive the repair of damaged DNA. Third, as a last resort, p53 can induce damaged cells to undergo programmed cell death (apoptosis), thereby eliminating damaged – and potentially dangerous – cells at risk for neoplastic transformation. Due to its critical importance in maintaining genetic stability, p53 has been called the "gatekeeper" or "guardian" of the genome.

Given the crucial role of p53 in maintaining genomic stability, it is perhaps not surprising to find that the gene encoding p53 is the most commonly altered gene in human cancers, being mutated or deleted in half of all tumors. Moreover, many cancers involve cellular or viral oncogenes that target and inactivate p53. For example, the simian virus 40 (SV40) large T-antigen (Mietz et al. 1992; Jiang et al. 1993), the adenoviral E1A, E1B, and E4orf6 proteins (Yew and Berk 1992; Dobner et al. 1996; Steegenga et al. 1996; Somasundaram and El-Deiry 1997), and the E6 oncoprotein from human papilomavirus (Band et al. 1993) all inhibit p53. Loss of functional p53 creates an environment that is permissive for genome instability, and allows cells with DNA damage (i.e., mutations and chromosomal aberrations) to continue replicating, which, left unchecked, can contribute to tumorigenesis.

The biological effects of p53 are predominantly carried out by its ability to transcriptionally regulate – either through activation or repression – the expression of specific target genes (although p53 can also perform functions that are independent of its transcriptional activity, some examples of which are provided in this chapter). To date, more than 150 p53 target genes have been identified; these genes act at essentially every step involved in carcinogenesis, providing an explanation for how p53 is capable of exerting such extensive restraints on tumor formation. In general, the p53 target genes that have been most well characterized are those involved in cell cycle arrest, such as *p21* (recently renamed *CDKN1A*), and those that induce apoptosis, such as *BAX*, *PUMA* (or *BBC3*), and *NOXA* (or *PMAIP1*).

p53 is a tetrameric protein that contains four functional domains and possesses the hallmarks of a classical transcription factor. The N-terminus of the protein contains a prototypical acidic transactivation domain, which interacts with components of the basal transcription machinery and promotes the transcription of genes harboring p53-binding elements in their promoters. The central core domain is involved in sequence-specific DNA binding and is the location of the majority of oncogenic p53 mutations. The oligomerization domain contains nuclear localization signals and is involved in tetramerization of the protein. Lastly, the basic C-terminal domain is a negative regulatory domain that can inhibit DNA binding by the core domain.

The activity of p53 is modulated by the coordinated interplay of covalent modifications within the N- and C-terminal domains and a suite of interacting protein partners, which function to keep p53 levels and activity under extremely tight control. In normal cells (i.e., those that are unstressed or undamaged), p53 is maintained at a very low level and in a relatively inactive form, held in check by interaction with its primary negative regulator, MDM2. MDM2 binds the N-terminal domain of p53 and restricts its function in three ways. First, MDM2 translocates p53 from the nucleus to the cytoplasm, thus preventing p53 from accessing DNA. Second, binding of MDM2 to p53 results in the concealment of its transcriptional activation domain, thereby suppressing p53-mediated transactivation. Third, MDM2, which is an E3 ubiquitin ligase, promotes the ubiquitination of p53 and targets it for degradation by the 26S proteasome. The continual degradation of p53 results in an extremely short half-life for the protein, in the range of mere minutes.

In response to a variety of cellular stress stimuli – such as hypoxia, DNA damage (induced by either UV, IR, or chemical agents), X-ray irradiation, or oncogene activation (for example, *ras*, *myc*, or E2F) – p53 undergoes substantial post-translational modification and becomes functionally active. The critical event leading to p53 activation is phosphorylation of its N-terminal domain, which inhibits MDM2 binding, resulting in the rapid accumulation of p53 in the nucleus. Post-translational modifications in the C-terminal domain, including not only phosphorylation but also acetylation, sumoylation, and methylation, have diverse affects on p53 stability and function. For example, acetylation of C-terminal residues has been shown to protect p53 from ubiquitination, to potentiate its interaction with other transcription factors, and to induce a conformational change in the protein that exposes the DNA binding domain, allowing it to activate or repress target genes (Appella and Anderson 2001). Different genotoxic stresses activate p53 through distinct pathways and result in post-translational modification of distinct subsets of residues, but the net result of these post-translational modifications is an increase in not only the stability of the protein but also its biological activity.

A Role for p53 in Inhibiting Angiogenesis

In addition to its well-known functions in regulating cell-autonomous effects (i.e., cell cycle arrest, DNA repair, and apoptosis), the tumor suppressive role of p53 is also mediated through more complex host–tumor interactions, in particular angiogenesis. Several lines of evidence support the notion that p53 limits tumor vascularization. First, clinical studies involving a variety of cancers have demonstrated that tumors carrying p53 mutations are more highly vascularized than tumors harboring wild-type p53. For example, prostate tumors expressing mutated p53 have significantly greater microvessel density (MVD), a semi-quantitative measure of tumor vascularization, than tumors expressing wild-type p53 (Yu et al. 1997; Takahashi et al. 1998). Similar correlations have been observed between p53 status and MVD in colon cancer (Kang et al. 1997; Takahashi et al. 1998; Faviana et al. 2002), head and neck tumors (Gasparini et al. 1993) and breast cancer (Gasparini et al. 1994). Of particular clinical interest is that even early stage node-negative breast cancers harboring p53 mutations appear to have higher MVD than tumors with wild-type p53 and correlate with poor prognosis (Gasparini et al. 1994). Normally, node-negative breast cancers have a favorable prognosis, but the increased angiogenic potential provided by early loss of p53 in these cancers may be sufficient to render them much more aggressive.

In addition to the clinical evidence, experimental studies in human cell lines and mouse models have also shown connections between p53 and angiogenesis. Initial clues came from studies showing that p53 was able to perform tumor suppressor functions independent of its anti-proliferative and pro-apoptotic effects and could result in avascular, dormant tumors in vivo (Holmgren, Jackson and Arbiser 1998). Further evidence came from reports showing that overexpression of wild-type p53 could inhibit differentiation of human umbilical vein endothelial cells (HUVECs) into capillary-like structures in vitro and neovascularization in vivo (Riccioni et al. 1998). Finally, additional experiments using mouse models have shown that p53-deficient cell lines show a less pronounced and slower response to anti-angiogenic therapy compared with p53 wild-type cell lines, indicating anti-angiogenic therapy is sensitive to p53 status (Yu et al. 2002).

The molecular basis by which p53 interacts with and inhibits the regulatory pathways of angiogenesis have recently begun to be elucidated. These studies have defined three basic mechanisms by which p53 inhibits angiogenesis: (1) inhibition of hypoxia-sensing systems, (2) downregulation of pro-angiogenesis genes, and (3) upregulation of anti-angiogenesis pathways. The overall combination of these effects dramatically dampens the angiogenic output of tumor cells and tilts the tumor microenvironment in the host substantially toward angiogenesis suppression.

Inhibition of Hypoxia-Sensing Systems

As described in earlier chapters (see Chapters 6 and 8), the key regulator of the cellular response to oxygen deprivation is hypoxia inducible factor 1 (HIF-1). HIF-1 is a heterodimeric transcription factor composed of two subunits, HIF-1α and HIF-1β. The HIF-1β subunit is constitutively expressed, whereas the levels of HIF-1α are intricately regulated in response to cellular oxygen levels. Under normoxic conditions, key oxygen sensors called prolyl hydroxylases (PHDs) use molecular oxygen as a substrate to hydroxylate HIF-1α on one of two conserved proline residues (Fig. 9.1). The hydroxylated motif on HIF-1α serves as a binding site for an E3 ubiquitin ligase called the von Hippel–Lindau (VHL) protein, which tags HIF-1α for proteolysis by the proteosome complex. By contrast, under hypoxic conditions PHD activity is low, allowing HIF-1α protein levels to increase. The functional HIF-1α/HIF-1β heterodimer then binds its cognate DNA binding sites, termed hypoxia responsive elements (HREs), located in the promoters of target genes. HIF-1 transcriptionally activates a number of genes required for response to hypoxia, including vascular endothelial growth factor (*VEGF*), a potent angiogenic gene required for both developmental and tumor angiogenesis (Forsythe et al. 1996; Carmeliet et al. 1998; Iyer et al. 1998; Ryan, Lo and Johnson 1998) (and see Chapter 6).

The p53 tumor suppressor inhibits the HIF-1 pathway by directly binding to HIF-1α and targeting the protein for degradation (Ravi et al. 2000) (see Fig. 9.1). Because HIF-1 is a master regulator of the hypoxia-induced response, inhibiting HIF-1 will have major effects on tumor angiogenesis. Notably, the ability of p53 to inhibit the HIF-1 system is mediated by its physical interaction with HIF-1α and does not require its transcriptional activity.

The ability of p53 to inhibit HIF-1 activity does not occur under normal physiological conditions (Rempe et al. 2007). Rather, it most likely occurs only in the

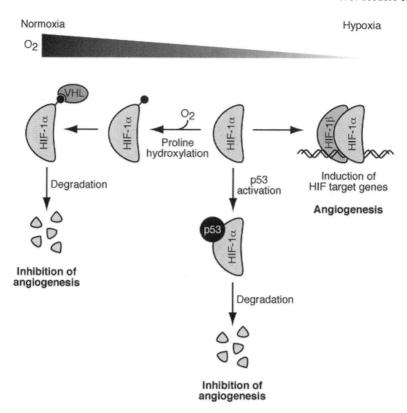

Fig. 9.1 The p53 tumor suppressor protein limits angiogenesis by inhibiting the central regulator of hypoxia, HIF-1. HIF-1 is a dimeric transcription factor comprised of HIF-1β, a constitutively expressed nuclear protein, and HIF-1α, whose levels are dependent on the oxygen levels in the cell. Under normal oxygen conditions (normoxia), the levels of HIF-1α are kept low by von Hippel–Lindau (VHL)-mediated protein degradation. Conversely, under low oxygen conditions (hypoxia), the levels of HIF-1α are stabilized, allowing activation of HIF-1 target genes that mediate angiogenesis. Upon oncogene activation, p53 directly binds HIF-1α and targets the protein for degradation, thus inhibiting angiogenesis

extreme hypoxic environment of a tumor or when accompanied by other forms of genotoxic stress (i.e., conditions under which p53 is activated). Evidence in support of this model has shown that inhibition of HIF-1 by p53 only occurs when p53 becomes stabilized in tumor cells by stimuli such as DNA damage (Kaluzova et al. 2004) or acidosis and nutrient deprivation that occur within tumors (Pan et al. 2004). Thus, one of the roles of p53 in tumor suppression may be to act as a final checkpoint in allowing angiogenesis to progress, much as it does for cell division.

Downregulation of Pro-angiogenic Factors

Much of the focus on the ability of p53 to act as a tumor suppressor has been on its role as a transcriptional activator. However, p53-dependent gene activation does not appear to occur significantly under conditions of extreme hypoxia (Koumenis et al. 2001), suggesting that p53-mediated transcriptional repression may be particularly important under certain circumstances, such as when a tumor becomes larger and low oxygen levels are sustained for long periods of time. The transcriptional repression of pro-angiogenic genes by p53 may, therefore, represent a mechanism of last resort to curtail tumor angiogenesis. In this regard, to date p53 has been shown to directly repress the expression of four genes encoding pro-angiogenic factors: *VEGF*, cyclooxygenase-2 (*COX-2*), fibroblast growth factor 2 (*FGF2*), and FGF-binding protein (*FGF-BP*) (Table 9.1). As discussed below, the mechanisms by which p53 mediates transcriptional repression of these genes can vary.

VEGF

p53 inhibits *VEGF* expression during hypoxia by binding the transcription factor Sp1 and inhibiting its ability to bind the *VEGF* promoter and activate *VEGF* transcription (Pal, Datta and Mukhopadhyay 2001). As noted above, p53 also indirectly modulates *VEGF* expression by inhibiting another transcriptional activator of *VEGF*, HIF-1. Thus, p53 employs redundant mechanisms to inhibit one of the most potent pro-angiogenic factors known.

Mutations in p53 have been associated with increased *VEGF* expression in a number of human cancers including lung (Fontanini et al. 1997), bladder (Crew et al. 1997), and colorectal (Takahashi et al. 1998) carcinomas. The correlation between p53 status and VEGF expression appears to have important prognostic value, as breast cancer prognosis can be predicted with greater accuracy using VEGF expression and p53 status as prognostic markers than either VEGF or p53 status alone (Gasparini et al. 1997; Obermair et al. 1997; Linderholm et al. 2000; Linderholm et al. 2001). Finally, the ability of wild-type p53 to inhibit angiogenesis has been linked to suppression of VEGF in human leiomyosarcoma and synovial sarcoma (Zhang et al. 2000a).

Table 9.1 p53-Regulated genes implicated in angiogenesis

p53-Downregulated genes	p53-Upregulated genes
VEGF (vascular endothelial growth factor)	TSP-1/THBS1 (thrombospondin-1)
COX-2/PTGS2 (cyclooxygenase-2)	BAI1 (brain-specific angiogenesis inhibitor 1)
FGF2/bFGF (basic fibroblast growth factor)	EPHA2 (ephrin receptor A2)
FGFBP1/bFGF-BP (basic fibroblast growth factor-binding protein)	EFNA1 (ephrin-A1)
	SERPIN5B (maspin)
	COL18A1 (α1 collagen 18)
	COL4A1 (α1 collagen 4)
	P4HA2 (α [II] 4-prolyl hydroxylase)

COX-2

COX-2 (also known as PTGS2) is an enzyme that converts arachidonic acid to prostaglandin H2, an intermediate that is subsequently converted to numerous other molecules known as prostanoids, which are key players in inflammation. Interestingly, the prostanoids produced by COX-2 can also stimulate the expression of pro-angiogenic factors (Tsujii et al. 1998; Williams et al. 2000). Thus, by directly repressing the *COX-2* gene, p53 may inhibit a significant pathway of prostanoid-mediated angiogenesis. p53-mediated repression of *COX-2* occurs by a mechanism whereby p53 inhibits TATA box-binding protein (TBP) from binding to the *COX-2* promoter (Subbaramaiah et al. 1999). Although the precise mechanism is not yet clear, previous studies have shown that p53 suppresses a number of promoters that contain TATA elements by directly binding to TBP and interfering with its ability to stably bind the TATA box (Seto et al. 1992; Ragimov et al. 1993).

COX-2 is upregulated in many types of human cancers (Masferrer et al. 2000), consistent with an important role for this enzyme in promoting tumor angiogenesis. In some cases, COX-2 overexpression has been associated with altered p53 status (for example, Erkinheimo et al., 2004). Notably, inhibition of COX-2 has been shown to suppress tumor formation in various animal models of carcinogenesis (Oshima et al. 1996; Chulada et al. 2000). These observations have generated significant interest in the use of COX-2 inhibitors as potential cancer therapeutics.

FGF2 and FGF-BP

FGF2 (also known as basic FGF or bFGF) is a potent pro-angiogenic cytokine present in the basement membranes and subendothelial ECM of blood vessels. FGF2 is held in an inactive form in the ECM through binding to heparan sulfates and proteoglycans present in the ECM and is liberated during angiogenesis from these ECM reservoirs. Release of FGF2 from the ECM requires the action of a secreted protein called FGF-BP (also called bFGF-BP). p53 represses expression of *FGF2* through direct repression of the *FGF2* core promoter (Ueba et al. 1994), although the precise mechanism is not yet clear as the *FGF2* promoter does not contain a TATA box. Moreover, p53 directly represses expression of the *FGF-BP* gene (Sherif et al. 2001). Thus, similar to regulation of VEGF, p53 uses redundant approaches to suppress a potent pro-angiogenic factor.

In addition to directly repressing transcription of pro-angiogenic genes, p53 may also inhibit production of pro-angiogenic factors through post-transcriptional mechanisms. In particular, a proteomics-based approach has identified a number of secreted factors induced or repressed by p53 (Khwaja et al. 2006). Among the repressed pro-angiogenic factors identified were known direct targets of p53, including VEGF and transforming growth factor-beta (TGF-β), as well as previously unidentified targets CYR61, FGF4, and the cytokine interleukin-8. However, p53 did not appear to modulate the mRNA levels of these genes, suggesting that p53 may increase the levels of these proteins by post-translational mechanisms such as enhancing their stability or secretion. Such secondary effects caused by p53 activation may also be significant in mediating changes in the tumor microenvironment and underscores the notion that not all p53-dependent effects are transcriptionally based.

Transcriptional Activation of Anti-Angiogenic Factors

p53 has been shown to upregulate a number of genes that inhibit angiogenesis (see Table 9.1). Unlike transcriptional repression by p53, which can occur by a variety of mechanisms, activation by p53 is strictly dependent on binding of p53 to a cognate DNA sequence motif in the promoter of its target gene. Anti-angiogenic factors upregulated by p53 are, in most cases, factors that are secreted into the ECM. The biological importance of these p53-induced factors in limiting tumor growth likely depends on both tumor type and location. As discussed below, several anti-angiogenic factors that are stimulated in response to p53 also require proteolytic cleavage in order to release a biologically active angiogenesis inhibitor.

Thrombospondin-1 (TSP-1 or THBS1)

One of the first p53 target genes identified was *TSP-1*; interestingly, it was also the first naturally occurring angiogenesis inhibitor to be discovered (Good et al. 1990; Tolsma et al. 1993; Dameron et al. 1994; Weinstat-Saslow et al. 1994). *TSP-1* expression is reciprocally regulated by tumor suppressor genes and oncogenes: for instance, *TSP-1* expression is upregulated by the p53 and PTEN tumor suppressors, but downregulated by a number of oncogenes, including *v-src* (Slack and Bornstein 1994), *c-jun* (Dejong et al. 1999), *myc* (Tikhonenko, Black and Linial 1996; Janz et al. 2000), and *ras* (Rak et al. 2000; Watnick et al. 2003). TSP-1 is a large, 450-kDa glycoprotein that is secreted into the ECM. The anti-angiogenic activity of TSP-1 has been localized to two of its three so-called thrombospondin type 1 repeats (TSRs), a motif that is present in over 70 human proteins. TSP-1 has been shown to potently inhibit angiogenesis through a number of different mechanisms. For example, TSP-1 negatively regulates endothelial cell proliferation and migration both in vitro and in vivo (Hsu et al. 1996; Jimenez et al. 2000; Nor et al. 2000). Many of these inhibitory effects are mediated by direct binding of TSP-1 to endothelial cells via interaction between the TSRs and the cell surface receptor, CD36 (Dawson et al. 1997; Jimenez et al. 2000). TSP-1 also directly activates the multifunctional cytokine TGF-β1, a secreted factor that plays a role in a variety of biological functions, including inhibition of angiogenesis. TGF-β1 is secreted in a latent form that is activated by TSP-1 in the ECM (Crawford et al. 1998). Notably, TGF-β1 has been shown to have potent tumor suppressive properties in several types of human cancers (Derynck, Akhurst and Balmain 2001).

TSP-1 expression has been shown to correlate with p53 status in a variety of cancers, including prostate cancer (Kwak et al. 2002), advanced epithelial ovarian carcinoma (Alvarez et al. 2001), and melanoma (Grant et al. 1998). However, in other cancers, such a correlation has not been found (Kawahara et al. 1998; Tokunaga et al. 1998; Grossfeld et al. 2002), suggesting that regulation of TSP-1 by p53 may be cell-type or tissue-type specific. In some cases, loss of p53 and the resulting decrease in TSP-1 has been shown to correlate with increased tumor angiogenesis (Grant et al. 1998; Alvarez et al. 2001). Fibroblasts from patients with Li–Fraumeni syndrome, a cancer predisposition disease, show a loss of p53 function that correlates with a reduction in TSP-1 protein expression and a switch from an inhibitory to stimulatory angiogenic phenotype (Stellmach et al. 1996; Volpert, Dameron and Bouck 1997). These results strongly suggest that loss of p53 function contributes, at least in part, to the development of an angiogenic phenotype by decreasing TSP-1 expression.

Brain-Specific Angiogenesis Inhibitor 1 (BAI1)

Expressed almost exclusively in the brain, *BAI1* was originally identified in a screen for p53-target genes in glioblastoma cells (Tokino et al. 1994), and subsequent studies verified that expression of *BAI1* could be induced directly by wild-type p53 (Nishimori et al. 1997). The *BAI1* gene product is a large, seven-pass transmembrane protein, with extended extracellular and cytoplasmic regions, that belongs to the adhesion-type family of G-protein-coupled receptors. The N-terminal extracellular region of BAI1 contains five TSRs, which bear homology to the TSRs that are found in TSP-1. BAI1 is cleaved at a conserved G-protein-coupled receptor proteolytic cleavage site within the extracellular domain to generate a soluble 120-kDa fragment containing the five TSRs. This fragment has been shown to inhibit endothelial cell migration and proliferation in vitro and to inhibit angiogenesis in vivo in a mouse model; because of these anti-angiogenic properties, the N-terminal fragment was dubbed vasculostatin (Kaur et al. 2005). The fragment also suppresses the growth of glioma tumor xenografts in mice. BAI1 was the first transmembrane protein identified that harbored a releasable proteolytic fragment with anti-angiogenic and anti-neoplastic properties. Interestingly, an earlier study had identified a secreted activity in glioblastoma cells that could potently inhibited angiogenesis and was also stimulated by p53 (Van Meir et al. 1994). This factor was called glioma-derived angiogenesis inhibitory factor (GD-AIF), but thus far, the identity of the protein has not been determined. It is tempting to speculate that this activity may be vasculostatin.

Ephrin Signaling

Another p53-inducible gene that has been implicated in regulation of angiogenesis is the *EPHA2* gene (Dohn, Jiang and Chen 2001; Brantley et al. 2002). EPHA2 is a member of a family of transmembrane receptor tyrosine kinases, called the ephrin receptors, which, together with their ligands (ephrins), are thought to play important roles in angiogenesis (Dodelet and Pasquale 2000; Pasquale 2005). Like most ephrin receptors, EPHA2 signaling is decidedly complex and has been shown to have either an oncogenic or a tumor suppressor effect depending on physiological context. In cancer cells, the *EPHA2* gene is typically overexpressed and functions as a potent oncogene (Walker-Daniels et al. 1999; Easty and Bennett 2000; Ogawa et al. 2000;

Zelinski et al. 2001; Miyazaki et al. 2003). In normal cells, however, EPHA2 is expressed at low levels and acts as a negative regulator of cell growth (Coffman et al. 2003; Kinch and Carles-Kinch 2003). These different activities appear to depend on the ability of EPHA2 to bind its ligand, ephrin-A1, which is anchored to the membrane of adjacent cells; in malignant cells, unstable cell–cell contacts prevent EPHA2 from binding ephrin-A1. Adenoviral-mediated delivery of ephrin-A1 has been shown to decrease the tumorigenic potential of EPHA2-overexpressing breast cancer cells in vivo (Noblitt et al. 2004). Interestingly, both the EPHA2 receptor and ephrin-A1 are upregulated in response to p53, suggesting that modulation of signaling through the ephrin pathway may represent another mechanism by which p53 disrupts angiogenesis (Dohn et al. 2001; Brantley et al. 2002).

SERPINB5/Maspin

The *SERPINB5* gene encodes a 42-kDa protein, commonly called maspin, that belongs to the serine protease inhibitor (serpin) superfamily. Serpins play a number of important biological functions, including regulating cell adhesion and differentiation. Maspin was initially identified as a candidate tumor suppressor gene involved in breast cancer based on its reduced expression in mammary tumor cell lines compared to normal mammary epithelial cells, and subsequent studies revealed that expression of maspin in breast tumor cells could inhibit tumor cell invasion and metastasis (Zou et al. 1994). Maspin is also downregulated in several other types of cancers, and clinical studies have associated loss of maspin expression with the progression and poor prognosis (Khalkhali-Ellis 2006). The ability of maspin to inhibit tumor cell invasion and metastasis appears to derive, at least in part, from its potential to inhibit angiogenesis. Maspin inhibits endothelial cell migration in vitro and blocks neovascularization in an animal model (Zhang et al. 2000b). p53 induces maspin expression by binding the p53-response element present in the promoter, indicating maspin is a direct p53 target gene (Zou et al. 2000). Interestingly, several studies have found correlations between maspin expression, p53 status, and MVD in colon cancers (Song et al. 2002).

Anti-angiogenic Collagens

A relatively recently identified class of potent, endogenous angiogenesis inhibitors are those that are derived from proteolytic fragments of certain types of collagen, an abundant insoluble fibrous protein present in the ECM and connective tissue. Most anti-angiogenic collagens are constitutively expressed in vascular basement membranes; these include type IV collagens, the main constituent of basement membranes, as well as type XVIII collagen (Kalluri 2003). These collagens can be proteolytically processed by matrix metalloproteases, serine proteases, or cysteine proteases to produce anti-angiogenic peptides such as endostatin, which is derived from $\alpha 1$ collagen 18, and tumstatin, canstatin, and arresten, which are derived, respectively, from $\alpha 3$, $\alpha 2$, and $\alpha 1$ collagen 4. These peptides exert their effects by interacting with specific receptors on the endothelial cell surface and inhibiting angiogenesis by, for example, reducing endothelial cell proliferation or migration, or increasing endothelial cell apoptosis. Collagen-derived anti-angiogenic peptides have generated significant therapeutic interest as angiogenesis inhibitors for the treatment of cancer, but recent evidence has begun to suggest that these molecules are also part of the body's naturally occurring tumor suppressor mechanisms. An understanding of these mechanisms first requires an introduction to the collagen biosynthesis pathway.

The collagen family of proteins is characterized by the presence of so-called collagen repeats, which comprise several copies of the amino acid sequence glycine-X-Y, in which X is often a proline residue and Y is frequently a 4-hydroxyproline residue. To create a mature collagen molecule, the collagen repeats from three separate collagen α chains wind around one another to form a rigid triple helix structure. Formation of this triple helix requires hydrogen bonding between the 4-hydroxyproline residues; without these modified amino acid residues, collagen molecules are unstable and do not form.

Proline hydroxylation is the rate-limiting step in collagen biosynthesis. The two enzymes that post-translationally modify prolines within the collagen repeats are called α[I] and α[II] prolyl 4-hydroxylase (hereafter referred to as α(I)PH and α(II)PH). The α(I)PH isoenzyme is ubiquitously expressed and is the predominant collagen prolyl hydroxlase activity in connective tissues. By contrast, the α(II)PH isoform has a much more restricted expression pattern and is mostly expressed in chondrocytes and capillary endothelial cells (Nissi et al. 2001). The prolyl 4-hydroxylases that modify collagens are catalytically very similar to the PHDs involved in HIF-1α hydroxylation mentioned above in that they require molecular oxygen, as well as ascorbic acid, Fe^{2+}, and α-ketoglutarate, as cofactor for catalytic activity. However, the collagen prolyl 4-hydroxylases differ from PHDs in their subcellular localization: prolyl 4-hydroxylases are localized to the endoplasmic reticulum where collagens are assembled, whereas PHDs reside primarily in the cytoplasm. Loss of collagen prolyl 4-hydroxylase enzymatic activity, which can occur when its essential cofactor ascorbic acid (vitamin C) is lacking in the diet, causes scurvy, highlighting the importance of prolyl hydroxylation in collagen biosynthesis.

Upon activation, the p53 tumor suppressor initiates a three-pronged transcriptional program that stimulates cells to produce and secrete collagen-derived angiogenesis inhibitors (Fig. 9.2). First, p53 directly upregulates expression of at least two anti-angiogenic collagen genes, COL18A1 (encoding α1 collagen 18) (Miled et al. 2005) and COL4A1 (encoding α1 collagen 4) (Wei et al. 2006). Second, p53 also directly induces expression of α(II)PH (Teodoro et al. 2006). Upregulation of α(II)PH by p53 has been shown to result in an increase in biosynthesis of α1 collagen 18 and α3 collagen 4 (Teodoro et al. 2006). As stated above, these two collagens possess potent anti-angiogenic activity in their C-terminal proteolytic fragments, also known as non-collagen 1 (NC1) domains. Thus, p53 increases the expression of not only anti-angiogenic collagen genes themselves, but also the rate-limiting prolyl 4-hydroxylase enzyme required for collagen biosynthesis. Lastly, p53 also increases the proteolytic processing of the mature collagens into anti-angiogenic peptides

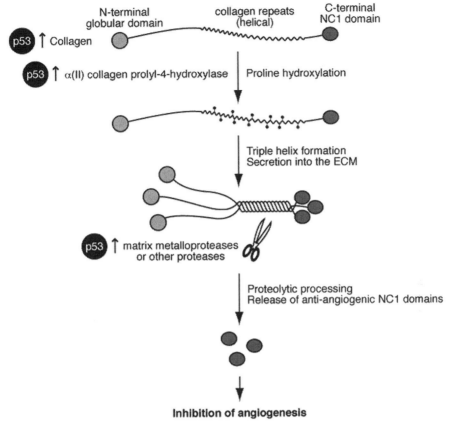

Fig. 9.2 The p53 tumor suppressor protein limits angiogenesis by activating a transcriptional program culminating in the secretion of endogenous collagen-derived angiogenesis inhibitors

(Teodoro et al. 2006). Although this p53-activated proteolytic activity remains to be identified, there are several candidate proteases known to be transcriptionally activated by p53, such as matrix metalloprotease 2 (MMP2) (Bian and Sun 1997), which could mediate this effect.

The identification of an elaborate p53-induced transcriptional program involved in the biosynthesis and processing of collagen-derived anti-angiogenic fragments suggests that the shedding of such fragments at the tumor–host interface is likely to contribute to the general p53-dependent mechanism of inhibiting tumor vascularization and growth. Notably, in addition to α3 collagen 4 and α1 collagen 18, there have been five other collagens identified to date that contain domains with demonstrated anti-angiogenic activity (Table 9.2); whether or not p53 also increases biosynthesis of these proteins, and their processing into anti-angiogenic fragments, remains to be determined. Although it is possible that the collagen-derived angiogenesis inhibitors will have tissue-specific and/or cancer-type-specific

Table 9.2 Collagen-derived anti-angiogenic factors

Collagen type	Anti-angiogenic peptide
α1 collagen 4	Arresten
α2 collagen 4	Canstatin
α3 collagen 4	Tumstatin
α6 collagen 4	As yet unnamed
α1 collagen 8	Vastatin
α1 collagen 15	Restin
α1 collagen 18	Endostatin

expression patterns, the additive effects of these inhibitors could have extremely powerful tumor suppression properties.

As stated above, type IV collagens are the most abundant component of vascular basement membranes. Notably, of the six type IV collagens, four have been reported to possess domains that are anti-angiogenic (see Table 9.2). The presence of anti-angiogenic collagens in the basement membrane is thought to maintain endothelial cells in a quiescent (non-dividing) state (Kalluri 2003). In order for angiogenesis to occur, endothelial or cancer cells must proteolytically degrade the vascular basement membrane by secreting matrix metalloproteases or other ECM-degrading enzymes. However, this process would also liberate vast amounts of collagen-derived angiogenesis inhibitors, and unless tumor cells under these conditions express sufficient pro-angiogenic factors to overcome the release of angiogenesis inhibitors, neovascularization will not occur.

It is interesting to note that small molecule inhibitors of matrix metalloproteases were once regarded as ideal drug targets to prevent metastasis. Unfortunately, such inhibitors are proved unsuccessful for treating cancer and, in some tumor types, even resulted in accelerated tumor growth during clinical trials (Coussens, Fingleton and Matrisian 2002; Fingleton 2006). One possible explanation for the ineffectiveness of these inhibitors is that by inhibiting matrix metalloproteases, they also inhibit the production of collagen-derived anti-angiogenic peptides, and thus may actually promote angiogenesis rather than inhibiting the process.

Clinical implications of p53-mediated Upregulation of Endogenous Angiogenesis Inhibitors

Collagen-Derived Angiogenesis Inhibitors May Contribute to the Body's Natural Tumor Suppressor Mechanisms

Although activation of p53 can lead to the production of collagen-derived angiogenesis inhibitors, whether or not these factors are effective in limiting tumor growth in vivo remains to be determined. Several lines of evidence suggest that increasing biosynthesis of endogenous angiogenesis inhibitors could potentially have dramatic impact on tumor incidence and growth. Perhaps the most intriguing piece of evidence has come from an interesting observation made in individuals with trisomy 21, also known as Down syndrome. In particular, certain common pediatric cancers such as neuroblastoma, which typically represents approximately 30% of childhood solid tumors, are only very rarely observed in individuals with Down syndrome. Likewise, in older individuals, prevalent cancers, such as breast cancer, are completely absent in Down's patients. The extremely low incidence of solid tumors in Down's individuals has led to the proposal that chromosome 21 harbors a potent tumor suppressor activity. Indeed, studies using mouse models have identified two candidate tumor suppressor genes, *Dscr1* (Down syndrome candidate region 1) (Minami et al. 2004) and *Ets2* (Sussan et al. 2008), present on chromosome 21.

Interestingly, the gene encoding α1 collagen 18, *COL18A1*, is also located on chromosome 21, and it has been proposed that increased dosage of its C-terminal anti-angiogenic fragment, endostatin, could help explain the reduced solid tumor incidence in individuals with Down syndrome (Folkman and Kalluri 2004; Sund et al. 2005). Consistent with this proposal, serum levels of endostatin are approximately 30% higher in Down's individuals compared to the general population (Zorick et al. 2001). Experiments in mice have demonstrated that an increase in endostatin levels as little as 1.7-fold results in significantly slower rates of tumor growth (Sund et al. 2005), suggesting that even a modest increase in the dosage of a collagen-derived anti-angiogenic peptide could lead to dramatically reduced tumor growth rates. Conversely, mice deficient in either the *Col4a3* or *Col18a1* gene exhibit increased rates of tumor growth (Sund et al. 2005). Collectively, these observations suggest that collagen-derived angiogenesis inhibitors may have physiological relevance in limiting tumor formation and growth.

Endogenous Angiogenesis Inhibitors May Mediate Long-Range Host–Tumor Interactions

Because anti-angiogenic peptides are secreted they are excellent candidates for mediating long-range effects associated with host–tumor interactions. For example, the p53-dependent production of anti-angiogenic factors may explain a rare and poorly understood phenomenon known as the radiation abscopal effect, in which ionizing radiation directed toward an unaffected region causes regression of a distal tumor outside the field of irradiation (Fig. 9.3). This effect is mediated by a soluble factor(s) produced at the site of irradiation that is able to inhibit tumor growth. Although originally thought to be due to an immune response directed against the tumor, it has since been demonstrated that the radiation abscopal effect is dependent on p53 (Camphausen et al. 2003), which is perhaps not surprising as X-ray irradiation, and the subsequent DNA damage it produces, is known to activate the p53 pathway. It is possible, then, that the radiation abscopal effect is due to p53-dependent production of collagen-derived angiogenesis inhibitors or other soluble anti-angiogenic factors.

The p53-mediated production of secreted collagen-derived angiogenesis inhibitors may also be relevant to abscopal effects that occur following surgical removal of a tumor (see Fig. 9.3). It has been reported that primary tumors can

Radiation abscopal effect

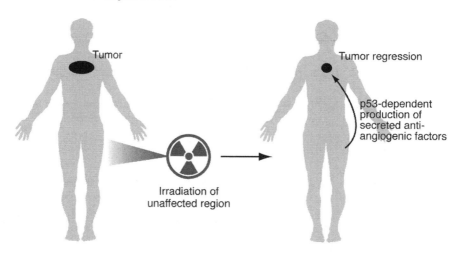

Surgical abscopal effect

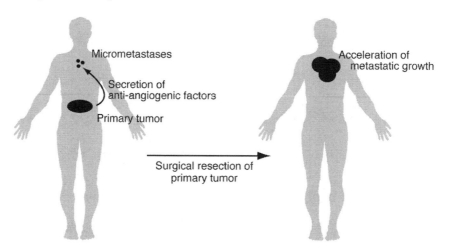

Fig. 9.3 p53-Induced production of endogenous angiogenesis inhibitors may mediate long-range host–tumor interactions. (*Top*) The radiation abscopal effect is mediated by soluble factors, perhaps endogenous anti-angiogenic factors, that are produced at the site of irradiation and are able to inhibit tumor growth. (*Bottom*) The p53-mediated production of secreted collagen-derived angiogenesis inhibitors may also be relevant to abscopal effects that occur following surgical removal of a tumor

inhibit the growth of a distant metastasis through inhibition of angiogenesis (Prehn 1991; O'Reilly et al. 1994; Sckell et al. 1998). In these situations, surgical removal of the primary tumor results in dramatically increased metastatic growth. However, when the primary tumor is irradiated, angiogenesis at a distal site is inhibited and growth of the metastases is limited (Hartford et al. 2000). Interestingly, in this same study, irradiation of the primary tumor was shown to lead to an increase in serum endostatin levels, consistent with the notion that p53-dependent production of collagen-derived angiogenesis inhibitors plays a role in this abscopal effect.

A Potential Role for Endogenous Angiogenesis Inhibitors in Promoting Tumor Dormancy

The p53-mediated production and secretion of anti-angiogenic factors may also help explain how small tumors are maintained in a dormant state for long periods of time. For instance, almost all individuals are thought to carry small microscopic growths of transformed cells – termed in situ carcinomas – in the thyroid, and yet thyroid cancer is a relatively rare type of malignancy (Harach, Franssila and Wasenius 1985; Black and Welch 1993). Similarly, approximately 40% of women between the ages of 40 and 50 harbor small malignant mammary cell foci; however, only 1% of the female population is diagnosed with breast cancer (Nielsen et al. 1987; Black and Welch 1993). It has been proposed that production of anti-angiogenic factors by in situ carcinomas limits their growth and prevents the majority of these tumors from becoming life threatening (Folkman and Kalluri 2004).

In some genetically well-characterized tumor types, such as colorectal cancer, the acquisition of p53 mutations is known to be a relatively late event in the progression from early to late-stage tumors (Baker et al. 1990). Loss of p53 function could, therefore, represent a turning point in which a small incipient tumor toggles the angiogenic switch to an "on state" and begins to rapidly grow due to neoangiogenesis. This model is supported by two experimental findings: first, reversal of the angiogenic switch requires either p53 or TSP-1 expression (Giuriato et al. 2006); and second, p53 expression has been shown to induce tumor dormancy by limiting angiogenesis (Holmgren et al. 1998; Gautam et al. 2002). Thus, part of the role of p53 may be to isolate small, non-vascularized microtumors by stimulating the constant production of angiogenesis inhibitors, thereby greatly hindering the angiogenic output of the tumor cells and limiting tumor growth (Fig. 9.4). Upon mutation of p53 this angiogenic checkpoint is lost, and tumor angiogenesis – and therefore tumor growth – proceeds unabated.

An important question in the field of cancer biology is: What are the molecular mechanisms that drive small benign growths to become highly vascularized, rapidly growing cancers? The goals of future research in this area are to understand the molecular events that control the angiogenic switch and how small in situ carcinomas can be maintained in dormant states for years or even decades. Once a clear understanding of the process is gained, it may then be possible to devise therapies that revert large tumors back into a dormant state. Moreover, current cancer diagnoses generally occur after the tumor has reached a dangerously large size. As better biomarkers are discovered that allow cancer to be detected at earlier stages, administration of anti-angiogenic therapy may be an effective method of maintaining tumors in a small, asymptomatic state.

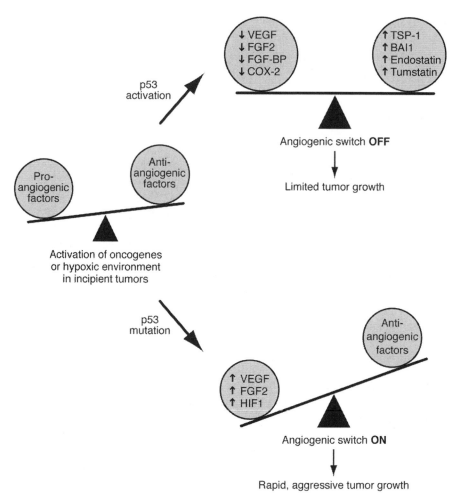

Fig. 9.4 p53 regulates the angiogenic switch in small, incipient tumors. Upon activation, p53 stimulates the constant production of angiogenesis inhibitors, thereby greatly hindering the angiogenic output of the tumor cells and limiting tumor growth. Tumors in which p53 is mutated have greater angiogenic potential due to both increased production of pro-angiogenic factors and decreased synthesis of anti-angiogenic factors. Under these conditions, the angiogenic switch is turned on and tumor growth proceeds unabated

p53-Induced Angiogenesis Inhibitors as Potential Cancer Therapeutics

In the early 1970s, Judah Folkman proposed that targeting angiogenesis in tumor tissues could be a therapeutic approach to preventing tumor progression. To date, more than 30 angiogenesis inhibitors are in clinical trials, representing one of the most promising avenues of cancer drug discovery. In particular, endogenous p53-induced angiogenesis inhibitors possess several important properties for therapeutic applications: they are generally non-toxic, they are secreted and function extracellularly, and often the biologically active portion of these molecules is a relatively small peptide. These ideal properties increase the possibility that endogenous p53-induced anti-angiogenic factors may make their way into the clinic as therapeutic treatments for cancer. The first endogenous angiogenesis inhibitor to enter clinical trials was endostatin. Although proven safe to use, recombinant human endostatin had only minimal efficacy when tested in clinical trials for advanced neuroendocrine tumors (Herbst et al. 2002; Kulke et al. 2006). Despite setbacks, there remains interest in further clinical trials for endostatin and other endogenous angiogenesis inhibitors such as tumstatin. One limitation of the endostatin trials was that the therapy was conducted as a monotherapy. However, successful trials with other angiogenesis inhibitors have generally been conducted in combination with conventional cancer therapeutics and may be a more feasible approach. In support of this notion, a modified form of endostatin called "Endostar" has been approved, in combination with chemotherapy, for treatment of non-small cell lung cancer in China (Jia and Kling 2006).

The limited success of endostatin has also prompted speculation that a more successful therapeutic approach may involve targeting multiple anti-angiogenic pathways. In this regard, one of the most promising angiogenesis inhibitors to be developed is Avastin (also known as bevacizumab), a monoclonal antibody that targets and inhibits the pro-angiogenic factor VEGF. Avastin was approved in 2004 in the United States for the treatment of metastatic colon cancer, and is now a frontline therapy for several types of malignancies. However, results of clinical trials with Avastin have not been overwhelming (Yang et al. 2003). One possibility yet to be addressed is whether agents that block pro-angiogenic factors, such as Avastin, can synergize with endogenous anti-angiogenic factors such as endostatin or tumstatin. Cocktail therapies containing a variety of anti-angiogenesis inhibitors targeting several pathways may provide significantly broader anti-cancer effects and dramatically improve the efficacy of current anti-angiogenesis approaches.

An additional strategy that may have potential in future therapies is to mobilize endogenous anti-angiogenic factors from their storage pools in the ECM by activating wild-type p53. The feasibility of this approach stems from the recent discovery of a family of small molecule MDM2 antagonists called Nutlins, which inhibit the p53-MDM2 interaction and thereby lead to activation of p53. One of these family members, Nutlin-3, has been shown to induce the expression of p53-regulated genes and to exhibit potent anti-proliferative activity in cells with functional p53. Nutlin-3 also inhibits the growth of human tumor xenografts in nude mice (Vassilev et al. 2004). Currently, there is interest in utilizing molecules such as Nutlin-3 as sensitizers for cytotoxic cancer therapies such as chemotherapy or radiation. It may be worthwhile to also test if these molecules also sensitize tumors to anti-angiogenic therapy in vivo.

The Role of p53 Status in Anti-angiogenic Therapies

It is well established that loss of p53 – which occurs in more than half of all human tumors – can diminish the therapeutic benefits of conventional chemotherapies such as radiation and other DNA damaging agents by reducing the cellular apoptosis response. With the recent development of angiogenesis inhibitors for cancer treatment, one of the most pressing clinical issues is whether the p53 status of tumors similarly influences the efficacy of drugs targeting tumor angiogenesis. Indeed, a number of studies have indicated that loss of p53 may reduce tumor responsiveness to anti-angiogenic treatments. In one study, for example, mice bearing tumors derived from p53$^{-/-}$ human colorectal cancer cells were more resistant than mice bearing isogenic p53$^{+/+}$ tumors to an anti-angiogenic therapy involving an antibody, DC101, targeting the VEGF receptor (Yu et al. 2002). This resistance could be due, at least in part, to one or more of the p53-dependent mechanisms discussed above.

There are several additional reasons why tumors carrying p53 mutations may be somewhat refractory to anti-angiogenic therapy. Hypoxia-induced apoptosis, for example, appears to be at least partially dependent on p53 (Graeber et al. 1994), and when grown under hypoxic conditions, cells harboring p53 mutations rapidly overtake wild-type p53 counterparts, demonstrating the selective advantage that p53 null cells have under hypoxic conditions (Graeber et al. 1996). However, even if loss of p53 diminishes the efficacy of anti-angiogenic therapies, this does not necessarily reduce the potential of these drugs for treating cancer. For example, even though the p53-negative tumors described above became less sensitive to the DC101 antibody, it is important to note that these tumors still responded to treatment (Yu et al. 2002).

Conclusions

Inhibition of angiogenesis is now widely recognized as an important component of the p53 tumor suppressor pathway. p53 has been shown to inhibit angiogenesis by interfering with central regulators of hypoxia that mediate angiogenesis, inhibiting production of pro-angiogenic factors, and directly increasing the production of endogenous angiogenesis inhibitors. The combination of these effects allows p53 to efficiently shut down the angiogenic potential of cancer cells. Inactivation of p53 during tumorigenesis reverses these effects and provides a potent stimulus for tumor angiogenesis; as a result, tumors carrying p53 mutations are more vascularized, often more aggressive and frequently correlate with poor prognosis for treatment. Thus, the loss of functional p53 during tumorigenesis likely represents an essential step in the switch to an angiogenic phenotype that is displayed by tumors. p53-induced angiogenesis inhibitors represent novel therapies for the treatment of cancer, although clinical data suggest that maximal therapeutic benefit may require these inhibitors to be used in conjunction with other therapies. Future directions of research should attempt to find optimal combinations of conventional chemotherapies and anti-angiogenic therapies.

References

Alvarez, A. A., Axelrod, J. R., Whitaker, R. S., Isner, P. D., Bentley, R. C., Dodge, R. K., and Rodriguez, G. C (2001) Thrombospondin-1 expression in epithelial ovarian carcinoma: Association with p53 status, tumor angiogenesis, and survival in platinum-treated patients. Gynecol. Oncol. 82:273–278.

Appella, E. and Anderson, C. W (2001) Post-translational modifications and activation of p53 by genotoxic stresses. Eur. J. Biochem. 268:2764–2772.

Baker, S. J., Preisinger, A. C., Jessup, J. M., Paraskeva, C., Markowitz, S., Willson, J. K., Hamilton, S., and Vogelstein, B (1990) p53 gene mutations occur in combination with 17p allelic deletions as late events in colorectal tumorigenesis. Cancer Res. 50:7717–7722.

Band, V., Dalal, S., Delmolino, L., and Androphy, E. J (1993) Enhanced degradation of p53 protein in HPV-6 and BPV-1 E6-immortalized human mammary epithelial cells. EMBO J. 12: 1847–1852.

Bian, J. and Sun, Y (1997) Transcriptional activation by p53 of the human type IV collagenase (gelatinase A or matrix metalloproteinase 2) promoter. Mol. Cell. Biol. 17:6330–6338.

Black, W. C. and Welch, H. G (1993) Advances in diagnostic imaging and overestimations of disease prevalence and the benefits of therapy. N. Engl. J. Med. 328:1237–1243.

Brantley, D. M., Cheng, N., Thompson, E. J., Lin, Q., Brekken, R. A., Thorpe, P. E., Muraoka, R. S., Cerretti, D. P., Pozzi, A., Jackson, D., Lin, C., and Chen, J (2002) Soluble Eph A receptors inhibit tumor angiogenesis and progression in vivo. Oncogene 21:7011–7026.

Camphausen, K., Moses, M. A., Menard, C., Sproull, M., Beecken, W. D., Folkman, J., and O'Reilly, M. S (2003) Radiation abscopal antitumor effect is mediated through p53. Cancer Res. 63:1990–1993.

Carmeliet, P., Dor, Y., Herbert, J. M., Fukumura, D., Brusselmans, K., Dewerchin, M., Neeman, M., Bono, F., Abramovitch, R., Maxwell, P., Koch, C. J., Ratcliffe, P., Moons, L., Jain, R. K., Collen, D., and Keshert, E (1998) Role of HIF-1alpha in hypoxia-mediated apoptosis, cell proliferation and tumour angiogenesis. Nature 394:485–490.

Chulada, P. C., Thompson, M. B., Mahler, J. F., Doyle, C. M., Gaul, B. W., Lee, C., Tiano, H. F., Morham, S. G., Smithies, O., and Langenbach, R (2000) Genetic disruption of Ptgs-1, as well as Ptgs-2, reduces intestinal tumorigenesis in Min mice. Cancer Res. 60: 4705–4708.

Coffman, K. T., Hu, M., Carles-Kinch, K., Tice, D., Donacki, N., Munyon, K., Kifle, G., Woods, R., Langermann, S., Kiener, P. A., and Kinch, M. S (2003) Differential EphA2 epitope display on normal versus malignant cells. Cancer Res. 63:7907–7912.

Coussens, L. M., Fingleton, B., and Matrisian, L. M (2002) Matrix metalloproteinase inhibitors and cancer: Trials and tribulations. Science 295:2387–2392.

Crawford, S. E., Stellmach, V., Murphy-Ullrich, J. E., Ribeiro, S. M., Lawler, J., Hynes, R. O., Boivin, G. P., and Bouck, N (1998) Thrombospondin-1 is a major activator of TGF-beta1 in vivo. Cell 93:1159–1170.

Crew, J. P., O'Brien, T., Bradburn, M., Fuggle, S., Bicknell, R., Cranston, D., and Harris, A. L (1997) Vascular endothelial growth factor is a predictor of relapse and stage progression in superficial bladder cancer. Cancer Res. 57:5281–5285.

Dameron, K. M., Volpert, O. V., Tainsky, M. A., and Bouck, N (1994) Control of angiogenesis in fibroblasts by p53 regulation of thrombospondin-1. Science 265:1582–1584.

Dawson, D. W., Pearce, S. F., Zhong, R., Silverstein, R. L., Frazier, W. A., and Bouck, N. P (1997) CD36 mediates the In vitro inhibitory effects of thrombospondin-1 on endothelial cells. J. Cell Biol. 138:707–717.

Dejong, V., Degeorges, A., Filleur, S., Ait-Si-Ali, S., Mettouchi, A., Bornstein, P., Binetruy, B., and Cabon, F (1999) The Wilms' tumor gene product represses the transcription of thrombospondin 1 in response to overexpression of c-Jun. Oncogene 18:3143–3151.

Derynck, R., Akhurst, R. J., and Balmain, A (2001) TGF-beta signaling in tumor suppression and cancer progression. Nat. Genet. 29:117–129.

Dobner, T., Horikoshi, N., Rubenwolf, S., and Shenk, T (1996) Blockage by adenovirus E4orf6 of transcriptional activation by the p53 tumor suppressor. Science 272:1470–1473.

Dodelet, V. C. and Pasquale, E. B (2000) Eph receptors and ephrin ligands: Embryogenesis to tumorigenesis. Oncogene 19:5614–5619.

Dohn, M., Jiang, J., and Chen, X (2001) Receptor tyrosine kinase EphA2 is regulated by p53-family proteins and induces apoptosis. Oncogene 20:6503–6515.

Easty, D. J. and Bennett, D. C (2000) Protein tyrosine kinases in malignant melanoma. Melanoma Res. 10:401–411.

Erkinheimo, T. L., Lassus, H., Finne, P., van Rees, B. P., Leminen, A., Ylikorkala, O., Haglund, C., Butzow, R., and Ristimaki, A (2004) Elevated cyclooxygenase-2 expression is associated with altered expression of p53 and SMAD4, amplification of HER-2/neu, and poor outcome in serous ovarian carcinoma. Clin. Cancer Res. 10:538–545.

Faviana, P., Boldrini, L., Spisni, R., Berti, P., Galleri, D., Biondi, R., Camacci, T., Materazzi, G., Pingitore, R., Miccoli, P., and Fontanini, G (2002) Neoangiogenesis in colon cancer: Correlation between vascular density, vascular endothelial growth factor (VEGF) and p53 protein expression. Oncol Rep. 9:617–620.

Fingleton, B (2006) Matrix metalloproteinases: Roles in cancer and metastasis. Front. Biosci. 11:479–491.

Folkman, J. and Kalluri, R (2004) Cancer without disease. Nature 427:787.

Fontanini, G., Vignati, S., Lucchi, M., Mussi, A., Calcinai, A., Boldrini, L., Chine, S., Silvestri, V., Angeletti, C. A., Basolo, F., and Bevilacqua, G (1997) Neoangiogenesis and p53 protein in lung cancer: Their prognostic role and their relation with vascular endothelial growth factor (VEGF) expression. Br. J. Cancer 75:1295–1301.

Forsythe, J. A., Jiang, B. H., Iyer, N. V., Agani, F., Leung, S. W., Koos, R. D., and Semenza, G. L (1996) Activation of vascular endothelial growth factor gene transcription by hypoxia-inducible factor 1. Mol. Cell. Biol. 16:4604–4613.

Gabellini, C., Del Bufalo, D., and Zupi, G (2006) Involvement of RB gene family in tumor angiogenesis. Oncogene 25:5326–5332.

Gasparini, G., Weidner, N., Maluta, S., Pozza, F., Boracchi, P., Mezzetti, M., Testolin, A., and Bevilacqua, P (1993) Intratumoral microvessel density and p53 protein: Correlation with metastasis in head-and-neck squamous-cell carcinoma. Int. J. Cancer 55:739–744.

Gasparini, G., Weidner, N., Bevilacqua, P., Maluta, S., Dalla Palma, P., Caffo, O., Barbareschi, M., Boracchi, P., Marubini, E., and Pozza, F (1994) Tumor microvessel density, p53 expression, tumor size, and peritumoral lymphatic vessel invasion are relevant prognostic markers in node-negative breast carcinoma. J. Clin. Oncol. 12:454–466.

Gasparini, G., Toi, M., Gion, M., Verderio, P., Dittadi, R., Hanatani, M., Matsubara, I., Vinante, O., Bonoldi, E., Boracchi, P., Gatti, C., Suzuki, H., and Tominaga, T (1997) Prognostic significance of vascular endothelial growth factor protein in node-negative breast carcinoma. J. Natl. Cancer Inst. 89:139–147.

Gautam, A., Densmore, C. L., Melton, S., Golunski, E., and Waldrep, J. C (2002) Aerosol delivery of PEI-p53 complexes inhibits B16-F10 lung metastases through regulation of angiogenesis. Cancer Gene Ther. 9:28–36.

Giuriato, S., Ryeom, S., Fan, A. C., Bachireddy, P., Lynch, R. C., Rioth, M. J., van Riggelen, J., Kopelman, A. M., Passegue, E., Tang, F., Folkman, J., and Felsher, D. W (2006) Sustained regression of tumors upon MYC inactivation requires p53 or thrombospondin-1 to reverse the angiogenic switch. Proc. Natl. Acad. Sci. USA 103:16266–16271.

Good, D. J., Polverini, P. J., Rastinejad, F., Le Beau, M. M., Lemons, R. S., Frazier, W. A., and Bouck, N. P (1990) A tumor suppressor-dependent inhibitor of angiogenesis is immunologically and functionally indistinguishable from a fragment of thrombospondin. Proc. Natl. Acad. Sci. USA 87:6624–6628.

Graeber, T. G., Peterson, J. F., Tsai, M., Monica, K., Fornace, A. J., Jr., and Giaccia, A. J (1994) Hypoxia induces accumulation of p53 protein, but activation of a G1-phase checkpoint by low-oxygen conditions is independent of p53 status. Mol. Cell. Biol. 14: 6264–6277.

Graeber, T. G., Osmanian, C., Jacks, T., Housman, D. E., Koch, C. J., Lowe, S. W., and Giaccia, A. J (1996) Hypoxia-mediated selection of cells with diminished apoptotic potential in solid tumours. Nature 379:88–91.

Grant, S. W., Kyshtoobayeva, A. S., Kurosaki, T., Jakowatz, J., and Fruehauf, J. P (1998) Mutant p53 correlates with reduced expression of thrombospondin-1, increased angiogenesis, and metastatic progression in melanoma. Cancer Detect. Prev. 22:185–194.

Grossfeld, G. D., Carroll, P. R., Lindeman, N., Meng, M., Groshen, S., Feng, A. C., Hawes, D., and Cote, R. J (2002) Thrombospondin-1 expression in patients with pathologic stage T3 prostate cancer undergoing radical prostatectomy: Association with p53 alterations, tumor angiogenesis, and tumor progression. Urology 59:97–102.

Harach, H. R., Franssila, K. O., and Wasenius, V. M (1985) Occult papillary carcinoma of the thyroid. A "normal" finding in Finland. A systematic autopsy study. Cancer 56:531–538.

Hartford, A. C., Gohongi, T., Fukumura, D., and Jain, R. K (2000) Irradiation of a primary tumor, unlike surgical removal, enhances angiogenesis suppression at a distal site: Potential role of host-tumor interaction. Cancer Res. 60:2128–2131.

Herbst, R. S., Hess, K. R., Tran, H. T., Tseng, J. E., Mullani, N. A., Charnsangavej, C., Madden, T., Davis, D. W., McConkey, D. J., O'Reilly, M. S., Ellis, L. M., Pluda, J., Hong, W. K., and Abbruzzese, J. L (2002) Phase I study of recombinant human endostatin in patients with advanced solid tumors. J. Clin. Oncol. 20:3792–3803.

Holmgren, L., Jackson, G., and Arbiser, J (1998) p53 induces angiogenesis-restricted dormancy in a mouse fibrosarcoma. Oncogene 17:819–824.

Hsu, S. C., Volpert, O. V., Steck, P. A., Mikkelsen, T., Polverini, P. J., Rao, S., Chou, P., and Bouck, N. P (1996) Inhibition of angiogenesis in human glioblastomas by chromosome 10 induction of thrombospondin-1. Cancer Res. 56:5684–5691.

Iyer, N. V., Kotch, L. E., Agani, F., Leung, S. W., Laughner, E., Wenger, R. H., Gassmann, M., Gearhart, J. D., Lawler, A. M., Yu, A. Y., and Semenza, G. L (1998) Cellular and developmental control of O2 homeostasis by hypoxia-inducible factor 1 alpha. Genes Dev. 12: 149–162.

Janz, A., Sevignani, C., Kenyon, K., Ngo, C. V., and Thomas-Tikhonenko, A (2000) Activation of the myc oncoprotein leads to increased turnover of thrombospondin-1 mRNA. Nucleic Acids Res. 28:2268–2275.

Jia, H. and Kling, J (2006) China offers alternative gateway for experimental drugs. Nat. Biotechnol. 24:117–118.

Jiang, D., Srinivasan, A., Lozano, G., and Robbins, P. D (1993) SV40 T antigen abrogates p53-mediated transcriptional activity. Oncogene 8:2805–2812.

Jimenez, B., Volpert, O. V., Crawford, S. E., Febbraio, M., Silverstein, R. L., and Bouck, N (2000) Signals leading to apoptosis-dependent inhibition of neovascularization by thrombospondin-1. Nat. Med. 6:41–48.

Kalluri, R (2003) Basement membranes: Structure, assembly and role in tumour angiogenesis. Nat. Rev. Cancer 3:422–433.

Kaluzova, M., Kaluz, S., Lerman, M. I., and Stanbridge, E. J (2004) DNA damage is a prerequisite for p53-mediated proteasomal degradation of HIF-1alpha in hypoxic cells and downregulation of the hypoxia marker carbonic anhydrase IX. Mol. Cell. Biol. 24:5757–5766.

Kang, S. M., Maeda, K., Onoda, N., Chung, Y. S., Nakata, B., Nishiguchi, Y., and Sowa, M (1997) Combined analysis of p53 and vascular endothelial growth factor expression in colorectal carcinoma for determination of tumor vascularity and liver metastasis. Int. J. Cancer 74:502–507.

Kaur, B., Brat, D. J., Devi, N. S., and Van Meir, E. G (2005) Vasculostatin, a proteolytic fragment of brain angiogenesis inhibitor 1, is an antiangiogenic and antitumorigenic factor. Oncogene 24:3632–3642.

Kawahara, N., Ono, M., Taguchi, K., Okamoto, M., Shimada, M., Takenaka, K., Hayashi, K., Mosher, D. F., Sugimachi, K., Tsuneyoshi, M., and Kuwano, M (1998) Enhanced expression of thrombospondin-1 and hypovascularity in human cholangiocarcinoma. Hepatology 28: 1512–1517.

Khalkhali-Ellis, Z (2006) Maspin: The new frontier. Clin. Cancer Res. 12:7279–7283.

Khwaja, F. W., Svoboda, P., Reed, M., Pohl, J., Pyrzynska, B., and Van Meir, E. G (2006) Proteomic identification of the wt-p53-regulated tumor cell secretome. Oncogene 25:7650–7661.

Kinch, M. S. and Carles-Kinch, K (2003) Overexpression and functional alterations of the EphA2 tyrosine kinase in cancer. Clin. Exp. Metastasis 20:59–68.

Koumenis, C., Alarcon, R., Hammond, E., Sutphin, P., Hoffman, W., Murphy, M., Derr, J., Taya, Y., Lowe, S. W., Kastan, M., and Giaccia, A (2001) Regulation of p53 by hypoxia: Dissociation of transcriptional repression and apoptosis from p53-dependent transactivation. Mol. Cell. Biol. 21:1297–1310.

Kulke, M. H., Bergsland, E. K., Ryan, D. P., Enzinger, P. C., Lynch, T. J., Zhu, A. X., Meyerhardt, J. A., Heymach, J. V., Fogler, W. E., Sidor, C., Michelini, A., Kinsella, K., Venook, A. P., and Fuchs, C. S (2006) Phase II study of recombinant human endostatin in patients with advanced neuroendocrine tumors. J. Clin. Oncol. 24:3555–3561.

Kwak, C., Jin, R. J., Lee, C., Park, M. S., and Lee, S. E (2002) Thrombospondin-1, vascular endothelial growth factor expression and their relationship with p53 status in prostate cancer and benign prostatic hyperplasia. BJU Int. 89:303–309.

Li F. P., Fraumeni J. F., Jr., Mulvihill J. J., Blattner W. A., Dreyfus M. G., Tucker M. A., and Miller R. W (1988) A cancer family syndrome in twenty-four kindreds. Cancer Res 48:5358–5362.

Linderholm, B., Lindh, B., Tavelin, B., Grankvist, K., and Henriksson, R (2000) p53 and vascular-endothelial-growth-factor (VEGF) expression predicts outcome in 833 patients with primary breast carcinoma. Int. J. Cancer 89:51–62.

Linderholm, B. K., Lindahl, T., Holmberg, L., Klaar, S., Lennerstrand, J., Henriksson, R., and Bergh, J (2001) The expression of vascular endothelial growth factor correlates with mutant p53 and poor prognosis in human breast cancer. Cancer Res. 61:2256–2260.

Masferrer, J. L., Leahy, K. M., Koki, A. T., Zweifel, B. S., Settle, S. L., Woerner, B. M., Edwards, D. A., Flickinger, A. G., Moore, R. J., and Seibert, K (2000) Antiangiogenic and antitumor activities of cyclooxygenase-2 inhibitors. Cancer Res. 60:1306–1311.

Mietz, J. A., Unger, T., Huibregtse, J. M., and Howley, P. M (1992) The transcriptional transactivation function of wild-type p53 is inhibited by SV40 large T-antigen and by HPV-16 E6 oncoprotein. EMBO J. 11:5013–5020.

Miled, C., Pontoglio, M., Garbay, S., Yaniv, M., and Weitzman, J. B (2005) A genomic map of p53 binding sites identifies novel p53 targets involved in an apoptotic network. Cancer Res. 65:5096–5104.

Minami, T., Horiuchi, K., Miura, M., Abid, M. R., Takabe, W., Noguchi, N., Kohro, T., Ge, X., Aburatani, H., Hamakubo, T., Kodama, T., and Aird, W. C (2004) Vascular endothelial growth factor- and thrombin-induced termination factor, Down syndrome critical region-1, attenuates endothelial cell proliferation and angiogenesis. J. Biol. Chem. 279:50537–50554.

Miyazaki, T., Kato, H., Fukuchi, M., Nakajima, M., and Kuwano, H (2003) EphA2 overexpression correlates with poor prognosis in esophageal squamous cell carcinoma. Int. J. Cancer 103: 657–663.

Mukhopadhyay, D., Tsiokas, L., and Sukhatme, V. P. (1995a) Wild-type p53 and v-Src exert opposing influences on human vascular endothelial growth factor gene expression. Cancer Res. 55:6161–6165.

Mukhopadhyay, D., Tsiokas, L., Zhou, X. M., Foster, D., Brugge, J. S., and Sukhatme, V. P. (1995b) Hypoxic induction of human vascular endothelial growth factor expression through c-Src activation. Nature 375:577–581.

Nielsen, M., Thomsen, J. L., Primdahl, S., Dyreborg, U., and Andersen, J. A (1987) Breast cancer and atypia among young and middle-aged women: A study of 110 medicolegal autopsies. Br. J. Cancer 56:814–819.

Nishimori, H., Shiratsuchi, T., Urano, T., Kimura, Y., Kiyono, K., Tatsumi, K., Yoshida, S., Ono, M., Kuwano, M., Nakamura, Y., and Tokino, T (1997) A novel brain-specific p53-target gene, BAI1, containing thrombospondin type 1 repeats inhibits experimental angiogenesis. Oncogene 15:2145–2150.

Nissi, R., Autio-Harmainen, H., Marttila, P., Sormunen, R., and Kivirikko, K. I (2001) Prolyl 4-hydroxylase isoenzymes I and II have different expression patterns in several human tissues. J. Histochem. Cytochem. 49:1143–1153.

Noblitt, L. W., Bangari, D. S., Shukla, S., Knapp, D. W., Mohammed, S., Kinch, M. S., and Mittal, S. K (2004) Decreased tumorigenic potential of EphA2-overexpressing breast cancer cells following treatment with adenoviral vectors that express EphrinA1. Cancer Gene Ther. 11:757–766.

Nor, J. E., Mitra, R. S., Sutorik, M. M., Mooney, D. J., Castle, V. P., and Polverini, P. J (2000) Thrombospondin-1 induces endothelial cell apoptosis and inhibits angiogenesis by activating the caspase death pathway. J. Vasc. Res. 37:209–218.

O'Reilly, M. S., Holmgren, L., Shing, Y., Chen, C., Rosenthal, R. A., Moses, M., Lane, W. S., Cao, Y., Sage, E. H., and Folkman, J (1994) Angiostatin: A novel angiogenesis inhibitor that mediates the suppression of metastases by a Lewis lung carcinoma. Cell 79:315–328.

Obermair, A., Kucera, E., Mayerhofer, K., Speiser, P., Seifert, M., Czerwenka, K., Kaider, A., Leodolter, S., Kainz, C., and Zeillinger, R (1997) Vascular endothelial growth factor (VEGF) in human breast cancer: Correlation with disease-free survival. Int. J. Cancer 74:455–458.

Ogawa, K., Pasqualini, R., Lindberg, R. A., Kain, R., Freeman, A. L., and Pasquale, E. B (2000) The ephrin-A1 ligand and its receptor, EphA2, are expressed during tumor neovascularization. Oncogene 19:6043–6052.

Oshima, M., Dinchuk, J. E., Kargman, S. L., Oshima, H., Hancock, B., Kwong, E., Trzaskos, J. M., Evans, J. F., and Taketo, M. M (1996) Suppression of intestinal polyposis in Apc delta716 knockout mice by inhibition of cyclooxygenase 2 (COX-2). Cell 87:803–809.

Pal, S., Datta, K., and Mukhopadhyay, D (2001) Central role of p53 on regulation of vascular permeability factor/vascular endothelial growth factor (VPF/VEGF) expression in mammary carcinoma. Cancer Res. 61:6952–6957.

Pan, Y., Oprysko, P. R., Asham, A. M., Koch, C. J., and Simon, M. C (2004) p53 cannot be induced by hypoxia alone but responds to the hypoxic microenvironment. Oncogene 23:4975–4983.

Pasquale, E. B (2005) Eph receptor signalling casts a wide net on cell behaviour. Nat. Rev. Mol. Cell Biol. 6:462–475.

Pelengaris, S., Littlewood, T., Khan, M., Elia, G., and Evan, G (1999) Reversible activation of c-Myc in skin: Induction of a complex neoplastic phenotype by a single oncogenic lesion. Mol. Cell 3:565–577.

Prehn, R. T (1991) The inhibition of tumor growth by tumor mass. Cancer Res. 51:2–4.

Ragimov, N., Krauskopf, A., Navot, N., Rotter, V., Oren, M., and Aloni, Y (1993) Wild-type but not mutant p53 can repress transcription initiation in vitro by interfering with the binding of basal transcription factors to the TATA motif. Oncogene 8:1183–1193.

Rak, J., Mitsuhashi, Y., Sheehan, C., Tamir, A., Viloria-Petit, A., Filmus, J., Mansour, S. J., Ahn, N. G., and Kerbel, R. S (2000) Oncogenes and tumor angiogenesis: Differential modes of vascular endothelial growth factor up-regulation in ras-transformed epithelial cells and fibroblasts. Cancer Res. 60:490–498.

Ravi, R., Mookerjee, B., Bhujwalla, Z. M., Sutter, C. H., Artemov, D., Zeng, Q., Dillehay, L. E., Madan, A., Semenza, G. L., and Bedi, A (2000) Regulation of tumor angiogenesis by p53-induced degradation of hypoxia-inducible factor 1alpha. Genes Dev. 14:34–44.

Rempe, D. A., Lelli, K. M., Vangeison, G., Johnson, R. S., and Federoff, H. J (2007) In cultured astrocytes, p53 and MDM2 do not alter hypoxia-inducible factor-1alpha function regardless of presence of DNA damage. J. Biol. Chem. 282:16187–16201.

Riccioni, T., Cirielli, C., Wang, X., Passaniti, A., and Capogrossi, M. C (1998) Adenovirus-mediated wild-type p53 overexpression inhibits endothelial cell differentiation in vitro and angiogenesis in vivo. Gene Ther. 5:747–754.

Ryan, H. E., Lo, J., and Johnson, R. S (1998) HIF-1 alpha is required for solid tumor formation and embryonic vascularization. EMBO J. 17:3005–3015.

Saez, E., Rutberg, S. E., Mueller, E., Oppenheim, H., Smoluk, J., Yuspa, S. H., and Spiegelman, B. M (1995) c-fos is required for malignant progression of skin tumors. Cell 82: 721–732.

Sckell, A., Safabakhsh, N., Dellian, M., and Jain, R. K (1998) Primary tumor size-dependent inhibition of angiogenesis at a secondary site: An intravital microscopic study in mice. Cancer Res. 58:5866–5869.

Seto, E., Usheva, A., Zambetti, G. P., Momand, J., Horikoshi, N., Weinmann, R., Levine, A. J., and Shenk, T (1992) Wild-type p53 binds to the TATA-binding protein and represses transcription. Proc. Natl. Acad. Sci. USA 89:12028–12032.

Sherif, Z. A., Nakai, S., Pirollo, K. F., Rait, A., and Chang, E. H (2001) Downmodulation of bFGF-binding protein expression following restoration of p53 function. Cancer Gene Ther. 8:771–782.

Slack, J. L. and Bornstein, P (1994) Transformation by v-src causes transient induction followed by repression of mouse thrombospondin-1. Cell Growth Differ. 5:1373–1380.

Somasundaram, K. and El-Deiry, W. S (1997) Inhibition of p53-mediated transactivation and cell cycle arrest by E1A through its p300/CBP-interacting region. Oncogene 14:1047–1057.

Song, S. Y., Lee, S. K., Kim, D. H., Son, H. J., Kim, H. J., Lim, Y. J., Lee, W. Y., Chun, H. K., and Rhee, J. C (2002) Expression of maspin in colon cancers: Its relationship with p53 expression and microvessel density. Dig. Dis. Sci. 47:1831–1835.

Soussi T., Ishioka C., Claustres M., and Beroud C (2006) Locus-specific mutation databases: Pitfalls and good practice based on the p53 experience. Nat Rev Cancer 6:83–90.

Steegenga, W. T., van Laar, T., Riteco, N., Mandarino, A., Shvarts, A., van der Eb, A. J., and Jochemsen, A. G (1996) Adenovirus E1A proteins inhibit activation of transcription by p53. Mol. Cell. Biol. 16:2101–2109.

Stellmach, V., Volpert, O. V., Crawford, S. E., Lawler, J., Hynes, R. O., and Bouck, N (1996) Tumour suppressor genes and angiogenesis: The role of TP53 in fibroblasts. Eur. J. Cancer 32A:2394–2400.

Subbaramaiah, K., Altorki, N., Chung, W. J., Mestre, J. R., Sampat, A., and Dannenberg, A. J (1999) Inhibition of cyclooxygenase-2 gene expression by p53. J. Biol. Chem. 274: 10911–10915.

Sund, M., Hamano, Y., Sugimoto, H., Sudhakar, A., Soubasakos, M., Yerramalla, U., Benjamin, L. E., Lawler, J., Kieran, M., Shah, A., and Kalluri, R (2005) Function of endogenous inhibitors of angiogenesis as endothelium-specific tumor suppressors. Proc. Natl. Acad. Sci. USA 102:2934–2939.

Sussan, T. E., Yang, A., Li, F., Ostrowski, M. C., and Reeves, R. H (2008) Trisomy represses Apc(Min)-mediated tumours in mouse models of Down's syndrome. Nature 451:73–75.

Takahashi, Y., Bucana, C. D., Cleary, K. R., and Ellis, L. M (1998) p53, vessel count, and vascular endothelial growth factor expression in human colon cancer. Int. J. Cancer 79:34–38.

Teodoro, J. G., Parker, A. E., Zhu, X., and Green, M. R (2006) p53-mediated inhibition of angiogenesis through up-regulation of a collagen prolyl hydroxylase. Science 313: 968–971.

Tikhonenko, A. T., Black, D. J., and Linial, M. L (1996) Viral Myc oncoproteins in infected fibroblasts down-modulate thrombospondin-1, a possible tumor suppressor gene. J. Biol. Chem. 271:30741–30747.

Tokino, T., Thiagalingam, S., el-Deiry, W. S., Waldman, T., Kinzler, K. W., and Vogelstein, B (1994) p53 tagged sites from human genomic DNA. Hum. Mol. Genet. 3:1537–1542.

Tokunaga, T., Nakamura, M., Oshika, Y., Tsuchida, T., Kazuno, M., Fukushima, Y., Kawai, K., Abe, Y., Kijima, H., Yamazaki, H., Tamaoki, N., and Ueyama, Y (1998) Alterations in tumour suppressor gene p53 correlate with inhibition of thrombospondin-1 gene expression in colon cancer cells. Virchows Arch. 433:415–418.

Tolsma, S. S., Volpert, O. V., Good, D. J., Frazier, W. A., Polverini, P. J., and Bouck, N (1993) Peptides derived from two separate domains of the matrix protein thrombospondin-1 have anti-angiogenic activity. J. Cell Biol. 122:497–511.

Tsujii, M., Kawano, S., Tsuji, S., Sawaoka, H., Hori, M., and DuBois, R. N (1998) Cyclooxygenase regulates angiogenesis induced by colon cancer cells. Cell 93:705–716.

Ueba, T., Nosaka, T., Takahashi, J. A., Shibata, F., Florkiewicz, R. Z., Vogelstein, B., Oda, Y., Kikuchi, H., and Hatanaka, M (1994) Transcriptional regulation of basic fibroblast growth factor gene by p53 in human glioblastoma and hepatocellular carcinoma cells. Proc. Natl. Acad. Sci. USA 91:9009–9013.

Van Meir, E. G., Polverini, P. J., Chazin, V. R., Su Huang, H. J., de Tribolet, N., and Cavenee, W. K (1994) Release of an inhibitor of angiogenesis upon induction of wild type p53 expression in glioblastoma cells. Nat. Genet. 8:171–176.

Vassilev, L. T., Vu, B. T., Graves, B., Carvajal, D., Podlaski, F., Filipovic, Z., Kong, N., Kammlott, U., Lukacs, C., Klein, C., Fotouhi, N., and Liu, E. A (2004) In vivo activation of the p53 pathway by small-molecule antagonists of MDM2. Science 303:844–848.

Volpert, O. V., Dameron, K. M., and Bouck, N (1997) Sequential development of an angiogenic phenotype by human fibroblasts progressing to tumorigenicity. Oncogene 14:1495–1502.

Walker-Daniels, J., Coffman, K., Azimi, M., Rhim, J. S., Bostwick, D. G., Snyder, P., Kerns, B. J., Waters, D. J., and Kinch, M. S (1999) Overexpression of the EphA2 tyrosine kinase in prostate cancer. Prostate 41:275–280.

Watnick, R. S., Cheng, Y. N., Rangarajan, A., Ince, T. A., and Weinberg, R. A (2003) Ras modulates Myc activity to repress thrombospondin-1 expression and increase tumor angiogenesis. Cancer Cell 3:219–231.

Wei, C. L., Wu, Q., Vega, V. B., Chiu, K. P., Ng, P., Zhang, T., Shahab, A., Yong, H. C., Fu, Y., Weng, Z., Liu, J., Zhao, X. D., Chew, J. L., Lee, Y. L., Kuznetsov, V. A., Sung, W. K., Miller, L. D., Lim, B., Liu, E. T., Yu, Q., Ng, H. H., and Ruan, Y (2006) A global map of p53 transcription-factor binding sites in the human genome. Cell 124:207–219.

Weinstat-Saslow, D. L., Zabrenetzky, V. S., VanHoutte, K., Frazier, W. A., Roberts, D. D., and Steeg, P. S (1994) Transfection of thrombospondin 1 complementary DNA into a human breast carcinoma cell line reduces primary tumor growth, metastatic potential, and angiogenesis. Cancer Res. 54:6504–6511.

Williams, C. S., Tsujii, M., Reese, J., Dey, S. K., and DuBois, R. N (2000) Host cyclooxygenase-2 modulates carcinoma growth. J. Clin. Invest. 105:1589–1594.

Yang, J. C., Haworth, L., Sherry, R. M., Hwu, P., Schwartzentruber, D. J., Topalian, S. L., Steinberg, S. M., Chen, H. X., and Rosenberg, S. A (2003) A randomized trial of bevacizumab, an anti-vascular endothelial growth factor antibody, for metastatic renal cancer. N. Engl. J. Med. 349:427–434.

Yew, P. R. and Berk, A. J (1992) Inhibition of p53 transactivation required for transformation by adenovirus early 1B protein. Nature 357:82–85.

Yu, E. Y., Yu, E., Meyer, G. E., and Brawer, M. K (1997) The relation of p53 protein nuclear accumulation and angiogenesis in human prostatic carcinoma. Prostate Cancer Prostatic Dis. 1:39–44.

Yu, J. L., Rak, J. W., Coomber, B. L., Hicklin, D. J., and Kerbel, R. S (2002) Effect of p53 status on tumor response to antiangiogenic therapy. Science 295:1526–1528.

Zelinski, D. P., Zantek, N. D., Stewart, J. C., Irizarry, A. R., and Kinch, M. S (2001) EphA2 overexpression causes tumorigenesis of mammary epithelial cells. Cancer Res. 61:2301–2306.

Zhang, L., Yu, D., Hu, M., Xiong, S., Lang, A., Ellis, L. M., and Pollock, R. E (2000a) Wild-type p53 suppresses angiogenesis in human leiomyosarcoma and synovial sarcoma by transcriptional suppression of vascular endothelial growth factor expression. Cancer Res. 60:3655–3661.

Zhang, M., Volpert, O., Shi, Y. H., and Bouck, N (2000b) Maspin is an angiogenesis inhibitor. Nat Med 6:196–199.

Zorick, T. S., Mustacchi, Z., Bando, S. Y., Zatz, M., Moreira-Filho, C. A., Olsen, B., and Passos-Bueno, M. R (2001) High serum endostatin levels in Down syndrome: Implications for improved treatment and prevention of solid tumours. Eur. J. Hum. Genet. 9:811–814.

Zou, Z., Anisowicz, A., Hendrix, M. J., Thor, A., Neveu, M., Sheng, S., Rafidi, K., Seftor, E., and Sager, R (1994) Maspin, a serpin with tumor-suppressing activity in human mammary epithelial cells. Science 263:526–529.

Zou, Z., Gao, C., Nagaich, A. K., Connell, T., Saito, S., Moul, J. W., Seth, P., Appella, E., and Srivastava, S (2000) p53 regulates the expression of the tumor suppressor gene maspin. J. Biol. Chem. 275:6051–6054.

Chapter 10
Ink4a Locus: Beyond Cell Cycle

Greg H. Enders

Cast of Characters

p16 is an established suppressor of both "liquid" and solid tumors, with the latter being the most prominent. Major human cancer types with regular inactivation of p16 include melanoma, adenocarcinoma of the breast, squamous cell carcinomas of the lung, pancreatic adenocarcinomas, and colorectal carcinomas (Baylin et al. 1998; Pollack, Pearson, and Hayward 1996). In pancreatic adenocarcinoma, the frequency of p16 inactivation approaches 100% (Caldas et al. 1994; Schutte et al. 1997). Mechanisms of inactivation run the gamut from large deletions to point mutations and promoter methylation (Baylin et al. 1998). Germ line p16 mutations in humans are now known to predispose to melanoma (Kamb et al. 1994b), pancreatic adenocarcinoma (Goldstein et al. 1995; Vasen et al. 2000), and hepatocellular carcinoma (Chaubert et al. 1997). The Ink4a locus is unusual in encoding a second protein, p19[Arf] (Arf), from an *alternative reading frame* (Liggett et al. 1996; Quelle et al. 1995). Arf is a tumor suppressor in its own right, acting through p53 and other targets (Clurman and Groudine 1998; Kamijo et al. 1997; Pomerantz et al. 1998; Zhang et al. 1998; Korgaonkar et al. 2002; Weber et al. 2000). Whereas Arf appears to be the dominant tumor suppressor in the mouse, p16 is in humans (Clurman and Groudine 1998; Quelle et al. 1997). Many mutations selectively inactivate p16, sparing Arf (Haber 1997; Koh et al. 1995; Ranade et al. 1995).

Introduction

p16 Is a Cdk Inhibitor and Tumor Suppressor

p16[Ink4a] was discovered as a binding partner and *inhibitor* of cyclin-dependent *kinase 4* (Cdk4) and the closely related enzyme Cdk6 (Serrano et al.1993). These biochemical properties immediately provoked the hypothesis that p16 might exert

G.H. Enders (✉)
Department of Medicine, Fox Chase Cancer Center, Philadelphia, PA, USA
e-mail: greg.enders@fccc.edu

A. Thomas-Tikhonenko (ed.), *Cancer Genome and Tumor Microenvironment*,
DOI 10.1007/978-1-4419-0711-0_10, © Springer Science+Business Media, LLC 2010

important constraints on cell proliferation, given evidence that Cdk4 and 6 act as gatekeepers for cell cycle entry. Shortly thereafter, the Ink4a locus was identified independently as a locus mutated in multiple human cancer cell lines and as a gene mutated frequently in familial melanoma, pointing to a major tumor suppressor role (Kamb et al. 1994a,b; Nobori et al. 1994). p16 arrests cells in G1 phase, prior to DNA replication, in a manner dependent on the retinoblastoma tumor suppressor protein (pRb) (Lukas et al. 1995; Koh et al. 1995; Medema et al. 1995; Serrano et al. 1995). p16 and pRb thus comprise upstream and downstream elements, respectively, of a tumor suppressor pathway. Reflecting the broad role of this pathway, p16 is frequently inactivated in sporadic human tumors of several types (Pollack, Pearson, and Hayward 1996). Moreover, knock-out mice are tumor prone, providing formal proof of p16's tumor suppressor activity (Serrano et al. 1996; Sharpless et al. 2001). This straightforward story of p16 as a major tumor suppressor and cell cycle inhibitor remains unchallenged. However, more recent studies have suggested additional complexity to the biology of p16, touching on several major, topical issues in cancer biology and including tumor progression and microenvironment.

Mechanism of Cell Cycle Inhibition

Although p16 specifically binds Cdk4 and 6, Cdk2 complexes are also inhibited, indirectly but potently (McConnell et al. 1999; Mitra et al. 1999; Parry et al. 1999). p16 binding displaces cyclin D from Cdk 4 and 6, freeing up a large pool of p21 and p27 Cdk inhibitors to bind to Cdk2 complexes. Inhibition of these Cdks activates proteins of the pRb family (Sherr 1996). The latter proteins repress transcription of E2F-dependent genes, which encode a host of proteins involved in cell replication (Weinberg 1995).

Tumor Biology

Induction in Settings of Sustained Proliferation

Whereas many tumor suppressors, such as pRb, are constitutively expressed, p16 regulation is more like that of p53. p16 expression is low or undetectable in most tissues during development and early adulthood in the mouse (Krishnamurthy et al. 2004; Zindy et al. 1997). Consistent with this observation, absence of p16 has no obvious effect during these stages (Serrano et al. 1996). p16 levels accumulate during aging in several tissues as well as in pre-neoplastic and neoplastic states (Krishnamurthy et al. 2004). This pattern of regulation is consistent with the notion that p16 is foremost a tumor suppressor, with limited roles in development or tissue homeostasis. p16 is routinely induced as cells approach replicative senescence in tissue culture, and p16 clearly contributes to such senescence (Alcorta et al. 1996; Brenner et al. 1998; Erickson et al. 1998; Jarrard et al. 1999; Reznikoff et al. 1996). In addition, p16 and Arf are induced by experimental states of acute oncogenic activation in vitro, where these proteins collaborate to impose a senescence-like state

(Serrano et al. 1997). Given this evidence, a major theme in p16 biology is that it limits the long-term proliferative capacity of cells. However, given that senescence has been experimentally defined in vitro, the relevance of these observations to physiologic settings of tumor suppression in vivo has remained uncertain. This state of affairs has underscored a need for studies of the tumor biology of p16, the focus of this chapter.

The Promoter

The p16 promoter has not been extensively mapped, but is known to respond to a number of experimental conditions and specific transcription factors (Wang et al. 2001). Ultraviolet irradiation induces p16 in skin, and gamma irradiation induces p16 in a variety of cell types after a lag period in vitro (Robles and Adami 1998; Wang et al. 1996). The relatively slow kinetics suggests that this induction may not be direct (Furth et al. 2006). Transcription factors JunB (Passegue and Wagner 2000), Ets1 and 2 (Ohtani et al. 2001), and Sp1 (Wu et al. 2007; Xue et al. 2004) contribute to p16 expression but may not account for the full program of p16 expression in vivo (Krishnamurthy et al. 2004). In addition, p16 and Arf expression are repressed by the polycomb group transcription factor Bmi1 (Jacobs et al. 1999). Bmi1 is viewed as an "architectural" factor, acting on chromatin structure rather than through a defined enhancer, which helps to account for the difficulty in mapping specific binding sites in promoters. Technical challenges in studying p16 promoter function include the delayed kinetics of induction by known stimuli and the frequent inactivation of p16 and/or disruption of its regulation (e.g., by promoter methylation) in transfectable cell lines.

Heterogeneous Expression in Tumors

Although p16 is induced in early neoplasia, expression is often heterogeneous in neoplastic cells (Dai et al. 2000; Wang et al. 2000). One possibility to account for this pattern is positive feedback regulation. For example, low levels of c-Myc have been shown to foster accumulation of p16 (Guney et al. 2006). Another factor may be restriction of expression based on the natural history and/or functional potential of such cells. Expression in human colon is consistent with restriction to cells with features of stem cells or their immediate products among the transit amplifying cells (Dai et al. 2000; Furth et al. 2006). That is, early neoplasms such as aberrant crypt foci or adenomas often show preferential expression at the base of the epithelial crypts, where stem cells are known to reside in normal colon (Dai et al. 2000). Moreover, p16 is frequently induced near the crypt base in patients with chronic ulcerative colitis, a pre-neoplastic condition associated with repetitive epithelial damage and regeneration (Furth et al. 2006). Crypt fission is known to occur. Presumably, proliferation of stem cells or their immediate products is required for such a process. p16 induction has also recently been observed in tumor models in vivo in settings of sustained proliferative arrest with features of senescence (Xue et al. 2007; Ventura et al. 2007). Here again, p16 induction appears to be heterogeneous.

Stem Cell Regulator?

This circumstantial evidence for function in a stem cell lineage in solid tumors of the colon dovetails with genetic evidence for p16 function in hematopoietic stem cells. Bmi1-null stem cells show reduced long-term replicative potential, a phenotype partially rescued by Ink4a/Arf deletion (Jacobs et al. 1999; Lessard and Sauvageau 2003; Park et al. 2003). Recent experiments, returned to in a later section, have shown that some neural tissues and aging pancreatic islets have greater capacity for regeneration in the absence of p16, pointing to p16 regulation of the proliferative capacity of progenitor cells in this tissue (Krishnamurthy et al. 2006; Molofsky et al. 2006). This notion has taken on added interest of late with evidence that long-term growth of some solid tumors may be driven by tumor stem cells (Clarke et al. 2006).

Genetic Dissection of p16 Function In Vivo

Spontaneous Tumorigenesis

Absence of p16 predisposes humans and mice to tumor development. As mentioned, humans with p16 mutations show increased incidence of melanoma, pancreatic adenocarcinoma, and hepatocellular carcinoma. However, even rare individuals with homozygous, apparently inactivating mutations in p16 have been known to live well into middle age. Thus, p16 does not appear to be a major gatekeeper of tumor initiation, despite being inactivated early and often in gastrointestinal malignancies. Mice null for both p16 and Arf routinely die of lymphomas and sarcomas within the first year of life. Those with selective loss of p16 are also prone to these tumor types but typically live beyond a year. These mice have a broadened tumor spectrum, but in general humans and mice null for p16 evince fewer tumors and at later ages than mice null for p53, adenomatous polyposis coli (APC), and some other tumor suppressors.

Inhibition of Tumor Progression

Absence of p16 accelerates progression of tumors initiated by independent lesions in several tissue types. Combined p16 absence and mutation of APC in Min (multiple intestinal neoplasia) mice yields more rapid growth of colon tumors associated with histological features of malignancy, marked by pockets of necrosis and a honeycombed pattern of epithelial growth ("cribriforming"). p16 absence alone partially recapitulated this phenotype (Gibson et al. 2005). Mutation of the Ink4a/Arf locus or overexpression of Cdk4 fosters accelerated growth of gliomas, when combined with activation of the epidermal growth factor, consistent with substantial evidence from human clinical samples that p16 restrains growth of these tumors (Holland et al. 1998). The most dramatic phenotype associated to date with p16 absence occurs in a mouse model of pancreatic cancer that utilizes conditional activation of an activated Kras allele from the endogenous promoter (Hingorani et al. 2003). In these animals, malignant disease occurred in only a minority of animals of advanced age, whereas Ink4a/Arf deficiency yielded the rapid onset of invasive and metastatic disease (Aguirre et al. 2003). Although absence of Arf may contribute to this phenotype, a substantial body of evidence implicates p16, led by the near universal inactivation of p16 in human pancreatic adenocarcinomas. Thus, in each of these instances, p16 limits progression of tumors initiated by mutations in other genes.

Increased Vascularity in the Absence of p16

Some of the human solid tumors with frequent inactivation of p16, such as gliomas and colorectal carcinomas, are known to be quite vascular. For colon tumors, compelling evidence has been obtained that vascularity plays a limiting role in tumor progression. From the adenoma stage to malignancy these tumors display abundant, well-developed, and fine-arborizing vessels, consistent with new vessel formation (angiogenesis) (Skinner et al. 1995). This vascularity is accompanied by high levels of vascular endothelial growth factor (VEGF) (Wong et al. 1999). Moreover, antibodies directed against VEGF add efficacy to combined modality treatment of advanced colorectal carcinoma (Hurwitz et al. 2004). The mechanism(s) underlying the clinical benefit remains a matter of speculation. One possibility is that the anti-VEGF treatment reduces vessel leakiness, improving tumor vessel blood flow and perfusion with the concurrently administered cytotoxic agents. However, the simplest interpretation is probably that VEGF promotes human colorectal carcinoma growth and that the antibodies antagonize it. Absence of p16 from esophageal squamous cell carcinomas was associated with high levels of VEGF expression and poor survival (Takeuchi et al. 2004). The most compelling experimental evidence obtained thus far for effects of p16 on the tumor microenvironment may be the increased vascularity seen in p16-null colon tumors (Gibson et al. 2005, 2003), so we address this setting in detail (Fig. 10.1).

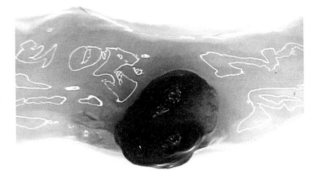

Fig. 10.1 Increased vascularity in a p16-null Min mouse colon tumor. Gross image through a dissecting microscope of a tumor following longitudinal dissection of the colon. Note the dramatic *red* coloration of the tumor, reflecting increased vascularity (and possibly vascular permeability), compared to surrounding tissue

Min colon tumors in Ink4a/Arf-null mice are more vascular than their Ink4a/Arf-wild-type counterparts (Gibson et al. 2003). The implication is that augmented angiogenesis may play a role in the more rapid progression of these tumors and that p16 may suppress this phenotype. Again, p16 absence alone partially recapitulated the vascular phenotype, whereas absence of Arf alone had no apparent effect (Gibson et al. 2005). p16-null tumors in these contexts had higher numbers of functional blood vessels, red blood cells, and hemoglobin. One can envision p16 suppressing angiogenesis in this context from within either the neoplastic cells or the vascular response cells. However, p16 expression assessed by immunohistological staining is most prominent in the neoplastic cells (Dai et al. 2000) (Cooper and Enders, unpublished data). In preliminary data, subcutaneous implants containing the angiogenic factor, basic fibroblast growth factor, did not recruit more vessels in the Ink4a/Arf-null background than in a wild-type background (Gibson et al. 2003). Moreover, VEGF levels were higher in p16-null tumors, providing genetic evidence that angiogenic signaling was increased by the absence of p16 in a tumor developing in situ. The mechanisms underlying this effect remain to be defined, but we will return to potential pathways below.

Increased Long-Term Proliferative Capacity in Some p16-Null Tissues

Recent studies have further defined a role for p16 in limiting long-term proliferation of cell types in vivo. As touched on earlier, hematopoietic stem cells from older mice have shown reduced capacity to repopulate the hematopoietic system following transfer to lethally irradiated mice. In contrast, Ink4a-null cells maintain this capacity longer (Janzen et al. 2006). p16 is induced during aging of progenitor cells in the subventricular zone (SVZ) of the brain (Molofsky et al. 2006). SVZ cells from older p16-null mice show increased formation of multipotent neurospheres in culture and proliferation in vivo. Similar effects were seen in the olfactory bulb, but not in other neural tissues, pointing to tissue specificity. Pancreatic islets express p16 throughout adulthood, suggesting a particularly sustained role for p16 in this tissue (Nielsen et al. 1999). Regeneration of islets can be assessed following toxin-mediated injury. Older mice show a decline in islet regeneration which is rescued in part by p16 absence (Krishnamurthy et al. 2006). Conversely, modestly elevated p16 expression in transgenic mice, comparable to that seen with aging, reduced islet regeneration. These results provide in vivo evidence that p16 constrains long-term proliferation of some cell types. This regulation is at least in part cell autonomous, because it can be seen in p16-null hematopoietic stem cells transplanted into p16-wild-type mice. On the other hand, interaction of stem or progenitor cells with the microenvironment might represent a key element of the regulation by p16, given the abundant evidence that proliferation of stem and progenitor cells in vivo is affected by intimate contacts with their microenvironment or "niche."

p16 Response Pathways Revisited: Potential
Non-cell-autonomous Effects

Repression of VEGF

This phenotype of increased vascularity and VEGF expression in p16-null tumors might be indirect or relatively direct. For example, absence of p16 might act indirectly by allowing evolution of a genetically unstable clone with increased angiogenic signaling. Alternatively, p16 may directly inhibit angiogenic signaling (Fig. 10.2). Evidence for potential direct effects has emerged. Ectopic expression of p16 in glioma cell lines reduces the vascularity of xenografts (Harada et al. 1999). p16 expression can acutely inhibit VEGF secretion from such lines in vitro. p16 appeared to be more potent than p21 or p53 in reducing VEGF transcript levels, after normalizing for cell cycle inhibition (Harada et al. 1999). Similarly, acute p16 expression in vitro can inhibit VEGF expression from human squamous cell carcinoma cell lines (Takeuchi et al. 2004) and human colorectal carcinoma cells (Gibson et al. 2005). The response pathway connecting p16 to VEGF expression has not been defined but might proceed through the canonical retinoblastoma (pRb) pathway. Expression of the pRb-related protein p130 reduced VEGF levels and angiogenesis in human lung carcinoma cell lines (Claudio et al. 2001).

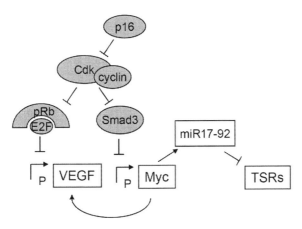

Fig. 10.2 Putative p16 response pathways inhibiting angiogenic signaling. p16 inhibits Cdk4/6 complexes, resulting in a net activation of pRb and SMAD3 as transcriptional repressors. The pRb family proteins repress transcription of E2F-responsive genes, potentially including VEGF. SMAD3 inhibits expression of myc. Myc, in turn, can augment VEGF expression, possibly through translational and transcriptional effects, and can drive expression of the microRNA 17-92, an antagonist of expression of thrombospondin repeat (TSR) proteins with anti-angiogenic properties, such as TSP1

Myc as a Target

Until recently, pRb family members have been the only known substrates for Cdk4/6 kinases, the Cdks bound by p16. Recently, SMAD3 has emerged as an alternative substrate (Matsuura et al. 2004). Cdk-dependent phosphorylation of SMAD3 can abrogate its ability to repress myc transcription. These observations suggest that myc may be downregulated by p16, through activation of SMAD3 as a myc repressor. Myc has potent angiogenic properties (see Chapter 9). Myc can induce VEGF (Knies-Bamforth et al. 2004; Baudino et al. 2002). Myc also inhibits expression of angiogenesis inhibitors, in part through induction of the miRNA17-92 (Dews et al. 2006; Thomas-Tikhonenko et al. 2004). Thus, p16-mediated repression of myc might mediate some of p16's effects on VEGF and angiogenic signaling.

COX-2 and "Stressed" Cells

Another potential candidate for regulation by p16 is COX-2. COX-2 is thought to be angiogenic. Mammary epithelial cells with epigenetic silencing of the p16 promoter have been found to express higher levels of COX-2 (Crawford et al. 2004). COX-2 here may be a marker of "stressed" cells with broadly heightened angiogenic signaling and/or a mediator itself (Tsujii et al. 1998). Although stress is an ill-defined term, it is often used in this context to refer to cells driven to proliferate in settings of tissue regeneration and inflammation, often accompanied by increased metabolic demands, production of reactive oxygen species, and DNA damage. These cells may display increased angiogenic signaling. One model to account for p16's apparent repression of angiogenesis despite heterogeneous expression is that p16 may be preferentially induced in stressed cells prone to angiogenic signaling.

Angiogenic Signaling and the Stem Cell Niche

Although treated here separately, p16 effects on angiogenic signaling and stem cell function may be interrelated. For example, evidence has been obtained that VEGF can help mold the stem cell niche (Keith and Simon 2007). It makes some intuitive sense that a function of stem cells may be to direct formation of new vessels when stem cell proliferation is stimulated and new tissue may be formed.

Conclusions

p16 function can no longer be effectively captured by a simple linear diagram depicting inhibition of Cdk4 and 6. Like p53, p16 is a potent cell cycle inhibitor whose expression is kept in tight check until conditions of sustained proliferation develop, often in settings of replicative stress that prefigure or mediate neoplastic growth. Furthermore, p16 appears, directly and/or indirectly, to repress certain extracellular signaling, such as expression of VEGF, with substantial non-cell-autonomous impact. These observations put p16 function in context and deepen our understanding of p16 as a tumor suppressor.

References

Aguirre, A. J., N. Bardeesy, M. Sinha, L. Lopez, D. A. Tuveson, J. Horner, M. S. Redston, and R. A. DePinho (2003) Activated Kras and Ink4a/Arf deficiency cooperate to produce metastatic pancreatic ductal adenocarcinoma. *Genes Dev* 17 (24):3112–26.

Alcorta, D.A., Y. Xiong, D. Phelps, G. Hannon, D. Beach, and J.C. Barret (1996) Involvement of the cyclin-dependent kinase inhibitor p16(INK4a) in replicative senescence of normal human fibroblasts. *PNAS* 93:13742–7.

Baudino, T. A., C. McKay, H. Pendeville-Samain, J. A. Nilsson, K. H. Maclean, E. L. White, A. C. Davis, J. N. Ihle, and J. L. Cleveland (2002) c-Myc is essential for vasculogenesis and angiogenesis during development and tumor progression. *Genes Dev* 16 (19):2530–43.

Baylin, S. B., J. G. Herman, J. R. Graff, P. M. Vertino, and J.-P. Issa (1998) Alterations in DNA methylation: a fundamental aspect of neoplasia. *Adv Can Res* 72:141–96.

Brenner, A. J., M. R. Stampfer, and C. M. Aldaz (1998) Increased p16 expression with first senescence arrest in human mammary epithelial cells and extended growth capacity with p16 inactivation. *Oncogene* 17 (2):199–205.

Caldas, C., S. A. Hahn, L. T. da Costa, M. S. Redston, M. Schutte, A. B. Seymour, C. L. Weinstein, R. H. Hruban, C. J. Yeo, and S. E. Kern (1994) Frequent somatic mutations and homozygous deletions of the p16 (MTS1) gene in pancreatic adenocarcinoma. *Nature Genetics* 8:27–32.

Chaubert, P., R. Gayer, A. Zimmermann, C. Fontolliet, B. Stamm, F. Bosman, and P. Shaw (1997) Germ-line mutations of the p16INK4(MTS1) gene occur in a subset of patients with hepatocellular carcinoma. *Hepatology* 25 (6):1376–81.

Clarke, M. F., J. E. Dick, P. B. Dirks, C. J. Eaves, C. H. Jamieson, D. L. Jones, J. Visvader, I. L. Weissman, and G. M. Wahl (2006) Cancer Stem Cells–Perspectives on Current Status and Future Directions: AACR Workshop on Cancer Stem Cells. *Cancer Res* 66 (19):9339–44.

Claudio, P. P., P. Stiegler, C. M. Howard, C. Bellan, C. Minimo, G. M. Tosi, J. Rak, A. Kovatich, P. De Fazio, P. Micheli, M. Caputi, L. Leoncini, R. Kerbel, G. G. Giordano, and A. Giordano (2001) RB2/p130 gene-enhanced expression down-regulates vascular endothelial growth factor expression and inhibits angiogenesis in vivo. *Cancer Res* 61 (2):462–8.

Clurman, B. E. and M. Groudine (1998) The CDKN2A tumor-suppressor locus–a tale of two proteins [editorial; comment]. *New England Journal of Medicine* 338 (13):910–12.

Crawford, Y. G., M. L. Gauthier, A. Joubel, K. Mantei, K. Kozakiewicz, C. A. Afshari, and T. D. Tlsty (2004) Histologically normal human mammary epithelia with silenced p16(INK4a) overexpress COX-2, promoting a premalignant program. *Cancer Cell* 5 (3):263–73.

Dai, C. Y., E. E. Furth, R. Mick, J. Koh, T. Takayama, Y. Niitsu, and G. H. Enders (2000) p16(INK4a) expression begins early in human colon neoplasia and correlates inversely with markers of cell proliferation. *Gastroenterology* 119 (4):929–42.

Dews, M., A. Homayouni, D. Yu, D. Murphy, C. Sevignani, E. Wentzel, E. E. Furth, W. M. Lee, G. H. Enders, J. T. Mendell, and A. Thomas-Tikhonenko (2006) Augmentation of tumor angiogenesis by a Myc-activated microRNA cluster. *Nat Genet* 38 (9):1060–5.

Erickson, S., O. Sangfelt, M. Heyman, J. Castro, S. Einhorn, and D. Grander (1998) Involvement of the Ink4 proteins p16 and p15 in T-lymphocyte senescence. *Oncogene* 17 (5):595–602.

Furth, E. E., K. S. Gustafson, C. Y. Dai, S. L. Gibson, P. Menard-Katcher, T. Chen, J. Koh, and G. H. Enders (2006) Induction of the tumor-suppressor p16(INK4a) within regenerative epithelial crypts in ulcerative colitis. *Neoplasia* 8 (6):429–36.

Gibson, S. L., C. Y. Dai, H.-W. Lee, R. A. DePinho, M. S. Gee, W. M. F. Lee, E. E. Furth, C. Brensinger, and G. H. Enders (2003) Inhibition of colon tumor progression by the Ink4a/Arf locus. *Cancer Research* 63 (4):742–6.

Gibson, S. L., A. Boquoi, T. Chen, N. E. Sharpless, C. Brensinger, and G. H. Enders (2005) p16(Ink4a) inhibits histologic progression and angiogenic signaling in min colon tumors. *Cancer Biol Ther* 4 (12):1389–94.

Goldstein, A. M., M. C. Fraser, J. P. Struewig, C. J. Hussussian, K. Ranade, D. P. Zametkin, L. S. Fontaine, S. M. Organic, N. C. Dracopoli, W. H. Clark, and M. A. Tucker (1995) Increased risk of pancreatic cancer in melanoma-prone kindreds with p16INK4 mutations. *New Engl J Med* 333:970–4.

Guney, I., S. Wu, and J. M. Sedivy (2006) Reduced c-Myc signaling triggers telomere-independent senescence by regulating Bmi-1 and p16(INK4a). *Proc Natl Acad Sci U S A* 103 (10):3645–50.

Haber, D (1997) Splicing into senescence: the curious case of p16 and p19ARF. *Cell* 91:555–8.

Harada, H., K. Nakagawa, S. Iwata, M. Saito, Y. Kumon, S. Sakaki, K. Sato, and K. Hamada (1999) Restoration of wild-type p16 down-regulates vascular endothelial growth factor expression and inhibits angiogenesis in human gliomas. *Cancer Res* 59 (15):3783–9.

Hingorani, S. R., E. F. Petricoin, A. Maitra, V. Rajapakse, C. King, M. A. Jacobetz, S. Ross, T. P. Conrads, T. D. Veenstra, B. A. Hitt, Y. Kawaguchi, D. Johann, L. A. Liotta, H. C. Crawford, M. E. Putt, T. Jacks, C. V. Wright, R. H. Hruban, A. M. Lowy, and D. A. Tuveson (2003) Preinvasive and invasive ductal pancreatic cancer and its early detection in the mouse. *Cancer Cell* 4 (6):437–50.

Holland, E. C., W. P. Hively, R. A. DePinho, and H. E. Varmus (1998) A constitutively active epidermal growth factor receptor cooperates with disruption of G1 cell-cycle arrest pathways to induce glioma-like lesions in mice. *Genes Dev* 12 (23):3675–85.

Hurwitz, H., L. Fehrenbacher, W. Novotny, T. Cartwright, J. Hainsworth, W. Heim, J. Berlin, A. Baron, S. Griffing, E. Holmgren, N. Ferrara, G. Fyfe, B. Rogers, R. Ross, and F. Kabbinavar (2004) Bevacizumab plus irinotecan, fluorouracil, and leucovorin for metastatic colorectal cancer. *N Engl J Med* 350 (23):2335–42.

Jacobs, J. J., K. Kieboom, S. Marino, R. A. DePinho, and M. van Lohuizen (1999) The oncogene and Polycomb-group gene bmi-1 regulates cell proliferation and senescence through the ink4a locus. *Nature* 397 (6715):164–8.

Janzen, V., R. Forkert, H. E. Fleming, Y. Saito, M. T. Waring, D. M. Dombkowski, T. Cheng, R. A. DePinho, N. E. Sharpless, and D. T. Scadden (2006) Stem-cell ageing modified by the cyclin-dependent kinase inhibitor p16INK4a. *Nature* 443 (7110):421–6.

Jarrard, D. F., S. Sarkar, Y. Shi, T. R. Yeager, G. Magrane, H. Kinoshita, N. Nassif, L. Meisner, M. A. Newton, F. M. Waldman, and C. A. Reznikoff (1999) p16/pRb pathway alterations are required for bypassing senescence in human prostate epithelial cells. *Cancer Res* 59 (12): 2957–64.

Kamb, A., N. A. Gruis, J. Weaver-Feldhaus, Q. Liu, K. Harshman, S. V. Tavtigian, E. Stockert, R. S. Day, B. E. Johnson, and M. H. Skolnick (1994a) A cell cycle regulator potentially involved in genesis of many tumor types. *Science* 264:436–40.

Kamb, A., Shattuck-Eidens, D., Eeles, R., Liu, Q., Gruis, N.A., Ding, W., Hussey, C., Tran, T., Miki, Y., Weaver-Feldhaus, J., McClure, M., Aitken, J.F., Anderson, D.E., Bergman, W., Frants, R., Goldgar, D.E., Green, A., MacLennan, R., Martin, N.G., Meyer, L.J., Youl, P., Zone, J.J., Skolnick, M.H., and Cannon-Albright, L.A (1994b) Analysis of the p16 gene (cdkN2) as a candidate for the chromosome 9p melanoma susceptibility locus. *Nature Genetics* 8:22–26.

Kamijo, T., F. Zindy, M. F. Roussel, D. E. Quelle, J. R. Downing, R. A. Ashburn, G. Grosveld, and C. J. Sherr (1997) Tumor suppression at the mouse INK4a locus mediated by the alternative reading frame product p19ARF. *Cell* 91 (5):649–660.

Keith, B. and M. C. Simon (2007) Hypoxia-inducible factors, stem cells, and cancer. *Cell* 129 (3):465–72.

Knies-Bamforth, U. E., S. B. Fox, R. Poulsom, G. I. Evan, and A. L. Harris (2004) c-Myc interacts with hypoxia to induce angiogenesis in vivo by a vascular endothelial growth factor-dependent mechanism. *Cancer Res* 64 (18):6563–70.

Koh, J., G. H. Enders, B. D. Dynlacht, and E. Harlow (1995) Tumor-derived p16 alleles encoding proteins defective in cell cycle inhibition. *Nature* 375 (8 June):506–10.

Korgaonkar, C., L. Zhao, M. Modestou, and D. E. Quelle (2002) ARF function does not require p53 stabilization or Mdm2 relocalization. *Mol Cell Biol* 22 (1):196–206.

Krishnamurthy, J., C. Torrice, M. R. Ramsey, G. I. Kovalev, K. Al-Regaiey, L. Su, and N. E. Sharpless (2004) Ink4a/Arf expression is a biomarker of aging. *J Clin Invest* 114 (9): 1299–307.

Krishnamurthy, J., M. R. Ramsey, K. L. Ligon, C. Torrice, A. Koh, S. Bonner-Weir, and N. E. Sharpless (2006) p16INK4a induces an age-dependent decline in islet regenerative potential. *Nature* 443 (7110):453–7.

Lessard, J. and G. Sauvageau (2003) Bmi-1 determines the proliferative capacity of normal and leukaemic stem cells. *Nature* 423 (6937):255–60.

Liggett, W. H., Jr., D. A. Sewell, J. Rocco, S. A. Ahrendt, W. Koch, and D. Sidransky (1996) p16 and p16 beta are potent growth suppressors of head and neck squamous carcinoma cells in vitro. *Cancer Research* 56 (18):4119–23.

Lukas, J., D. Parry, L. Aagarrd, D. J. Mann, J. Bartkova, M. Strauss, G. Peters, and J. Bartek (1995) Retinoblastoma-protein-dependent inhibition by the tumor-suppressor p16. *Nature* 375 (8 June):503–6.

Matsuura, I., N. G. Denissova, G. Wang, D. He, J. Long, and F. Liu (2004) Cyclin-dependent kinases regulate the antiproliferative function of Smads. *Nature* 430 (6996):226–31.

McConnell, B. B., F. J. Gregory, F. J. Stott, E. Hara, and G. Peters (1999) Induced expression of p16(INK4a) inhibits both CDK4- and CDK2-associated kinase activity by reassortment of cyclin-CDK-inhibitor complexes [In Process Citation]. *Mol Cell Biol* 19 (3):1981–9.

Medema, R. H., R. E. Herrera, F. Lam, and R. A. Weinberg (1995) Growth suppression by p16ink4 requires functional retinoblastoma protein. *Proc. Natl. Acad. Sci. USA* 92:6289–93.

Mitra, J., C. Y. Dai, K. Somasundaram, W. S. El-Deiry, K. Satyamoorthy, M. Herlyn, and G. H. Enders (1999) Induction of p21(WAF1/CIP1) and inhibition of Cdk2 mediated by the tumor suppressor p16(INK4a). *Mol Cell Biol* 19 (5):3916–28.

Molofsky, A. V., S. G. Slutsky, N. M. Joseph, S. He, R. Pardal, J. Krishnamurthy, N. E. Sharpless, and S. J. Morrison (2006) Increasing p16INK4a expression decreases forebrain progenitors and neurogenesis during ageing. *Nature* 443 (7110):448–52.

Nielsen, G. P., A. O. Stemmer-Rachamimov, J. Shaw, J. E. Roy, J. Koh, and D. N. Louis (1999) Immunohistochemical survey of p16INK4A expression in normal human adult and infant tissues. *Lab Invest* 79 (9):1137–43.

Nobori, T., K. Miura, D. J. Wu, A. Lois, K., Takabayashi, and D. A. Carson (1994) Deletions of the cyclin-dependent kinase-4 inhibitor gene in multiple human cancers. *Nature* 368:753–6.

Ohtani, N., Z. Zebedee, T. J. Huot, J. A. Stinson, M. Sugimoto, Y. Ohashi, A. D. Sharrocks, G. Peters, and E. Hara (2001) Opposing effects of Ets and Id proteins on p16INK4a expression during cellular senescence. *Nature* 409 (6823):1067–70.

Park, I. K., D. Qian, M. Kiel, M. W. Becker, M. Pihalja, I. L. Weissman, S. J. Morrison, and M. F. Clarke (2003) Bmi-1 is required for maintenance of adult self-renewing haematopoietic stem cells. *Nature* 423 (6937):302–5.

Parry, D., D. Mahony, K. Wills, and E. Lees (1999) Cyclin D-CDK subunit arrangement is dependent on the availability of competing INK4 and p21 class inhibitors. *Mol Cell Biol* 19 (3):1775–83.

Passegue, E. and E. F. Wagner (2000) JunB suppresses cell proliferation by transcriptional activation of p16(INK4a) expression. *Embo J* 19 (12):2969–79.

Pollack, P.M., J.V. Pearson, and N.K. Hayward (1996) Compilation of somatic mutations of the CDKN2 gene in human cancers: Non-random distribution of base substitutions. *Genes, Chromosomes and Cancer* 15:77–88.

Pomerantz, J., N. Schreiber-Agus, N. J. Liegeois, A. Silverman, L. Alland, L. Chin, J. Potes, K. Chen, I. Orlow, H. W. Lee, H. Cordon-Cardo, and R. A. DePinho (1998) The Ink4a tumor suppressor gene product, p19Arf, interacts with MDM2 and neutralizes MDM2's inhibition of p53. *Cell* 92 (6):713–23.

Quelle, D. E., F. Zindy, R. A. Ashmun, and C. J. Sherr (1995) Alternative reading frames of the INK4a tumor suppressor gene encode two unrelated proteins capable of inducing cell cycle arrest. *Cell* 83 (6):993–1000.

Quelle, D. E., M. Cheng, R. A. Ashmun, and C. J. Sherr (1997) Cancer-associated mutations at the INK4a locus cancel cell cycle arrest by p16INK4a but not by the alternative reading frame protein p19ARF. *Proc Natl Acad Sci U S A* 94 (2):669–73.

Ranade, K., C. J. Hussussian, R. S. Sikorski, H. E. Varmus, A. M. Goldstein, M. A. Tucker, M. Serrano, G. J. Hannon, D. Beach, and N. C. Dracopoli (1995) Mutations associated with familial melanoma impair p16INK4 function [letter]. *Nature Genetics* 10 (1):114–16.

Reznikoff, C. A., T.R. Yeager, C. D. Belair, E. Savelia, J. A. Puthenveetil, and W. M. Stadler (1996) Elevated p16 at senescence and loss of p16 at immortalization in human papillomovirus 16 E6, but not E7, transformed human uroepithelial cells. *Canc Res* 56:2886–90.

Robles, S. J. and G. R. Adami (1998) Agents that cause DNA double strand breaks lead to p16INK4a enrichment and the premature senescence of normal fibroblasts. *Oncogene* 16 (9):1113–23.

Schutte, M., R. H. Hruban, J. Geradts, R. Maynard, W. Hilgers, S. K. Rabindran, C. A. Moskaluk, S. A. Hahn, I. Schwarte-Waldhoff, W. Schmiegel, S. B. Baylin, S. E. Kern, and J. G. Herman (1997) Abrogation of the Rb/p16 tumor-suppressive pathway in virtually all pancreatic carcinomas. *Cancer Res* 57 (15):3126–30.

Serrano, M., G. J. Hannon, and D. Beach (1993) A new regulatory motif in cell-cycle control causing specific inhibition of cyclin D/CDK4. *Nature* 366 (6456):704–7.

Serrano, M., E. Gomez-Lahoz, R. A. DePinho, D. Beach, and D. Bar-Sagi (1995) Inhibition of ras-induced proliferation and cellular transformation by p16INK4. *Science* 267 (5195):249–52.

Serrano, M., H. Lee, L. Chin, C. Cordon-Cardo, D. Beach, and R. A. DePinho (1996) Role of the INK4a locus in tumor suppression and cell mortality. *Cell* 85 (1):27–37.

Serrano, M., A. W. Lin, M. E. McCurrach, D. Beach, and S. W. Lowe (1997) Oncogenic ras provokes premature cell senescence associated with accumulation of p53 and p16INK4a. *Cell* 88 (5):593–602.

Sharpless, N. E., N. Bardeesy, K. H. Lee, D. Carrasco, D. H. Castrillon, A. J. Aguirre, E. A. Wu, J. W. Horner, and R. A. DePinho (2001) Loss of p16Ink4a with retention of p19Arf predisposes mice to tumorigenesis. *Nature* 413 (6851):86–91.

Sherr, C. J (1996) Cancer cell cycles. *Science* 274:1672–7.

Skinner, S. A., G. M. Frydman, and P. E. O'Brien (1995) Microvascular structure of benign and malignant tumors of the colon in humans. *Dig Dis Sci* 40 (2):373–84.

Takeuchi, H., S. Ozawa, C. H. Shih, N. Ando, Y. Kitagawa, M. Ueda, and M. Kitajima (2004) Loss of p16INK4a expression is associated with vascular endothelial growth factor expression in squamous cell carcinoma of the esophagus. *Int J Cancer* 109 (4):483–90.

Thomas-Tikhonenko, A., I. Viard-Leveugle, M. Dews, P. Wehrli, C. Sevignani, D. Yu, S. Ricci, W. el-Deiry, B. Aronow, G. Kaya, J. H. Saurat, and L. E. French (2004) Myc-transformed epithelial cells down-regulate clusterin, which inhibits their growth in vitro and carcinogenesis in vivo. *Cancer Res* 64 (9):3126–36.

Tsujii, M., S. Kawano, S. Tsuji, H. Sawaoka, M. Hori, and R. N. DuBois (1998) Cyclooxygenase regulates angiogenesis induced by colon cancer cells [published erratum appears in *Cell* 1998 Jul 24;94(2):following 271]. *Cell* 93 (5):705–16.

Vasen, H. F., N. A. Gruis, R. R. Frants, P. A. van Der Velden, E. T. Hille, and W. Bergman (2000) Risk of developing pancreatic cancer in families with familial atypical multiple mole melanoma associated with a specific 19 deletion of p16 (p16-Leiden). *Int J Cancer* 87 (6):809–11.

Ventura, A., D. G. Kirsch, M. E. McLaughlin, D. A. Tuveson, J. Grimm, L. Lintault, J. Newman, E. E. Reczek, R. Weissleder, and T. Jacks (2007) Restoration of p53 function leads to tumour regression in vivo. *Nature* 445 (7128):661–5.

Wang, X. Q., B. G. Gabrielli, A. Milligan, J. L. Dickinson, T. M. Antalis, and K. A. Ellem (1996) Accumulation of p16CDKN2A in response to ultraviolet irradiation correlates with late S-G(2)-phase cell cycle delay. *Cancer Res* 56 (11):2510–14.

Wang, Q. S., A. Papanikolaou, P. R. Nambiar, and D. W. Rosenberg (2000) Differential expression of p16(INK4a) in azoxymethane-induced mouse colon tumorigenesis. *Mol Carcinog* 28 (3):139–47.

Wang, W., J. Wu, Z. Zhang, and T. Tong (2001) Characterization of regulatory elements on the promoter region of p16(INK4a) that contribute to overexpression of p16 in senescent fibroblasts. *J Biol Chem* 276 (52):48655–61.

Weber, J. D., J. R. Jeffers, J. E. Rehg, D. H. Randle, G. Lozano, M. F. Roussel, C. J. Sherr, and G. P. Zambetti (2000) p53-independent functions of the p19(ARF) tumor suppressor. *Genes Dev* 14 (18):2358–65.

Weinberg, R. A. (1995) The retinoblastoma protein and cell cycle control. *Cell* 81:323–30.

Wong, M. P., N. Cheung, S. T. Yuen, S. Y. Leung, and L. P. Chung (1999) Vascular endothelial growth factor is up-regulated in the early pre- malignant stage of colorectal tumour progression. *Int J Cancer* 81 (6):845–50.

Wu, J., L. Xue, M. Weng, Y. Sun, Z. Zhang, W. Wang, and T. Tong (2007) Sp1 is essential for p16 expression in human diploid fibroblasts during senescence. *PLoS ONE* 2 (1):e164.

Xue, L., J. Wu, W. Zheng, P. Wang, J. Li, Z. Zhang, and T. Tong (2004) Sp1 is involved in the transcriptional activation of p16(INK4) by p21(Waf1) in HeLa cells. *FEBS Lett* 564 (1-2): 199–204.

Xue, W., L. Zender, C. Miething, R. A. Dickins, E. Hernando, V. Krizhanovsky, C. Cordon-Cardo, and S. W. Lowe (2007) Senescence and tumour clearance is triggered by p53 restoration in murine liver carcinomas. *Nature* 445 (7128):656–60.

Zhang, Y., Y. Xiong, and W. G. Yarbrough (1998) ARF promotes MDM2 degradation and stabilizes p53: ARF-INK4a locus deletion impairs both the Rb and p53 tumor suppression pathways. *Cell* 92 (6):725–34.

Zindy, F., D. E. Quelle, M. F. Roussel, and C. J. Sherr (1997) Expression of the p16INK4a tumor suppressor versus other INK4 family members during mouse development and aging. *Oncogene* 15 (2):203–11.

Part IV
Gaining New Ground:
Metastasis and Stromal Cell Interactions

Chapter 11
Nm23 as a Metastasis Inhibitor

Rajeev Kaul, Masanao Murakami, Pankaj Kumar, and Erle S. Robertson

Cast of Characters

Nm23 was first cloned from a murine melanoma cell line wherein its expression correlated inversely with metastatic potential (Steeg et al. 1988). While it is abundantly expressed in aggressive neuroblastoma, the NB alleles typically encode the S120G substitution, which is likely to be a hypomorphic variant with reduced function (Chang et al. 1994, 1996). Mutations in other members of Nm23 family proteins, although not complete loss of function, are thought to be hypomorphic as well. Furthermore, in colorectal cancers, the allelic deletions of Nm23-H1 gene have been associated with a more aggressive behavior of cancers in some studies (Campo et al. 1994) and loss of heterozygocity of Nm23-H1 gene contributes to the metastasis potential of hepatocellular carcinoma (Ye et al. 1998). The molecular mechanisms underlying the biological activity of Nm23 are delineated below.

Introduction

The spread of cancer cells to distant organs by metastasis is one of the major causes of death in cancer patients. In the United States, most of cancer-related deaths are a consequence of metastatic disease rather than because of the primary tumor itself (Kauffman et al. 2003). Clinical studies in cancers suggest that dissemination to the secondary site is frequently an early clinical event (Kauffman et al. 2003). Further, many studies support a role for the interaction of a cancer cell with its microenvironment that involves multiple processes operating in parallel at the secondary site influencing metastasis (Nicolson 1988). Several genes have been identified that contribute toward the ability of cancer cells to metastasize. The Nm23 gene was discovered on the basis of its reduced expression in highly metastatic cell lines (Steeg et al. 1988) and is one of the best characterized metastasis suppressor gene.

E.S. Robertson (✉)
Department of Microbiology and Tumor Virology Program, Abramson Comprehensive Cancer Center, University of Pennsylvania School of Medicine, Philadelphia, PA, USA
e-mail: erle@mail.med.upenn.edu

A. Thomas-Tikhonenko (ed.), *Cancer Genome and Tumor Microenvironment*,
DOI 10.1007/978-1-4419-0711-0_11, © Springer Science+Business Media, LLC 2010

234   R. Kaul et al.

Nm23 Discovery and the Nm23 Gene Family

The first Nm23 gene was discovered by Steeg et al. in 1989 on the basis of its reduced expression in the highly metastatic murine myeloma cell lines, as compared to their nonmetastatic counterparts. The Nm23 family of proteins can be separated into two groups based on their sequence homology (Lacombe et al. 2000). The group I possesses the classic enzymatic activity of a nucleoside diphosphate (NDP) kinase and includes Nm23 members H1–H4 which share 58–88% identity (Fig. 11.1). The protein products of the group II genes which include Nm23-H5 to H8 are more divergent as the sequences share only 25–45% identity with the first group of proteins and between each other. However, only one product of the group II genes, Nm23-H6, has been demonstrated to catalyze the NDP kinase reaction (Tee et al. 2006).

Nm23-H1 shows reduced expression in a highly metastatic melanoma cell line and is therefore regarded as a putative metastasis suppression gene (Steeg et al. 1988). Nm23-H2 is highly homologous to Nm23-H1 and is identical to the transcriptional regulator PuF (Postel et al. 1993). It is thought to play a role in regulation of transcription of the c-Myc proto-oncogene (Postel et al. 1993, Stahl et al. 1991). The third gene, Nm23-H3, also known as DR-Nm23 shares about 70% identity with the first two genes. It inhibits differentiation and induces apoptosis of granulocytes (Venturelli et al. 1995). The fourth gene, Nm23-H4, encodes a

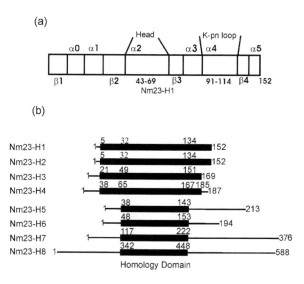

Fig. 11.1 (a) The structure of Nm23-H1 shows the four beta-sheets, the five alpha-helical regions, and two regions referred to as the head and the K-pn loop. (b) Nm23-H1 protein family members can be divided into two groups based on sequence homology. The groups I comprises of Nm23-H1 to H4 genes encode proteins which possess NDP kinase enzymatic activity and share 58–88% identity with each other. Group II comprises Nm23-H5 to H8 which are more divergent and share only 25–45% identity with the first group proteins and between each other. The homologous regions in the different Nm23 family members are highlighted.

protein with an amino terminal pre-sequence that has some characteristics consistent with import into mitochondria (Milon et al. 1997). Nm23-H5 is expressed almost exclusively in testis and may be involved in spermatogenesis (Munier et al. 1998). Nm23-H6 also exhibits functional NDP kinase activity and is highly expressed in heart, placenta, skeletal muscle, and some cancer cell lines (Mehus et al. 1999, Tsuiki et al. 1999). Nm23-H7 has been suggested to be involved in the development of colon and gastric carcinoma possibly in a type-specific manner (Seifert et al. 2005). Nm23-H8 is similar to dyenin intermediate chain from sea urchin (IC3) and *Ciona intestinalis* IC3, which suggests its distinctiveness from other Nm23 proteins (Padma et al. 2001). Nm23-LV is a recently described long variant of the Nm23 protein family which contains part of Nm23-H1 and the complete Nm23-H2 protein. It is expressed as a result of read-through transcripts that start in the Nm23-H1 open reading frame and continue in the neighboring Nm23-H2 gene and contain exons 1–4 of Nm23-H1 and exons 2–5 of Nm23-H2 (Valentijn et al. 2006).

Nm23 Structure

On the basis of X-ray structure, Nm23 was determined to be a hexamer made of identical subunits with a novel mononucleotide-binding fold (Dumas et al. 1992). Each subunit was found to contain an alpha/beta domain with a four stranded, antiparallel beta-sheet. Subsequently it was found that each hexamer was in fact consisting of two kinds of polypeptide chains, A and B (Gilles et al. 1991). These chains by random association (A6, A5B ... AB5, B6) form hexameric isoenzymes differing in their isoelectric point. Sequence determination showed that the chain A corresponds to Nm23-H1 protein whereas chain B is Nm23-H2 (Gilles et al. 1991). NDP kinase activity of the molecule is located within the region involved in protein–protein interaction with the oligomers. The protein–protein interaction which is a dimeric interaction is conserved among all NDP kinases. X-ray structure of Nm23-H2 also revealed it to be a hexamer and indicated that two serine residues that are phosphorylated, Ser44 and Ser122, are on the surface of the hexamer in contrast to Ser120 which is buried (Webb et al. 1995). The crystal structure analysis confirmed that Nm23-H1 and Nm23-H2 are very similar and that they bind their nucleotide substrates in a similar manner suggesting that they are interchangeable as phosphate transferase enzymes (Chen et al. 2003b). However, the available structural data shed little light on its mechanism or the relationship between the enzymatic activity and the alternative functions. Indeed previous attempts investigating the relationship between structure and function by studying point mutants of Nm23-H1 showed no significant change in structure (Giraud et al. 2006, Kim et al. 2003).

Nm23 Promoter Characterization

The mapping of 2.1 kb Nm23-H1 promoter has identified three regions involved in its differential expression levels in human breast carcinoma cell lines, which include a 195 bp NheI–XbaI fragment responsible for basal expression levels, a 248 bp AvrII–NheI fragment which contribute to the elevated Nm23-H1 expression observed in the high expressing cell lines, and a 544 bp AvrII fragment containing an inhibitory element (Ouatas et al. 2002). A common transcription initiation site for Nm23-H1 has been reported to be located at −136 upstream from the first ATG codon in placenta tissue, breast, colorectal, prostate tumor cell lines and in the primary colorectal tumor; however, multiple transcription start sites were identified in tumor cell lines, and colorectal tumor (Chen et al. 1994). The Nm23-H1 promoter has no TATA box, but it contains a number of sequences which may bind known transcriptional regulatory elements (de la Rosa et al. 1996). The analysis of the 248 bp AvrII–NheI fragment revealed the presence of the transcription factor-binding sites for MAF/Ets, CTF/NF1, and ACAAAG enhancer which are important for transcriptional regulation of Nm23-H1 gene (Ouatas et al. 2002). The Nm23-H1 gene also contains a putative p53-binding site about 5 kb upstream of the transcription start site (Rahman-Roblick et al. 2007). Also, there are two CpG islands in the Nm23-H1 promoter (Hartsough et al. 2001). The promoter sequence of Nm23-H2 has also been sequenced and was found to have no significant sequence homology with Nm23-H1 promoter suggesting that the two genes might be regulated differently, and/or in a cell-type-specific manner (Okada et al. 1996, Seifert et al. 1995).

Nm23 Gene Mutations

Reduced expression of Nm23-H1 is associated with high potential of metastasis in most cancers but its expression is increased in aggressive neuroblastoma. The Nm23-H1 sequence analysis from different cases of neuroblastoma shows that S120G substitution is present in advanced tumors but not in limited stage tumors indicating that the mutation in Nm23-H1 could be a feature of advanced neuroblastoma (Chang et al. 1994). Indeed recombinant Nm23-H1 protein containing the S120G mutation exhibited reduced hexameric and increased dimeric oligomerization relative to the wild type and also has lower phosphotransferase activity coupled with a significant decrease in the enzyme stability (Chang et al. 1996). The same mutation also affects protein folding (Lascu et al. 1997) and suppresses desensitization of muscarinic potassium current which are important in transmembrane signaling (Otero et al. 1999). The proline at position 96 and histidine at position 120 but not serine at 44 position are also important for cell motility functions (MacDonald et al. 1996). Mutations in other members of Nm23 family proteins such as position histidine 118 in Nm23-H2, serine at position 61 in DR-Nm23 are also known to affect biochemical activities including effects on apoptosis, differentiation, and metastasis potential of cells (Hamby et al. 2000, Negroni et al. 2000). The carboxy terminal half (76–152) of Nm23-H1 is known for its transactivation ability with amino acids from position 109 to 152 absolutely required for this transactivation (Cho et al. 2001). The point mutation of proline at position 96 and serine at position 120 but not histidine at position 118 affects anti-metastasis potential of Nm23-H1 without affecting its transactivation potential suggesting that transactivation potential of Nm23 is likely to be related to its kinase activity but not to its metastasis suppressor activity. However, the double mutant P96S/S120G of Nm23-H1 abrogates its NDPK activity as well as the motility-suppressive ability (Zhou et al. 2007). The k-pn (killer of prune mutation in drosophila *awd* gene)-type proline-96 to serine (P96S) and neuroblastoma-type serine-120 to glycine (S120G) mutations of Nm23-H1 are also known to abrogate its inhibitory activity on colo-nization and invasion probably because of structural changes resulting in reduced hexameric and increased dimeric oligomerization (Kim et al. 2003). In general, however, cancers containing overexpressed mutated Nm23-H1 proteins are rare events which, even if present, rarely leads to its inactivation (Cipollini et al. 2000, Wang et al. 1997a). Whereas, loss of expression of Nm23-H1 is a common feature of aggressive, poorly differentiated tumors (Fujimoto et al. 1998, Hartsough and Steeg 1998).

Nm23 Allelic Variations

Genetic polymorphism has become a useful tool for identifying candidate genes associated with disease. For Nm23-H1 gene, two bi-allelic polymorphic restriction sites, EcoRI and BgIII, have been described (Varesco et al. 1992, Yague et al. 1991). The correlation between tumor stage or metastatic status of cancer and Nm23 muta-tions or allelic loss or loss of heterozygocity at the Nm23 locus has been extensively studied (Bosnar et al. 1997, Mandai et al. 1995). In colorectal cancers, the allelic deletions of Nm23-H1 gene have been associated with a more aggressive behav-ior of cancers in some studies (Campo et al. 1994), whereas no correlation was detected between allelic deletion and tumor size, location, or differentiation in other studies (Seifert et al. 1997, Xu et al. 1995). It has also been suggested that Nm23-H1 protein expression in the early stages of sporadic colon cancer may have a role in suppressing metastasis, whereas at the later stages both reduced Nm23-H1 protein expression and loss of heterozygocity of the Nm23-H1 gene may play a role in colon cancer progression and metastasis (Kapitanovic et al. 2004). Loss of heterozygocity of Nm23-H1 gene has been shown to have some relationship with the metastasis potential of hepatocellular carcinoma and has been suggested to be of some help to predict its recurrence and metastasis (Ye et al. 1998). A recent study on lung cancer has shown a significant association between the EcoR1 polymorphisms of Nm23-H1 gene and the susceptibility and severity of disease (Hsieh et al. 2007). Therefore, studies on Nm23-H1 gene in hepatocellular carcinoma, colorectal cancer and human breast cancer tissues, and cell lines have indeed suggested that genomic alteration of Nm23-H1 is a rare event (Bafico et al. 1993, Cipollini et al. 2000, Fujimoto et al. 1998).

Nm23 Sub-cellular Localization

Both Nm23-H1 and Nm23-H2 are principally found in the cytosol and in the endo-plasmic reticulum with some cells exhibiting nuclear staining with the possibility that this may be cell cycle dependent (Bosnar et al. 2004) as the sub-cellular local-ization of proteins is directly related to their functions. Initially based upon the surface expression detection of Nm23-H1 and Nm23-H2 by flow cytometry, an extracellular role for these proteins was suggested in addition to their reported intracellular functions (Urano et al. 1993). The subsequent discovery of a role for Nm23-H2 in transcriptional activation of c-myc proto-oncogene suggested its nuclear localization in addition to cytoplasm. Indeed, in addition to its intense and homogenous cytoplasmic expression, Nm23-H2 is also detected in the centromere region whereas the distribution of Nm23-H2 in interphase nuclei exhibits a pattern of uniformly dispersed punctate dots with reduced staining of the nucleoli (Kraeft et al. 1996).The association of Nm23-H1 and Nm23-H2 with cytoskeletal proteins and their identical co-localization pattern with microtubules have been reported (Pinon et al. 1999). In addition, there was a report of the centrosomal localiza-tion of Nm23-H1 in association with Aurora-A (Du and Hannon 2002). Nm23-R1 and Nm23-R2, the rat homologue of human Nm23-H1 and Nm23-H2, are also associated with the intermediate filaments suggesting a possible function in poly-merization of intermediate filament proteins (Roymans et al. 2000). Nm23-H1/R1 are also present in the centrosome of different dividing and non-dividing human and rat cell types, suggesting that the presence of Nm23-H1 homologues in centrosome is a general event (Roymans et al. 2001). Nm23-H4 localizes specifically in mito-chondria and associates with mitochondrial membranes where its amino terminal extension is cleaved resulting in NDP kinase activity (Kowluru et al. 2002, Milon et al. 2000). However, cell surface expression of Nm23 proteins is only observed on tumor cells and not on normal cells (Okabe-Kado et al. 2002). Nm23-H1 is expressed on the surface of myeloid leukemia lines but not lymphoid lines, while Nm23-H2 is only expressed on erythroleukemia lines suggesting that the surface expression of Nm23 proteins is likely to be related to cellular lineage and the differ-entiation stage of leukemia cells (Okabe-Kado et al. 2002). Immuno-histochemical studies on breast cancer tissues also show that strong staining intensity and nuclear localization of Nm23 protein can be a useful marker of breast cancer progression (Ismail et al. 2008). Both Nm23-H1 and Nm23-H2 occupy similar locations in cells of different origin and differentiation status suggesting that even if Nm23 proteins have different functions in different cells types, they may perform them at similar cellular locations (Bosnar et al. 2004).

Nm23 Expression Levels

The level of Nm23-H1 protein in normal serum is lower than 10 ng/ml, while that in the different tumors vary from about 0 to 1000 ng/ml. Tumor cell lines that over-express Nm23 also secrete this protein into extracellular environment. Exogenously added Nm23-H1 protein does not affect the growth or survival of various leukemia and lymphoma cell lines. However, Nm23-H1 protein inhibits the survival of adher-ent normal peripheral blood mononuclear cells (PBMNC) at 100–1000 ng/ml, and slightly stimulates the survival of non-adherent PBMNC (Okabe-Kado and Kasukabe 2003). Also, in gastric cancer cells Nm23-H1 levels are significantly higher both at the mRNA and protein levels in free-floating cells than that in adherent cells (Iizuka et al. 2001). These studies suggest that Nm23-H1 may act as a molecular switch between the free-floating and adherent states of cancer cells.

Nm23 and Cell Cycle

Nm23 gene expression and protein localization are also related to the growth state of the cells with Nm23-H1 mRNA reaching a maximum abundance in the S-phase. It is absent or only present at very low levels during G0/G1 phase, whereas Nm23-H2 is present in growth-arrested cells but is upregulated following serum growth stimulation (Caligo et al. 1995). Both Nm23-H1 and Nm23-H2 colocalize with microtubules in cells at interphasic possibly interacting indirectly with microtubules. In dividing cells, both are distributed with a punctuate pattern and do not colocalize with the mitotic spindle suggesting a role for these enzymes in some nucleotide channeling processes where they can locally furnish triphosphonucleotides (Pinon et al. 1999). Both Nm23-H1 and Nm23-H2 are transiently localized in the nucleus late in the G1 phase of the cycle and are excluded from the nuclei during S-phase (Bosnar et al. 2004).

Nm23 in a Mouse Model

Propagation of human tumors in the athymic nude mouse has been widely used as a model for studying human cancer biology and therapeutics. The expression of Nm23 mRNA and Nm23 antigen in human uveal melanomas is correlated closely with reduced metastatic behavior in experimental mice (Ma et al. 1996). Also, the critical EBV latent antigens EBNA1 and EBNA3C were shown to interact with Nm23-H1. Using the nude mice model we investigated functional significance of this interaction and evaluated the metastatic and tumorigenic potential of EBV latent nuclear antigens. These studies showed that the expression of Nm23-H1 affected the growth of cancer cells and suppressed their metastatic potential in nude mice. Our studies establishes this system as a useful functional model for studying the biological consequences of interaction between Nm23-H1 and latent viral proteins (Kaul et al. 2007).

Nm23-H1 in Various Cancers

Nm23-H1 is involved in the pathogenesis on many different cancers. Its involvement is summarized in the Table 11.1 and detailed in subsequent paragraphs.

Table 11.1 Association of Nm23-H1 with metastasis in different human cancers

Cancer type	Correlation with metastasis	References	Comments
Anal canal carcinoma	Negative	Indinnimeo (2000)	
Astrocytoma	Negative	Nasser (2006), Martin (1998)	
Bladder and renal cancer	Negative	Chow (2000)	
Breast cancer	Negative	Yamaguchi (1998), Charpin (1998)	
Colorectal carcinoma	Negative	Tannapfel (1995)	
Endometrial and cervical carcinoma	Negative	Chen (2001)	Low expression
Ewing tumor	Positive	Aryee (1995)	
Gall bladder, bile duct	Negative	Lee (1994)	High expression – aggressive
Gastric cancer	Negative	Wang (2004), Lacombe et al. (1991)	Low expression – poor prognosis
Glioma	Negative	Nasser (2006)	
Head and neck cancer	Positive	Pavelic (2000)	Not associate with malignancy
Hepatocellular carcinoma	Negative	Bei (1998), Nakayama (1992)	High expression
Laryngeal cancer	Positive	Wang et al.(1996)	
Leukemia	Positive	Okabe-Kado (2002), Yokoyama (1996)	Low expression – metastasis
Lung cancer	Negative	Ayabe (2004), Okabe-Kado (2003)	High expression – poor prognosis
Lymphoma	Positive	Niitsu (1999), Subramania (2001), Murakami (2005)	Low expression – poor survival
Melanoma	Positive	Steeg (1988)	In non-Hodgkin
Meningioma	Positive	Wang (1997)	
Nasopharyngeal cancer	Negative	Liu (2008)	High expression – benign tumors
Neuroblastoma	Positive	Leone (1993)	
Esophageal	Negative	Tomita (2001)	
Oral cancer	Negative	Khan (2001), Wang (2004)	
Ovarian carcinoma	Negative	Okabe-Kado (2003), Yi (2003), Gao (2004)	
Pancreatic cancer	Positive	Nakamori (1993)	
Prostrate carcinoma	Negative ?	Prowatke (2000), Konishi (1993)	Early stage – high expression
Rheumatoid arthritis	Negative	Dooley (1996)	Primary tumor is positive
Testicular seminoma	Not correlate	Hori (1997)	
Thyroid carcinoma	Negative	Zafon (2001)	

Breast Cancer

The cohort study revealed no correlation between the expression of Nm23-H1 protein/mRNA and breast carcinoma cancer grade and carcinogenesis. However, lymph node metastatic potential has been shown to clearly have an inverse correlation with Nm23-H1. In addition, several studies have shown inverse relationship between Nm23-H1 expression and metastasis/cell invasion in an in vitro system using breast carcinoma cell lines and also in vivo mice experiments (Kaul et al. 2007, Leone et al. 1993a, Murakami et al. 2005, Steeg et al. 1993, Subramanian et al. 2001).

Melanoma

Melanoma is a malignant tumor of melanocytes and is potentially the most dangerous form of skin cancer. Nm23-H1 was originally identified from a melanoma cell line (Steeg et al. 1988). Although extensive studies have established Nm23-H1 as a putative metastasis suppressor, conflicting data do exist as to its role in melanoma progression. Nm23-H1 expression though is significantly reduced in the oral melanomas (Korabiowska et al. 2005).

Gall Bladder

Most gallbladder cancers are adenocarcinomas and about 75% gall bladder cancers are categorized as nonpapillary adenocarcinoma. Nm23-H1 protein expression is absent or weak in most of the poorly differentiated cases. The low expression of Nm23-H1 is generally associated with reduced patient survival (Lee and Pirdas-Zivcic 1994).

Lung Cancer

Histologically, the most frequent type of lung cancer is the non-small cell lung carcinoma which constitutes about 80% of the total lung cancers. The second frequent type is the small cell lung carcinoma which is about 15% of all lung cancers. There is controversy regarding the role of Nm23-H1 in metastasis in lung cancer. Some reports suggest that association of Nm23-H1 with anti-metastatic potential in lung cancer is significant (Kawakubo et al. 1997, Lai et al. 1996, Ohta et al. 2000), whereas others suggest a contrary view (Higashiyama et al. 1992 and Tomita et al. 2001b). Nm23-H1 expression might, however, be associated with micro-metastasis in the lung cancer and low expression of Nm23-H1 may be associated with distant metastasis and a poor 5 years survival score (Ayabe et al. 2004).

Anal Canal Carcinoma

Most anal canal carcinomas come from the squamous cells where growth start off as a benign pre-cancerous condition but over time can develop into a more serious malignant condition. In anal canal carcinoma, significant association has been reported between Nm23-H1 and the depth of lesion invasion and also with the lymph node involvement. However, Nm23-H1 has rarely been detected in cases with metastatic lesions (Indinnimeo et al. 1999).

Oral Cancer

Increased Nm23-H1 expression is associated with low lymph node metastasis at an early T stage (Wang et al. 2004). Low levels of Nm23-H1 expression in oral squamous cell carcinoma indicate a poor survival outcome of patients (Wang et al. 2008).

Astrocytoma

Astrocytoma is the tumor of astrocytes which are star-shaped cells of the central nervous system. Astrocytoma is a major type of brain tumors in the childhood. Nm23-H1 has not been detected in most astrocytomas including high- or low-grade astrocytoma cultures (Kimberly 1998).

Glioma

The gliomas are the most common primary tumors of the central nervous system. About 77% of the malignant brain tumors are gliomas. Though Nm23-H1 is detected in the gliomas, it does not correlate with the malignancy state or invasiveness (Nasser et al. 2006). No significant correlations are seen between Nm23-H1 expression and the pathological grade of tumor (Nasser et al. 2006). The endogenous Nm23-H1 expression in gliomas has been found to be inversely correlated with their migratory abilities in one study (Jung et al. 2006). Interestingly little or no Nm23 expression was observed in the adjacent non-tumorous cerebral tissues. This suggests that high levels of Nm23 expression might correlate with extraneural metastatic potential in astrocytic neoplasms (Nawashiro et al. 1996).

Neuroblastoma

Neuroblastoma commonly occurs in infants and young children. It is rarely found in children older than 10 years. Regional (state III) and metastatic (stage IV) childhood neuroblastomas show elevated Nm23 RNA levels as compared to localized tumors. Elevated Nm23 RNA levels were also associated with significant reduction in patient survival rate (Leone et al. 1993b). The most frequent genetic abnormality detected in neuroblastomas is the gain of chromosome 17q which is correlated with

N-myc amplification (Bown et al. 1999). The Nm23 genes are located at the edge of the common region of chromosome 17q and the expression of Nm23-H1 and Nm23-H2 is increased by this gain of 17q in neuroblastoma (Godfried et al. 2002).

Bladder and Renal Cancer

Urothelial carcinoma is the most common and accounts for more than 90% of all bladder cancers. Squamous cell carcinomas are about 4% of bladder carcinomas followed by adenocarcinomas. Nearly all squamous cell carcinomas and adenocarcinomas of the bladder carcinomas are invasive. There are contrasting results with studies regarding the association of Nm23 expression and metastasis of these cancers. Some studies have shown that reduced or low levels of Nm23-H1 significantly correlate with the occurrence of tumor metastasis or poor patient survival (Chow et al. 2000), while other studies showed that reduced Nm23 mRNA levels are not associated with the metastatic status of either bladder or renal cancer (Kanayama et al. 1994). Moreover, in vitro studies also show that there is no difference of Nm23-H1 protein levels between human bladder cancer cell line T24 and its more aggressive lineage-related variant, T24T (Seraj et al. 2000).

Leukemia

Nm23-H1 is expressed on the cell surface of myeloid leukemia cell lines but not on lymphoid cell lines, while Nm23-H2 is only expressed on erythroleukemia cell lines (Okabe-Kado et al. 2002). Surface expression of Nm23-H1 and Nm23-H2 proteins is decreased during in vitro erythroid and granulocyte differentiation. The surface expression of Nm23 proteins is related to cellular lineage and differentiation stage of leukemia line cells (Okabe-Kado et al. 2002).

Lymphoma

The concentration of Nm23-H1 is significantly higher in patients with malignant lymphoma, especially in aggressive non-Hodgkin's lymphoma (Niitsu et al. 1999). The patients with aggressive non-Hodgkin's lymphoma having higher Nm23-H1 levels have worse overall and progression-free survival rates than those with lower Nm23-H1 levels (Niitsu et al. 2001). Epstein–Barr virus (EBV), a ubiquitous human herpesvirus known to primarily infect B cells may also be a factor in Hodgkins and Non-Hodgkins lymphoma. The EBV-infected lymphoblastoid cells which express the critical nuclear antigens EBNA3C and EBNA1 has an interaction and interestingly induces translocation of Nm23-H1 to the nucleus (Murakami et al. 2005, Subramanian, Cotter et al. 2001). The direct correlation between EBV antigen linked to Nm23-H1 and invasiveness and metastasis of these lymphomas is still to be resolved. However, studies in nude mice suggest a string correlation (Kaul et al. 2007).

Meningioma

The expression of Nm23-H1 protein is sex-dependent and detected on tumor progression in female, but not in male patients. RT-PCR results confirm that Nm23-H1 expression is higher in benign tumors than in their normal counterpart. Nm23-H1 may play an important role in the progression of meningiomas particularly in female patients (Wang et al. 1997b).

Nasopharyngeal Carcinoma

Nasopharyngeal carcinoma (NPC) is an EBV-associated malignancy and is the most common epithelial malignant neoplasm especially in Southern China. Nm23-H1 expression was shown to be related with tumor progression in nasopharyngeal carcinoma especially intracranial invasion (Liu et al. 2008). There is an inverse correlation between Nm23-H1 expression and lymph node metastasis (Huang et al. 2001).

Pancreatic Cancer

Nm23 expression in human pancreatic cancer is positively associated with lymph node metastasis or perineural invasion and with poor prognosis (Nakamori et al. 1993). In contrast, early stage pancreatic cancer samples exhibit stronger Nm23-H1 immunoreactivity than either the normal controls or advanced tumor stages (Friess et al. 2001).

Colorectal Carcinoma

More than 95% of colorectal cancers are adenocarcinomas. The stage of a colorectal cancer depends on how deeply it invades into these layers. In some cases, colorectal cancers of TNM (tumor, node, metastases) stage 0–II showed high ratio of Nm23-H1 and Nm23-H2 expressions. This suggests that Nm23-H1 and Nm23-H2 expressions are linked to early stages of cancer. However, the loss of Nm23-H1 expression is seen in more advanced TNM stages III and IV (Martinez et al. 1995).

Endometrial and Cervical Carcinoma

Endometrial and cervical carcinomas represent most common cancers of the female genital tract. In cervical cancer and its precursor lesions, Nm23-H1 has been analyzed in a number of studies with conflicting results (Chen et al. 2001, Lee and Gad 1998, Marone et al. 1996, Wang et al. 2003a). Regarding cervical intraepithelial neoplasia (CIN) lesions, some studies have reported a definite inverse metastatic effect for Nm23-H1 and the CIN grade (Lee and Gad 1998, Marone et al. 1996,

Morimura et al. 1998), whereas other reports indicate increased Nm23-H1 expression with high-grade CIN (Wang et al. 2003a). No in vitro studies are available on the possible interactions between HPV and the Nm23 gene family (Branca et al. 2006). The high Nm23-H1 expression in cervical cancer cells induces their proliferation resulting in the progression from low-grade stage to a higher grade intraepithelial neoplasia with characteristics of invasive carcinoma involving deep stromal invasion (Wang et al. 2003b), and lower rates of lymph node metastasis and better prognosis (Yalcinkaya et al. 2006). Decreased Nm23-H1 expression is markedly associated with progression from CIN2, to CIN3, and associated with poor prognosis in cervical cancer. Therefore, downregulation of Nm23-H1 expression is probably orchestrated by mechanisms independent of virus-encoding oncoproteins. There is no evidence of direct interactions between HPV-coding oncoproteins and Nm23-H1, and there is no plausible explanation linking this downregulation with HR-HPV. However, Nm23-H1 seems to be a marker of progressive cervical cancer (Branca et al. 2006).

Ewing Tumor

Ewing tumor, also known as Ewing's sarcoma, is an aggressive bone tumor in children. This is one of the tumors in which the Nm23-H1 expression level is high (Aryee et al. 1995). When the metastasis is limited to the lung, the prognosis is better as compared to bone marrow metastasis.

Gastric Cancer

The expression of the Nm23 gene in gastric carcinoma is significantly correlated with aggressive tumor growth, tumor progression, and poor prognosis (Muller et al. 1998, Nesi et al. 2001). About half (52%) of the gastric carcinoma samples show reduction of Nm23-H1 immunoreactivity in the metastatic regional lymph nodes, as compared to the primary tumor. Moreover, 71% of the gastric carcinoma samples showed weaker Nm23-H1 expression in the liver metastasis than in the primary tumor. These results suggest that the expression of Nm23-H1 is linked with development and pathogenesis of gastric carcinomas, and the decrease expression of Nm23 correlate tightly with metastasis (Nakayama et al. 1993, Yeung et al. 1998).

Rheumatoid Arthritis

Up to 30-fold decreased expression of the Nm23-H1 is seen in 90% of rheumatoid arthritis tissues (Dooley et al. 1996). There are three stages of RA progression and in the early stage, the decreased expression of Nm23-H1 may be related to the local invasiveness of the lesions (Dooley et al. 1996).

Esophageal

There is an inverse correlation between Nm23-H1 expression and the lymphatic vessel invasion in cases of esophageal cancer, whereas no correlation is seen between Nm23-H1 expression and blood vessel invasion (Tomita et al. 2001a).

Testicular Seminoma

The immuno-histochemical expression of both the Nm23-H1 and Nm23-H2 gene products is not associated with the metastatic status or the invasive status of testicular seminoma (Hori et al. 1997).

Thyroid Carcinoma

The thyroid gland contains mainly two types of cells: thyroid follicular cells and parafollicular cells. The patients with follicular carcinoma show a significant inverse association between metastatic disease and the expression of Nm23-H1. Significant differences are found in the survival curves according to Nm23-H1 immunoreactivity (Zafon et al. 2001).

Hepatocellular Carcinoma

There are some conflicting reports which involve the relationship between Nm23-H1 expression and the prognosis in hepatocellular carcinoma patients. The relationship between Nm23-H1 expression (mRNA and protein) at primary sites and the rate of intrahepatic metastases shows a significant inverse correlation with intrahepatic metastasis and TNM (tumor, node, metastases) stage. Patients with Nm23-H1 negative tumors or a low Nm23-H1 expression had a greater relative risk of death compared with those with Nm23-H1 positive tumors (Nanashima et al. 2004). The other studies also reported an inverse association between the expression of Nm23-H1 and the metastatic potential (Boissan and Lacombe 2006). However, there are some studies which could not identify any correlation between Nm23-H2 mRNA abundance and intrahepatic metastasis (Iizuka et al. 1995), or between the level of Nm23-H1 expression and the metastatic potential of hepatocellular carcinoma (Cui et al. 2005, Lin et al. 1998, Shimada et al. 1998). Several in vitro studies have shown an inverse relationship between Nm23-transfected metastatic hepatoma cells and their metastatic potential (Fujimoto et al. 1998, Lin et al. 1995).

Ovarian Carcinoma

Strong expression of Nm23-H1 is associated with decreased overall survival and also significantly correlates with mortality in ovarian cancer patients (Youn et al. 2008). The expression of Nm23 (mRNA and protein) negatively correlates with lymph node metastasis in ovarian carcinomas (Yi et al. 2003). Moreover, the expression of Nm23-H1 also correlates closely with the reduced metastatic behavior in experimental animals (Gao et al. 2004).

Prostate Carcinoma

There is no known correlation between Nm23-H1 expression and the metastatic status with pathological parameters of primary prostate carcinomas (Prowatke et al. 2007). However, primary tumors corresponding to the metastases show positive immunostaining for Nm23-H1 (Konishi et al. 1993). This is indicative of an inverse relationship between Nm23-H1 expression and metastatic status.

Nm23 Functions and Biochemical Activities

NDP Kinase Activity

NDP kinases are a ubiquitous family of enzyme involved in the high energy transfer necessary to produce nucleoside triphosphates pools at the expense of ATP. Human NDP kinase 1 or Nm23-H1 removes the terminal phosphate from nucleoside triphosphate to autophosphorylate its own histidine 118, then transfers the phosphate to NDP to recreate NTP (Fig. 11.2) (Wallet et al. 1990). Studies in drosophila *awd* gene, a homolog of human Nm23, have shown that NDP kinase activity of the protein is necessary for its biological function but is not sufficient for its full functionality (Xu et al. 1996). The histidine 118-mutated Nm23-H1 protein lacking NDPK activity displays decreased invasiveness and colonization in soft agar

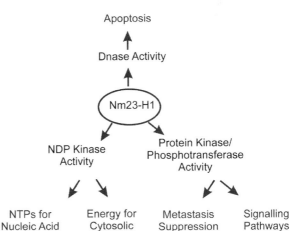

Fig. 11.2 Major biochemical activities of Nm23-H1 and their regulated functions are shown

suggesting that the metastasis-suppressing function of Nm23-H1 is independent of the NDPK enzymatic activity (Lee and Lee 1999). Nm23-H1 and Nm23-H2 can be phosphorylated on S122 by casein kinase II and affect their NDPK activity (Biondi et al. 1996). Nm23 proteins can also phosphorylate geranyl and farnesyl pyrophosphates to give triphosphates which could alter isoprenoid metabolism (Wagner and Vu 2000). Moreover, Nm23-H1 interacts with and phosphorylates the kinase suppressor of Ras, which is a putative scaffold protein for the MAPK pathway, via a histidine-dependent pathway (Hartsough et al. 2002). The regulation of the myosin light chain phosphorylation by Nm23-H1 has been demonstrated as having a potential role in cell migration (Suzuki et al. 2004). The most important roles for NDP kinase is to provide NTPs for nucleic acid synthesis and to the cytosol (Lacombe et al. 2000). Numerous reports suggest that NDP kinase activity may also provide phosphorylation energy to cytosolic structures, such as the translation apparatus (Sastre-Garau et al. 1992, Sonnemann and Mutzel 1995), G-proteins, microtubules (Biggs et al. 1990, Pinon et al. 1999), and chaperons (Leung and Hightower 1997). However, the evidence for such i'nteractions has generally been controversial and further work is needed.

DNase Activity

Studies from the Lieberman laboratory has shown that Nm23-H1 has a DNA-nicking activity. It can act as a granzyme A-activated DNase which can be activated during cytotoxic T lymphocyte (CTL)-mediated apoptosis. This results in translocation of Nm23-H1 to nucleus where it acts as a DNase to nick chromosomal DNA (Fan et al. 2003). It is therefore believed that loss of Nm23-H1 expression in tumors can allow for resistance of the tumors to immune surveillance by CTL and natural killer (NK) cells. Nm23-H1 has also been shown to have a 3'–5' exonuclease activity by virtue of its ability to excise single nucleotides in a stepwise manner from the 3' terminus of DNA (Ma et al. 2004). In addition, Nm23-H5, Nm23-H7, and Nm23-H8 also contain 3'–5' exonuclease activity (Yoon et al. 2005).This activity is believed to play an important role in DNA repair and represents a plausible candidate mediator of the metastasis suppressor properties of the Nm23-H1 molecule (Kaetzel et al. 2006).

Protein Kinase or Phosphotransferase Activity

Other than DNA-binding and NDPK activities, Nm23 proteins are also capable of transferring a phosphate group to other proteins specifically on serine and threonine residues (Engel et al. 1995). Nm23-H1 can also transfer phosphate from its catalytic histidine to histidine or aspartate or glutamate residues on membrane proteins. However, the transfer of phosphate from Nm23-H1 to aspartates or glutamates on other proteins like aldolase A and C correlates better with the suppression of motility than does the transfer to histidines (Wagner et al. 1997). The Nm23-H1 protein mutated at positions 96 and 120 has very little of phosphotransferase activity (Wagner and Vu 2000). The purified native Nm23-H1 protein does not phosphorylate other proteins because Nm23-H1 requires glyceraldehyde-3-phosphate dehydrogenase (GAPDH) as a binding partner to activate its phosphotransferase function (Engel et al. 1998). Nm23-H1 is also associated with AMP-activated protein kinase complex that responds to cellular energy status by switching off ATP-consuming pathways and switching on ATP-generating pathways when ATP is limiting (Crawford et al. 2005). The attempts to identify other physiologically relevant substrates of Nm23 phosphotransferase activity have not been successful. This is probably because of their being present in low concentrations (Wagner and Vu 2000). The phosphotransferase activity of Nm23 proteins may provide an alternate mechanism by which they can affect metastasis.

Interaction of Nm23 with Cellular Antigens

Association with Structural Proteins

For cancer cells to migrate and metastasize, it must first detach itself from the neighboring cells and the intercellular material to which it is anchored. The process involves changes in the cellular internal skeleton and associated structural proteins. The association of Nm23 proteins with structural proteins has been studied in context of several different human cancers. Nm23-H1 plays a role in inhibition of cell migration by regulating the phosphorylation of myosin light chain (Suzuki et al. 2004). DR-Nm23 gene expression is associated with increased expression of vimentin, collagen type IV, and integrin in cells characterized by increased differentiation in neuroblastoma (Amendola et al. 1997). Impairment of Nm23-H1 expression is an early event in the progression of colorectal metastasis that precedes E-cadherin transcriptional silencing in the majority of sporadic colorectal carcinomas (Garinis et al. 2003). Nm23-H1 also correlates negatively with matrix metalloproteinase-2 expression (Ohba et al. 2005). RpS3 which is a component of the 40S ribosomal subunit of eukaryotes interacts with Nm23-H1 and reduces matrix metalloproteinase-9 (MMP-9) expression resulting in reduction of invasive potential of cells (Kim and Kim 2006). EBV nuclear antigen EBNA3C can modulate Nm23-H1 activity leading to upregulation of expression of MMP-9 (Kuppers et al. 2005). Nm23-beta which is a murine homolog of human Nm23-H1 is known to inhibit transcription of MMP-2 by interference with transactivator Y-box protein-1 (Cheng et al. 2002). However, Nm23-H1 has also been shown to inhibit the invasive activity of oral squamous cell carcinoma by suppression of cell motility without altering the MMP-2 and MMP-9 status (Khan et al. 2001).

Nm23 Association with Cellular Enzymes

The association of Nm23 proteins with other cellular proteins depends on the cell type and the state of differentiation. In hepatocellular carcinoma the expression of Nm23-H1 has been found to be associated with the enzyme heparanase in relation to metastasis and recurrence of hepatocellular carcinoma (Duenas-Gonzalez et al. 1996). In pancreatic beta cells the mitochondrial isoform of Nm23 Nm23-H4 complexes with mitochondrial succinyl-CoA synthetase (Kowluru et al. 2002). In human fibroblasts, Nm23-H1 interacts with Aurora-A which is a centrosome-associated kinase and both localize at the centrosome throughout the cell cycle irrespective of the integrity of the microtubule network in normal human fibroblasts (Du and Hannon 2002). Cellular methylation imbalance is known to be associated with tumor progression. S-Adenosylhomocysteine, which is an inhibitor of cellular methyltransferases, has been found to be highly correlated to the expression of Nm23-H1 and may play an important role in inhibition of metastasis through DNA hypomethylation (Yang and Hu 2006). Recently, Nm23-H1 has been shown to interact with Dbl-1, a proto-oncogene, and blocks its ability to function as a guanidine exchange factor for a critical Rho-GTPase family member Cdc42 (Murakami et al. 2008a). Furthermore, Nm23-H1 directly interacts with Cdc42 and the pleckstrin homology domain of oncoprotein Dbl-1. This results in suppression of cell migration (Fig. 11.3) (Murakami et al. 2008b).

Association with Transcriptional and Growth Factors

Nm23-H1 can be referred to as a master transcriptional regulator that regulates different signaling pathways involved in tumorigenesis and invasiveness of cancer. Numerous studied have shown its association with other transcriptional as well as growth factors. Nm23-H1 interacts directly with p53 and positively regulates its function through the stimulation of the nuclear translocation of p53, including p53-induced apoptosis and cell cycle arrest (Jung et al. 2007). However, no correlation has been found between Nm23-H1 and p53 expression levels in breast cancer tissue (Huang et al. 2004). Vascular endothelial growth factor (VEGF) expression is inversely correlated with Nm23-H1 expression in young breast cancer patients; however, no significant correlation of VEGF and Nm23-H1 expressions exists with differentiation of the tumor (Huang et al. 2004). Nm23-H1 interacts with the estrogen receptor alpha and alters the expression of estrogen-responsive genes (Curtis et al. 2007). Nm23-H2 has been shown to be involved in activation of the c-MYC gene. The mechanism of activation seems to involve binding of Nm23 to DNA although there is no definite proof of a direct DNA–Nm23-H1 binding in vivo (Postel et al. 2000). Interestingly, c-MYC is also known to upregulate Nm23-H1 and Nm23-H2 (Godfried et al. 2002, Schuhmacher et al. 2001). The C-terminal half of both Nm23-H1 and Nm23-H2 exhibits strong transactivation activities whereas the full-length Nm23-H1 and its N-terminal do not (Chae et al. 1998). The ErbB2

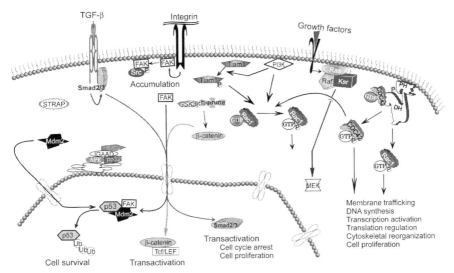

Fig. 11.3 This schematic shows the related Nm23-H1 associations and their effect on cell signaling. In a high motility cell environment, several stimulations such as oncoproteins activate small GTPase proteins. They induce a variety of biological processes including membrane trafficking, translation regulation, transcription activation, DNA synthesis, and cytoskeleton reorganization. A response to stimulation from growth factor receptor also induces kinase suppressor of Ras (Ksr), a scaffold protein for the mitogen-activated protein kinase (MAPK) cascade. MAPK activates several transcription factors. The signal from TGF-beta also shows many transactivation by translocation of Smad2/3 to the nucleus. Cell survival related to p53-dependent apoptosis signal accumulated FAK and p53. Shuttling of p53 from the cytoplasm to nucleus is linked to ubiquitination and degradation by a complex of Mdm2 and FAK. Nm23-H1 interacts with numerous cellular proteins and these interactions show anti-metastatic-related regulation by inhibition of the kinase activities which include reduced phosphorylation of MAPK, Cdc42, Tiam1, and FAK. However, interaction with h-prune showed induction of cell migration by rescue GSK3-beta activity on the beta-catenin. Moreover Nm23-H1 shows stabilization of Smad7 by interacting with STRAP. Stabilized Smad7 inhibits activation of Smad2/3. Nm23-H1 or STRAP or both can disrupt p53-Mdm2 complex which allows for p53 will induced apoptosis. Cytotoxic T lymphocyte release granzyme A, B, and perforin which results in killing of abnormal cells. Perforin forms pores in the membrane of the target cell and granzymes enter the target cell from these pores. Once inside, granzyme A activates DNA-nicking ability of Nm23-H1 by releasing it from the SET complex

gene which is involved in growth regulation and has a role in the initial phases of cell proliferation show a tight association between regulation of its expression by serum factors and Nm23-H1 (Tommasi et al. 2003). Nm23-H1 is also downregulated with another tumor suppressor protein PTEN (phosphatase and tensin homolog) and metastasis suppressor protein KAI-1 specifically in non-small cell lung carcinomas (Goncharuk et al. 2004). The positive expression of sialylated carbohydrate antigens and the reduced expression of Nm23-H1 gene are significantly associated with lymph node involvement in cases of breast cancer indicating their association in the metastatic processes in human breast cancer (Ding and Wu 2004).

Nm23- and DNA-Binding Activities

Although there is no definite evidence of a direct DNA–Nm23-H1 binding in vivo (Postel et al. 2000), the method of in vivo cross-linking followed by ChIP has been used to identify the DNA sequences that may interact with Nm23. The results showed that Nm23-h1 associates with or is in close proximity of the promoters of platelet-derived growth factor A, c-myc, myeloperoxidase, CD11b, p53, WT1, CCR5, ING1, and Nm23-H1 genes (Cervoni et al. 2006). Interestingly, TRF1, which is a telomeric-binding protein, interacts with Nm23-H2 resulting in an increase in affinity of telomerase for its substrate (Nosaka et al. 1998). Since Nm23-H2 is known to bind DNA and also forms a hetero-hexameric complex with Nm23-H1, it is possible that interaction of Nm23-H1 with DNA may be indirectly linked to some of its functions.

Nm23 Association with Viral Proteins

The first demonstration of a specific interaction between Nm23-H1 and any viral oncoprotein was with the EBV latent antigen EBNA3C (Subramanian et al. 2001). Subsequent studies have showed that Nm23-H1 may have intrinsic transcription activities in EBV-infected cells which can be modulated in the presence of the essential EBV latent antigen EBNA3C (Subramanian and Robertson 2002). EBV latent antigen EBNA1 also associates with Nm23-H1, and these antigens can induce Nm23-H1 translocation to nucleus. These viral antigens also rescue the cells from Nm23-H1-mediated suppression of cell migration (Murakami et al. 2005). Further EBNA3C and Nm23-H1 can also cooperate to regulate expression of different proteins including matrix metalloproteinase-9 which is involved in degradation of all components of the basement membrane (Kuppers et al. 2005), and alpha V integrin which is one of the major signaling pathway proteins in cancer development and progression (Choudhuri et al. 2006). Nm23-H1 also regulates the expression of COX-2, a mediator of inflammation which is a key molecule in prostaglandin synthase pathway (Kaul et al. 2006). The down regulation of Nm23-H1 in cervical cancers has not been shown to be associated with human papilloma virus oncoproteins in vivo (Branca et al. 2006), however, E7 protein of HPV-16 has been shown to interact with Nm23-H1 as well as Nm23-H2 resulting in their functional inactivation in vitro (Mileo et al. 2006).

Regulation of Nm23 Expression

Methylation of DNA promoters is an important mechanism for gene regulation. There are two CpG islands present in the promoter of Nm23-H1 and studies have shown that DNA methylation inhibitors can directly or indirectly cause both elevation of Nm23-H1 expression and decrease in cellular motility which can affect the metastatic potential (Hartsough et al. 2001). Three transcription factor-binding sites including MAF/Ets, CTF/NF1 half site, and the ACAAAG enhancer have been identified located within the Nm23-H1 gene promoter (Ouatas et al. 2002). A functional negative thyroid hormone response element is present in the promoter region of the Nm23-H1 gene, and indeed expression of Nm23-H1 is inhibited by thyroid hormone T3 (Lin et al. 2000). The Nm23-H1 gene contains a putative p53-binding site approximately 5 kb upstream of the transcription start site (Rahman-Roblick et al. 2007). Also, p53 was shown to regulate the expression of Nm23-H1 at protein and mRNA levels although the effect is cell type dependent (Chen et al. 2003a). The stimulation by Vitamin D3, a known differentiative agent and modulator of normal and malignant cell proliferation, decreases Nm23-H1 and Nm23-H2 expression in the monocytes (Caligo et al. 1996). The effect is probably at the transcription level as Vitamin D3 is known to act by inhibiting transcription of other genes such as c-myc (Simpson et al. 1987). The expression of Nm23-H1 has been shown to be reduced by tumor necrosis factor-alpha and interferon-gamma (Parhar et al. 1995). Amplification and overexpression of PRUNE has also been suggested as a mechanism for inhibition of Nm23-H1 activity (Forus et al. 2001).

The upregulation of Nm23-H1 has been found to be associated with other intra and extracellular factors. For example, the cellular proto-oncogene c-myc can upregulate Nm23-H1 and Nm23-H2 expressions (Godfried et al. 2002). The expression of Nm23-H1 mRNA is upregulated by all-trans retinoic acid and downregulated by treatment with epidermal growth factor (Liu et al. 2000). The non-specific cyclo-oxygenase inhibitor indomethacin also elevates Nm23-H1 expression in breast cancer cells (Natarajan et al. 2002). The glucocorticoids dexamethasone and medroxyprogesterone acetate elevate Nm23-H1 expression in human breast carcinoma cells (Ouatas et al. 2003a). The effect of medroxyprogesterone acetate on Nm23-H1 expression has also been validated in pulmonary metastasis in vivo (Palmieri et al. 2005). The carotenoid lycopene, which is known to inhibit metastasis, upregulates Nm23-H1 both at mRNA and protein levels in hepatocarcinoma cells (Huang et al. 2005). Keratinocyte growth factor which is an important regulator of epidermal homeostasis and repair has been identified as a regulator of Nm23-H1 gene and subsequent studies have suggested Nm23-H1 to be one of the regulators of epidermal homeostasis (Braun et al. 2007). Human PRUNE gene, a member of DHH phosphoesterase family which is highly expressed in dorsal root ganglia and in the ganglia of cranial nerves, interacts with Nm23-H1 protein and is a negative regulator of the Nm23-H1 protein (Fig. 11.3) (Reymond et al. 1999). Recently, it was reported that phosphorylation of Nm23-H1 by casein kinase I induces its complex formation with h-prune (Garzia et al. 2006, 2008).

Nm23 Regulates the Expression and Activity of Other Cellular Factors

Nm23 proteins exert their effect either by regulating the expression of other proteins at transcriptional levels or by modifying their functions through regulation of post-translational modifications. N-acetylglucosaminyltransferase V also known

as GnT-V is a key enzyme in the processing of multiantennary N-glycans during
the synthesis of glycoproteins. It is associated with alterations in cell surface glycoproteins commonly associated with changes in growth, adhesion, and migration
of cells. The overexpression of Nm23-H1 downregulates the transcription as well
as the functional activity of GnT-V (Guo et al. 2000). Nm23-H1 modulates the
expression of the Rb2/p130 gene by stimulating its promoter in neuronal cells and
also modulates their function by promoting phosphorylation of these proteins mak-
ing them active as negative regulators of cell cycle (Lombardi et al. 2001). Nm23
recognizes nuclease-hypersensitive elements as substrates for DNA cleavage in the
promoter of platelet-derived growth factor (Ma et al. 2002). The inhibitory interaction of Nm23-H1 and Nm23-H2 with PDGF promoter has been suggested as
a possible mechanism for biological actions of Nm23-H1 as PDGF is a protein
implicated in both tumorigenesis and metastasis. In fact initially Nm23-H2 was
identified as a sequence-specific DNA-binding protein with affinity for a nuclease-
hypersensitive element of the c-MYC gene promoter (Postel et al. 1993). This may
be another mechanism by which the Nm23 family of proteins can regulate other
cellular targets. The altered expression level of Nm23-H1 in breast cancer cells
influences the binding properties, stability, and function of the Ksr1 (kinase suppressor of ras 1) which is a scaffold protein (Salerno et al. 2005). Nm23-H2 binds
to and negatively regulates the Lbc proto-oncogene which is a transforming gene
in leukemic cells (Iwashita et al. 2004). Interestingly, Nm23-H1 suppresses tumor
cell motility by downregulating the lysophosphatidic acid receptor EDG2, and this
downregulation of the EDG2 receptor is critical for suppression of cell motility
(Horak et al. 2007a). Nm23-H1 increases expression of beta-Catenin, E-Cadherin
and TIMP-1 and decreases the expression of MMP-2, CD44v6, and VEGF in human
non-small lung cancer cell (Che et al. 2006).

Nm23-Regulated Signaling Pathways

Studies on the interaction of Nm23-H1 and the kinase suppressor of Ras have
shown that Nm23-H1 can phosphorylate kinase suppressor of Ras, which is
an important scaffold molecule in MAPK signaling (Hartsough et al. 2002).
Nm23-H1 gene might inhibit the invasion and metastasis of lung cancer cells
by downregulating PKC signaling pathway (Nie et al. 2006). Nm23-H1 physically interacts with serine–threonine kinase receptor-associated protein and the
association results in modification of biochemical activities of Nm23-H1 including autophosphorylation, phosphotransferase, and NDP kinase activities. This also
affects STRAP (serine–threonine kinase receptor-associated protein)-induced inhibition of TGF-beta-pathway-mediated apoptosis and growth inhibition (Seong
et al. 2007). Nm23-H1 and STRAP are also important in the regulation of a
p53-induced signaling pathway and act as positive regulators of p53 activity by
dissociating Mdm2 which is a known negative regulator of p53 (Fig. 11.3) (Jung
et al. 2007).

Nm23 and Tumorigenicity

A widely accepted definition of a metastasis suppressor gene states that such a gene when expressed can inhibit the spread of cancer cells to secondary sites without affecting tumorigenicity (Lombardi 2006). Re-expression of a metastasis suppressor gene in a metastatic tumor cell line results in a significant reduction in metastatic behavior with no effect on tumorigenicity (Steeg et al. 2003). Nm23-H1, however, has also been shown to affect the growth rate of EBV latent proteins expressing cancer cells in addition to suppressing their metastasis potential (Kaul et al. 2006). Since Nm23-H1 does not appear to affect growth of tumors on its own (Tseng et al. 2001), it is possible that interaction with viral proteins can play role in affecting the tumorigenicity potential of Nm23-H1.

Nm23 Effects on Cell Growth and Differentiation

Nm23-H1 protein level has been associated with increasing levels of proliferating cell nuclear antigen (PCNA) expression in human prostate cancer (Igawa et al. 1996). Since PCNA was originally identified as an antigen that is expressed in the nuclei of cells during the DNA synthesis phase of the cell cycle, this observation points to a link between Nm23-H1 and cell growth. In fact, overexpression of Nm23-H1 in human breast carcinoma cells leads to the formation of basement membrane and growth arrest suggesting its role in mammary development and differentiation (Howlett et al. 1994). On other hand, murine homolog of Nm23-H2 has been identified as a differentiation-inhibiting factor or I-factor in mouse myeloid leukemia cells (Okabe-Kado et al. 1995a), which is also capable of inhibiting erythroid differentiation of human leukemic cells (Okabe-Kado et al. 1995a). The differentiation inhibitory activity of Nm23 protein is independent of its enzyme activity and requires the presence of N-terminal peptides (Okabe-Kado et al. 1995b). Increased expression of DR-Nm23 also known as Nm23-H3 contributes to differentiation arrest and suppresses granulocyte differentiation of myeloid precursor cells (Venturelli et al. 1995). Moreover, the nucleoside diphosphate kinase activity of DR-Nm23 is also not required for inhibition of differentiation and induction of apoptosis in myeloid precursor cells (Venturelli et al. 2000). Nm23-H1 is involved in inhibition of progesterone-induced oocyte maturation and growth through regulation of MAPK cascade (Kim et al. 2000).

The amount of Nm23-H1 protein is known to vary during the induced differentiation of leukemia cell lines suggesting that Nm23-H1 plays an important role to maintain the proliferation of immature leukemic cells and may also play a role in the early stages of their differentiation (Yamashiro et al. 1994). The bone marrow progenitors of blood cells contain the highest intracellular levels of both Nm23-H1 and Nm23-H2 followed by lower levels in more mature bone marrow cells, whereas peripheral blood leukocytes had the lowest expression of Nm23-H1. This suggests a function of Nm23-H1 in early hematopoiesis and its downregulation upon differentiation (Willems et al. 1998). Nm23-H1 also modulates the expression of the

Rb2/p130 gene which is a known negative regulator of cell cycle progression also implicated in the maintenance of the differentiated state (Lombardi et al. 2001). It has also been shown that the levels of extracellular Nm23-H1 protein in plasma have a modulating effect on the terminal stages of normal hematopoietic differentiation (Willems et al. 2002). Therefore, the fairly high concentrations of Nm23 constitutively present in plasma could have a physiologic role in supporting erythropoiesis and inhibiting excessive macrophage formation. These point to a likely function of Nm23 proteins related to cell growth and differentiation which may be dependent on cell type independent of other functions associated with Nm23-H1.

Nm23-H1- and Apoptosis-Related Activities

Nm23 family members have a common NDPK activity which is important for cell proliferation (Keim et al. 1992), development (Biggs et al. 1990), and differentiation (Willems et al. 1998). DR-Nm23, one of the Nm23 family member, when transfected to several neuroblastoma cell lines showed growth arrest and increased expression of vimentin, collagen type IV, and integrin-beta1 (Amendola et al. 1997). The study using myeloid precursor 32Dc13 cell line, in which DR-Nm23 was transfected, showed that DR-Nm23 contributes to differentiation arrest and induces an apoptosis in myeloid cell (Venturelli et al. 1995). However, the exact mechanism remains unclear. Necrosis is unprogramed cell death which is caused by atypical body conditions including infection and cancer. Apoptosis is programmed cell death that can occur through two principal signaling pathways. The intrinsic pathway is triggered by the p53 tumor suppressor in response to several cell stresses, such as DNA damage. The extrinsic pathway is triggered by activation of pro-apoptotic receptors which is independent of p53. However, both pathways merge at the activation point of caspase 3, 6, and 7. The granzymes which induce apoptosis are serine protease and are most abundant in CTL and NK cells. Granzyme A induces caspase-independent pathway of apoptosis, although DNA is damaged (Beresford et al. 1999, Shresta et al. 1999). Granzyme B triggers apoptosis through caspase-dependent and independent pathways which involve direct cleavage of downstream caspase substrates (Sarin et al. 1997). If target cells are resistant to granzyme B or caspases, these cells are typically susceptible to granzymeA (Beresford et al. 1999). Nm23-H1 has been identified as granzyme A-activated DNase (GAAD) and its specific inhibitor (IGAAD) is SET. Nm23-H1 binds to SET and is released by granzyme A cleavage of SET, removing the inhibitor (Fan et al. 2003). Then Nm23-H1 moves to the nucleus where it can nick DNA (Fig. 11.3) (Fan et al. 2003). The $3'$–$5'$ exonuclease TREX1 binds to SET and NM23-H1 works with TREX1 in concert to degrade DNA (Chowdhury et al. 2006). Silencing Nm23-H1 or TREX1 inhibits DNA damage and death of cells (Chowdhury et al. 2006). Since cells with silenced Nm23-H1 are less sensitive to GzmA-induced cell death, the loss of Nm23-H1 expression in tumors may provide some resistance to immune surveillance by CTL and NK cells as well as promote their growth.

Nm23 and Tumor Metastasis

The Nm23 genes were discovered on the basis of their reduced expression in highly metastatic cell lines. Several studies have demonstrated the suppressive effect of Nm23 overexpression on the metastatic aggressiveness of melanoma and breast carcinoma cells in vivo (Howlett et al. 1994, Leone et al. 1993a). It was initially hypothesized that the mechanism of action of Nm23 in metastasis suppression involves diminished signal transduction downstream of a nuclear hormone receptor (Ouatas et al. 2003b). Importantly, the histidine protein kinase activity of Nm23 underlies its suppression of metastasis function. Mutational analyses of Nm23-H1 have shown that substitution mutants P96S and S120G do not inhibit motility and invasion. Transfection of Nm23-H1 into the human MDA-MB-435 breast carcinoma cell lines suppresses the metastatic potential of these cells (Leone et al. 1993a). The levels of Nm23-H1 in cell lines and xenografts also show an inverse correlation with their metastatic potential in nude mice. Although Nm23-H2 was initially suspected to not be involved in metastasis suppression, subsequent studies suggested that both Nm23-H1 and Nm23-H2 can suppress metastasis (Baba et al. 1995). Decreased expression of Nm23-H2 gene homolog is in fact associated with metastatic potential of rat mammary–adenocarcinoma cells (Fukuda et al. 1996). Studies in human breast cancer patients have also shown that high levels of Nm23 are associated with excellent survival probabilities (Heimann et al. 1998). However, the Nm23 expression cannot predict outcome in lymph node negative breast carcinoma patients (Russell et al. 1997). Nm23-H1 loss of heterozygocity is also related to the metastasis potential of hepatocellular carcinoma and can help to predict recurrence and metastasis (Ye et al. 1998). However Nm23 appears to be a suppressor of systemic, but not lymphatic, metastasis in primary non-small cell lung cancer (Graham et al. 2002). Nm23-H1 plays more important role in switching the initial metastases formation than in influencing the later metastases spread, as the negative expressions of Nm23-H1 in solid tumors of oral squamous cell carcinoma induce the formation of high metastatic cellular subpopulations (Yang et al. 2003). Human prune is a phosphoesterase DHH family appertaining protein which has cyclic nucleotide phosphodiesterase activity. Nm23-H1 interacts with human prune and this interaction has also been associated with incidence of higher metastasis in breast cancer cases (Fig. 11.3) (D'Angelo et al. 2004). Further the phosphorylation of Nm23-H1 by casein kinase I induces its complex formation with h-prune and promotes cell motility (Garzia et al. 2008).

Nm23-H1 may also act as metastasis promoter in certain tumor types. Overexpression of Nm23-H1 have been found in 14–30% of advanced neuroblastomas, and studies have confirmed that Nm23-H1 does not behave as a metastasis suppressor in human neuroblastomas derived from NB69 cells (Almgren et al. 2004). Also several studies have found that overexpression of Nm23-H1 protein may indicate poor survival for cervical cancer patients (Chen et al. 2001, Wang et al. 2003b). Cancer cells overexpressing Nm23 are more sensitive to the alkylating agent cisplatin resulting in more pronounced inhibition of pulmonary metastasis whereas reduced expression of intracellular Nm23-H1 is associated with cisplatin resistance via the prevention of both nuclear and mitochondrial DNA damages (Ferguson et al. 1996, Iizuka et al. 2000). Nm23-H1 also suppresses the metastatic potential of prostate carcinoma cells (Lim et al. 1998). Nm23 genes may affect suppression of metastasis through phospholipid-mediated signaling resulting in higher levels of phosphodiester compounds relative to phosphomonoester compounds and also cellular pH regulation (Bhujwalla et al. 1999). Downregulation of lysophosphatidic acid receptor EDG2 by Nm23-H1 is critical for motility suppression and is important for the suppression of in vivo metastasis (Horak et al. 2007b). Nm23-H1 can also exert its role in regulation of metastasis by its interaction or regulation of intracytoplasmic cellular structural proteins. Nm23-R1, the murine homolog of Nm23-H1 has been shown to associate with intermediate filaments (Roymans et al. 2000). ARF6 which is a member of the ARF family of proteins recruits Nm23-H1 and induces disassembly of adherens junctions thus facilitating endocytosis of E-cadherin and down regulation of Rac1 activity and thus contributing to the regulation of migratory potential of cell (Palacios et al. 2002). Although Nm23-H1 expression is divergent in various malignant tumors, its reduced expression seems to be related to increased metastatic potential in most cancer cell types.

Conclusions

Nm23-H1 is associated with tumor metastasis. Although the expression of Nm23-H1 is variable in different malignant tumor types, most of the clinical and in vitro data suggest that its overexpression is related to reduced metastatic potential in most of the cancer cell types. Moreover, it is clear that the biological role of Nm23-H1 goes way beyond what are expected of a simple metastasis suppressor gene. Its role in cell cycle progression and its recently discovered DNase activity along with phosphotransferase activity that enables it to function as protein kinase have enabled it to regulate a much wider range of downstream functions. Its association with viral latent antigens resulting in modulations of its activities has added an entirely new dimension to its biological significance in viral-related cancers.

References

Almgren, M. A., K. C. Henriksson, J. Fujimoto, and C. L. Chang (2004) Nucleoside diphosphate kinase A/nm23-H1 promotes metastasis of NB69-derived human neuroblastoma. Mol Cancer Res 2:387–94.

Amendola, R., R. Martinez, A. Negroni, D. Venturelli, B. Tanno, B. Calabretta, and G. Raschella (1997) DR-nm23 gene expression in neuroblastoma cells: relationship to integrin expression, adhesion characteristics, and differentiation. J Natl Cancer Inst 89:1300–10.

Aryee, D. N., T. Strobel, K. Kos, M. Salzer-Kuntschik, A. Zoubek, M. Veron, I. M. Ambros, F. Traincart, H. Gadner, and H. Kovar (1995) High nm23-H1/NDPK-A expression in Ewing tumors: paradoxical immunohistochemical reactivity and lack of prognostic significance. Int J Cancer 64:104–11.

Ayabe, T., M. Tomita, Y. Matsuzaki, H. Ninomiya, M. Hara, T. Shimizu, M. Edagawa, T. Onitsuka, and M. Hamada (2004) Micrometastasis and expression of nm23 messenger RNA of lymph nodes from lung cancer and the postoperative clinical outcome. Ann Thorac Cardiovasc Surg 10:152–9.

Baba, H., T. Urano, K. Okada, K. Furukawa, E. Nakayama, H. Tanaka, K. Iwasaki, and H. Shiku (1995) Two isotypes of murine nm23/nucleoside diphosphate kinase, nm23-M1 and nm23-M2, are involved in metastatic suppression of a murine melanoma line. Cancer Res 55: 1977–81.

Bafico, A., L. Varesco, L. De Benedetti, M. A. Caligo, V. Gismondi, S. Sciallero, H. Aste, G. B. Ferrara, and G. Bevilacqua (1993) Genomic PCR-SSCP analysis of the metastasis associated NM23-H1 (NME1) gene: a study on colorectal cancer. Anticancer Res 13:2149–54.

Beresford, P. J., Z. Xia, A. H. Greenberg, and J. Lieberman (1999) Granzyme A loading induces rapid cytolysis and a novel form of DNA damage independently of caspase activation. Immunity 10:585–94.

Bhujwalla, Z. M., E. O. Aboagye, R. J. Gillies, V. P. Chacko, C. E. Mendola, and J. M. Backer (1999) Nm23-transfected MDA-MB-435 human breast carcinoma cells form tumors with altered phospholipid metabolism and pH: a 31P nuclear magnetic resonance study in vivo and in vitro. Magn Reson Med 41:897–903.

Biggs, J., E. Hersperger, P. S. Steeg, L. A. Liotta, and A. Shearn (1990) A Drosophila gene that is homologous to a mammalian gene associated with tumor metastasis codes for a nucleoside diphosphate kinase. Cell 63:933–40.

Biondi, R. M., M. Engel, M. Sauane, C. Welter, O. G. Issinger, L. Jimenez de Asua, and S. Passeron (1996) Inhibition of nucleoside diphosphate kinase activity by in vitro phosphorylation by protein kinase CK2. Differential phosphorylation of NDP kinases in HeLa cells in culture. FEBS Lett 399:183–7.

Boissan, M. and M. L. Lacombe (2006) Nm23/NDP kinases in hepatocellular carcinoma. J Bioenerg Biomembr 38:169–75.

Bosnar, M. H., K. Pavelic, R. Hrascan, Z. Zeljko, I. Krhen, Z. Marekoyic, S. Krizanac, and J. Pavelic (1997) Loss of heterozygosity of the nm23-H1 gene in human renal cell carcinomas. J Cancer Res Clin Oncol 123:485–8.

Bosnar, M. H., J. De Gunzburg, R. Bago, L. Brecevic, I. Weber, and J. Pavelic (2004) Subcellular localization of A and B Nm23/NDPK subunits. Exp Cell Res 298:275–84.

Bown, N., S. Cotterill, M. Lastowska, S. O'Neill, A. D. Pearson, D. Plantaz, M. Meddeb, G. Danglot, C. Brinkschmidt, H. Christiansen, G. Laureys, F. Speleman, J. Nicholson, A. Bernheim, D. R. Betts, J. Vandesompele, and N. Van Roy (1999) Gain of chromosome arm 17q and adverse outcome in patients with neuroblastoma. N Engl J Med 340:1954–61.

Branca, M., C. Giorgi, M. Ciotti, D. Santini, L. Di Bonito, S. Costa, A. Benedetto, D. Bonifacio, P. Di Bonito, P. Paba, L. Accardi, L. Mariani, M. Ruutu, C. Favalli, and K. Syrjanen (2006) Down-regulated nucleoside diphosphate kinase nm23-H1 expression is unrelated to high-risk human papillomavirus but associated with progression of cervical intraepithelial neoplasia and unfavourable prognosis in cervical cancer. J Clin Pathol 59:1044–51.

Braun, S., C. Mauch, P. Boukamp, and S. Werner (2007) Novel roles of NM23 proteins in skin homeostasis, repair and disease. Oncogene 26:532–42.

Caligo, M. A., G. Cipollini, L. Fiore, S. Calvo, F. Basolo, P. Collecchi, F. Ciardiello, S. Pepe, M. Petrini, and G. Bevilacqua (1995) NM23 gene expression correlates with cell growth rate and S-phase. Int J Cancer 60:837–42.

Caligo, M. A., G. Cipollini, M. Petrini, P. Valentini, and G. Bevilacqua (1996) Down regulation of NM23.H1, NM23.H2 and c-myc genes during differentiation induced by 1,25 dihydroxyvitamin D3. Leuk Res 20:161–7.

Campo, E., R. Miquel, P. Jares, F. Bosch, M. Juan, A. Leone, J. Vives, A. Cardesa, and J. Yague (1994) Prognostic significance of the loss of heterozygosity of Nm23-H1 and p53 genes in human colorectal carcinomas. Cancer 73:2913–21.

Cervoni, L., L. Egistelli, M. Eufemi, A. S. d'Abusco, F. Altieri, I. Lascu, C. Turano, and A. Giartosio (2006) DNA sequences acting as binding sites for NM23/NDPK proteins in melanoma M14 cells. J Cell Biochem 98:421–8.

Chae, S. K., N. S. Lee, K. J. Lee, and E. Kim (1998) Transactivation potential of the C-terminus of human Nm23-H1. FEBS Lett 423:235–8.

Chang, C. L., X. X. Zhu, D. H. Thoraval, D. Ungar, J. Rawwas, N. Hora, J. R. Strahler, S. M. Hanash, and E. Radany (1994) Nm23-H1 mutation in neuroblastoma. Nature 370:335–6.

Chang, C. L., J. R. Strahler, D. H. Thoraval, M. G. Qian, R. Hinderer, and S. M. Hanash (1996) A nucleoside diphosphate kinase A (nm23-H1) serine 120–>glycine substitution in advanced stage neuroblastoma affects enzyme stability and alters protein-protein interaction. Oncogene 12:659–67.

Che, G., J. Chen, L. Liu, Y. Wang, L. Li, Y. Qin, and Q. Zhou (2006) Transfection of nm23-H1 increased expression of beta-Catenin, E-Cadherin and TIMP-1 and decreased the expression of MMP-2, CD44v6 and VEGF and inhibited the metastatic potential of human non-small cell lung cancer cell line L9981. Neoplasma 53:530–7.

Chen, H. C., L. Wang, and S. Banerjee (1994) Isolation and characterization of the promoter region of human nm23-H1, a metastasis suppressor gene. Oncogene 9:2905–12.

Chen, H. Y., C. T. Hsu, W. C. Lin, H. D. Tsai, and W. C. Chang (2001) Prognostic value of nm23 expression in stage IB1 cervical carcinoma. Jpn J Clin Oncol 31:327–32.

Chen S. L., Y. S. Wu, H. Y. Shieh, C. C. Yen, J. J. Shen, and K. H. Lin (2003a) P53 is a regulator of the metastasis suppressor gene Nm23-H1. Mol Carcinog 36:204–14.

Chen, Y., S. Gallois-Montbrun, B. Schneider, M. Veron, S. Morera, D. Deville-Bonne, and J. Janin (2003b) Nucleotide binding to nucleoside diphosphate kinases: X-ray structure of human NDPK-A in complex with ADP and comparison to protein kinases. J Mol Biol 332:915–26.

Cheng, S., M. A. Alfonso-Jaume, P. R. Mertens, and D. H. Lovett (2002) Tumour metastasis suppressor, nm23-beta, inhibits gelatinase A transcription by interference with transactivator Y-box protein-1 (YB-1). Biochem J 366:807–16.

Cho, S. J., N. S. Lee, Y. S. Jung, H. Lee, K. J. Lee, E. Kim, and S. K. Chae (2001) Identification of structural domains affecting transactivation potential of Nm23. Biochem Biophys Res Commun 289:738–43.

Choudhuri, T., S. C. Verma, K. Lan, and E. S. Robertson (2006) Expression of alpha V integrin is modulated by Epstein-Barr virus nuclear antigen 3C and the metastasis suppressor Nm23-H1 through interaction with the GATA-1 and Sp1 transcription factors. Virology 351:58–72.

Chow, N. H., H. S. Liu, and S. H. Chan (2000) The role of nm23-H1 in the progression of transitional cell bladder cancer. Clin Cancer Res 6:3595–9.

Chowdhury, D., P. J. Beresford, P. Zhu, D. Zhang, J. S. Sung, B. Demple, F. W. Perrino, and J. Lieberman (2006) The exonuclease TREX1 is in the SET complex and acts in concert with NM23-H1 to degrade DNA during granzyme A-mediated cell death. Mol Cell 23:133–42.

Cipollini, G., A. Moretti, C. Ghimenti, P. Viacava, G. Bevilacqua, and M. A. Caligo (2000) Mutational analysis of the NM23.H1 gene in human breast cancer. Cancer Genet Cytogenet 121:181–5.

Crawford, R. M., K. J. Treharne, O. G. Best, R. Muimo, C. E. Riemen, and A. Mehta (2005) A novel physical and functional association between nucleoside diphosphate kinase A and AMP-activated protein kinase alpha1 in liver and lung. Biochem J 392:201–9.

Cui, J., B. W. Dong, P. Liang, X. L. Yu, and D. J. Yu (2005) Construction and clinical significance of a predictive system for prognosis of hepatocellular carcinoma. World J Gastroenterol 11: 3027–33.

Curtis, C. D., V. S. Likhite, I. X. McLeod, J. R. Yates, and A. M. Nardulli (2007) Interaction of the tumor metastasis suppressor nonmetastatic protein 23 homologue H1 and estrogen receptor alpha alters estrogen-responsive gene expression. Cancer Res 67:10600–7.

D'Angelo, A., L. Garzia, A. Andre, P. Carotenuto, V. Aglio, O. Guardiola, G. Arrigoni, A. Cossu, G. Palmieri, L. Aravind, and M. Zollo (2004) Prune cAMP phosphodiesterase binds nm23-H1 and promotes cancer metastasis. Cancer Cell 5:137–49.

de la Rosa, A., B. Mikhak, and P. S. Steeg (1996) Identification and characterization of the promoter for the human metastasis suppressor gene nm23-H1. Arch Med Res 27: 395–401.

Ding, K. F. and J. M. Wu (2004) [Expression of sialylated carbohydrate antigens and nm23-H1 gene in prognosis of breast cancer]. Zhejiang Da Xue Xue Bao Yi Xue Ban 33:326–30, 339.

Dooley, S., I. Herlitzka, R. Hanselmann, A. Ermis, W. Henn, K. Remberger, T. Hopf, and C. Welter (1996) Constitutive expression of c-fos and c-jun, overexpression of ets-2, and reduced expression of metastasis suppressor gene nm23-H1 in rheumatoid arthritis. Ann Rheum Dis 55:298–304.

Du, J. and G. J. Hannon (2002) The centrosomal kinase Aurora-A/STK15 interacts with a putative tumor suppressor NM23-H1. Nucleic Acids Res 30:5465–75.

Duenas-Gonzalez, A., M. M. Abad-Hernandez, J. Garcia-Mata, J. I. Paz-Bouza, J. J. Cruz-Hernandez, and R. Gonzalez-Sarmiento (1996) Analysis of nm23-H1 expression in breast cancer. Correlation with p53 expression and clinicopathologic findings. Cancer Lett 101: 137–42.

Dumas, C., I. Lascu, S. Morera, P. Glaser, R. Fourme, V. Wallet, M. L. Lacombe, M. Veron, and J. Janin (1992) X-ray structure of nucleoside diphosphate kinase. EMBO J 11:3203–8.

Engel, M., M. Veron, B. Theisinger, M. L. Lacombe, T. Seib, S. Dooley, and C. Welter (1995) A novel serine/threonine-specific protein phosphotransferase activity of Nm23/nucleoside-diphosphate kinase. Eur J Biochem 234:200–7.

Engel, M., M. Seifert, B. Theisinger, U. Seyfert, and C. Welter (1998) Glyceraldehyde-3-phosphate dehydrogenase and Nm23-H1/nucleoside diphosphate kinase A. Two old enzymes combine for the novel Nm23 protein phosphotransferase function. J Biol Chem 273:20058–65.

Fan, Z., P. J. Beresford, D. Y. Oh, D. Zhang, and J. Lieberman (2003) Tumor suppressor NM23-H1 is a granzyme A-activated DNase during CTL-mediated apoptosis, and the nucleosome assembly protein SET is its inhibitor. Cell 112:659–72.

Ferguson, A. W., U. Flatow, N. J. MacDonald, F. Larminat, V. A. Bohr, and P. S. Steeg (1996) Increased sensitivity to cisplatin by nm23-transfected tumor cell lines. Cancer Res 56:2931–5.

Forus, A., A. D'Angelo, J. Henriksen, G. Merla, G. M. Maelandsmo, V. A. Florenes, S. Olivieri, B. Bjerkehagen, L. A. Meza-Zepeda, F. del Vecchio Blanco, C. Muller, F. Sanvito, J. Kononen, J. M. Nesland, O. Fodstad, A. Reymond, O. P. Kallioniemi, G. Arrigoni, A. Ballabio, O. Myklebost, and M. Zollo (2001) Amplification and overexpression of PRUNE in human sarcomas and breast carcinomas-a possible mechanism for altering the nm23-H1 activity. Oncogene 20:6881–90.

Friess, H., X. Z. Guo, A. A. Tempia-Caliera, A. Fukuda, M. E. Martignoni, A. Zimmermann, M. Korc, and M. W. Buchler (2001) Differential expression of metastasis-associated genes in papilla of vater and pancreatic cancer correlates with disease stage. J Clin Oncol 19:2422–32.

Fujimoto, Y., T. Ohtake, H. Nishimori, K. Ikuta, M. Ohhira, M. Ono, and Y. Kohgo (1998) Reduced expression and rare genomic alteration of nm23-H1 in human hepatocellular carcinoma and hepatoma cell lines. J Gastroenterol 33:368–75.

Fukuda, M., A. Ishii, Y. Yasutomo, N. Shimada, N. Ishikawa, N. Hanai, N. Nagata, T. Irimura, G. L. Nicolson, and N. Kimura (1996) Decreased expression of nucleoside diphosphate kinase alpha isoform, an nm23-H2 gene homolog, is associated with metastatic potential of rat mammary-adenocarcinoma cells. Int J Cancer 65:531–7.

Gao, Q. L., D. Ma, L. Meng, S. X. Wang, C. Y. Wang, Y. P. Lu, A. L. Zhang, and J. Li (2004) Association between Nm23-H1 gene expression and metastasis of ovarian carcinoma. Ai Zheng 23:650–4.

Garinis, G. A., E. N. Manolis, N. E. Spanakis, G. P. Patrinos, G. Peros, and P. G. Menounos (2003) High frequency of concomitant nm23-H1 and E-cadherin transcriptional inactivation in primary non-inheriting colorectal carcinomas. J Mol Med 81:256–63.

Garzia, L., A. D'Angelo, A. Amoresano, S. K. Knauer, C. Cirulli, C. Campanella, R. H. Stauber, C. Steegborn, A. Iolascon, and M. Zollo (2008) Phosphorylation of nm23-H1 by CKI induces its complex formation with h-prune and promotes cell motility. Oncogene 27:1853–64.

Garzia, L., C. Roma, N. Tata, D. Pagnozzi, P. Pucci, and M. Zollo (2006) H-prune-nm23-H1 protein complex and correlation to pathways in cancer metastasis. J Bioenerg Biomembr 38: 205–13.

Gilles, A. M., E. Presecan, A. Vonica, and I. Lascu (1991) Nucleoside diphosphate kinase from human erythrocytes. Structural characterization of the two polypeptide chains responsible for heterogeneity of the hexameric enzyme. J Biol Chem 266:8784–9.

Giraud, M. F., F. Georgescauld, I. Lascu, and A. Dautant (2006) Crystal structures of S120G mutant and wild type of human nucleoside diphosphate kinase A in complex with ADP. J Bioenerg Biomembr 38:261–4.

Godfried, M. B., M. Veenstra, P. v Sluis, K. Boon, R. v Asperen, M. C. Hermus, B. D. v Schaik, T. P. Voute, M. Schwab, R. Versteeg, and H. N. Caron (2002) The N-myc and c-myc downstream pathways include the chromosome 17q genes nm23-H1 and nm23-H2. Oncogene 21: 2097–101.

Goncharuk, V. N., A. del-Rosario, L. Kren, S. Anwar, C. E. Sheehan, J. A. Carlson, and J. S. Ross (2004) Co-downregulation of PTEN, KAI-1, and nm23-H1 tumor/metastasis suppressor proteins in non-small cell lung cancer. Ann Diagn Pathol 8:6–16.

Graham, A. N., P. Maxwell, K. Mulholland, A. H. Patterson, N. Anderson, K. G. McManus, H. Bharucha, and J. A. McGuigan (2002) Increased nm23 immunoreactivity is associated with selective inhibition of systemic tumour cell dissemination. J Clin Pathol 55:184–9.

Guo, H. B., F. Liu, J. H. Zhao, and H. L. Chen (2000) Down-regulation of N-acetylglucosaminyltransferase V by tumorigenesis- or metastasis-suppressor gene and its relation to metastatic potential of human hepatocarcinoma cells. J Cell Biochem 79: 370–85.

Hamby, C. V., R. Abbi, N. Prasad, C. Stauffer, J. Thomson, C. E. Mendola, V. Sidorov, and J. M. Backer (2000) Expression of a catalytically inactive H118Y mutant of nm23-H2 suppresses the metastatic potential of line IV Cl 1 human melanoma cells. Int J Cancer 88:547–53.

Hartsough, M. T. and P. S. Steeg (1998) Nm23-H1: genetic alterations and expression patterns in tumor metastasis. Am J Hum Genet 63:6–10.

Hartsough, M. T., S. E. Clare, M. Mair, A. G. Elkahloun, D. Sgroi, C. K. Osborne, G. Clark, and P. S. Steeg (2001) Elevation of breast carcinoma Nm23-H1 metastasis suppressor gene expression and reduced motility by DNA methylation inhibition. Cancer Res 61:2320–7.

Hartsough, M. T., D. K. Morrison, M. Salerno, D. Palmieri, T. Ouatas, M. Mair, J. Patrick, and P. S. Steeg (2002) Nm23-H1 metastasis suppressor phosphorylation of kinase suppressor of Ras via a histidine protein kinase pathway. J Biol Chem 277:32389–99.

Heimann, R., D. J. Ferguson, and S. Hellman (1998) The relationship between nm23, angiogenesis, and the metastatic proclivity of node-negative breast cancer. Cancer Res 58:2766–71.

Higashiyama, M., O. Doi, H. Yokouchi, K. Kodama, S. Nakamori, R. Tateishi, and N. Kimura (1992) Immunohistochemical analysis of nm23 gene product/NDP kinase expression in pulmonary adenocarcinoma: lack of prognostic value. Br J Cancer 66:533–6.

Horak, C. E., J. H. Lee, A. G. Elkahloun, M. Boissan, S. Dumont, T. K. Maga, S. Arnaud-Dabernat, D. Palmieri, W. G. Stetler-Stevenson, M. L. Lacombe, P. S. Meltzer, and P. S. Steeg (2007a) Nm23-H1 suppresses tumor cell motility by down-regulating the lysophosphatidic acid receptor EDG2. Cancer Res 67:7238–46.

Horak, C. E., A. Mendoza, E. Vega-Valle, M. Albaugh, C. Graff-Cherry, W. G. McDermott, E. Hua, M. J. Merino, S. M. Steinberg, C. Khanna, and P. S. Steeg (2007b) Nm23-H1 suppresses metastasis by inhibiting expression of the lysophosphatidic acid receptor EDG2. Cancer Res 67:11751–9.

Hori, K., K. Uematsu, H. Yasoshima, K. Sakurai, A. Yamada, and M. Ohya (1997) Immunohistochemical analysis of the nm23 gene products in testicular seminoma. Pathol Int 47:288–92.

Howlett, A. R., O. W. Petersen, P. S. Steeg, and M. J. Bissell (1994) A novel function for the nm23-H1 gene: overexpression in human breast carcinoma cells leads to the formation of basement membrane and growth arrest. J Natl Cancer Inst 86:1838–44.

Hsieh, Y. S., Y. L. Lee, S. F. Yang, J. S. Yang, W. Chen, S. C. Chen, and C. M. Shih (2007) Association of EcoRI polymorphism of the metastasis-suppressor gene NME1 with susceptibility to and severity of non-small cell lung cancer. Lung Cancer 58:191–5.

Huang, G. W., W. N. Mo, G. Q. Kuang, H. T. Nong, M. Y. Wei, M. Sunagawa, and T. Kosugi (2001) Expression of p16, nm23-H1, E-cadherin, and CD44 gene products and their significance in nasopharyngeal carcinoma. Laryngoscope 111:1465–71.

Huang, Z. H., G. Q. Su, Q. G. Mao, Q. Z. Wang, Z. Li, J. L. Yu, and Y. F. Fan (2004) [Expressions of vascular endothelial growth factor and nm23-H1 gene and their relation to the prognosis of breast cancer in young women]. Di Yi Jun Yi Da Xue Xue Bao 24:1398–401.

Huang, C. S., M. K. Shih, C. H. Chuang, and M. L. Hu (2005) Lycopene inhibits cell migration and invasion and upregulates Nm23-H1 in a highly invasive hepatocarcinoma, SK-Hep-1 cells. J Nutr 135:2119–23.

Igawa, M., S. Urakami, H. Shiina, T. Ishibe, T. Usui, and G. W. Chodak (1996) Association of nm23 protein levels in human prostates with proliferating cell nuclear antigen expression at autopsy. Eur Urol 30:383–7.

Iizuka, N., M. Oka, T. Noma, A. Nakazawa, K. Hirose, and T. Suzuki (1995) NM23-H1 and NM23-H2 messenger RNA abundance in human hepatocellular carcinoma. Cancer Res 55: 652–7.

Iizuka, N., A. Tangoku, S. Hazama, S. Yoshino, N. Mori, and M. Oka (2001) Nm23-H1 gene as a molecular switch between the free-floating and adherent states of gastric cancer cells. Cancer Lett 174:65–71.

Indinnimeo, M., C. Cicchini, A. Stazi, E. Giarnieri, M. R. Limiti, C. Ghini, and A. Vecchione (1999) Correlation between nm23-H1 overexpression and clinicopathological variables in human anal canal carcinoma. Oncol Rep 6:1353–6.

Ismail, N. I., G. Kaur, H. Hashim, and M. S. Hassan (2008) Nuclear localization and intensity of staining of nm23 protein is useful marker for breast cancer progression. Cancer Cell Int 8:6.

Iwashita, S., M. Fujii, H. Mukai, Y. Ono, and M. Miyamoto (2004) Lbc proto-oncogene product binds to and could be negatively regulated by metastasis suppressor nm23-H2. Biochem Biophys Res Commun 320:1063–8.

Jung, S., Y. W. Paek, K. S. Moon, S. C. Wee, H. H. Ryu, Y. I. Jeong, H. S. Sun, Y. H. Jin, K. K. Kim, and K. Y. Ahn (2006) Expression of Nm23 in gliomas and its effect on migration and invasion in vitro. Anticancer Res 26:249–58.

Jung, H., H. A. Seong, and H. Ha (2007) NM23-H1 tumor suppressor and its interacting partner STRAP activate p53 function. J Biol Chem 282:35293–307.

Kaetzel, D. M., Q. Zhang, M. Yang, J. R. McCorkle, D. Ma, and R. J. Craven (2006) Potential roles of 3′–5′ exonuclease activity of NM23-H1 in DNA repair and malignant progression. J Bioenerg Biomembr 38:163–7.

Kanayama, H., H. Takigawa and S. Kagawa (1994) Analysis of nm23 gene expressions in human bladder and renal cancers. Int J Urol 1:324–31.

Kapitanovic, S., T. Cacev, M. Berkovic, M. Popovic-Hadzija, S. Radosevic, S. Seiwerth, S. Spaventi, K. Pavelic, and R. Spaventi (2004) nm23-H1 expression and loss of heterozygosity in colon adenocarcinoma. J Clin Pathol 57:1312–18.

Kauffman, E. C., V. L. Robinson, W. M. Stadler, M. H. Sokoloff, and C. W. Rinker-Schaeffer (2003) Metastasis suppression: the evolving role of metastasis suppressor genes for regulating cancer cell growth at the secondary site. J Urol 169:1122–33.

Kaul, R., S. C. Verma, M. Murakami, K. Lan, T. Choudhuri, and E. S. Robertson (2006) Epstein-Barr virus protein can upregulate cyclo-oxygenase-2 expression through association with the suppressor of metastasis Nm23-H1. J Virol 80:1321–31.

Kaul, R., M. Murakami, T. Choudhuri, and E. S. Robertson (2007) Epstein-Barr virus latent nuclear antigens can induce metastasis in a nude mouse model. J Virol 81:10352–61.

Kawakubo, Y., Y. Sato, T. Koh, H. Kono, and T. Kameya (1997) Expression of nm23 protein in pulmonary adenocarcinomas: inverse 1orrelation to tumor progression. Lung Cancer 17: 103–13.

Keim, D., N. Hailat, R. Melhem, X. X. Zhu, I. Lascu, M. Veron, J. Strahler, and S. M. Hanash (1992) Proliferation-related expression of p19/nm23 nucleoside diphosphate kinase. J Clin Invest 89:919–24.

Khan, M. H., M. Yasuda, F. Higashino, S. Haque, T. Kohgo, M. Nakamura, and M. Shindoh (2001) nm23-H1 suppresses invasion of oral squamous cell carcinoma-derived cell lines without modifying matrix metalloproteinase-2 and matrix metalloproteinase-9 expression. Am J Pathol 158:1785–91.

Kim, S. H. and J. Kim (2006) Reduction of invasion in human fibrosarcoma cells by ribosomal protein S3 in conjunction with Nm23-H1 and ERK. Biochim Biophys Acta 1763:823–32.

Kim, S. Y., J. E. Ferrell, Jr., S. K. Chae, and K. J. Lee (2000) Inhibition of progesterone-induced Xenopus oocyte maturation by Nm23. Cell Growth Differ 11:485–90.

Kim, Y. I., S. Park, D. I. Jeoung, and H. Lee (2003) Point mutations affecting the oligomeric structure of Nm23-H1 abrogates its inhibitory activity on colonization and invasion of prostate cancer cells. Biochem Biophys Res Commun 307:281–9.

Kimberly, M., andrew, King., Kevin, O'Neill., Apsara, Kandanearatchi., Krishanthi Liyanage., and Geoffrey, J Pilkington., (1998) Expression of the candidate invasion suppressor gene, nm23, in human brain tumors. Neuropathology 18:315–20.

Konishi, N., S. Nakaoka, T. Tsuzuki, K. Matsumoto, Y. Kitahori, Y. Hiasa, T. Urano, and H. Shiku (1993) Expression of nm23-H1 and nm23-H2 proteins in prostate carcinoma. Jpn J Cancer Res 84:1050–4.

Korabiowska, M., J. F. Honig, J. Jawien, J. Knapik, J. Stachura, C. Cordon-Cardo, and G. Fischer (2005) Relationship of nm23 expression to proliferation and prognosis in malignant melanomas of the oral cavity. In Vivo 19:1093–6.

Kowluru, A., M. Tannous, and H. Q. Chen (2002) Localization and characterization of the mitochondrial isoform of the nucleoside diphosphate kinase in the pancreatic beta cell: evidence for its complexation with mitochondrial succinyl-CoA synthetase. Arch Biochem Biophys 398:160–9.

Kraeft, S. K., F. Traincart, S. Mesnildrey, J. Bourdais, M. Veron, and L. B. Chen (1996) Nuclear localization of nucleoside diphosphate kinase type B (nm23-H2) in cultured cells. Exp Cell Res 227:63–9.

Kuppers, D. A., K. Lan, J. S. Knight, and E. S. Robertson (2005) Regulation of matrix metalloproteinase 9 expression by Epstein-Barr virus nuclear antigen 3C and the suppressor of metastasis Nm23-H1. J Virol 79:9714–24.

Lacombe, M. L., L. Milon, A. Munier, J. G. Mehus, and D. O. Lambeth (2000) The human Nm23/nucleoside diphosphate kinases. J Bioenerg Biomembr 32:247–58.

Lai, W. W., M. H. Wu, J. J. Yan, and F. F. Chen (1996) Immunohistochemical analysis of nm23-H1 in stage I non-small cell lung cancer: a useful marker in prediction of metastases. Ann Thorac Surg 62:1500–4.

Lascu, I., S. Schaertl, C. Wang, C. Sarger, A. Giartosio, G. Briand, M. L. Lacombe, and M. Konrad (1997) A point mutation of human nucleoside diphosphate kinase A found in aggressive neuroblastoma affects protein folding. J Biol Chem 272:15599–602.

Lee, C. S. and J. Gad (1998) nm23-H1 protein immunoreactivity in intraepithelial neoplasia and invasive squamous cell carcinoma of the uterine cervix. Pathol Int 48:806–11.

Lee, C. S. and A. Pirdas-Zivcic (1994) nm23-H1 protein immunoreactivity in cancers of the gallbladder, extrahepatic bile ducts and ampulla of Vater. Pathology 26:448–52.

Lee, H. Y. and H. Lee (1999) Inhibitory activity of nm23-H1 on invasion and colonization of human prostate carcinoma cells is not mediated by its NDP kinase activity. Cancer Lett 145:93–9.

Leone, A., U. Flatow, K. VanHoutte, and P. S. Steeg (1993a) Transfection of human nm23-H1 into the human MDA-MB-435 breast carcinoma cell line: effects on tumor metastatic potential, colonization and enzymatic activity. Oncogene 8:2325–33.

Leone, A., R. C. Seeger, C. M. Hong, Y. Y. Hu, M. J. Arboleda, G. M. Brodeur, D. Stram, D. J. Slamon, and P. S. Steeg (1993b) Evidence for nm23 RNA overexpression, DNA amplification and mutation in aggressive childhood neuroblastomas. Oncogene 8:855–65.

Leung, S. M. and L. E. Hightower (1997) A 16-kDa protein functions as a new regulatory protein for Hsc70 molecular chaperone and is identified as a member of the Nm23/nucleoside diphosphate kinase family. J Biol Chem 272:2607–14.

Lim, S., H. Y. Lee, and H. Lee (1998) Inhibition of colonization and cell-matrix adhesion after nm23-H1 transfection of human prostate carcinoma cells. Cancer Lett 133:143–9.

Lin, L. I., P. H. Lee, C. M. Wu, and J. K. Lin (1998) Significance of nm23 mRNA expression in human hepatocellular carcinoma. Anticancer Res 18:541–6.

Lin, K. H., Y. W. Lin, H. F. Lee, W. L. Liu, S. T. Chen, K. S. Chang, and S. Y. Cheng (1995) Increased invasive activity of human hepatocellular carcinoma cells is associated with an over-expression of thyroid hormone beta 1 nuclear receptor and low expression of the anti-metastatic nm23 gene. Cancer Lett 98:89–95.

Lin, K. H., H. Y. Shieh, and H. C. Hsu (2000) Negative regulation of the antimetastatic gene Nm23-H1 by thyroid hormone receptors. Endocrinology 141:2540–7.

Liu, F., H. L. Qi, and H. L. Chen (2000) Effects of all-trans retinoic acid and epidermal growth factor on the expression of nm23-H1 in human hepatocarcinoma cells. J Cancer Res Clin Oncol 126:85–90.

Liu, S. J., Y. M. Sun, D. F. Tian, Y. C. He, L. Zeng, Y. He, C. Q. Ling, and S. H. Sun (2008) Downregulated NM23-H1 expression is associated with intracranial invasion of nasopharyngeal carcinoma. Br J Cancer 98:363–9.

Iizuka, N., K. Miyamoto, A. Tangoku, H. Hayashi, S. Hazama, S. Yoshino, K. Yoshimura, K. Hirose, H. Yoshida, and M. Oka (2000) Downregulation of intracellular nm23-H1 prevents cisplatin-induced DNA damage in oesophageal cancer cells: possible association with Na(+), K(+)-ATPase. Br J Cancer 83:1209–15.

Lombardi, D (2006) Commentary: nm23, a metastasis suppressor gene with a tumor suppressor gene aptitude? J Bioenerg Biomembr 38:177–80.

Lombardi, D., E. Palescandolo, A. Giordano, and M. G. Paggi (2001) Interplay between the antimetastatic nm23 and the retinoblastoma-related Rb2/p130 genes in promoting neuronal differentiation of PC12 cells. Cell Death Differ 8:470–6.

Ma, D., G. P. Luyten, T. M. Luider, M. J. Jager, and J. Y. Niederkorn (1996) Association between NM23-H1 gene expression and metastasis of human uveal melanoma in an animal model. Invest Ophthalmol Vis Sci 37:2293–301.

Ma, D., Z. Xing, B. Liu, N. G. Pedigo, S. G. Zimmer, Z. Bai, E. H. Postel, and D. M. Kaetzel (2002) NM23-H1 and NM23-H2 repress transcriptional activities of nuclease-hypersensitive elements in the platelet-derived growth factor-A promoter. J Biol Chem 277:1560–7.

Ma, D., J. R. McCorkle, and D. M. Kaetzel (2004) The metastasis suppressor NM23-H1 possesses 3′–5′ exonuclease activity. J Biol Chem 279:18073–84.

MacDonald, N. J., J. M. Freije, M. L. Stracke, R. E. Manrow, and P. S. Steeg (1996) Site-directed mutagenesis of nm23-H1. Mutation of proline 96 or serine 120 abrogates its motility inhibitory activity upon transfection into human breast carcinoma cells. J Biol Chem 271:25107–16.

Mandai, M., I. Konishi, T. Komatsu, T. Mori, S. Arao, H. Nomura, Y. Kanda, H. Hiai, and M. Fukumoto (1995) Mutation of the nm23 gene, loss of heterozygosity at the nm23 locus and K-ras mutation in ovarian carcinoma: correlation with tumour progression and nm23 gene expression. Br J Cancer 72:691–5.

Marone, M., G. Scambia, G. Ferrandina, C. Giannitelli, P. Benedetti-Panici, S. Iacovella, A. Leone, and S. Mancuso (1996) Nm23 expression in endometrial and cervical cancer: inverse correlation with lymph node involvement and myometrial invasion. Br J Cancer 74:1063–8.

Martinez, J. A., S. Prevot, B. Nordlinger, T. M. Nguyen, Y. Lacarriere, A. Munier, I. Lascu, J. C. Vaillant, J. Capeau, and M. L. Lacombe (1995) Overexpression of nm23-H1 and nm23-H2 genes in colorectal carcinomas and loss of nm23-H1 expression in advanced tumour stages. Gut 37:712–20.

Mehus, J. G., P. Deloukas, and D. O. Lambeth (1999) NME6: a new member of the nm23/nucleoside diphosphate kinase gene family located on human chromosome 3p21.3. Hum Genet 104:454–9.

Mileo, A. M., E. Piombino, A. Severino, A. Tritarelli, M. G. Paggi, and D. Lombardi (2006) Multiple interference of the human papillomavirus-16 E7 oncoprotein with the functional role of the metastasis suppressor Nm23-H1 protein. J Bioenerg Biomembr 38:215–25.

Milon, L., M. F. Rousseau-Merck, A. Munier, M. Erent, I. Lascu, J. Capeau, and M. L. Lacombe (1997) nm23-H4, a new member of the family of human nm23/nucleoside diphosphate kinase genes localised on chromosome 16p13. Hum Genet 99:550–7.

Milon, L., P. Meyer, M. Chiadmi, A. Munier, M. Johansson, A. Karlsson, I. Lascu, J. Capeau, J. Janin, and M. L. Lacombe (2000) The human nm23-H4 gene product is a mitochondrial nucleoside diphosphate kinase. J Biol Chem 275:14264–72.

Morimura, Y., K. Yanagida, T. Hashimoto, Y. Takano, F. Watanabe, H. Yamada, and A. Sato (1998) Evaluation of immunostaining for MIB1 and nm23 products in uterine cervical adenocarcinoma. Tohoku J Exp Med 185:185–97.

Muller, W., A. Schneiders, G. Hommel, and H. E. Gabbert (1998) Expression of nm23 in gastric carcinoma: association with tumor progression and poor prognosis. Cancer 83:2481–7.

Munier, A., C. Feral, L. Milon, V. P. Pinon, G. Gyapay, J. Capeau, G. Guellaen, and M. L. Lacombe (1998) A new human nm23 homologue (nm23-H5) specifically expressed in testis germinal cells. FEBS Lett 434:289–94.

Murakami, M., K. Lan, C. Subramanian, and E. S. Robertson (2005) Epstein-Barr virus nuclear antigen 1 interacts with Nm23-H1 in lymphoblastoid cell lines and inhibits its ability to suppress cell migration. J Virol 79:1559–68.

Murakami, M., P. I. Meneses,.J. S. Knight, K. Lan, R. Kaul, S. C. Verma, and E. S. Robertson (2008a) Nm23-H1 modulates the activity of the guanine exchange factor Dbl-1. Int J Cancer 123(3):500–10.

Murakami M., P. I. Meneses, K. Lan, and E. S. Robertson (2008b) The suppressor of metastasis Nm23-H1 interacts with the Cdc42 Rho family member and the pleckstrin homology domain of oncoprotein Dbl-1 to suppress cell migration. Cancer Biol Therapy 7(5):677–88.

Nakamori, S., O. Ishikawa, H. Ohhigashi, M. Kameyama, H. Furukawa, Y. Sasaki, H. Inaji, M. Higashiyama, S. Imaoka, T. Iwanaga, and et al. (1993) Expression of nucleoside diphosphate kinase/nm23 gene product in human pancreatic cancer: an association with lymph node metastasis and tumor invasion. Clin Exp Metastasis 11:151–8.

Nakayama, H., W. Yasui, H. Yokozaki, and E. Tahara (1993) Reduced expression of nm23 is associated with metastasis of human gastric carcinomas. Jpn J Cancer Res 84:184–90.

Nanashima, A., H. Yano, H. Yamaguchi, K. Tanaka, S. Shibasaki, Y. Sumida, T. Sawai, H. Shindou, and T. Nakagoe (2004) Immunohistochemical analysis of tumor biological factors in hepatocellular carcinoma: relationship to clinicopathological factors and prognosis after hepatic resection. J Gastroenterol 39:148–54.

Nasser, J. A., A. Falavigna, F. Ferraz, G. Duigou, and J. Bruce (2006) Transcription analysis of TIMP-1 and NM23-H1 genes in glioma cell invasion. Arq Neuropsiquiatr 64:774–80.

Natarajan, K., N. Mori, D. Artemov, and Z. M. Bhujwalla (2002) Exposure of human breast cancer cells to the anti-inflammatory agent indomethacin alters choline phospholipid metabolites and Nm23 expression. Neoplasia 4:409–16.

Nawashiro, H., Y. Ozeki, K. Takishima, K. Shima, and H. Chigasaki (1996) Immunohistochemical analysis of the nm23 gene product (NDP kinase) expression in astrocytic neoplasms. Acta Neurochir (Wien) 138:445–50.

Negroni, A., D. Venturelli, B. Tanno, R. Amendola, S. Ransac, V. Cesi, B. Calabretta, and G. Raschella (2000) Neuroblastoma specific effects of DR-nm23 and its mutant forms on differentiation and apoptosis. Cell Death Differ 7:843–50.

Nesi, G., D. Palli, L. M. Pernice, C. Saieva, M. Paglierani, K. C. Kroning, S. Catarzi, C. A. Rubio, and A. Amorosi (2001) Expression of nm23 gene in gastric cancer is associated with a poor 5-year survival. Anticancer Res 21:3643–9.

Nicolson, G. L (1988) Cancer metastasis: tumor cell and host organ properties important in metastasis to specific secondary sites. Biochim Biophys Acta 948:175–224.

Nie, Q., Q. H. Zhou, W. Zhu, L. X. Liu, J. K. Fu, D. B. Li, Y. Li, and G. W. Che (2006) [nm23-H1 gene inhibits lung cancer cell invasion through down-regulation of PKC signal pathway]. Zhonghua Zhong Liu Za Zhi 28:334–6.

Niitsu, N., J. Okabe-Kado, T. Kasukabe, Y. Yamamoto-Yamaguchi, M. Umeda, and Y. Honma (1999) Prognostic implications of the differentiation inhibitory factor nm23-H1 protein in the plasma of aggressive non-Hodgkin's lymphoma. Blood 94:3541–50.

Niitsu, N., J. Okabe-Kado, M. Okamoto, T. Takagi, T. Yoshida, S. Aoki, M. Hirano, and Y. Honma
   (2001) Serum nm23-H1 protein as a prognostic factor in aggressive non-Hodgkin lymphoma.
   Blood 97:1202–10.
Nosaka, K., M. Kawahara, M. Masuda, Y. Satomi, and H. Nishino (1998) Association of nucleoside
   diphosphate kinase nm23-H2 with human telomeres. Biochem Biophys Res Commun 243:
   342–8.
Ohba, K., Y. Miyata, S. Koga, S. Kanda, and H. Kanetake (2005) Expression of nm23-H1 gene
   product in sarcomatous cancer cells of renal cell carcinoma: correlation with tumor stage and
   expression of matrix metalloproteinase-2, matrix metalloproteinase-9, sialyl Lewis X, and c-
   erbB-2. Urology 65:1029–34.
Ohta, Y., H. Nozawa, H. Tanaka, M. Oda, and Y. Watanabe (2000) Increased vascular endothelial
   growth factor and vascular endothelial growth factor-c and decreased nm23 expression associ-
   ated with microdissemination in the lymph nodes in stage I non-small cell lung cancer. J Thorac
   Cardiovasc Surg 119:804–13.
Okabe-Kado, J. and T. Kasukabe (2003) Physiological and pathological relevance of extracellular
   NM23/NDP kinases. J Bioenerg Biomembr 35:89–93.
Okabe-Kado, J.,T. Kasukabe, H. Baba, T. Urano, H. Shiku, and Y. Honma (1995a) Inhibitory action
   of nm23 proteins on induction of erythroid differentiation of human leukemia cells. Biochim
   Biophys Acta 1267:101–6.
Okabe-Kado, J., T. Kasukabe, M. Hozumi, Y. Honma, N. Kimura, H. Baba, T. Urano, and H. Shiku
   (1995a) A new function of Nm23/NDP kinase as a differentiation inhibitory factor, which does
   not require it's kinase activity. FEBS Lett 363:311–15.
Okabe-Kado, J., T. Kasukabe, and Y. Honma (2002) Expression of cell surface NM23 proteins
   of human leukemia cell lines of various cellular lineage and differentiation stages. Leuk Res
   26:569–76.
Okada, K., T. Urano, H. Baba, K. Furukawa, and H. Shiku (1996) Independent and differential
   expression of two isotypes of human Nm23: analysis of the promoter regions of the nm23-H1
   and H2 genes. Oncogene 13:1937–43.
Otero, A. S., M. B. Doyle, M. T. Hartsough, and P. S. Steeg (1999) Wild-type NM23-H1, but not its
   S120 mutants, suppresses desensitization of muscarinic potassium current. Biochim Biophys
   Acta 1449:157–68.
Ouatas, T., S. E. Clare, M. T. Hartsough, A. De La Rosa, and P. S. Steeg (2002) MMTV-associated
   transcription factor binding sites increase nm23-H1 metastasis suppressor gene expression in
   human breast carcinoma cell lines. Clin Exp Metastasis 19:35–42.
Ouatas, T.,D. Halverson, and P. S. Steeg (2003a) Dexamethasone and medroxyprogesterone acetate
   elevate Nm23-H1 metastasis suppressor gene expression in metastatic human breast carcinoma
   cells: new uses for old compounds. Clin Cancer Res 9:3763–72.
Ouatas, T., M. Salerno, D. Palmieri, and P. S. Steeg (2003b) Basic and translational advances in
   cancer metastasis: Nm23. J Bioenerg Biomembr 35:73–9.
Padma, P., A. Hozumi, K. Ogawa, and K. Inaba (2001) Molecular cloning and characterization of a
   thioredoxin/nucleoside diphosphate kinase related dynein intermediate chain from the ascidian,
   Ciona intestinalis. Gene 275:177–83.
Palacios, F., J. K. Schweitzer, R. L. Boshans, and C. D'Souza-Schorey (2002) ARF6-GTP recruits
   Nm23-H1 to facilitate dynamin-mediated endocytosis during adherens junctions disassembly.
   Nat Cell Biol 4:929–36.
Palmieri, D., D. O. Halverson, T. Ouatas, C. E. Horak, M. Salerno, J. Johnson, W. D. Figg,
   M. Hollingshead, S. Hursting, D. Berrigan, S. M. Steinberg, M. J. Merino, and P. S. Steeg
   (2005) Medroxyprogesterone acetate elevation of Nm23-H1 metastasis suppressor expression
   in hormone receptor-negative breast cancer. J Natl Cancer Inst 97:632–42.
Parhar, R. S., Y. Shi, M. Zou, N. R. Farid, P. Ernst, and S. T. al-Sedairy (1995) Effects of cytokine-
   mediated modulation of nm23 expression on the invasion and metastatic behavior of B16F10
   melanoma cells. Int J Cancer 60:204–10.
Pinon, V. P., G. Millot, A. Munier, J. Vassy, G. Linares-Cruz, J. Capeau, F. Calvo, and M. L.
   Lacombe (1999) Cytoskeletal association of the A and B nucleoside diphosphate kinases of

interphasic but not mitotic human carcinoma cell lines: specific nuclear localization of the B subunit. Exp Cell Res 246:355–67.

Postel, E. H., S. J. Berberich, S. J. Flint, and C. A. Ferrone (1993) Human c-myc transcription factor PuF identified as nm23-H2 nucleoside diphosphate kinase, a candidate suppressor of tumor metastasis. Science 261:478–80.

Postel, E. H., S. J. Berberich, J. W. Rooney, and D. M. Kaetzel (2000) Human NM23/nucleoside diphosphate kinase regulates gene expression through DNA binding to nuclease-hypersensitive transcriptional elements. J Bioenerg Biomembr 32:277–84.

Prowatke, I., F. Devens, A. Benner, E. F. Grone, D. Mertens, H. J. Grone, P. Lichter, and S. Joos (2007) Expression analysis of imbalanced genes in prostate carcinoma using tissue microarrays. Br J Cancer 96:82–8.

Rahman-Roblick, R., U. J. Roblick, U. Hellman, P. Conrotto, T. Liu, S. Becker, D. Hirschberg, H. Jornvall, G. Auer, and K. G. Wiman (2007) p53 targets identified by protein expression profiling. Proc Natl Acad Sci U S A 104:5401–6.

Reymond, A., S. Volorio, G. Merla, M. Al-Maghtheh, O. Zuffardi, A. Bulfone, A. Ballabio, and M. Zollo (1999) Evidence for interaction between human PRUNE and nm23-H1 NDPKinase. Oncogene 18:7244–52.

Roymans, D., R. Willems, K. Vissenberg, C. De Jonghe, B. Grobben, P. Claes, I. Lascu, D. Van Bockstaele, J. P. Verbelen, C. Van Broeckhoven, and H. Slegers (2000) Nucleoside diphosphate kinase beta (Nm23-R1/NDPKbeta) is associated with intermediate filaments and becomes upregulated upon cAMP-induced differentiation of rat C6 glioma. Exp Cell Res 261:127–38.

Roymans, D., K. Vissenberg, C. De Jonghe, R. Willems, G. Engler, N. Kimura, B. Grobben, P. Claes, J. P. Verbelen, C. Van Broeckhoven, and H. Slegers (2001) Identification of the tumor metastasis suppressor Nm23-H1/Nm23-R1 as a constituent of the centrosome. Exp Cell Res 262:145–53.

Russell, R. L., K. R. Geisinger, R. R. Mehta, W. L. White, B. Shelton, and T. E. Kute (1997) nm23–relationship to the metastatic potential of breast carcinoma cell lines, primary human xenografts, and lymph node negative breast carcinoma patients. Cancer 79:1158–65.

Salerno, M., D. Palmieri, A. Bouadis, D. Halverson, and P. S. Steeg (2005) Nm23-H1 metastasis suppressor expression level influences the binding properties, stability, and function of the kinase suppressor of Ras1 (KSR1) Erk scaffold in breast carcinoma cells. Mol Cell Biol 25:1379–88.

Sarin, A., M. S. Williams, M. A. Alexander-Miller, J. A. Berzofsky, C. M. Zacharchuk, and P. A. Henkart (1997) Target cell lysis by CTL granule exocytosis is independent of ICE/Ced-3 family proteases. Immunity 6:209–15.

Sastre-Garau, X., L. Ovtracht, I. Lascu, M. L. Lacombe, M. Veron, K. Bourdache, and J. P. Thiery (1992) [Ultrastructural immunocytochemical localization of diphosphate kinase/Nm23 in human cancer cells]. Bull Cancer 79:465–70.

Schuhmacher, M., F. Kohlhuber, M. Holzel, C. Kaiser, H. Burtscher, M. Jarsch, G. W. Bornkamm, G. Laux, A. Polack, U. H. Weidle, and D. Eick (2001) The transcriptional program of a human B cell line in response to Myc. Nucleic Acids Res 29:397–406.

Seifert, M., T. Seib, M. Engel, S. Dooley, and C. Welter (1995) Characterization of the human nm23-H2 promoter region and localization of the microsatellite D17S396. Biochem Biophys Res Commun 215:910–14.

Seifert, M., B. Theisinger, M. Engel, T. Seib, G. Seitz, M. Stolte, K. Hilgert, and C. Welter (1997) Isolation and characterization of new microsatellites at the nm23-H1 and nm23-H2 gene loci and application for loss of heterozygosity (LOH) analysis. Hum Genet 100:515–19.

Seifert, M., C. Welter, Y. Mehraein, and G. Seitz (2005) Expression of the nm23 homologues nm23-H4, nm23-H6, and nm23-H7 in human gastric and colon cancer. J Pathol 205:623–32.

Seong, H. A., H. Jung, and H. Ha (2007) NM23-H1 tumor suppressor physically interacts with serine-threonine kinase receptor-associated protein, a transforming growth factor-beta (TGF-beta) receptor-interacting protein, and negatively regulates TGF-beta signaling. J Biol Chem 282:12075–96.

Seraj, M. J., M. A. Harding, J. J. Gildea, D. R. Welch, and D. Theodorescu (2000) The relationship of BRMS1 and RhoGDI2 gene expression to metastatic potential in lineage related human bladder cancer cell lines. Clin Exp Metastasis 18:519–25.

Shimada, M., K. Taguchi, H. Hasegawa, T. Gion, K. Shirabe, M. Tsuneyoshi, and K. Sugimachi (1998) Nm23-H1 expression in intrahepatic or extrahepatic metastases of hepatocellular carcinoma. Liver 18:337–42.

Shresta, S., T. A. Graubert, D. A. Thomas, S. Z. Raptis, and T. J. Ley (1999) Granzyme A initiates an alternative pathway for granule-mediated apoptosis. Immunity 10:595–605.

Simpson, R. U., T. Hsu, D. A. Begley, B. S. Mitchell, and B. N. Alizadeh. (1987) Transcriptional regulation of the c-myc protooncogene by 1,25-dihydroxyvitamin D3 in HL-60 promyelocytic leukemia cells. J Biol Chem 262:4104–8.

Sonnemann, J. and R. Mutzel (1995) Cytosolic nucleoside diphosphate kinase associated with the translation apparatus may provide GTP for protein synthesis. Biochem Biophys Res Commun 209:490–6.

Stahl, J. A., A. Leone, A. M. Rosengard, L. Porter, C. R. King, and P. S. Steeg (1991) Identification of a second human nm23 gene, nm23-H2. Cancer Res 51:445–9.

Steeg, P. S., G. Bevilacqua, L. Kopper, U. P. Thorgeirsson, J. E. Talmadge, L. A. Liotta, and M. E. Sobel. (1988) Evidence for a novel gene associated with low tumor metastatic potential. J Natl Cancer Inst 80:200–4.

Steeg, P. S., A. de la Rosa, U. Flatow, N. J. MacDonald, M. Benedict, and A. Leone (1993) Nm23 and breast cancer metastasis. Breast Cancer Res Treat 25:175–87.

Steeg, P. S., T. Ouatas, D. Halverson, D. Palmieri, and M. Salerno (2003) Metastasis suppressor genes: basic biology and potential clinical use. Clin Breast Cancer 4:51–62.

Subramanian, C. and E. S. Robertson (2002) The metastatic suppressor Nm23-H1 interacts with EBNA3C at sequences located between the glutamine- and proline-rich domains and can cooperate in activation of transcription. J Virol 76:8702–9.

Subramanian, C., M. A. Cotter, 2nd, and E. S. Robertson (2001) Epstein-Barr virus nuclear protein EBNA-3C interacts with the human metastatic suppressor Nm23-H1: a molecular link to cancer metastasis. Nat Med 7:350–5.

Suzuki, E., T. Ota, K. Tsukuda, A. Okita, K. Matsuoka, M. Murakami, H. Doihara, and N. Shimizu (2004) nm23-H1 reduces in vitro cell migration and the liver metastatic potential of colon cancer cells by regulating myosin light chain phosphorylation. Int J Cancer 108:207–11.

Tee, Y. T., G. D. Chen, L. Y. Lin, J. L. Ko, and P. H. Wang (2006) Nm23-H1: a metastasis-associated gene. Taiwan J Obstet Gynecol 45:107–13.

Tomita, M., T. Ayabe, Y. Matsuzaki, M. Edagawa, M. Maeda, T. Shimizu, M. Hara, and T. Onitsuka (2001a) Expression of nm23-H1 gene product in esophageal squamous cell carcinoma and its association with vessel invasion and survival. BMC Cancer 1:3.

Tomita, M., T. Ayabe, Y. Matsuzaki, and T. Onitsuka (2001b) Expression of nm23-H1 gene product in mediastinal lymph nodes from lung cancer patients. Eur J Cardiothorac Surg 19: 904–7.

Tommasi, S., V. Fedele, A. Crapolicchio, A. Bellizzi, A. Paradiso, and S. J. Reshkin (2003) ErbB2 and the antimetastatic nm23/NDP kinase in regulating serum induced breast cancer invasion. Int J Mol Med 12:131–4.

Tseng, Y. H., D. Vicent, J. Zhu, Y. Niu, A. Adeyinka, J. S. Moyers, P. H. Watson, and C. R. Kahn (2001) Regulation of growth and tumorigenicity of breast cancer cells by the low molecular weight GTPase Rad and nm23. Cancer Res 61:2071–9.

Tsuiki, H., M. Nitta, A. Furuya, N. Hanai, T. Fujiwara, M. Inagaki, M. Kochi, Y. Ushio, H. Saya, and H. Nakamura (1999) A novel human nucleoside diphosphate (NDP) kinase, Nm23-H6, localizes in mitochondria and affects cytokinesis. J Cell Biochem 76:254–69.

Urano, T., K. Furukawa, and H. Shiku (1993) Expression of nm23/NDP kinase proteins on the cell surface. Oncogene 8:1371–6.

Valentijn, L. J., J. Koster, and R. Versteeg (2006) Read-through transcript from NM23-H1 into the neighboring NM23-H2 gene encodes a novel protein, NM23-LV. Genomics 87:483–9.

Varesco, L., M. A. Caligo, P. Simi, D. M. Black, V. Nardini, L. Casarino, M. Rocchi, G. Ferrara, E. Solomon, and G. Bevilacqua (1992) The NM23 gene maps to human chromosome band 17q22 and shows a restriction fragment length polymorphism with BglII. Genes Chromosomes Cancer 4:84–8.

Venturelli, D., R. Martinez, P. Melotti, I. Casella, C. Peschle, C. Cucco, G. Spampinato, Z. Darzynkiewicz, and B. Calabretta (1995) Overexpression of DR-nm23, a protein encoded by a member of the nm23 gene family, inhibits granulocyte differentiation and induces apoptosis in 32Dc13 myeloid cells. Proc Natl Acad Sci U S A 92:7435–9.

Venturelli, D., V. Cesi, S. Ransac, A. Engelhard, D. Perrotti, and B. Calabretta (2000) The nucleoside diphosphate kinase activity of DRnm23 is not required for inhibition of differentiation and induction of apoptosis in 32Dc13 myeloid precursor cells. Exp Cell Res 257:265–71.

Wagner, P. D. and N. D. Vu (2000) Histidine to aspartate phosphotransferase activity of nm23 proteins: phosphorylation of aldolase C on Asp-319. Biochem J 346 Pt 3:623–30.

Wagner, P. D. and N. D. Vu (2000) Phosphorylation of geranyl and farnesyl pyrophosphates by Nm23 proteins/nucleoside diphosphate kinases. J Biol Chem 275:35570–6.

Wagner, P. D., P. S. Steeg, and N. D. Vu (1997) Two-component kinase-like activity of nm23 correlates with its motility-suppressing activity. Proc Natl Acad Sci U S A 94:9000–5.

Wallet, V., R. Mutzel, H. Troll, O. Barzu, M. Wurster, M. Veron, and M. L. Lacombe (1990) Dictyostelium nucleoside diphosphate kinase highly homologous to Nm23 and Awd proteins involved in mammalian tumor metastasis and Drosophila development. J Natl Cancer Inst 82:1199–202.

Wang, Q., M. Guo, and L.Sun.(1996)[Study on expression of nm23-H1 gene in laryngeal cancer tissues]. Zhonghua Er Bi Yan Hou Ke Za Zhi 31:198–200.

Wang, G., C. Du, and Q. Lin (1997a) [The correlation between lung cancer lymph node metastasis and nm23-H1 gene mutation, mRNA expression]. Zhonghua Jie He He Hu Xi Za Zhi 20:340–3.

Wang, S. W., H. F. Yam, L. Yang, H. K. Ng, S. L. Wang, B. Q. Wu, Z. H. Wang, S. B. Chew-Cheng, and E. C. Chew (1997b) Expression of nm23-H1 in human meningioma cells. Anticancer Res 17:3569–73.

Wang, P. H., H. Chang, J. L. Ko, and L. Y. Lin (2003a) Nm23-H1 immunohistochemical expression in multisteps of cervical carcinogenesis. Int J Gynecol Cancer 13:325–30.

Wang, P. H., J. L. Ko, H. Chang, and L. Y. Lin (2003b) Clinical significance of high nm23-H1 expression in intraepithelial neoplasia and early-stage squamous cell carcinoma of the uterine cervix. Gynecol Obstet Invest 55:14–19.

Wang, Y. F., K. C. Chow, S. Y. Chang, J. H. Chiu, S. K. Tai, W. Y. Li, and L. S. Wang (2004) Prognostic significance of nm23-H1 expression in oral squamous cell carcinoma. Br J Cancer 90:2186–93.

Wang, Y. F., J. Y. Chen, S. Y. Chang, J. H. Chiu, W. Y. Li, P. Y. Chu, S. K. Tai, and L. S. Wang (2008) Nm23-H1 expression of metastatic tumors in the lymph nodes is a prognostic indicator of oral squamous cell carcinoma. Int J Cancer 122:377–86.

Webb, P. A., O. Perisic, C. E. Mendola, J. M. Backer, and R. L. Williams (1995) The crystal structure of a human nucleoside diphosphate kinase, NM23-H2. J Mol Biol 251:574–87.

Willems, R., D. R. Van Bockstaele, F. Lardon, M. Lenjou, G. Nijs, H. W. Snoeck, Z. N. Berneman, and H. Slegers (1998) Decrease in nucleoside diphosphate kinase (NDPK/nm23) expression during hematopoietic maturation. J Biol Chem 273:13663–8.

Willems, R., H. Slegers, I. Rodrigus, A. C. Moulijn, M. Lenjou, G. Nijs, Z. N. Berneman, and D. R. Van Bockstaele (2002) Extracellular nucleoside diphosphate kinase NM23/NDPK modulates normal hematopoietic differentiation. Exp Hematol 30:640–8.

Xu, W., J. Bai, and D. Yang (1995) [Correlation study of allelic gene deletion of nm23-H1 and human colorectal carcinoma metastasis]. Zhonghua Zhong Liu Za Zhi 17:263–5.

Xu, J., L. Z. Liu, X. F. Deng, L. Timmons, E. Hersperger, P. S. Steeg, M. Veron, and A. Shearn (1996) The enzymatic activity of Drosophila AWD/NDP kinase is necessary but not sufficient for its biological function. Dev Biol 177:544–57.

Yague, J., M. Juan, A. Leone, M. Romero, A. Cardesa, J. Vives, P. S. Steeg, and E. Campo (1991)

BglII and EcoRI polymorphism of the human nm23-H1 gene (NME1). Nucleic Acids Res 19:6663.

Yalcinkaya, U., S. Ozuysal, T. Bilgin, I. Ercan, O. Saraydaroglu, and D. Demir (2006) Nm23 expression in node-positive and node-negative endometrial cancer. Int J Gynaecol Obstet 95:35–9.

Yamashiro, S., T. Urano, H. Shiku, and K. Furukawa (1994) Alteration of nm23 gene expression during the induced differentiation of human leukemia cell lines. Oncogene 9:2461–8.

Yang, T. H. and M. L. Hu (2006) Intracellular levels of S-adenosylhomocysteine but not homocysteine are highly correlated to the expression of nm23-H1 and the level of 5-methyldeoxycytidine in human hepatoma cells with different invasion activities. Nutr Cancer 55:224–31.

Yang, Z., Y. Wen, and P. Pu (2003) [The regulation of nm23-H1/NDPK-A in different processes of regional lymph node metastases of oral squamous cell carcinomas]. Hua Xi Kou Qiang Yi Xue Za Zhi 21:263–6.

Ye, Y., Y. Yu, D. Wan, Z. Tang, J. Lu, and L. He (1998) [The relationship between nm23-H1 loss of heterozygosity and metastasis in hepatocellular carcinoma]. Zhonghua Wai Ke Za Zhi 36:161–3.

Yeung, P., C. S. Lee, P. Marr, M. Sarris, and D. Fenton-Lee (1998) Nm23 gene expression in gastric carcinoma: an immunohistochemical study. Aust N Z J Surg 68:180–2.

Yi, S., H. Guangqi, and H. Guoli (2003) The association of the expression of MTA1, nm23H1 with the invasion, metastasis of ovarian carcinoma. Chin Med Sci J 18:87–92.

Yoon, J. H., P. Singh, D. H. Lee, J. Qiu, S. Cai, T. R. O'Connor, Y. Chen, B. Shen, and G. P. Pfeifer (2005) Characterization of the 3′ –> 5′ exonuclease activity found in human nucleoside diphosphate kinase 1 (NDK1) and several of its homologues. Biochemistry 44:15774–86.

Youn, B. S.,D. S. Kim, J. W. Kim, Y. T. Kim, S. Kang, and N. H. Cho (2008) NM23 as a prognostic biomarker in ovarian serous carcinoma. Mod Pathol 21(7):885-92.

Zafon, C., G. Obiols, J. Castellvi, N. Tallada, P. Galofre, E. Gemar, J. Mesa, and R. Simo (2001) nm23-H1 immunoreactivity as a prognostic factor in differentiated thyroid carcinoma. J Clin Endocrinol Metab 86:3975–80.

Zhou, Q., X. Yang, D. Zhu, L. Ma, W. Zhu, Z. Sun, and Q. Yang (2007) Double mutant P96S/S120G of Nm23-H1 abrogates its NDPK activity and motility-suppressive ability. Biochem Biophys Res Commun 356:348–53.

Chapter 12
HGF/c-MET Signaling in Advanced Cancers

Mandira Ray, JG Garcia, and Ravi Salgia

Cast of Characters

Papillary renal carcinoma (RCCP) is histologically and genetically distinct from other forms of inherited renal carcinoma (e.g., von Hippel–Lindau disease, which is caused by inactivation of the VHL gene – see Chapter 6). RCCP genes map to several loci; one of each on 7q31.1-q34 encodes the c-Met oncoprotein (Schmidt et al. 1997). In the original publication, missense mutations in the tyrosine kinase domain of the MET gene were found both in the germlines of affected patients and in a subset of sporadic papillary renal carcinomas. Additionally, tumors from RCCP patients commonly show trisomy of chromosome 7 harboring non-random duplication of the mutant MET allele (Zhuang et al. 1998). Since its initial discovery, the MET gene has been found to have an important role in a wide variety of malignancies, including lung cancer, head and neck cancers, and gastric cancers. The following chapter focuses on the role of c-Met receptor and its cognate ligand HGF in advanced stages of cancer progression.

Introduction

As a unique member of RTKs, c-MET and its ligand hepatocyte growth factor, also known as scatter factor (HGF/SF), are pivotal for normal development, tissue regeneration, angiogenesis, growth, and cell motility/migration. c-MET overexpression, amplification, or mutations in the tyrosine kinase domain, juxtamembrane domain, and semaphorin domain alter the normal biological function leading to deregulated or prolonged tyrosine kinase activity. Moreover, the disruptions of the cytoskeleton promote an invasive phenotype in c-MET-activated malignant cells. Herein, the structure and biological function of the c-Met pathway will be highlighted. Alternations in this pathway that allow for tumor growth in a variety of malignancies including lung cancer will be discussed. By inhibiting the MET pathway and

R. Salgia (✉)
Department of Medicine, University of Chicago, 5841 South Maryland Ave, Chicago, IL, USA
e-mail: rsalgia@medicine.bsd.uchicago.edu

A. Thomas-Tikhonenko (ed.), *Cancer Genome and Tumor Microenvironment*,
DOI 10.1007/978-1-4419-0711-0_12, © Springer Science+Business Media, LLC 2010

downstream signaling in these cells and also affecting angiogenesis, targeted therapies to prevent tumor growth and invasion can be developed to be used alone or in combination with standard therapies. A brief overview of potential therapies in pre-clinical and clinical studies will be given at the end of the chapter.

MET Structure

As a prototypic member of a sub-family of RTKs which also include Ron and Sea, MET receptor tyrosine kinase is a high-affinity α-β heterodimeric receptor for hepatocyte growth factor/scatter factor (HGF/SF), which is produced by mesenchymal and epithelial cells to stimulate mobility (or scatter) (Jeffers et al. 1996). Historically, MET was first described as an in vitro-activated oncogene after human osteogenic sarcoma (HOS) line was treated with the chemical carcinogen N-methyl-N′-nitro-N-nitrosoguanidine (Cooper et al. 1984). The MET gene is 120 kb in length, is on chromosome 7 band 7q21-q31, and consists of 21 exons that are separated by 20 introns (Liu 1998). MET transcription yields a 150 kDa polypeptide which is initially partially glycosylated to produce a 170 kDa precursor protein. This precursor molecule is additionally glycosylated and then cleaved into a 50 kDa α chain and a 140 kDa β-chain, linked by disulfide bonds (Liu 1998). The MET β-chain contains structural components such as a semaphorin (Sema) domain, a PSI domain (found within plexins, semaphorins, and integrins), four IPT repeats (found within immunoglobulins, plexins and transcription factors), a transmembrane domain, a juxtamembrane (JM) domain, a tyrosine kinase (TK) domain, and a carboxy-terminal tail region (Sattler and Salgia 2007) (Fig. 12.1). Together, MET and HGF are crucial for normal development, and disruption of their regulation is implicated in cancer growth (Bottaro et al. 1991).

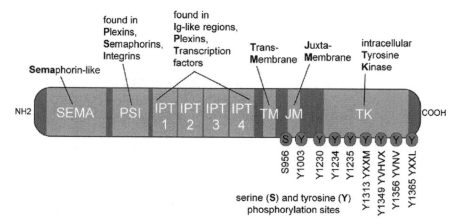

Fig. 12.1 Domain structure of the β-chain of the c-Met receptor

HGF Structure

The ligand for MET is hepatocyte growth factor (HGF). Originally discovered as a potent mitogen for hepatocytes, HGF is disulfide-linked heterodimer composed of 62 kDa α-subunit (heavy) consisting of a 27 amino acid N-terminal hairpin domain followed by four canonical kringle domains. These domains, which are important for protein–protein interactions, are 80 amino acid double-looped structures stabilized by 3 internal disulfide bridges (Comoglio 1993; Maulik et al. 2002b). The high-affinity binding domain for MET is found within the first kringle domain. HGF is kept near the vicinity of target cells by the low-affinity interaction between the hairpin loop and the second domain binding sites for heparin sulfate proteoglycans(Maulik et al. 2002b). HGF is a plasminogen-related growth factor, and the gene encoding HGF is about 70 kb on chromosome 7q21.1 with 18 exons and 17 introns (Seki et al. 1991). HGF contains six domains and binds to this sema domain which is located in the cystein-rich Met-related sequence (MRS) (Maulik et al. 2002b; Gherardi et al. 2006). The sema domain is a 500 amino acid extracellular domain that is found in all semaphorins. Semaphorins are proteins that control cell dissociation and repulsive events, similar to those seen during neural development (Tamagnone and Comoglio 2000).

Biological Activity of the MET Pathway

When bound by HGF, specific tyrosine residues within the intracellular MET region are autophosphorylated. Specifically, Tyr1234 and Tyr1235 residing in the activation group of the tyrosine kinase domain activated MET. The tyrosine phosphorylation results in activation of adaptor proteins (Grb2, Shc, c-Cbl) and signal transducers (PI-3-Kinase, STATs, ERK1 and 2, and FAK) similar to other RTKs; however, signaling dependent on MET differs because there is a distinct multisubstrate docking site at the C-terminal region of the receptor and utilization of a unique adaptor protein called Gab1 (Fig. 12.2) (Christensen et al. 2005). Phosphorylation of Tyr1349 and Tyr1356 within the C-terminus activates this multisubstrate docking site which thought to be crucial in MET-mediated mechanisms (Furge et al. 2000). Interestingly, Gab1 is necessary for a cell growth, differentiation, tissue maintenance, and repair in the majority of MET-dependent pathways (Gu and Neel 2003). This increased cellular proliferation and motility in tumor cells can lead to metastasis.

The MET pathway is integral for the development of cytoskeleton, a network of proteins located in the cytoplasm of eukaryotic cells that are crucial for cell structure, durability, growth, motility, and proliferation (Maulik et al. 2002b). A major component of cytoskeleton is actin filaments, which are bound to each other and to the cell via numerous accessory proteins such as integrins, focal adhesion proteins FAK and paxillin, GTP-binding proteins, Crk and CRKL adaptor proteins, and non-receptor kinases such as PI3-K and cadherin/catenin complexes (Maulik et al. 2002b).

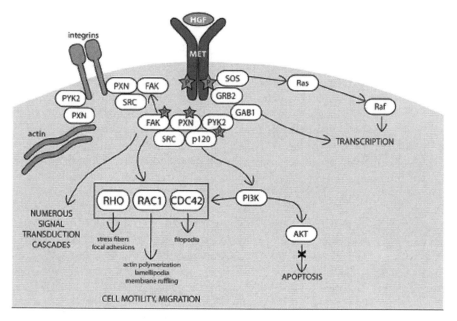

Fig. 12.2 Signaling pathways downstream of c-Met receptor.

Defined as cell surface heterodimeric receptors, integrins bind to the extracellular matrix and affect cell anchorage and adhesion, thereby controlling cell motility and potential invasion (Hynes 1992). In certain cell populations, MET signaling utilizes the PI3-K mechanism to stimulate cell adhesion on laminins 1 and 5, fibronectin, and vitronectin which enhances invasion using multiple integrins including β1, β3, β4, and β5. By activating integrin clustering, HGF signaling encourages invasion by enhancing the binding between integrins to their ligands (Trusolino et al. 1998). Finally, a monoclonal antibody against integrin α2 blocks the MET pathway-mediated cell migration in Madin–Darby canin kidney cells, further suggesting the importance of integrins for tumor metastasis (Lai et al. 2000).

In addition to actin filaments and integrins, focal adhesion kinases (FAK) also assist in cell structure and cell signaling. HGF and activation MET can promote formation of these focal adhesions (Matsumoto et al. 1995). Interestingly, in oral squamous carincoma cells, tyrosine phosphorylation of focal adhesion kinase (p125FAK) by HGF has been implicated in the migration and invasion of these malignant cells (Matsumoto et al. 1994). Overexpression of FAK stimulates cell migration mediated by HGF. Furthermore, if FAK is mutated so it is unable to activate PI3-K, cell proliferation by HGF is inhibited (Matsumoto et al. 1994). By inhibiting this phosphorylation with herbimycin A, cell spreading and migration are halted (Matsumoto et al. 1994). p125FAK, composed of a 125 kDA protein, and the N-terminus is an integrin binding protein while the C-terminus focal adhesion targeting and paxillin-binding domain (Schaller and Sasaki 1997). Paxillin is a 68 kDa

structure, and tyrosine phosphorylated in response to HGF. Intriguingly, by binding to paxillin, oncogenes such as BCR/ABL and E6 may initiate cell proliferation (Parr et al. 2001).

By providing a structural link between extracellular matrix and actin skeleton, paxillin is a crucial element within focal adhesions of the actin cytoskeleton and provides multiple docking sites for a wide variety of signaling and structural proteins including tyrosine kinase receptors (Salgia et al. 1999; Hagel et al. 2002). Overexpression of paxillin has been associated with an aggressive tumor phenotypes (Kurayoshi et al. 2006). Increased paxillin allows for oncogene binding and transformation. Furthermore, somatic mutations within paxillin, such as A127T, are not only associated with MET amplification but also promote proliferative tumor growth and muscle invasion in non-small cell lung cancer cells; however, these paxillin mutations are not frequently seen in other tumor types (Jagadeeswaran et al. 2008). Because of the paxillin/MET overexpression is associated with tumor growth, this pathway is a new promising target in cancer therapy.

As members of the ras oncogene super family, small guanosine triphosphate GTP-binding proteins such as Rho, Rac, and Cdc42 are important for growth factor-mediated cell movement. These proteins are activated when bound to GTP. Specifically, assembly of stress fibers and focal adhesions incorporate Rho while Rac is required for actin polymerization. Finally, Cdc42 is involved with filopodia formation. Stimulation of Cdc42 and Rac results in Rho activation which can promote oncogenic transformation (Nobes and Hall 1999). Furthermore, recent evidence suggests patients with ras mutations confer a resistance to tyrosine kinase inhibitors targeting the epidermal growth factor pathway such as gefinitib and erlotinib (EGFR TK inhibitors) (Bergot et al. 2007). Because ras-mutated cells demonstrate an upregulation of MET and disrupting the HGF/SF signaling can suppress the ability of tumor cells to form metastasis, suggesting MET inhibitors could overcome resistance to EGFR TK inhibitors in patients with ras mutations (Furge et al. 2001).

Adapter proteins such as Crk and CRKL also are vital for MET-mediated cell motility and migration (Uemura et al. 1997). Both proteins are composed of SH2 and SH3 domains and attache to phosphorylated Gab1 (Grb2-associated binding protein-1), which is a large adapter protein that binds to MET via the Met-binding domain (MBD) and Grb2. Crk stimulated Gab1 in response to MET, but not other tyrosine kinases, suggesting the importance of sustained tyrosine phosphorylation of Gab1 in tumor invasion (Sakkab et al. 2000).

As a non-receptor tyrosine kinase, phosphoinositide 3-kinase (PI3-K) plays a significant role in mitogenesis, cell transformation, and other tyrosine kinase-mediated cellular events (Cantrell 2001). It is heterodimer containing a p85 regulatory subunit which is an adapter while the p110 catalytic subunit binds protein tyrosine kinases (Cantrell 2001). In human glioblastoma cells, the HGF-mediated protection against cell death can be suppressed by inhibitors of PI3-K such as LY249003 and wortmannin (Bowers et al. 2000).

Cytoplasmic proteins called catenins bind with transmembrane proteins E-cadherins. This complex aids the actin cytoskeleton to uphold cell–cell adhesions.

Tyrosine phosphorylation of β-catenin occurs via MET activation by HGF altering cell–cell adhesions (Nabeshima et al. 1998). When stimulated by HGF prostate cancer cells demonstrate E-cadherin, β-catenin and MET at sites of cell–cell contact, suggesting the importance of these complexes in cell adhesion and metastasis (Davies et al. 2001).

Previously, MET mutants have utilized mouse models to study the role of this pathway in context of the whole organisms. Recently, nematode *C. elegans* has proven to be an alternative model organism to study MET mutations (Siddiqui et al. 2008). Furthermore, mutant human MET forms correlated with significantly low fecundity and abnormal vulval development characterized by hyperplasia. In addition, carcinogens enhanced mutant MET function expressed in *C. elegans* transgenic animal models. The *C. elegans* model provides a rapid method to assess the role of specific gene mutations in the context of the whole organism.

Angiogenesis

Angiogenesis (formation of new blood vessels) plays a key role in cell growth normal cell proliferation is highly controlled through apoptosis or programmed cell death. When the delicate equilibrium between proliferation and apoptosis is disrupted, cells can accrue in excess numbers arising into tumors. Evidence suggests that oxygen and nutrients can diffuse into a tumor mass when it measures less than 0.5 mm in diameter; however, the proliferation and morphogenesis of vascular endothelial cells resulting in new blood vessels is required for a tumor mass beyond 0.5 mm in diameter (Fidler et al. 2002). HGF stimulates MET endothelial expression and promotes migration, proliferation, and invasion (Rosen et al. 1990, 1997) Vascular endothelial growth factor (VEGF), IL 8, and other pro-angiogenic factors are upregulated by HGF in tumor and smooth muscle cells while anti-angiogenic factors such as thrombospondin 1 are downregulated (Van Belle et al. 1998; Zhang et al. 2003). Two other critical pathways for biologic activity include the ERK, which controls mitogenesis, and phosphotidyllinositol-3-OH kinase (PI3K), which regulates MET-dependent cell survival and promotes angiogensis (Liu et al. 2007) (Xiao et al. 2001).

As the vasculature grows and interacts with smooth musculature, the network of vessels allows local and systemic to traffic oxygen, hormones, and nutrients needed for cell proliferation. In mature cells, angiogenesis is essential for tissue repair and hemostasis. Overt angiogenesis can result in not only malignancy but also atherosclerosis, arthritis, and diabetic retinopathy (Griffioen and Molema 2000). Growth factors promote the binding of cell surface molecules to the extracellular matrix enabling tissue stabilization. Interrupting tumor growth by limiting angiogenesis may be a potent inhibiting subsequent metastasis. Therapies disrupting this process have become increasing attractive targets in oncology.

Metastasis occurs as the tumor cells disrupt the extracellular milieu, thereby increasing motility through cytoskeletal remodeling and integrin-mediated responses by the attachment of cancer cells to the extracellular matrix. Proteases degrade the basal laminar components enabling motile cells to alter integrin-mediated pathways within the extracellular matrix (Jafri et al. 2003). By producing new capillaries, angiogenetic factors allow the tumor to grow and spread by entering the circulation via fragmented basement membranes (Maulik et al. 2002b). Tumor cells metastasize through lymphatic and circulatory vessels, and as the tumor adheres to the organ's capillary beds, the tumor invades the organ itself. Studies suggest that different cancers metastasize using different mechanisms. By understanding these pathways, targeted therapies may be developed (Cattley and Radinsky 2004).

HGF increases the expression of VEGF and initiates angiogenesis in a paracrine manner (Wojta et al. 1999). While VEGF inhibitors have been clinically useful to treat cancer, MET inhibitors are currently under development. Furthermore, in vitro studies suggest that while selective VEGF inhibitors such as PTK 787 block VEGF-induced angiogenesis, HGF can still induce angiogenesis independently, perhaps through the activation of mitogen-activated protein kinase (MAPK or ERKs) and PI3K (AKT) cascades (Sengupta et al. 2003). Both of these cascades have been implicated in the initiation of angiogenesis (Eliceiri et al. 1998). This finding suggests that while VEGF inhibitors like bevacizumab have already proved to have clinical activity, development of MET/HGF inhibitors may enhance treatment against tumor-expressing HGF by suppressing VEGF independent pathways.

Alterations of MET in Malignancies

While the complexities of MET and HGF are not fully understood, but both are expressed in most carcinomas. Uncontrolled MET activation in cell lines results in highly invasive and metastatic tumors. The importance of MET pathway in a variety of tumors is highlighted below.

Missense mutations of MET have been demonstrated in families with hereditary papillary renal cell carcinoma and the pathway's role in oncogenesis makes it an important novel drug target (Schmidt et al. 1998). Von Hippel–Landau tumor suppressor genes regulate cell-cycle cessation and the expression of various mRNAs such as for vascular endothelial growth factor. Malignant cells that are VHL negative possess decreased levels of tissue inhibitor metalloproteinase (TIMP) 1 and 2 but increased levels of matrix metalloproteinases 2 and 9, which promote an invasive phenotype. If renal cell carcinoma cells express the von Hippel–Landau (VHL) tumor suppressor gene, these malignant cells are immune to HGF signaling for invasion and branching (Koochekpour et al. 1999). Furthermore, germline missense mutations in exon 16 in the tyrosine kinase domain have been detected. Additionally, three MET gene mutations were found within the codons that are found in proto-oncogenes, c-KIT and RET, which targets naturally occurring mutations. This evidence proposes that missense mutations arise in activation of the MET protein and papillary renal carcinomas (Schmidt et al. 1997).

Importance of MET in Lung Cancer

As the leading cause of cancer-related mortality, lung cancer accounts for more deaths in the United States than breast, colon cancer, and prostate cancer combined (Jemal et al. 2007). While the earlier the stage of non-small lung cancer usually correlates with a better prognosis, there are certain discrepancies, suggesting stage alone is not a completely accurate predictor of survival. Even among patients that were resected, recurrence was noted on an average 41% of patients with a 11.5 month median time of recurrence after surgery. There was only a 8-month median survival after recurrence observed (Sugimura et al. 2007). Additionally, patients presenting with metastatic non-small cell lung cancer have a dismal 5-year survival rate of approximately 1%(Adebonojo et al. 1999).

In non-small cell lung carcinoma, adenocarcinomas have routinely expressed up to three times the normal levels of MET (Liu and Tsao 1993). In 42 samples analyzed, a quarter of the samples demonstrated significant MET overexpression; HGF was overexpressed 10–100-fold more than controls (Olivero et al. 1996). Moreover, resected tumors demonstrating MET expression were found to have a higher tumor stage and correlated with a poorer outcome than those tumor that did not (Ichimura et al. 1996). Out of 131 cases of small-sized lung adenocarcinomas, 69 possessed MET positive myofibroblasts and were associated with poor survival rate in all stages (Tokunou et al. 2001). Multivariate analysis suggests MET had a significant effect on the prognosis; a similar correlation with HGF was not appreciated (Takanami et al. 1996). However, evidence suggests that elevated HGF in non-small cell lung cancer may still predict a more aggressive tumor type (Siegfried et al. 1998). In addition, in non-small cell lung cancer, tumor MET and HGF elevation indicate a poor prognosis (Siegfried et al. 1997). Mutations in the juxtamembrane domain lead to augmented tumorigenicity, enhanced cell motility, and increased downstream signaling (Ma et al. 2003). This phenomenon allows for a enhanced response to small molecule inhibitors (Ma et al. 2005a). Carriers of these mutations may have altered risk for lung cancer.

Small cell lung cancer (SCLC) is a malignant neoplasm that carries an extremely poor prognosis. The 5-year survival is less than 10% (Murray et al. 2004). This tumor is classically located within the main stem bronchus. This aggressive tumor easily spreads to liver, adrenal glands, brain, and bone and often is metastatic upon presentation. In addition, certain paraneoplastic syndromes such as production of inappropriate antiuretic hormone (SIADH), ectopic Cushing's syndrome, and Lambert–Eaton myasthenia syndrome are found in SCLC (Ellison and Berl 2007). SCLC is either staged as limited or extensive stage. A third of patients have limited stage disease is confined to the thoracic cavity and is treated with standard chemotherapy with radiation while patients with extrathoracic disease are considered to be extensive stage and are treated with chemotherapy alone. While chemotherapy such as cisplatin and etoposide can achieve a partial or complete response, the rate of recurrent is high. There is a dire need for novel therapy because despite over two decades of research, the median survival remains at 8–10 months (Chute et al. 1999).

Evidence suggests MET pathway is overexpressed in both SCLC and non-small cell lung cancer (Maulik et al. 2002b). Activation of MET with HGF activates several pathways crucial for cell proliferation including cytoskeletal proteins such has paxillin and FAK. In addition, overexpression of MET is seen in 67% adenocarcinomas and 35% of SCLC (Ma et al. 2005a). Specifically, 10% of mutations occur outside the tyrosine kinase domain in the juxtamembrane domain or semaphorin domain, which binds HGF and is vital for receptor activation (Ma et al. 2003). It is hypothesized that HGF is manufactured by mesenchymal cells within the tumor, thereby acting on MET receptors on epithelial cells in a paracrine activation loop (Tokunou et al. 2001). HGF stimulation of H69 SCLC line resulted in cells with increased membrane ruffling, clustering, and filopodia formation, thus changing cell motility and furthering disease state (Maulik et al. 2002a). Additionally, when PHA-665752, a small molecule, ATP competitive inhibitor of the catalytic activity of the MET kinase, was added to these cell line nude mouse xenografts, angiogenesis was inhibited by greater than 85% (Puri et al. 2007).

Head and Neck Cancer

Furthermore, evidence suggests MET activation is selected during metastatic progression of head and neck squamous cell cancer (HNSCC) (Di Renzo et al. 2000). Additional studies indicate MET mutations found in lung metastasis from HNSCC predicted poor response to radiotherapy and decreased progression-free survival (Lorenzato et al. 2002). Moreover, MET expression and mutation correlates with resistance to radiotherapy in head and neck squamous cell carcinoma (Aebersold et al. 2001, 2003)

Gastrointestinal Malignancies

In gastric carcinoma, amplification of MET not only has been detected but also is associated with an advanced tumor stage and correlated with a poorer prognosis. Moreover, out of the gastric lines studied, 38% of the scirrhous gastric carcinoma tissues demonstrated MET amplification, suggesting MET may play a vital role in this tumor type's carcinogenesis (Kuniyasu et al. 1992). Additional studies indicate that in 16 out of 31 gastric carcinoma tissues, overexpression of 6.0 kb transcription of MET has been detected and additionally, associated with advanced tumor stage, lymph node metastases, and depth of invasion (Kuniyasu et al. 1993). Interestingly, no aberrant single-strand conformational polymorphism patterns were detected in 43 cell lines, indicating perhaps there are no genetic alterations in the kinase domain of the Met gene and the receptor structure is maintained; but instead, HGF-mediated stimulation and overexpression result in over-development and progression of gastric carcinoma (Park et al. 2000). Finally, a novel germline missense mutation P10009S has been detected in patients with gastric carcinoma (Lee et al. 2000).

Interestingly, while MET dysregulation was usually not found in primary colon cancer, it has been overexpressed in liver metastasis (Zeng et al. 2004). Similar findings have been reported in gastric cancer and breast cancer (Kaji et al. 1996; Beviglia et al. 1997). MET activation in cancer can occur through multiple different mechanisms. Elevated expression of MET has been identified in a wide variety of cancers including lung, breast, prostate, gastric and colorectal, pancreatic, and renal carcinoma (Maulik et al. 2002b). Tumor-secreted growth factors and activation of ras oncogenes upregulate MET expression in cancer (Furge et al. 2001). Alternatively, elevated tumor or plasma HGF is found in multiple cancers and is overexpressed in stroma cells, such as fibroblasts and endothelial cells, stimulated by tumor cell secreted cytokines and growth factors (Gohda et al. 1994). Ligand-independent activation of the pathway secondary to selected MET mutations or truncations, hypoxia-induced pathway activation, transactivation by EGFR receptors, or the loss of negative regulators, all partially bypass the need for HGF activation in the MET pathway (Christensen et al. 2005).

Receptor Tyrosine Kinases as Therapeutic Targets

Receptor tyrosine kinase (RTK)-targeted therapies has revolutionized the treatment of certain malignancies. They work by different mechanisms, including but not limited to the disruption of angiogenesis. For example, inhibiting cellular proliferation and tumor formation by BCR/ABL-expressing cells with imatinib has profoundly changed the treatment of chronic myelogenous leukemia (O'Brien et al. 2003). In these newly diagnosed patients, elevated levels of vascular endothelial growth factor (VEGF) are found in the bone marrow, and imatinib lowers the level of VEGF and interferes with tumor angiogenesis (Legros et al. 2004). Imatinib also blocks signaling via the tyrosine kinase receptor c-KIT pathway by binding to the ATP-binding pocket required for phosphorylation. This phenomenon, combined with decreased levels VEGF and angiogenesis, translated into a dramatic tumor response in patients with metastatic gastrointestinal stromal tumors, which were previously felt to be chemotherapy resistant (Joensuu et al. 2001; McAuliffe et al. 2007). Clearly, imatinib demonstrates how targeting RTKs may have a potent clinical impact in a wide variety of malignancies and highlights the need to investigate other tyrosine kinases such as MET.

Inhibition of the MET Pathway as Targeted Therapy

Multiple agents inhibiting the MET pathway have been investigated as possible therapeutic targets (Table 12.1). It is thought that inhibition of MET kinase activity reduces cell growth and induces G1 cell-cycle arrest and apoptosis. Small interference RNA (siRNA) against MET have decreased cell growth and augmented apoptosis in lung cancer cell lines by suppressing the MET pathway (Ma et al. 2005a). Small molecule inhibitors such as SU11274 are effective against activated MET cells but not with cells with activated ABL and JAK2 (Sattler

Table 12.1 List of current MET inhibitors in clinical trials

Compound	Mech. of inhibition	Phase of study	Tumor types	Company
AMG102	Anti-HGF Antibody	II	Renal cell carcinoma, malignant glioma	Amgen, Inc.
ARQ197 (small molecule)	MET	II	Pancreatic cancer	Arqule, Inc.
MetMAb	Anti-MET Antibody	I	Advanced solid tumors	Genentech, Inc.
PF02341066 (small molecule)	MET, ALK	I	Solid tumors, Anaplastic large-cell lymphomas	Pfizer, Inc.
SGX523 (small molecule)	MET	I	Advanced malignancies	SGX Pharmaceuticals
XL184 (small molecule)	MET, VEGFR2, RET	I	Advanced malignancies (lymphoma, cancer, thyroid cancer)	Exelixis, Inc.
		I / II	NSCLC (w/erlotinib)	
XL880 (small molecule)	MET, VEGFR2	II	HNSCC, gastric cancer, papillary renal cell carcinoma	Exelixis, Inc.

et al. 2003). Additional specific MET inhibitors include PHA66752 which inhibits MET-dependent effects in tumor cells. PHA665752 is a prototype ATP competitive inhibitor of the catalytic kinase activity of the MET pathways. It has also been active against several solid tumors (Christensen et al. 2003). When it is introduced to IL 3-dependent mutant c-MET BaF3 cells, it inhibited cell growth with an IC_{50} < 0.06 μmol/L, while SU11274 inhibited IL-3 independent cell growth in a dose-dependent manner with IC_{50} < 3 μmol/L suggesting PHA66752 was more potent (Sattler et al. 2003; Ma et al. 2005b).

Additionally, when mTOR inhibitor rapamycin was combined with PHA66752, it showed a cooperative inhibition to reduce growth of BaF3 cells and MET-expressing H441 non-small cell lung cell (NSCLC) cells (Ma et al. 2005b). Rapamycin (sirolimus) was approved in 1999 as an immunosuppressant to prevent transplant rejection; however, it also has antitumor activity in a multitude of cancers (Luo et al. 2003). Another innovative approach is utilizing a modified anti-HGF antibody to inhibit HGF binding to MET. AMG 102 potentiates the effect of temozolomide or docetaxel in U-87 MG (human glioblastoma-derived containing HGF/MET autocrine loop) cells (Jun et al. 2007). Multiple other inhibitors including PF2341066, XL880, XL184, ARQ197, and SGX523 are under clinical investigation

Phase I and Phase II trials. Moreover, antibodies against MET (known as MetMab) are in Phase I clinical trials in advanced solid tumors. Even though the trials are early, one also has to be very cautious. As an example, Phase I trial for SGX-523 have recently halted due to unexpected toxicity.

Anisomycin antibiotics inhibit HGF-mediated plasmin activation in canine kidney cells. These geldanamycin decrease MET expression and prevent HGF-mediated cell motility and subsequent invasion at nanomolar concentrations nine-order below their growth inhibitory concentrations. Furthermore, NIH3T3 cells altered by Met mutations convert to the normal phenotype when treated with gel-danamycins (Webb et al. 2000). Of note, geldanamycin downregulate tyrosine kinase pathways by decreasing the number of cell signaling pathways by direct inhi-bition of the heat shock protein 90 chaperone function, resulting in client protein destabilization (Neckers et al. 1999).

Evidence indicates that an engineered Met receptor that has impaired ability to bind to HGF will result in a loss of transforming activity, suggesting the pathway is ligand dependent (Michieli et al. 1999). As a competitive agonist of HGF, pro-HGF is the inactive precursor molecule that binds but does not activate the MET pathway. Therefore, these precursor molecules are potential HGF antagonists that may even-tually become clinically useful. For example, NK (N-terminal hairpin domain and Kringle domain) has four variants and NK2 is a naturally occurring alterative-sliced form of HGF that inhibits growth but stimulates the metastasis of melanoma cells in bitransgenic mice (Otsuka et al. 2000). As a truncated HGF consisting only of the α-chain, NK4 binds to MET without activating it. In the laboratory, alterated HGF motility and invasion of HT115 human colorectal cells has been observed when treated with NK4 (Parr et al. 2000). Furthermore, NK4 can inhibit paxillin phos-phorylation and decrease matrix invasion in prostate cancer (Jiang et al. 1999). NK inhibitors antagonize the binding of HGF and disrupting the autocrine or paracrine activation of the MET receptor. Alternatively, a phase I clinical trial with AMG 102, a fully humanized anti-HGF antibody, was found to enhance the efficacy of temozolomide or docetaxel in U-87 MG (human glioblastoma-derived containing HGF/MET autocrine loop) cells and phase I and phase II trials are underway (Jun et al. 2007).

While targeted therapies such as erlotinib are already utilized in clinical prac-tice, resistance is often observed in patients. However, evidence suggests that MET amplification occurs in such patients with acquired resistance to erlotinib, thus mak-ing MET inhibition a potential and important treatment target (Bean et al. 2007). XL184 is an orally bioavailable inhibitor of RET, MET & VEGFR2 that strongly inhibits cell proliferation. Recently, a phase I study demonstrated that 55 patients with advanced malignanices, including medullary thyroid cancer, tolerated XL 184 well. Overall, 22 patients achieved stable disease for greater than 3 months. Additionally, 12 patients were found to have stable disease for greater than 6 months. Three patients with medullary thyroid cancer were found to have a par-tial response. Therefore, this phase I study will be expanded to include an additional 20 medullary thyroid patients (Salgia et al. 2008).

Other Pre-clinical Targets

In vivo studies indicate that peptides derived from c-MET receptor tail bind and subsequently inhibit HGF-mediated phosphorylation in the C-MET pathway without altering other pathways, such as VEGF (Bardelli et al. 1999). These peptides inhibit kinase on A549 cells and decrease HGF-mediated invasive growth by half. Other promising peptides include those derived from the kinase activation loop with N-terminal sequence from the Antennapedia protein for internalization or located within carboxy-tail of c-MET (Bardelli et al. 1999).

Effector proteins such as Grb2 are able to activate c-MET and induce Ras-MAP kinase signaling which stimulates c-MET-mediated events such as cell proliferation, shape change, and motility (Atabey et al. 2001). Activated c-MET directly binds to Grb 2 via the multisubstrate docking site on Src homology 2 (SH2) domain. In addition, Grb 2 indirectly interacts with c-MET using SHC adaptor proteins (Atabey et al. 2001). Tripeptide-based inhibitors of Grb2/SH2 domain potentiates anti-motility agents, suggesting these compounds may become clinically important in decreasing metastasis.

Because of direct interaction with c-MET via Y1349 and Y1356, the tyrosine kinase c-Src is crucial for cell migration and subsequent transformation (Rahimi et al. 1998). In vivo, when c-Src lacks both kinase activity (K295R) and a regulatory tyrosine residue (Y527F), cells have significantly reduced c-Src kinase activity. Additionally, blockade of HGF-induced motility and colony growth are noted (Rahimi et al. 1998). It is hypothesized that this inhibition is secondary to decreased phosphorylation of paxillin and focal adhesion kinase and that did not interfere with Grb2 binding.

Similar to insulin receptor substrate-1, Gab1 is a member of adapter proteins containing an N-terminal pleckstrin homolog (PH) that binds the membrane lipid phosphatidylinositol 3,4,5-triphosate (PIP3), which holds 16 tyrosine phosphorylation sites and promotes sustained activation, possibly for branching morphogenesis (Gual et al. 2000). These sites bind SH2 domain possessing signal transducers and C-terminal proline-rich c-MET-binding domain (MBD) (Sachs et al. 2000). Furthermore, Gab1 can indirectly interact with c-MET via Gab2 because the SH3 domains of Grb2 are bound by MBD. If cells are treated with okadaic acid, a potent inhibitor of serine/threonine protein phosphatases PP1 and PP2, the activation of serine/threonine kinases PKC-α and PKC-β1 occurs and disrupts Gab1-SH2 signalizing, thus inhibiting HGF-induced pathways (Gual et al. 2001).

Wortmannin inhibits phosphotidyllinositol-3-OH kinase (PI3K), thus downregulating branching formation on collage matrix (Derman et al. 1995). Specifically in A549 non-small cell lung cancer cells, dominant negative Rac microinjections inhibit HGF-mediated spreading and actin reorganization (Graziani et al. 1993). Furthermore, microinjections of rhoGDI, an inhibitory GDP/GTP exchange protein for rho p21 small GTP-binding protein, inhibit HGF-mediated spreading and scattering (Takaishi et al. 1994).

Conclusions

c-MET and its ligand HGF are crucial for normal cell proliferation and motility; however, evidence indicates that c-MET stimulation enhances tumor angiogenesis, invasion, and metastasis in certain malignancies. Because of the importance of c-MET in cytoskeleton structure, activation of this pathway in cancer cells suggests a more aggressive and invasive phenotype of malignancy especially in lung cancer. Downregulating the c-MET pathway may prove to be an ideal target for clinical therapeutics leading to a spectacular inhibition of cancer growth and METastasis in a wide variety of malignancies. Multiple pre-clinical and clinical studies are utilizing multiple mechanisms to inhibit the c-MET pathway and interrupt tumor angiogenesis. These targeted therapies may be combined with standard or other novel therapies and further clinical trials are warranted.

References

Adebonojo SA, Bowser AN, Moritz DM, Corcoran PC (1999) Impact of revised stage classification of lung cancer on survival: a military experience. Chest 115:1507–1513.

Aebersold DM, Kollar A, Beer KT, Laissue J, Greiner RH, Djonov V (2001) Involvement of the hepatocyte growth factor/scatter factor receptor c-met and of Bcl-xL in the resistance of oropharyngeal cancer to ionizing radiation. Int J Cancer 96:41–54.

Aebersold DM, Landt O, Berthou S, Gruber G, Beer KT, Greiner RH, Zimmer Y (2003) Prevalence and clinical impact of Met Y1253D-activating point mutation in radiotherapy-treated squamous cell cancer of the oropharynx. Oncogene 22:8519–8523.

Atabey N, Gao Y, Yao ZJ, Breckenridge D, Soon L, Soriano JV, Burke TR Jr, Bottaro DP (2001) Potent blockade of hepatocyte growth factor-stimulated cell motility, matrix invasion and branching morphogenesis by antagonists of Grb2 Src homology 2 domain interactions. J Biol Chem 276:14308–14314.

Bardelli A, Longati P, Williams TA, Benvenuti S, Comoglio PM (1999) A peptide representing the carboxyl-terminal tail of the met receptor inhibits kinase activity and invasive growth. J Biol Chem 274:29274–29281.

Bean J, Brennan C, Shih JY, Riely G, Viale A, Wang L, Chitale D, Motoi N, Szoke J, Broderick S, Balak M, Chang WC, Yu CJ, Gazdar A, Pass H, Rusch V, Gerald W, Huang SF, Yang PC, Miller V, Ladanyi M, Yang CH, Pao W (2007) MET amplification occurs with or without T790M mutations in EGFR mutant lung tumors with acquired resistance to gefitinib or erlotinib. Proc Natl Acad Sci U S A 104:20932–20937.

Bergot E, Richard N, Zalcman G (2007) [Mechanisms of action of targeted therapies ... and mechanisms of resistance]. Rev Mal Respir 24:6S180–187.

Beviglia L, Matsumoto K, Lin CS, Ziober BL, Kramer RH (1997) Expression of the c-Met/HGF receptor in human breast carcinoma: correlation with tumor progression. Int J Cancer 74: 301–309.

Bottaro DP, Rubin JS, Faletto DL, Chan AM, Kmiecik TE, Vande Woude GF, Aaronson SA (1991) Identification of the hepatocyte growth factor receptor as the c-met proto-oncogene product. Science 251:802–804.

Bowers DC, Fan S, Walter KA, Abounader R, Williams JA, Rosen EM, Laterra J (2000) Scatter factor/hepatocyte growth factor protects against cytotoxic death in human glioblastoma via phosphatidylinositol 3-kinase- and AKT-dependent pathways. Cancer Res 60:4277–4283.

Cantrell DA (2001) Phosphoinositide 3-kinase signalling pathways. J Cell Sci 114:1439–1445

Cattley RC and Radinsky RR (2004) Cancer therapeutics: understanding the mechanism of action. Toxicol Pathol 32 Suppl 1:116–121.

Christensen JG, Schreck R, Burrows J, Kuruganti P, Chan E, Le P, Chen J, Wang X, Ruslim L, Blake R, Lipson KE, Ramphal J, Do S, Cui JJ, Cherrington JM, Mendel DB (2003) A selective small molecule inhibitor of c-Met kinase inhibits c-Met-dependent phenotypes in vitro and exhibits cytoreductive antitumor activity in vivo. Cancer Res 63:7345–7355.

Christensen JG, Burrows J, Salgia R (2005) c-Met as a target for human cancer and characterization of inhibitors for therapeutic intervention. Cancer Lett 225:1–26.

Chute JP, Chen T, Feigal E, Simon R, Johnson BE (1999) Twenty years of phase III trials for patients with extensive-stage small-cell lung cancer: perceptible progress. J Clin Oncol 17:1794–1801.

Comoglio PM (1993) Structure, biosynthesis and biochemical properties of the HGF receptor in normal and malignant cells. Exs 65:131–165.

Cooper CS, Park M, Blair DG, Tainsky MA, Huebner K, Croce CM, Vande Woude GF (1984) Molecular cloning of a new transforming gene from a chemically transformed human cell line. Nature 311:29–33.

Davies G, Jiang WG, Mason MD (2001) HGF/SF modifies the interaction between its receptor c-Met, and the E-cadherin/catenin complex in prostate cancer cells. Int J Mol Med 7:385–388.

Derman MP, Cunha MJ, Barros EJ, Nigam SK, Cantley LG (1995) HGF-mediated chemotaxis and tubulogenesis require activation of the phosphatidylinositol 3-kinase. Am J Physiol 268: F1211–1217.

Di Renzo MF, Olivero M, Martone T, Maffe A, Maggiora P, Stefani AD, Valente G, Giordano S, Cortesina G, Comoglio PM (2000) Somatic mutations of the MET oncogene are selected during metastatic spread of human HNSC carcinomas. Oncogene 19:1547–1555.

Eliceiri BP, Klemke R, Stromblad S, Cheresh DA (1998) Integrin alphavbeta3 requirement for sustained mitogen-activated protein kinase activity during angiogenesis. J Cell Biol 140: 1255–1263.

Ellison DH and Berl T (2007) Clinical practice. The syndrome of inappropriate antidiuresis. N Engl J Med 356:2064–2072.

Fidler IJ, Yano S, Zhang RD, Fujimaki T, Bucana CD (2002) The seed and soil hypothesis: vascularisation and brain metastases. Lancet Oncol 3:53–57.

Furge KA, Zhang YW, Vande Woude GF (2000) Met receptor tyrosine kinase: enhanced signaling through adapter proteins. Oncogene 19:5582–5589.

Furge KA, Kiewlich D, Le P, Vo MN, Faure M, Howlett AR, Lipson KE, Woude GF, Webb CP (2001) Suppression of Ras-mediated tumorigenicity and metastasis through inhibition of the Met receptor tyrosine kinase. Proc Natl Acad Sci U S A 98:10722–10727.

Gherardi E, Sandin S, Petoukhov MV, Finch J, Youles ME, Ofverstedt LG, Miguel RN, Blundell TL, Vande Woude GF, Skoglund U, Svergun DI (2006) Structural basis of hepatocyte growth factor/scatter factor and MET signalling. Proc Natl Acad Sci U S A 103:4046–4051.

Gohda E, Matsunaga T, Kataoka H, Takebe T, Yamamoto I (1994) Induction of hepatocyte growth factor in human skin fibroblasts by epidermal growth factor, platelet-derived growth factor and fibroblast growth factor. Cytokine 6:633–640.

Graziani A, Gramaglia D, dalla Zonca P, Comoglio PM (1993) Hepatocyte growth factor/scatter factor stimulates the Ras-guanine nucleotide exchanger. J Biol Chem 268:9165–9168.

Griffioen AW and Molema G (2000) Angiogenesis: potentials for pharmacologic intervention in the treatment of cancer, cardiovascular diseases, and chronic inflammation. Pharmacol Rev 52:237–268.

Gu H and Neel BG (2003) The "Gab" in signal transduction. Trends Cell Biol 13:122–130.

Gual P, Giordano S, Williams TA, Rocchi S, Van Obberghen E, Comoglio PM (2000) Sustained recruitment of phospholipase C-gamma to Gab1 is required for HGF-induced branching tubulogenesis. Oncogene 19:1509–1518.

Gual P, Giordano S, Anguissola S, Parker PJ, Comoglio PM (2001) Gab1 phosphorylation: a novel mechanism for negative regulation of HGF receptor signaling. Oncogene 20:156–166.

Hagel M, George EL, Kim A, Tamimi R, Opitz SL, Turner CE, Imamoto A, Thomas SM (2002) The adaptor protein paxillin is essential for normal development in the mouse and is a critical transducer of fibronectin signaling. Mol Cell Biol 22:901–915.

Hynes RO (1992) Integrins: versatility, modulation, and signaling in cell adhesion. Cell 69:11–25.

Ichimura E, Maeshima A, Nakajima T, Nakamura T (1996) Expression of c-met/HGF receptor in human non-small cell lung carcinomas in vitro and in vivo and its prognostic significance. Jpn J Cancer Res 87:1063–1069.

Jafri NF, Ma PC, Maulik G, Salgia R (2003) Mechanisms of metastasis as related to receptor tyrosine kinases in small-cell lung cancer. J Environ Pathol Toxicol Oncol 22:147–165.

Jagadeeswaran R, Surawska H, Krishnaswamy S, Janamanchi V, Mackinnon AC, Seiwert TY, Loganathan S, Kanteti R, Reichman T, Nallasura V, Schwartz S, Faoro L, Wang YC, Girard L, Tretiakova MS, Ahmed S, Zumba O, Soulii L, Bindokas VP, Szeto LL, Gordon GJ, Bueno R, Sugarbaker D, Lingen MW, Sattler M, Krausz T, Vigneswaran W, Natarajan V, Minna J, Vokes EE, Ferguson MK, Husain AN, Salgia R (2008) Paxillin is a target for somatic mutations in lung cancer: implications for cell growth and invasion. Cancer Res 68: 132–142.

Jeffers M, Rong S, Vande Woude GF (1996) Enhanced tumorigenicity and invasion-metastasis by hepatocyte growth factor/scatter factor-met signalling in human cells concomitant with induction of the urokinase proteolysis network. Mol Cell Biol 16:1115–1125.

Jemal A, Siegel R, Ward E, Murray T, Xu J, Thun MJ (2007) Cancer statistics, 2007. CA Cancer J Clin 57:43–66.

Jiang WG, Hiscox SE, Parr C, Martin TA, Matsumoto K, Nakamura T, Mansel RE (1999) Antagonistic effect of NK4, a novel hepatocyte growth factor variant, on in vitro angiogenesis of human vascular endothelial cells. Clin Cancer Res 5:3695–3703.

Joensuu H, Roberts PJ, Sarlomo-Rikala M, Andersson LC, Tervahartiala P, Tuveson D, Silberman S, Capdeville R, Dimitrijevic S, Druker B, Demetri GD (2001) Effect of the tyrosine kinase inhibitor STI571 in a patient with a metastatic gastrointestinal stromal tumor. N Engl J Med 344:1052–1056.

Jun HT, Sun J, Rex K, Radinsky R, Kendall R, Coxon A, Burgess TL (2007) AMG 102, a fully human anti-hepatocyte growth factor/scatter factor neutralizing antibody, enhances the efficacy of temozolomide or docetaxel in U-87 MG cells and xenografts. Clin Cancer Res 13: 6735–6742.

Kaji M, Yonemura Y, Harada S, Liu X, Terada I, Yamamoto H (1996) Participation of c-met in the progression of human gastric cancers: anti-c-met oligonucleotides inhibit proliferation or invasiveness of gastric cancer cells. Cancer Gene Ther 3:393–404.

Koochekpour S, Jeffers M, Wang PH, Gong C, Taylor GA, Roessler LM, Stearman R, Vasselli JR, Stetler-Stevenson WG, Kaelin WG Jr, Linehan WM, Klausner RD, Gnarra JR, Vande Woude GF (1999) The von Hippel-Lindau tumor suppressor gene inhibits hepatocyte growth factor/scatter factor-induced invasion and branching morphogenesis in renal carcinoma cells. Mol Cell Biol 19:5902–5912.

Kuniyasu H, Yasui W, Kitadai Y, Yokozaki H, Ito H, Tahara E (1992) Frequent amplification of the c-met gene in scirrhous type stomach cancer. Biochem Biophys Res Commun 189:227–232.

Kuniyasu H, Yasui W, Yokozaki H, Kitadai Y, Tahara E (1993) Aberrant expression of c-met mRNA in human gastric carcinomas. Int J Cancer 55:72–75.

Kurayoshi M, Oue N, Yamamoto H, Kishida M, Inoue A, Asahara T, Yasui W, Kikuchi A (2006) Expression of Wnt-5a is correlated with aggressiveness of gastric cancer by stimulating cell migration and invasion. Cancer Res 66:10439–10448.

Lai JF, Kao SC, Jiang ST, Tang MJ, Chan PC, Chen HC (2000) Involvement of focal adhesion kinase in hepatocyte growth factor-induced scatter of Madin-Darby canine kidney cells. J Biol Chem 275:7474–7480.

Lee JH, Han SU, Cho H, Jennings B, Gerrard B, Dean M, Schmidt L, Zbar B, Vande Woude GF (2000) A novel germ line juxtamembrane Met mutation in human gastric cancer. Oncogene 19:4947–4953.

Legros L, Bourcier C, Jacquel A, Mahon FX, Cassuto JP, Auberger P, Pagès G (2004) Imatinib mesylate (STI571) decreases the vascular endothelial growth factor plasma concentration in patients with chronic myeloid leukemia. Blood 104:495–501.

Liu Y (1998) The human hepatocyte growth factor receptor gene: complete structural organization and promoter characterization. Gene 215:159–169.

Liu C and Tsao MS (1993) In vitro and in vivo expressions of transforming growth factor-alpha and tyrosine kinase receptors in human non-small-cell lung carcinomas. Am J Pathol 142: 1155–1162.

Liu Z, Greco AJ, Hellman NE, Spector J, Robinson J, Tang OT, Lipschutz JH (2007) Intracellular signaling via ERK/MAPK completes the pathway for tubulogenic fibronectin in MDCK cells. Biochem Biophys Res Commun 353:793–798.

Lorenzato A, Olivero M, Patanè S, Rosso E, Oliaro A, Comoglio PM, Di Renzo MF (2002) Novel somatic mutations of the MET oncogene in human carcinoma metastases activating cell motility and invasion. Cancer Res 62:7025–7030.

Luo J, Manning BD, Cantley LC (2003) Targeting the PI3K-Akt pathway in human cancer: rationale and promise. Cancer Cell 4:257–262.

Ma PC, Kijima T, Maulik G, Fox EA, Sattler M, Griffin JD, Johnson BE, Salgia R (2003) c-MET mutational analysis in small cell lung cancer: novel juxtamembrane domain mutations regulating cytoskeletal functions. Cancer Res 63:6272–6281.

Ma PC, Jagadeeswaran R, Jagadeesh S, Tretiakova MS, Nallasura V, Fox EA, Hansen M, Schaefer E, Naoki K, Lader A, Richards W, Sugarbaker D, Husain AN, Christensen JG, Salgia R (2005a) Functional expression and mutations of c-Met and its therapeutic inhibition with SU11274 and small interfering RNA in non-small cell lung cancer. Cancer Res 65:1479–1488.

Ma PC, Schaefer E, Christensen JG, Salgia R (2005b) A selective small molecule c-MET Inhibitor, PHA665752, cooperates with rapamycin. Clin Cancer Res 11:2312–2319.

Matsumoto K, Matsumoto K, Nakamura T, Kramer RH (1994) Hepatocyte growth factor/scatter factor induces tyrosine phosphorylation of focal adhesion kinase (p125FAK) and promotes migration and invasion by oral squamous cell carcinoma cells. J Biol Chem 269:31807–31813.

Matsumoto K, Ziober BL, Yao CC, Kramer RH (1995) Growth factor regulation of integrin-mediated cell motility. Cancer Metastasis Rev 14:205–217.

Maulik G, Kijima T, Ma PC, Ghosh SK, Lin J, Shapiro GI, Schaefer E, Tibaldi E, Johnson BE, Salgia R (2002a) Modulation of the c-Met/hepatocyte growth factor pathway in small cell lung cancer. Clin Cancer Res 8:620–627.

Maulik G, Shrikhande A, Kijima T, Ma PC, Morrison PT, Salgia R (2002b) Role of the hepatocyte growth factor receptor, c-Met, in oncogenesis and potential for therapeutic inhibition. Cytokine Growth Factor Rev 13:41–59.

McAuliffe JC, Lazar AJ, Yang D, Steinert DM, Qiao W, Thall PF, Raymond AK, Benjamin RS, Trent JC (2007) Association of intratumoral vascular endothelial growth factor expression and clinical outcome for patients with gastrointestinal stromal tumors treated with imatinib mesylate. Clin Cancer Res 13:6727–6734.

Michieli P, Basilico C, Pennacchietti S, Maffè A, Tamagnone L, Giordano S, Bardelli A, Comoglio PM (1999) Mutant Met-mediated transformation is ligand-dependent and can be inhibited by HGF antagonists. Oncogene 18:5221–5231.

Murray N, Salgia R, Fossella FV (2004) Targeted molecules in small cell lung cancer. Semin Oncol 31:106–111.

Nabeshima K, Shimao Y, Inoue T, Itoh H, Kataoka H, Koono M (1998) Hepatocyte growth factor/scatter factor induces not only scattering but also cohort migration of human colorectal-adenocarcinoma cells. Int J Cancer 78:750–759.

Neckers L, Schulte TW, Mimnaugh E (1999) Geldanamycin as a potential anti-cancer agent: its molecular target and biochemical activity. Invest New Drugs 17:361–373.

Nobes CD and Hall A (1999) Rho GTPases control polarity, protrusion, and adhesion during cell movement. J Cell Biol 144:1235–1244.

O'Brien SG, Guilhot F, Larson RA, Gathmann I, Baccarani M, Cervantes F, Cornelissen JJ, Fischer T, Hochhaus A, Hughes T, Lechner K, Nielsen JL, Rousselot P, Reiffers J, Saglio G, Shepherd J, Simonsson B, Gratwohl A, Goldman JM, Kantarjian H, Taylor K, Verhoef G, Bolton AE, Capdeville R, Druker BJ; IRIS Investigators (2003) Imatinib compared with interferon and low-dose cytarabine for newly diagnosed chronic-phase chronic myeloid leukemia. N Engl J Med 348:994–1004.

Olivero M, Rizzo M, Madeddu R, Casadio C, Pennacchietti S, Nicotra MR, Prat M, Maggi G, Arena N, Natali PG, Comoglio PM, Di Renzo MF (1996) Overexpression and activation of hepatocyte growth factor/scatter factor in human non-small-cell lung carcinomas. Br J Cancer 74:1862–1868.

Otsuka T, Jakubczak J, Vieira W, Bottaro DP, Breckenridge D, Larochelle WJ, Merlino G (2000) Disassociation of met-mediated biological responses in vivo: the natural hepatocyte growth factor/scatter factor splice variant NK2 antagonizes growth but facilitates metastasis. Mol Cell Biol 20:2055–2065.

Park WS, Oh RR, Kim YS, Park JY, Shin MS, Lee HK, Lee SH, Yoo NJ, Lee JY (2000) Absence of mutations in the kinase domain of the Met gene and frequent expression of Met and HGF/SF protein in primary gastric carcinomas. Apmis 108:195–200.

Parr C, Hiscox S, Nakamura T, Matsumoto K, Jiang WG (2000) Nk4, a new HGF/SF variant, is an antagonist to the influence of HGF/SF on the motility and invasion of colon cancer cells. Int J Cancer 85:563–570.

Parr C, Davies G, Nakamura T, Matsumoto K, Mason MD, Jiang WG (2001) The HGF/SF-induced phosphorylation of paxillin, matrix adhesion, and invasion of prostate cancer cells were suppressed by NK4, an HGF/SF variant. Biochem Biophys Res Commun 285:1330–1337.

Puri N, Khramtsov A, Ahmed S, Nallasura V, Hetzel JT, Jagadeeswaran R, Karczmar G, Salgia R (2007) A selective small molecule inhibitor of c-Met, PHA665752, inhibits tumorigenicity and angiogenesis in mouse lung cancer xenografts. Cancer Res 67:3529–3534.

Rahimi N, Hung W, Tremblay E, Saulnier R, Elliott B (1998) c-Src kinase activity is required for hepatocyte growth factor-induced motility and anchorage-independent growth of mammary carcinoma cells. J Biol Chem 273:33714–33721.

Rosen EM, Meromsky L, Setter E, Vinter DW, Goldberg ID (1990) Purified scatter factor stimulates epithelial and vascular endothelial cell migration. Proc Soc Exp Biol Med 195:34–43.

Rosen EM, Lamszus K, Laterra J, Polverini PJ, Rubin JS, Goldberg ID (1997) HGF/SF in angiogenesis. Ciba Found Symp 212:215–226; discussion 227–219.

Sachs M, Brohmann H, Zechner D, Müller T, Hülsken J, Walther I, Schaeper U, Birchmeier C, Birchmeier W (2000) Essential role of Gab1 for signaling by the c-Met receptor in vivo. J Cell Biol 150:1375–1384.

Sakkab D, Lewitzky M, Posern G, Schaeper U, Sachs M, Birchmeier W, Feller SM (2000) Signaling of hepatocyte growth factor/scatter factor (HGF) to the small GTPase Rap1 via the large docking protein Gab1 and the adapter protein CRKL. J Biol Chem 275:10772–10778.

Salgia R, Li JL, Ewaniuk DS, Wang YB, Sattler M, Chen WC, Richards W, Pisick E, Shapiro GI, Rollins BJ, Chen LB, Griffin JD, Sugarbaker DJ (1999) Expression of the focal adhesion protein paxillin in lung cancer and its relation to cell motility. Oncogene 18:67–77.

Salgia RS, S. Hong, D.S. Ng, C.S. Frye, J. Janisch, L. Ratain, M.J. Kurzrock, R (2008) A phase I study of XL184, a RET, VEGFR2, and MET kinase inhibitor, in patients (pts) with advanced malignancies, including pts with medullary thyroid cancer (MTC). J Clin Oncol 26:2008 (May 20 suppl; abstr 3522).

Sattler M and Salgia R (2007) c-Met and hepatocyte growth factor: potential as novel targets in cancer therapy. Curr Oncol Rep 9:102–108.

Sattler M, Pride YB, Ma P, Gramlich JL, Chu SC, Quinnan LA, Shirazian S, Liang C, Podar K, Christensen JG, Salgia R (2003) A novel small molecule met inhibitor induces apoptosis in cells transformed by the oncogenic TPR-MET tyrosine kinase. Cancer Res 63:5462–5469.

Schaller MD and Sasaki T (1997) Differential signaling by the focal adhesion kinase and cell adhesion kinase beta. J Biol Chem 272:25319–25325.

Schmidt L, Duh FM, Chen F, Kishida T, Glenn G, Choyke P, Scherer SW, Zhuang Z, Lubensky I, Dean M, Allikmets R, Chidambaram A, Bergerheim UR, Feltis JT, Casadevall C, Zamarron A, Bernues M, Richard S, Lips CJ, Walther MM, Tsui LC, Geil L, Orcutt ML, Stackhouse T,

Lipan J, Slife L, Brauch H, Decker J, Niehans G, Hughson MD, Moch H, Storkel S, Lerman MI, Linehan WM, Zbar B (1997) Germline and somatic mutations in the tyrosine kinase domain of the MET proto-oncogene in papillary renal carcinomas. Nat Genet 16:68–73.

Schmidt L, Junker K, Weirich G, Glenn G, Choyke P, Lubensky I, Zhuang Z, Jeffers M, Vande Woude G, Neumann H, Walther M, Linehan WM, Zbar B (1998) Two North American families with hereditary papillary renal carcinoma and identical novel mutations in the MET proto-oncogene. Cancer Res 58:1719–1722.

Seki T, Hagiya M, Shimonishi M, Nakamura T, Shimizu S (1991) Organization of the human hepatocyte growth factor-encoding gene. Gene 102:213–219.

Sengupta S, Gherardi E, Sellers LA, Wood JM, Sasisekharan R, Fan TP (2003) Hepatocyte growth factor/scatter factor can induce angiogenesis independently of vascular endothelial growth factor. Arterioscler Thromb Vasc Biol 23:69–75.

Siddiqui SS, Loganathan S, Krishnaswamy S, Faoro L, Jagadeeswaran R, Salgia R (2008) C. elegans as a model organism for in vivo screening in cancer: effects of human c-Met in lung cancer affect C. elegans vulva phenotypes. Cancer Biol Ther 7.

Siegfried JM, Weissfeld LA, Singh-Kaw P, Weyant RJ, Testa JR, Landreneau RJ (1997) Association of immunoreactive hepatocyte growth factor with poor survival in resectable non-small cell lung cancer. Cancer Res 57:433–439.

Siegfried JM, Weissfeld LA, Luketich JD, Weyant RJ, Gubish CT, Landreneau RJ (1998) The clinical significance of hepatocyte growth factor for non-small cell lung cancer. Ann Thorac Surg 66:1915–1918.

Sugimura H, Nichols FC, Yang P, Allen MS, Cassivi SD, Deschamps C, Williams BA, Pairolero PC (2007) Survival after recurrent nonsmall-cell lung cancer after complete pulmonary resection. Ann Thorac Surg 83:409–417; discussion 417–408.

Takaishi K, Sasaki T, Kato M, Yamochi W, Kuroda S, Nakamura T, Takeichi M, Takai Y (1994) Involvement of Rho p21 small GTP-binding protein and its regulator in the HGF-induced cell motility. Oncogene 9:273–279.

Takanami I, Tanana F, Hashizume T, Kikuchi K, Yamamoto Y, Yamamoto T, Kodaira S (1996) Hepatocyte growth factor and c-Met/hepatocyte growth factor receptor in pulmonary adenocarcinomas: an evaluation of their expression as prognostic markers. Oncology 53: 392–397.

Tamagnone L and Comoglio PM (2000) Signalling by semaphorin receptors: cell guidance and beyond. Trends Cell Biol 10:377–383.

Tokunou M, Niki T, Eguchi K, Iba S, Tsuda H, Yamada T, Matsuno Y, Kondo H, Saitoh Y, Imamura H, Hirohashi S (2001) c-MET expression in myofibroblasts: role in autocrine activation and prognostic significance in lung adenocarcinoma. Am J Pathol 158:1451–1463.

Trusolino L, Serini G, Cecchini G, Besati C, Ambesi-Impiombato FS, Marchisio PC, De Filippi R (1998) Growth factor-dependent activation of alphavbeta3 integrin in normal epithelial cells: implications for tumor invasion. J Cell Biol 142:1145–1156.

Uemura N, Salgia R, Li JL, Pisick E, Sattler M, Griffin JD (1997) The BCR/ABL oncogene alters interaction of the adapter proteins CRKL and CRK with cellular proteins. Leukemia 11: 376–385.

Van Belle E, Witzenbichler B, Chen D, Silver M, Chang L, Schwall R, Isner JM (1998) Potentiated angiogenic effect of scatter factor/hepatocyte growth factor via induction of vascular endothelial growth factor: the case for paracrine amplification of angiogenesis. Circulation 97:381–390.

Webb CP, Hose CD, Koochekpour S, Jeffers M, Oskarsson M, Sausville E, Monks A, Vande Woude GF (2000) The geldanamycins are potent inhibitors of the hepatocyte growth factor/scatter factor-met-urokinase plasminogen activator-plasmin proteolytic network. Cancer Res 60: 342–349.

Wojta J, Kaun C, Breuss JM, Koshelnick Y, Beckmann R, Hattey E, Mildner M, Weninger W, Nakamura T, Tschachler E, Binder BR (1999) Hepatocyte growth factor increases expression of vascular endothelial growth factor and plasminogen activator inhibitor-1 in human keratinocytes and the vascular endothelial growth factor receptor flk-1 in human endothelial cells. Lab Invest 79:427–438.

Xiao GH, Jeffers M, Bellacosa A, Mitsuuchi Y, Vande Woude GF, Testa JR (2001) Anti-apoptotic signaling by hepatocyte growth factor/Met via the phosphatidylinositol 3-kinase/Akt and mitogen-activated protein kinase pathways. Proc Natl Acad Sci U S A 98: 247–252.

Zeng ZJ, Yang LY, Ding X, Wang W (2004) Expressions of cysteine-rich61, connective tissue growth factor and Nov genes in hepatocellular carcinoma and their clinical significance. World J Gastroenterol 10:3414–3418.

Zhang YW, Su Y, Volpert OV, Vande Woude GF (2003) Hepatocyte growth factor/scatter factor mediates angiogenesis through positive VEGF and negative thrombospondin 1 regulation. Proc Natl Acad Sci U S A 100:12718–12723.

Zhuang Z, Park WS, Pack S, Schmidt L, Vortmeyer AO, Pak E, Pham T, Weil RJ, Candidus S, Lubensky IA, Linehan WM, Zbar B, Weirich G (1998) Trisomy 7-harbouring non-random duplication of the mutant MET allele in hereditary papillary renal carcinomas. Nat Genet 20:66–69.

Chapter 13
Contribution of ADAMs and ADAMTSs to Tumor Expansion and Metastasis

Antoni Xavier Torres-Collado and M. Luisa Iruela-Arispe

Cast of Characters

Inactivating mutations in extracellular protease-encoding genes are a recent and somewhat surprising finding, since these enzymes were long believed to be promoting tumor cell detachment and invasion. However, in recent years several inhibitory roles in cancer progression have been attributed to matrix metalloproteinases and also members of the adamalysin family. In a recent comprehensive genetic screen of breast and colorectal cancer mutations, loss-of-function mutations were found in ADAM12 (Dyczynska et al. 2008), ADAMTS15, and ADAMTS18 (Sjöblom et al. 2006). Additionally, local copy number alterations involving deletions of ADAMTS20 were detected in glioblastoma multiforme (Cancer Genome Atlas Research Network 2008), and ADAM23, a possible tumor suppressor gene, is frequently silenced in gastric cancers by homozygous deletion or aberrant promoter hypermethylation (Takada et al. 2005). The mechanisms underlying the involvement of ADAM and ADAMTS proteins in tumor progression are reviewed below.

Introduction

Tumor expansion requires invasion of surrounding stroma, which is frequently associated with destruction of parenchyma and remodeling of the extracellular matrix. The process is greatly assisted by the catalytic activity of extracellular proteases which facilitate migration, mediate release of matrix-bound growth factors, and expose cryptic matrix sites for adhesion (Fig. 13.1). Thus it is intuitive to predict that extracellular proteases participate in the process of tumor expansion and metastatic spread, but in addition, they also partake in the regulation of tumor angiogenesis and in the process of immunological surveillance. Therefore, their net contribution to the process of tumorigenesis is broad and continuous.

M.L. Iruela-Arispe (✉)
Biomedical Research Building, UCLA, 615 Charles E. Young Drive South,
Los Angeles, CA, USA
e-mail: arispe@mbi.ucla.edu

A. Thomas-Tikhonenko (ed.), *Cancer Genome and Tumor Microenvironment*,
DOI 10.1007/978-1-4419-0711-0_13, © Springer Science+Business Media, LLC 2010

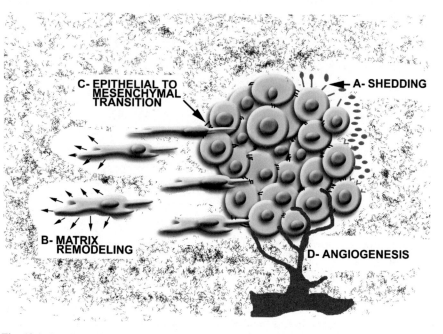

Fig. 13.1 Possible effects of ADAMs and ADAMTSs in cancer. Our understanding of the contribution of adamalysins to cancer progression and metastasis has expanded significantly in the last 5 years. These proteases provide both pro- and anti-tumor effects depending on the availability of substrates and on the dependency of these substrates for tumor growth. A – ADAMs promote shedding of a large number of membrane-anchored proteins, including growth factors. Consequently, ADAM-mediated activation of growth factors can increase signaling of cell surface receptors and enhance tumor cell proliferation. B – ADAMs and ADAMTSs are involved in the proteolytic remodeling of signaling molecules and in the release of growth factors from extracellular stores. C – Metastatic events and epithelial-to-mesenchymal transitions can be facilitated by adamalysins through cleavage of cell–cell adhesion molecules (e.g., E-cadherin). D – ADAM and ADAMTSs also modulate angiogenesis in a positive and negative manner

Approximately 2% of human genes code for proteases or protease inhibitors, representing a wide range of possible therapeutic targets for tumors and other pathologies (Overall and Kleifeld 2006; Turk 2006). The difficulty in therapeutic exploration has resided in the complex nature of the biological functions performed by these proteases, many involved in homeostatic physiology of tissues and the overlapping nature of their catalytic activities.

Proteases are frequently classified based on their enzymatic properties and include aspartic, metallo, cysteine, serine, and threonine proteases. Matrix metalloproteases (MMPs) have been without doubt a major focus of study in cancer biology. The family comprises two major groups: matrix metalloproteinases (MMPs) and adamalysins (ADAMs and ADAMTSs). The implication of MMPs in cancer progression has been extensively and elegantly reviewed (Egeblad and Werb 2002; Overall and Lopez-Otin 2002; Fingleton 2006; Overall and

Kleifeld 2006; Lopez-Otin and Matrisian 2007; Page-McCaw et al. 2007). This chapter will focus on a second, rapidly emerging group of extracellular enzymes: the adamalysins. Many of these enzymes have been identified and cloned only in the last 5 years, and yet, they have quickly become recognized as significant contributors to cancer progression and metastasis. Here, we will first provide a general overview of their molecular features and biological activities and will subsequently summarize the body of literature associated with ADAMs/ADAMTSs in cancer.

Adamalysins: ADAM and ADAMTS Proteases

The adamalysins comprise a group of extracellular enzymes with structural features that include disintegrin and metalloprotease domains. Two major subgroups of proteases are included in the adamalysin family: the membrane-anchored ADAMs (*A Disintegrin And Metalloprotease*) and the secreted ADAMTSs (*A Disintegrin And Metalloprotease with Thrombospondin repeats*). The presence of a zinc-dependent metalloprotease domain places these enzymes within the superfamily of metzincins that also includes matrixins (MMPs), astacins, and serralisins (Kaushal and Shah 2000). Adamalysins also display structural features (disintegrin domains) similar to the reprolysin family of snake venomases. However, the disintegrin domain of ADAMs and ADAMTSs does not appear to display functional analogy to that of snake venom proteases; that is, this region does not compete with endogenous matrix proteins for biding to integrins. In some circumstances, however, ADAMs and ADAMTSs have been shown to support binding and spreading of cells in an integrin-dependent manner. Adamalysins also interact with several extracellular proteins in the absence of catalysis and thus, participate in the formation, rather than in the destruction of the extracellular matrix. Although at first face this appears paradoxical, the activity of adamalysins is under tight regulatory control and their presence in the extracellular milieu does not necessarily translate into proteolytic activity.

The ADAM family of proteinases includes 38 distinct membrane-anchored proteins with multiple roles in cell–cell and/or cell–matrix interactions, in addition to their anticipated functions in processing and/or degradation of substrates (Wolfsberg et al. 1995a, 1995b; Primakoff and Myles 2000; Seals and Courtneidge 2003; Rocks et al. 2008). Members of this family have a unique structural organization including prodomain, metalloprotease, disintegrin-like, cysteine-rich, epidermal growth factor-like, transmembrane, and cytoplasmatic domains (Fig. 13.2).

ADAMTS comprises the secreted arm of the adamalysin family. The 19 members of this group display the same domain structure as ADAMs except for the transmembrane region. In addition, ADAMTSs show a variable number of thrombospondin (TSR) repeats in the C-terminal half of the protein. The TSR domains facilitate interaction with the extracellular matrix and, in some cases, convey independent functions once cleaved from the parental protein (Kuno and Matsushima 1998; Rodriguez-Manzaneque et al. 2000; Tang 2001; Luque et al. 2003; Lee et al. 2006).

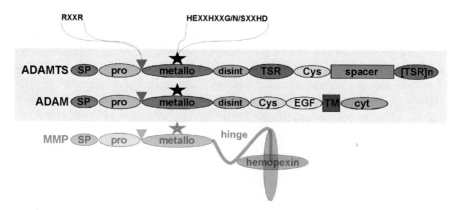

Fig. 13.2 Modular structure displayed by ADAMTS, ADAM, and MMPs. Red arrowhead represents the consensus furin-recognition site and the star the consensus sequence for the zinc motif in the catalytic domain. SP, signal peptide; pro, prodomain; metallo, matalloproteinase domain; disint, disintegrin-like domain; TSR, thrombospondin repeats; spacer, spacer region; Cys, cysteine-rich region; EGF, epidermal growth factor-like domain; TM, transmembrane region; cyt, cytoplasmatic tail; hinge, hinge region; hemopexin, hemopexin domain

Prototypical Structure of ADAMs and ADAMTS

All adamalysins have a signal peptide sequence (SP) that directs them to the secretory pathway. The SP is followed by a prodomain that keeps the enzyme in a zymogen state (latent). Removal of this region through proteolytic processing is generally mediated extracellularly by another enzyme and unveils the catalytic function of the adamalysins. Most adamalysins also have a furin-recognition site (RXXR sequence) that is targeted by furin-like proprotein convertases in the secretory pathway and that participates in the intracellular activation of some ADAMS (ADAMS9, 12, 15, and 17). The catalytic domain, also known as the metalloprotease domain, contains a zinc motif (HEXXHXXG/N/SXXHD) typical of reprolysins and a methionine in the sequence V/IMA/S, or "Met-turn," under the third histidine that facilitates the interaction with zinc.

The disintegrin domain follows the metalloprotease domain. While in snake venom proteases this domain binds to integrins through an RGD motif (Perutelli 1995), in adamalysins the disintegrin domain is frequently folded and not available for binding to cells (Takeda et al. 2006), but in some cases, other regions of the molecule might contain RGD repeats and interact with integrins. This domain is followed by a cysteine-rich region of unclear function.

The carboxy terminal half of ADAMs includes EGF-like structural domains, a transmembrane region and a cytoplasmic tail with SH3 binding sequences, and a variable number of phosphorylation sites indicative of signaling functions. Figure 13.2 shows the structural features of ADAMs in comparison to that of ADAMTSs and MMPs.

As mentioned previously, ADAMTSs lack the transmembrane region and the signaling features present in the intracellular domain of ADAM proteases; instead, they exhibit a spacer region followed by a variable number of TSR repeats. The number of TSR domains can range from none (e.g., ADAMTS4) to 14 (e.g., ADAMTS20 and the longer isoform of ADAMTS9) (Tortorella et al. 1999; Llamazares et al. 2003; Somerville et al. 2003). These domains interact with a variety of proteins that participate either as cofactors in their catalytic activity or facilitate the interaction of these molecules with the extracellular matrix (Kuno and Matsushima 1998; Rodriguez-Manzaneque et al. 2000; Lee et al. 2005; Torres-Collado et al. 2006). In addition, some members of the ADAMTS family have one or two additional C-terminal motifs such as mucin domains (e.g., ADAMTS7 and 12), GON domains (ADAMTS9 and 20), CUB domains (e.g., ADAMTS13), and/or PLAC domains (e.g., ADAMTS2, 3, 10, 12, 14, 17, and 19).

Contributions of ADAMs to Tumor Growth and Metastasis

ADAMs participate in diverse biological processes that range from fertilization (Eto et al. 2002) to adipogenesis (Masaki et al. 2005). This is not surprising considering their multidomain structure and their wide range of expression patterns during development and in the adult. Under pathological settings, however, ADAMs are better known for their function as inducible shedasses, that is, enzymes that mediate cleavage of cell surface proteins. In particular, ADAM17, also known as TACE (*T*NF-*a*lpha *C*onverting *E*nzyme), promotes the shedding and activation of many growth factors including TNF-alpha, TGF-alpha, and HB-EGF (Black et al. 1997; Moss et al. 1997; Sahin et al. 2004) and receptors such as Notch1 (Qi et al. 1999). Furthermore, ADAMs also mediate cleavage of cell–cell adhesion molecules and basement membrane proteins including type IV collagen, both critical events in the epithelial–mesenchymal transition of invasive carcinomas. Thus, it is not surprising that the academic and private sector have invested significant efforts to elucidate the specific contributions of ADAMs in tumor growth and metastatic events. Here, we will take a systematic analysis and summarize the current information available for ADAMs in cancer biology. Table 13.1 also provides a current overview of the expression of ADAMs and ADAMTSs in tumors.

No reports to date have indicated expression or function of ADAMs 1–7 in cancer. In contrast, ADAM8, also known as CD156, has been identified in various tumors including lung and renal carcinoma and its expression has been validated as a metastatic prognostic marker for renal cancer (Roemer et al. 2004). In agreement with these findings, ectopic expression of ADAM8 increased the migratory capability of tumor cells (Ishikawa et al. 2004) and therefore it might play a role in promoting invasion and metastasis. Additional studies have also found upregulation of ADAM8 and ADAM19 in primary brain tumors (astrocytomas). This increase was correlated with higher catalytic activity and invasiveness (Wildeboer et al. 2006).

ADAM9 protein levels were found increased in breast carcinoma when compared to normal tissue, and it also exhibited a positive correlation with levels of

Table 13.1 Expression of adamalysins in tumors, known substrates, and possible functions

Enzyme	Substrates	Natural inhibitors	Tumor type	Function/expression	Reference
ADAM8	CD23	NR	Lung carcinoma	Pro-migratory/higher expression in tumor compared to control	Ishikawa et al. (2004)
			Renal cell carcinoma	NR/higher expression in tumor compared to control	Roemer et al. (2004)
			Brain carcinoma	Pro-invasive/higher expression in tumor compared to control	Wildeboer et al. (2006)
ADAM9	HB-EGF, TNF-p75, APP, fibronectin, gelatin, c-kit, insulin β-chain, laminin	NR	Renal carcinoma	NR/higher expression in tumor compared to normal adjacent tissue	Fritzsche et al. (2008)
			Hepatic carcinoma and metastasis	NR/higher expression in tumor compared to normal tissue	Le Pabic et al. (2003), Tannapfel et al. (2003), Mazzocca et al. (2005)
			Gastric carcinoma	Pro-invasive/higher expression in tumor compared to normal tissue	Carl-McGrath et al. (2005)
			Melanoma	Proliferation/higher expression in tumor compared to normal tissue	Zigrino et al. (2005)
			Pancreatic carcinoma	NR/higher expression in tumor compared to normal tissue	Grützmann et al. (2003, 2004)
			Breast carcinoma	NR/higher expression in tumor compared to normal tissue	O'Shea et al. (2003)
			Prostate carcinoma	NR/higher expression in tumor compared to normal tissue	Karan et al. (2003)
ADAM10	L1	TIMP-1	Oral squamos cell carcinoma	Proliferative/higher expression in tumor compared to normal tissue	Ko et al. (2007)
			Uterine and ovarian carcinoma	Pro-migratory/higher expression in tumor compared to normal tissue	Fogel et al. (2003)
			Colorectal carcinoma	Pro-migratory, proliferative/ADAM10 expressed in invasive front of human colorectal tumors	Gavert et al. (2005)

ADAM	Substrate	Inhibitor	Tumor type	Expression	References
			Prostate carcinoma	NR/ADAM-10 protein was predominantly membrane bound in benign glands but showed marked nuclear localization in cancer cells	McCulloch et al. (2004)
ADAM12	HB-EGF	TIMP-3		NR/higher expression in tumor compared to normal tissue	Karan et al. (2003)
			Hepatic carcinoma	NR/higher expression in tumor compared to normal tissue	Le Pabic et al. (2003)
			Glioblastoma	Proliferative/higher expression in tumor compared to normal tissue	Kodama et al. (2004)
			Breast carcinoma	NR/higher expression in tumor compared to normal samples	Roy et al. (2004)
				Anti-proliferative/higher expression in tumor compared to normal tissues	Lendeckel et al. (2005)
			Gastric carcinoma	Anti-proliferative/higher expression in tumor compared to normal tissues	Carl-McGrath et al. (2005)
			NSCLC	NR/higher expression in tumor compared to normal tissue	Rocks et al. (2006)
ADAM15	Collagen IV and gelatin	NR	Prostate carcinoma	NR/higher expression in tumor compared to normal tissue	Kuefer et al. (2006)
			Breast carcinoma	Proliferative/higher expression in tumor compared to normal tissues	Lendeckel et al. (2005), Kuefer et al. (2006)
			Gastric carcinoma	Proliferative/higher expression in tumor compared to normal tissue	Carl-McGrath et al. (2005)
			Lung carcinoma	NR/higher expression in tumor compared to normal tissue	Schutz et al. (2005)
ADAM17	TNF-α, TGF-β, TNF-p75R, ErbB4, TRANCE, APP, Notch, L-selectin, CD44.	TIMP-2	Oral squamous carcinoma	NR/higher expression in tumor compared to normal tissue	Takamune et al. (2007)
			Breast carcinoma	Proliferative/higher expression in tumor compared to normal tissues	Lendeckel et al. (2005)

(continued)

300 A.X. Torres-Collado and M.L. Iruela-Arispe

Table 13.1 (continued)

Enzyme	Substrates	Natural inhibitors	Tumor type	Function/expression	Reference
			Ovarian carcinoma	NR/higher expression in tumor compared to normal tissue	Takada et al. (2005)
			Colon carcinoma	NR/higher expression in tumor compared to normal tissue	Blanchot-Jossic et al. (2005)
			Prostate carcinoma	NR/higher expression in tumor compared to normal tissue	Karan et al. (2003)
			Renal carcinoma	NR/higher expression in tumor compared to normal tissue	Roemer et al. (2004)
ADAM19	Neuregulin	NR	Brain carcinoma	Invasiveness/higher expression in tumor compared to normal tissue	Wildeboer et al. (2006)
			Renal carcinoma	NR/higher expression in tumor compared to normal tissue	Roemer et al. (2004)
ADAM23	Catalytically inactive NR		Breast carcinoma	NR/reduced in comparison with controls	Costa et al. (2004)
			Gastric carcinoma	NR/reduced in comparison with controls	Takada et al. (2005)
ADAM28	IGFBP-3	TIMP-3	Non-small cell carcinoma	NR/higher expression in tumor compared to normal tissue	Ohtsuka et al. (2006)
			Breast carcinoma	Proliferative/higher expression in tumor compared to normal tissue	Mitsui et al. (2006)

	Substrates	Inhibitor	Tumor type	Description	Reference
ADAMTS1	Agrecan, versican, Nidogen, thrombospondin, TFPI-2, HB-EGF, Amphiregulin	TIMP-3	Pancreatic carcinoma	Local invasion and lymph node metastasis/ higher expression of METH-1 showed significantly severe lymph node metastasis	Masui et al. (2001)
			Breast carcinoma	NR/reduced in comparison with controls	Porter et al. (2004)
			NSCLC	NR/reduced in comparison with controls	Rocks et al. (2006)
			Bone metastasis	NR/present in bone metastatic cells compared with non metastatic	Kang et al. (2003)
ADAMTS4	Agrecan, brevican, versican	TIMP-3	Glioblastoma	Increased invasive potential, brevican degradation/higher expression in tumor compared to control	Held-Feindt et al. (2006)
ADAMTS5	Agrecan, brevican	TIMP-3	Glioblastoma	Increased invasive potential, brevican degradation/higher expression in tumor compared to control	Nakada et al. (2005), Held-Feindt et al. (2006)
ADAMTS9	Agrecan, versican	NR	Nasopharyngeal carcinoma	NR/downregulated	Lo et al. (2007); Lung et al. (2008)

NR – Not reported

the oncoprotein HER2/neu (O'Shea et al. 2003). Also documented in the literature is a direct association between poor prognosis and levels of ADAM9 for pancreatic ductal carcinoma and renal cancer (Grützmann et al. 2003, 2004; Fritzsche et al. 2008). Enhanced expression of ADAM9 was also noted in metastatic renal cancer (Fritzsche et al. 2008). Another study using protein arrays found overexpression of ADAM9 in liver carcinomas when compared with normal liver tissue (Tannapfel et al. 2003). Interestingly, a soluble alternative splicing isoform of this protein is synthesized by activated stellate cells in the liver. This isoform has the ability to bind to α6β4 integrin on the surface of colon carcinoma cells, increasing their invasiveness in a manner that requires metalloproteinase activity (Mazzocca et al. 2005). While the fragment of ADAM9 lacks catalytic activity, additional studies have found that MMP2 is increased in colon metastasis from liver tumors when both ADAM9 and ADAM12 were expressed by stromal cells (Le Pabic et al. 2003). At this point, the relationship between ADAM9/12 and expression of MMP2 is unclear; but matrix metalloproteinases have been shown to frequently act in molecular cascades, imposing domino effects of sequential activations (Page-McCaw et al. 2007). Another link between ADAM9 and metastasis has been documented in lung. Both transcripts and protein for ADAM9 were increased in ECB-1 lung cancer cell lines with tropism for bone (Shintani et al. 2004). Furthermore, overexpression of ADAM9 in A549 lung cancer cells increases adhesion to brain tissue and the potential to induce brain metastasis when injected intravenously (Shintani et al. 2004). The mechanisms that regulate these pro-metastatic events are unclear; however, ADAM9 is known to cleave fibronectin and denatured collagen (Millichip et al. 1998; Roy et al. 2004) and also promote the shedding of HB-EGF and TNF-p75 receptors (Izumi et al. 1998), functions likely relevant to tumor invasion and spreading. In prostate cancer, expression of ADAM9 is regulated by 5alpha-dihydrotestosterone, insulin-like growth factor I, and epidermal growth factor (Shigemura et al. 2007).

ADAM10, also known as kuzbanian, is well known for its ability to cleave Notch1 and therefore participate in its activation (Qi et al. 1999). It is not surprising that ADAM10 has been found increased in leukemias, a tumor type where Notch1 deregulation is a direct contributor. In addition, overexpression of ADAM10 has been reported in multiple tumors (McCulloch et al. 2004). In oral squamous cell carcinoma, high levels of ADAM10 directly correlate with increase in APP, one of its substrates (Ko et al. 2007). ADAM10 expression in uterine and ovarian carcinomas has been directly linked to circulating serum levels of L1 and high risk of progression (Fogel et al. 2003). The same substrate is also apparently cleaved in the invasive front of colorectal cancers by ADAM10 (Gavert et al. 2005). L1 is a cell–cell adhesion molecule, member of the immunoglobulin superfamily that is also involved in the motility and invasion of lymphoma, lung carcinoma, and melanoma, cells where ADAM10 is frequently expressed (Gutwein et al. 2000; Mechtersheimer et al. 2001). Interestingly, ADAM9, 10, 12, and 15 were found to be overexpressed after gastric cell infection by *Helicobacter pylori*, suggesting a possible link between *H. pylori*-induced inflammation and gastric cancer (Cox et al. 2001; Yoshimura et al. 2002; Carl-McGrath et al. 2005). Considering that ADAM10 participates in the shedding of EGFR ligand, it is likely that ADAM10 mediates increased epithelial proliferation post-infection through enhanced EGFR activation. ADAM10 also contributes to E-cadherin and VE-cadherin shedding (Ito et al. 1999; Maretzky et al. 2005; Schulz et al. 2008). E-cadherins are homotypic cell–cell adhesion molecules present in epithelial cells that must be removed or downregulated during the process of invasion and epithelial-to-mesenchymal transitions. Therefore, expression of ADAM10 in carcinomas greatly facilitates the process of invasion and proliferation through the release of beta-catenin and consequent increase in cyclin D1 (Shtutman et al. 1999). It is extremely likely that these events are physiologically relevant, as genetic inactivation of ADAM10 results in growth arrest, apoptosis, and overexpression of full length E-cadherin (Maretzky et al. 2005).

In view of its role in pro-HB-EGF processing and activation, it is not surprising that ADAM12, also known as meltrin, has been found increased in a large number of tumors (Roy et al. 2004, Dyczynska et al. 2008). ADAM12 can be alternatively spliced into a secreted form where it facilitates activation of HB-EGF receptors in adjacent cells, both forms have been found increased in a large number of tumors including breast, brain, colon, and liver. Blockade of ADAM12 function by synthetic inhibitors in glioblastoma directly decreased the production of mature HB-EGF, suggesting that the link between ADAM12-HB-EGF might be of high relevance for tumor expansion (Kodama et al. 2004). Interestingly, the cysteine-rich domain of ADAM12 has been shown to support adhesion via syndecans which initiates signaling events leading to beta1 integrin activation, cell spreading, and consequent tumor expansion (Iba et al. 1999). Presence of ADAM12 in urine directly correlates with progression of breast carcinoma (Roy et al. 2004). In a recent comprehensive genetic screen of breast cancer mutations, three somatic inhibitory mutations were found in ADAM12. The mutations generate a protein that behaved in a dominant-negative manner, but it is unclear and unlikely that these are initiating transforming mutations (Dyczynska et al. 2008).

ADAM15 was found to be overexpressed in lung carcinomas, but without correlation with tumor stage or differentiation status, although higher expression was noted at the invasion front of several carcinomas (Schutz et al. 2005). Subsequent studies found that the protease was increased in malignant tumors where the highest levels of expression corresponded to adenocarcinomas of prostate and breast (Kuefer et al. 2006). ADAM15 was also implicated in metastasis of stomach and lung cancer. Interestingly, treatment of breast carcinoma cells with anti-ADAM15 antibodies efficiently reduced tumor growth (Lendeckel et al. 2005). Consistent with these findings, inactivation of ADAM15 in a prostate cancer model directly reduced tumorigenicity and inhibition of tumor cell migration. Moreover, downregulation of ADAM15 leads to inhibition of N-cadherin proteolysis and attenuation in CD44, αv, and MMP9 levels. N-cadherin and CD44 are known substrates for the protease; however, the link between ADAM15 and αv integrin and ADAM15 and MMP9 is unclear. Interestingly ADAM15 contains an RGD sequence and directly interacts with both αvβ3 and α5β1, perhaps in a manner that facilitates spreading of tumor cells (Zhang et al. 1998; Nath et al. 1999). ADAM15 also impacts angiogenesis presenting a paradoxical question to its overall effects in tumor growth. ADAM15 is expressed by activated endothelial cells and smooth muscle cells (Herren et al. 1997) and in vitro, it suppresses endothelial cell migration (Najy et al. 2008). More importantly, in vivo, the recombinant disintegrin domain (RDD) of ADAM15 inhibits angiogenesis and tumor growth (Trochon-Joseph et al. 2004). In support of these findings angiogenesis was significantly attenuated in ADAM15-deficient mice that were induced to develop retinopathy (Horiuchi et al. 2003)

ADAM17, also known as TACE, is by far the most studied of all the ADAM proteases. ADAM17 has been reported to cleave a variety of substrates, including TGFα, TGF-beta, TNF-p75 receptor, ErbB4, TRANCE, Notch, L-selectin, CD44, and HB-EGF (Gschwind et al. 2003; Ongusaha et al. 2004; Schafer et al. 2004; Blobel 2005; Zhang et al. 2006; Sahin and Blobel 2007). Many, if not all of these substrates, are involved in tumor invasion and growth (Borrell-Pages et al. 2003; Tanaka et al. 2005). For example, in ovarian cancer there is a direct correlation between levels of HB-EGF and expression of ADAM17. Moreover, the levels of the growth factor correlate with cancer prognosis (Tanaka et al. 2005). There is also strong correlation between EGFR and ADAM17 overexpression in colon carcinoma independently of tumor stage and differentiation (Blanchot-Jossic et al. 2005). In oral squamous cell carcinoma, presence of ADAM17 has been associated with cleavage of CD44 and metastasis (Takamune et al. 2007). ADAM17 was upregulated in a hypoxia-induced glioma invasion model and its pharmacological inactivation effectively blocked tumor cell invasion (Zheng et al. 2007). More importantly, inhibition in ADAM17-mediated shedding by either targeting the protein or its activity significantly reduces the size of tumors in xenograft assays, suggesting that ADAM17 is a relevant therapeutic target, particularly in those tumors that are driven by Erb2 activation (Borrell-Pages et al. 2003). Interestingly, in many circumstances, an inverse correlation was observed between the levels of ADAM17 and those of TIMP-3, its endogenous inhibitor, giving to the expression of the protease a prominent role in the pathogenesis of these cancers (Karan et al. 2003).

Although with the same prototypical structure as the other ADAMs, ADAM23 is an inactive metalloprotease. Through its disintegrin domain, it promotes cell adhesion and supports spreading. Binding is mediated by the integrin $\alpha v\beta 3$ in an RGD-independent manner (Sagane et al. 1998; Cal et al. 2000). Little is known about the role of ADAM23 in development and disease; however, its promoter appears to be frequently targeted for methylation. ADAM23 was silenced by methylation in a panel of breast carcinoma primary tumors and in several brain cell lines and is frequently methylated or deleted in gastric carcinomas (Takada et al. 2005). The investigators reported that primary tumors with a higher grade presented higher percentage of methylation in the 5′ upstream region of ADAM23 (Costa et al. 2004).

ADAM28 has been frequently found to be upregulated in lung cancer. Particularly, in non-small cell carcinoma, overexpression of membrane-anchored and soluble forms of ADAM28 displayed a positive correlation with tumor growth and lymph node metastasis (Ohtsuka et al. 2006). In the case of breast carcinoma, ADAM28 participates in the cleavage of insulin-like growth factor-binding protein 3 (IGBP-3) that accelerates tumor cell growth. Suppression of ADAM28 levels by iRNA reduces proliferation of breast cancer cell lines, supposedly through an IGBP-3-dependent mechanism (Mitsui et al. 2006).

ADAMTS and Tumor Progression

The first member of the ADAMTS family was identified in a screen for transcripts that were increased in murine cachexic colon adenocarcinomas (Kuno et al. 1997). Shortly thereafter, the human ADAMTS1 gene was cloned in a search for genes that contained the anti-angiogenic domain present in thrombospondin-1 (Vázquez et al. 1999). In the last decade 19 members of the ADAMTS family have been identified, all displaying similar domain structure, but exhibiting pleiotropic roles in development, homeostasis, and pathology. Here we have summarized the information pertinent to cancer biology.

ADAMTS1 behaves similarly to an early response gene and it is quickly upregulated during inflammation and other pathological insults, possibly through the regulatory control of TNF and IL1beta (Kalinski et al. 2007). Thus, it is not surprising to find the gene product increased in a variety of cancers. In particular, ADAMTS1 was found in breast, pancreatic, lung, colon, renal, and liver cancer, some of these with elevated metastatic activity (Masui et al. 2001; Kang et al. 2003; Kuno et al. 2004; Lind et al. 2006; Liu et al. 2006; Grigo et al. 2008). However, its specific contributions to tumor progression have not been fully elucidated. In pancreatic cancers, increased transcripts for ADAMTS1 were found to correlate with severe lymph node metastasis and retroperitoneal invasion and in fact, overall levels of ADAMTS1 were considered to be poor prognostic indicators in this tumor type (Masui et al. 2001). Nevertheless, other groups have also found that ADAMTS1 transcripts were decreased in breast carcinoma samples and in small cell lung carcinoma compared with normal tissue (Porter et al. 2004; Rocks et al. 2006). It is unclear how these studies compare in cancer stage and inflammatory cell infiltrate with previous published work. However, recent reports have indicated that ADAMTS1 might display multiple effects in different tumor cell compartments providing both pro- and anti-tumor growth activities.

Like other members of the family, the modular structure of ADAMTS1 is prone to multiple cell and protein interactions. Thus, while its metalloprotease domain promotes tumor growth and facilitates invasion, its C-terminal region including the spacer domain and the TSP repeats displays anti-tumoral and anti-metastatic effects through suppression of angiogenesis and sequestration of heparin-binding growth factors (Iruela-Arispe et al. 2003; Kuno et al. 2004; Lee et al. 2006; Liu et al. 2006).

Much of the pro-tumorigenic effect attributed to ADAMTS1 relies on its catalytic activity. ADAMTS1 was initially found to cleave aggrecan, versican, nidogen, and thrombospondin1 facilitating matrix remodeling and invasion (Kuno et al. 2000; Sandy et al. 2001; Rodriguez-Manzaneque et al. 2002; Canals et al. 2006; Lee et al. 2006). More recently, however, the protease has been noted to promote shedding of HB-EGF and amphiregulin with subsequent activation of EGF and

ErbB-2 receptors. The effect required enzymatic activity, as it was not found with catalytically inactive mutant protein (Liu et al. 2006). Thus, tumors in which growth is dependent on EGF receptors might benefit from increased expression of ADAMTS1. In fact, Massagué and colleagues identified ADAMTS1 as a significantly upregulated transcript in a subpopulation of breast tumor cells that successfully metastasized to the lung (Kang et al. 2003). Additional experiments will be required to ensure that increased EGF-mediated signaling is promoted by increased expression of ADAMTS1, but overall this prediction can explain the positive and negative associations of ADAMTS1 with tumor expansion.

The effects of ADAMTS1 in the suppression of angiogenesis were initially thought to rely entirely on the presence of three TSR repeats in the C-terminal region that harbor the anti-angiogenic motif identified in thrombospondin1 (Vazquez et al. 1999). In fact, structure–function analysis using this region was found to inhibit tumor growth via an anti-angiogenic activity that involved both suppression of endothelial cell proliferation and migration (Iruela-Arispe et al. 2003; Luque et al. 2003; Kuno et al. 2004). The C-terminal domain of ADAMTS1 was shown to bind and sequester VEGF165, impacting VEGF bioavailability with consequences to receptor phosphorylation, endothelial proliferation, and angiogenesis (Luque et al. 2003). Furthermore, it was recently reported that the catalytic activity of ADAMTS1 might also contribute to its angiostatic properties. Specifically, ADAMTS1 cleaves both throbospondin1 and 2 releasing anti-angiogenic peptides (Lee et al. 2006). In the absence of thrombospondin1, the vascular suppressive effect of ADAMTS1 in wound healing is attenuated (Lee et al. 2006). Supporting a role for ADAMTS1 as an endogenous inhibitor of angiogenesis, evaluation of the *adamts1*-null mouse revealed an increased capillary density in the ovary, a site of constitutive ADAMTS1 expression (Shozu et al. 2005).

In addition, aberrant methylation of the ADAMTS1 promoter has been reported in both non-small cell carcinoma and colorectal cancer (Lind et al. 2006; Choi et al. 2008). The relevance of hypermethylation is unclear at this point, but downregulation of ADAMTS1 in over 30% of lung cancer specimens has been attributed to this epigenetic modification (Choi et al. 2008).

ADAMTS4 and ADAMTS5 are upregulated in brain tumors, particularly glioblastoma (Nakada et al. 2005; Held-Feindt et al. 2006). Both proteases target and degrade secreted proteoglycans. Degradation of brevican, in particular, has been implicated in the process of tumor growth and invasion by glioblastoma cells (Nakada et al. 2005). Several growth factors contribute to the increase of these proteases in tumors. Specifically, TGFβ induces ADAMTS4, while interleukin-1 has been shown to increase ADAMTS5 in brain cancer (Held-Feindt et al. 2006).

Similar to ADAMTS1, ADAMTS8 also displays anti-angiogenic functions (Vázquez et al. 1999) and it was found decreased in brain, lung, pancreatic, and hepatocellular carcinoma (Masui et al. 2001; Dunn et al. 2004). Using dual-channel microarray analysis, ADAMTS8 was noted under-represented in 85% of non-small cell carcinomas, quite a significant number to be a random event (Dunn et al. 2004). Subsequently, it was reported that most of this suppression was due to hypermethylation of the ADAMTS8 promoter (Dunn et al. 2006).

ADAMTS9 is downregulated or absent in 73.9% of lymph metastasis from nasopharyngeal carcinoma, compared to higher expression in 32.6% found in primary tumors (Lung et al. 2008). Overexpression of the protease in cell lines resulted in reduction of tumor colony formation and growth (Lung et al. 2008). Similar findings were noted with esophageal squamous carcinoma (Lo et al. 2007). Using unbiased microcell-mediated chromosome transfer, ADAMTS9 was independently found to be critical for tumor suppression in this cancer type (Lo et al. 2007). The gene is silenced by promoter hypermethylation in esophageal carcinoma and de-repression of methylation results in tumor reduction (Lo et al. 2007). Together these findings have indicated that ADAMTS9 functions as a tumor suppressor gene with unknown mechanism.

Hypermethylation seems to also target and silence the ADAMTS18 promoter in several carcinomas (Jin et al. 2007). Moreover, ectopic expression of the protease led to a significant inhibition of both anchorage-dependent and anchorage-independent growth of carcinomas that originally lacked ADAMTS18 expression (Jin et al. 2007). Inactivating mutations in ADAMTS15 and 18 were also found in colorectal and breast tumor specimens (Sjoblom et al. 2006).

Conclusions

We have reviewed the structure of ADAMs and ADAMTSs and provided an updated summary of their contributions in tumor progression and metastasis. Metastatic events require the departure of tumor cells from the primary tumor mass, transit frequently through the bloodstream, and de novo settling in a new environment. The prominent contribution of ADAM and ADAMTS proteases in this process has been highlighted in many specific tumor types. It is anticipated that tumor expansion and invasion would be associated with degradation of the extracellular stroma, and therefore, presence of proteases is expected to mediate pro-tumorigenic events. However, the fact that proteases modulate tumor angiogenesis in a negative manner makes the interpretation of the expression data significantly more complex. In recent years several inhibitory roles in cancer progression have been attributed to MMPs, and it appears that a similar picture is emerging in the adamalysin family (Lopez-Otin and Matrisian 2007; Martin and Matrisian 2007). Particularly, in the case of ADAMTSs, it seems that many of these enzymes are either repressed through hypermethylation or mutated, suggesting more prominent roles in tumor suppression than tumor promotion. For example, both pro- and anti-tumor effects have been reported for ADAMTS1 with equally compelling experimental evidence, indicating that the final outcome of this enzyme in tumors is likely to be tumor specific and dependent on the microenvironmental factors particular to a tissue setting. Additional functional explorations of the proteolytic profile of adamalysins will likely shed light toward building comprehensive frameworks to better understand the net pro- and anti-tumorigenic activities of these enzymes.

References

Black RA, Rauch CT, Kozlosky CJ, Peschon JJ, Slack JL, Wolfson MF, Castner BJ, Stocking KL, Reddy P, Srinivasan S, Nelson N, Boiani N, Schooley KA, Gerhart M, Davis R, Fitzner JN, Johnson RS, Paxton RJ, March CJ, Cerretti DP (1997) A metalloproteinase disintegrin that releases tumour-necrosis factor-alpha from cells. Nature 385:729–733.

Blanchot-Jossic F, Jarry A, Masson D, Bach-Ngohou K, Paineau J, Denis MG, Laboisse CL, Mosnier JF (2005) Up-regulated expression of ADAM17 in human colon carcinoma: co-expression with EGFR in neoplastic and endothelial cells. J Pathol 207:156–163.

Blobel CP (2005) ADAMs: key components in EGFR signalling and development. Nat Rev Mol Cell Biol 6:32–43.

Borrell-Pages M, Rojo F, Albanell J, Baselga J, Arribas J (2003) TACE is required for the activation of the EGFR by TGF-alpha in tumors. Embo J 22:1114–1124.

Cal S, Freije JM, Lopez JM, Takada Y, Lopez-Otin C (2000) ADAM 23/MDC3, a human disintegrin that promotes cell adhesion via interaction with the alphavbeta3 integrin through an RGD-independent mechanism. Mol Biol Cell 11:1457–1469.

Canals F, Colome N, Ferrer C, Plaza-Calonge Mdel C, Rodriguez-Manzaneque JC (2006) Identification of substrates of the extracellular protease ADAMTS1 by DIGE proteomic analysis. Proteomics 6 Suppl 1:S28–35.

Cancer Genome Atlas Research Network (2008) Comprehensive genomic characterization defines human glioblastoma genes and core pathways. Nature 455:1061–1068.

Carl-McGrath S, Lendeckel U, Ebert M, Roessner A, Rocken C (2005) The disintegrin-metalloproteinases ADAM9, ADAM12, and ADAM15 are upregulated in gastric cancer. Int J Oncol 26:17–24.

Choi JE, Kim DS, Kim EJ, Chae MH, Cha SI, Kim CH, Jheon S, Jung TH, Park JY (2008) Aberrant methylation of ADAMTS1 in non-small cell lung cancer. Cancer Genet Cytogenet 187:80–84.

Costa FF, Verbisck NV, Salim AC, Ierardi DF, Pires LC, Sasahara RM, Sogayar MC, Zanata SM, Mackay A, O'Hare M, Soares F, Simpson AJ, Camargo AA (2004) Epigenetic silencing of the adhesion molecule ADAM23 is highly frequent in breast tumors. Oncogene 23: 1481–1488.

Cox JM, Clayton CL, Tomita T, Wallace DM, Robinson PA, Crabtree JE (2001) cDNA array analysis of cag pathogenicity island-associated Helicobacter pylori epithelial cell response genes. Infect Immun 69:6970–6980.

Dunn JR, Panutsopulos D, Shaw MW, Heighway J, Dormer R, Salmo EN, Watson SG, Field JK, Liloglou T (2004) METH-2 silencing and promoter hypermethylation in NSCLC. Br J Cancer 91:1149–1154.

Dunn JR, Reed JE, du Plessis DG, Shaw EJ, Reeves P, Gee AL, Warnke P, Walker C (2006) Expression of ADAMTS-8, a secreted protease with antiangiogenic properties, is downregulated in brain tumours. Br J Cancer 94:1186–1193.

Dyczynska E, Syta E, Sun D, Zolkiewska A (2008) Breast cancer-associated mutations in metalloprotease disintegrin ADAM12 interfere with the intracellular trafficking and processing of the protein. Int J Cancer 122:2634–2640.

Egeblad M and Werb Z (2002) New functions for the matrix metalloproteinases in cancer progression. Nat Rev Cancer 2:161–174.

Eto K, Huet C, Tarui T, Kupriyanov S, Liu HZ, Puzon-McLaughlin W, Zhang XP, Sheppard D, Engvall E, Takada Y (2002) Functional classification of ADAMs based on a conserved motif for binding to integrin alpha 9beta 1: implications for sperm-egg binding and other cell interactions. J Biol Chem 277:17804–17810.

Fingleton B (2006) Matrix metalloproteinases: roles in cancer and metastasis. Front Biosci 11: 479–491.

Fogel M, Gutwein P, Mechtersheimer S, Riedle S, Stoeck A, Smirnov A, Edler L, Ben-Arie A, Huszar M, Altevogt P (2003) L1 expression as a predictor of progression and survival in patients with uterine and ovarian carcinomas. Lancet 362:869–875.

Fritzsche FR, Wassermann K, Jung M, Tölle A, Kristiansen I, Lein M, Johannsen M, Dietel M, Jung K, Kristiansen G (2008) ADAM9 is highly expressed in renal cell cancer and is associated with tumour progression. BMC Cancer 8:179.

Gavert N, Conacci-Sorrell M, Gast D, Schneider A, Altevogt P, Brabletz T, Ben-Ze'ev A (2005) L1, a novel target of beta-catenin signaling, transforms cells and is expressed at the invasive front of colon cancers. J Cell Biol 168:633–642.

Grigo K, Wirsing A, Lucas B, Klein-Hitpass L, Ryffel GU (2008) HNF4 alpha orchestrates a set of 14 genes to down-regulate cell proliferation in kidney cells. Biol Chem 389:179–187.

Grützmann R, Foerder M, Alldinger I, Staub E, Brümmendorf T, Röpcke S, Li X, Kristiansen G, Jesnowski R, Sipos B, Löhr M, Lüttges J, Ockert D, Klöppel G, Saeger HD, Pilarsky C (2003) Gene expression profiles of microdissected pancreatic ductal adenocarcinoma. Virchows Arch 443:508–517.

Grützmann R, Lüttges J, Sipos B, Ammerpohl O, Dobrowolski F, Alldinger I, Kersting S, Ockert D, Koch R, Kalthoff H, Schackert HK, Saeger HD, Klöppel G, Pilarsky C (2004) ADAM9 expression in pancreatic cancer is associated with tumour type and is a prognostic factor in ductal adenocarcinoma. Br J Cancer 90:1053–1058.

Gschwind A, Hart S, Fischer OM, Ullrich A (2003) TACE cleavage of proamphiregulin regulates GPCR-induced proliferation and motility of cancer cells. Embo J 22:2411–2421.

Gutwein P, Oleszewski M, Mechtersheimer S, Agmon-Levin N, Krauss K, Altevogt P (2000) Role of Src kinases in the ADAM-mediated release of L1 adhesion molecule from human tumor cells. J Biol Chem 275:15490–15497.

Held-Feindt J, Paredes EB, Blömer U, Seidenbecher C, Stark AM, Mehdorn HM, Mentlein R (2006) Matrix-degrading proteases ADAMTS4 and ADAMTS5 (disintegrins and metalloproteinases with thrombospondin motifs 4 and 5) are expressed in human glioblastomas. Int J Cancer 118:55–61.

Herren B, Raines EW, Ross R (1997) Expression of a disintegrin-like protein in cultured human vascular cells and in vivo. Faseb J 11:173–180.

Horiuchi K, Weskamp G, Lum L, Hammes HP, Cai H, Brodie TA, Ludwig T, Chiusaroli R, Baron R, Preissner KT, Manova K, Blobel CP (2003) Potential role for ADAM15 in pathological neovascularization in mice. Mol Cell Biol 23:5614–5624.

Iba K, Albrechtsen R, Gilpin BJ, Loechel F, Wewer UM (1999) Cysteine-rich domain of human ADAM 12 (meltrin alpha) supports tumor cell adhesion. Am J Pathol 154:1489–1501.

Iruela-Arispe ML, Carpizo D, Luque A (2003) ADAMTS1: a matrix metalloprotease with angioinhibitory properties. Ann N Y Acad Sci 995:183–190.

Ishikawa N, Daigo Y, Yasui W, Inai K, Nishimura H, Tsuchiya E, Kohno N, Nakamura Y (2004) ADAM8 as a novel serological and histochemical marker for lung cancer. Clin Cancer Res 10:8363–8370.

Ito K, Okamoto I, Araki N, Kawano Y, Nakao M, Fujiyama S, Tomita K, Mimori T, Saya H (1999) Calcium influx triggers the sequential proteolysis of extracellular and cytoplasmic domains of E-cadherin, leading to loss of beta-catenin from cell-cell contacts. Oncogene 18:7080–7090.

Izumi Y, Hirata M, Hasuwa H, Iwamoto R, Umata T, Miyado K, Tamai Y, Kurisaki T, Sehara-Fujisawa A, Ohno S, Mekada E (1998) A metalloprotease-disintegrin, MDC9/meltrin-gamma/ADAM9 and PKCdelta are involved in TPA-induced ectodomain shedding of membrane-anchored heparin-binding EGF-like growth factor. Embo J 17:7260–7272.

Jin H, Wang X, Ying J, Wong AH, Li H, Lee KY, Srivastava G, Chan AT, Yeo W, Ma BB, Putti TC, Lung ML, Shen ZY, Xu LY, Langford C, Tao Q (2007) Epigenetic identification of ADAMTS18 as a novel 16q23.1 tumor suppressor frequently silenced in esophageal, nasopharyngeal and multiple other carcinomas. Oncogene 26:7490–7498.

Kalinski T, Krueger S, Sel S, Werner K, Ropke M, Roessner A (2007) ADAMTS1 is regulated by interleukin-1beta, not by hypoxia, in chondrosarcoma. Hum Pathol 38:86–94.

Kang Y, Siegel PM, Shu W, Drobnjak M, Kakonen SM, Cordón-Cardo C, Guise TA, Massagué J (2003) A multigenic program mediating breast cancer metastasis to bone. Cancer Cell 3: 537–549.

Karan D, Lin FC, Bryan M, Ringel J, Moniaux N, Lin MF, Batra SK (2003) Expression of ADAMs (a disintegrin and metalloproteases) and TIMP-3 (tissue inhibitor of metalloproteinase-3) in human prostatic adenocarcinomas. Int J Oncol 23:1365–1371.

Kaushal GP and Shah SV (2000) The new kids on the block: ADAMTSs, potentially multifunctional metalloproteinases of the ADAM family. J Clin Invest 105:1335–1337.

Ko SY, Lin SC, Wong YK, Liu CJ, Chang KW, Liu TY (2007) Increase of disintegrin metalloprotease 10 (ADAM10) expression in oral squamous cell carcinoma. Cancer Lett 245:33–43.

Kodama T, Ikeda E, Okada A, Ohtsuka T, Shimoda M, Shiomi T, Yoshida K, Nakada M, Ohuchi E, Okada Y (2004) ADAM12 is selectively overexpressed in human glioblastomas and is associated with glioblastoma cell proliferation and shedding of heparin-binding epidermal growth factor. Am J Pathol 165:1743–1753.

Kuefer R, Day KC, Kleer CG, Sabel MS, Hofer MD, Varambally S, Zorn CS, Chinnaiyan AM, Rubin MA, Day ML (2006) ADAM15 disintegrin is associated with aggressive prostate and breast cancer disease. Neoplasia 8:319–329.

Kuno K and Matsushima K (1998) ADAMTS-1 protein anchors at the extracellular matrix through the thrombospondin type I motifs and its spacing region. J Biol Chem 273:13912–13917.

Kuno K, Kanada N, Nakashima E, Fujiki F, Ichimura F, Matsushima K (1997) Molecular cloning of a gene encoding a new type of metalloproteinase-disintegrin family protein with thrombospondin motifs as an inflammation associated gene. J Biol Chem 272:556–562.

Kuno K, Okada Y, Kawashima H, Nakamura H, Miyasaka M, Ohno H, Matsushima K (2000) ADAMTS-1 cleaves a cartilage proteoglycan, aggrecan. FEBS Lett 478:241–245.

Kuno K, Bannai K, Hakozaki M, Matsushima K, Hirose K (2004) The carboxyl-terminal half region of ADAMTS-1 suppresses both tumorigenicity and experimental tumor metastatic potential. Biochem Biophys Res Commun 319:1327–1333.

Le Pabic H, Bonnier D, Wewer UM, Coutand A, Musso O, Baffet G, Clément B, Théret N (2003) ADAM12 in human liver cancers: TGF-beta-regulated expression in stellate cells is associated with matrix remodeling. Hepatology 37:1056–1066.

Lee NV, Rodriguez-Manzaneque JC, Thai SN, Twal WO, Luque A, Lyons KM, Argraves WS, Iruela-Arispe ML (2005) Fibulin-1 acts as a cofactor for the matrix metalloprotease ADAMTS-1. J Biol Chem 280:34796–34804.

Lee NV, Sato M, Annis DS, Loo JA, Wu L, Mosher DF, Iruela-Arispe ML (2006) ADAMTS1 mediates the release of antiangiogenic polypeptides from TSP1 and 2. Embo J 25:5270–5283.

Lendeckel U, Kohl J, Arndt M, Carl-McGrath S, Donat H, Rocken C (2005) Increased expression of ADAM family members in human breast cancer and breast cancer cell lines. J Cancer Res Clin Oncol 131:41–48.

Lind GE, Kleivi K, Meling GI, Teixeira MR, Thiis-Evensen E, Rognum TO, Lothe RA (2006) ADAMTS1, CRABP1, and NR3C1 identified as epigenetically deregulated genes in colorectal tumorigenesis. Cell Oncol 28:259–272.

Liu YJ, Xu Y, Yu Q (2006) Full-length ADAMTS-1 and the ADAMTS-1 fragments display pro- and antimetastatic activity, respectively. Oncogene 25:2452–2467.

Llamazares M, Cal S, Quesada V, Lopez-Otin C (2003) Identification and characterization of ADAMTS-20 defines a novel subfamily of metalloproteinases-disintegrins with multiple thrombospondin-1 repeats and a unique GON domain. J Biol Chem 278:13382–13389.

Lo PH, Leung AC, Kwok CY, Cheung WS, Ko JM, Yang LC, Law S, Wang LD, Li J, Stanbridge EJ, Srivastava G, Tang JC, Tsao SW, Lung ML (2007) Identification of a tumor suppressive critical region mapping to 3p14.2 in esophageal squamous cell carcinoma and studies of a candidate tumor suppressor gene, ADAMTS9. Oncogene 26:148–157.

Lopez-Otin C and Matrisian LM (2007) Emerging roles of proteases in tumour suppression. Nat Rev Cancer 7:800–808.

Lung HL, Lo PH, Xie D, Apte SS, Cheung AK, Cheng Y, Law EW, Chua D, Zeng YX, Tsao SW, Stanbridge EJ, Lung ML (2008) Characterization of a novel epigenetically-silenced, growth-suppressive gene, ADAMTS9, and its association with lymph node metastases in nasopharyngeal carcinoma. Int J Cancer 123:401–408.

Luque A, Carpizo DR, Iruela-Arispe ML (2003) ADAMTS1/METH1 inhibits endothelial cell proliferation by direct binding and sequestration of VEGF165. J Biol Chem 278:23656–23665.

Maretzky T, Reiss K, Ludwig A, Buchholz J, Scholz F, Proksch E, de Strooper B, Hartmann D, Saftig P (2005) ADAM10 mediates E-cadherin shedding and regulates epithelial cell-cell adhesion, migration, and beta-catenin translocation. Proc Natl Acad Sci U S A 102:9182–9187.

Martin MD and Matrisian LM (2007) The other side of MMPs: protective roles in tumor progression. Cancer Metastasis Rev 26:717–724.

Masaki M, Kurisaki T, Shirakawa K, Sehara-Fujisawa A (2005) Role of meltrin {alpha} (ADAM12) in obesity induced by high- fat diet. Endocrinology 146:1752–1763.

Masui T, Hosotani R, Tsuji S, Miyamoto Y, Yasuda S, Ida J, Nakajima S, Kawaguchi M, Kobayashi H, Koizumi M, Toyoda E, Tulachan S, Arii S, Doi R, Imamura M (2001) Expression of METH-1 and METH-2 in pancreatic cancer. Clin Cancer Res 7:3437–3443.

Mazzocca A, Coppari R, De Franco R, Cho JY, Libermann TA, Pinzani M, Toker A (2005) A secreted form of ADAM9 promotes carcinoma invasion through tumor-stromal interactions. Cancer Res 65:4728–4738.

McCulloch DR, Akl P, Samaratunga H, Herington AC, Odorico DM (2004) Expression of the disintegrin metalloprotease, ADAM-10, in prostate cancer and its regulation by dihydrotestosterone, insulin-like growth factor I, and epidermal growth factor in the prostate cancer cell model LNCaP. Clin Cancer Res 10:314–323.

Mechtersheimer S, Gutwein P, Agmon-Levin N, Stoeck A, Oleszewski M, Riedle S, Postina R, Fahrenholz F, Fogel M, Lemmon V, Altevogt P (2001) Ectodomain shedding of L1 adhesion molecule promotes cell migration by autocrine binding to integrins. J Cell Biol 155:661–673.

Millichip MI, Dallas DJ, Wu E, Dale S, McKie N (1998) The metallo-disintegrin ADAM10 (MADM) from bovine kidney has type IV collagenase activity in vitro. Biochem Biophys Res Commun 245:594–598.

Mitsui Y, Mochizuki S, Kodama T, Shimoda M, Ohtsuka T, Shiomi T, Chijiiwa M, Ikeda T, Kitajima M, Okada Y (2006) ADAM28 is overexpressed in human breast carcinomas: implications for carcinoma cell proliferation through cleavage of insulin-like growth factor binding protein-3. Cancer Res 66:9913–9920.

Moss ML, Jin SL, Milla ME, Bickett DM, Burkhart W, Carter HL, Chen WJ, Clay WC, Didsbury JR, Hassler D, Hoffman CR, Kost TA, Lambert MH, Leesnitzer MA, McCauley P, McGeehan G, Mitchell J, Moyer M, Pahel G, Rocque W, Overton LK, Schoenen F, Seaton T, Su JL, Becherer JD, et al. (1997) Cloning of a disintegrin metalloproteinase that processes precursor tumour-necrosis factor-alpha. Nature 385:733–736.

Najy AJ, Day KC, Day ML (2008) ADAM15 supports prostate cancer metastasis by modulating tumor cell-endothelial cell interaction. Cancer Res 68:1092–1099.

Nakada M, Miyamori H, Kita D, Takahashi T, Yamashita J, Sato H, Miura R, Yamaguchi Y, Okada Y (2005) Human glioblastomas overexpress ADAMTS-5 that degrades brevican. Acta Neuropathol 110:239–246.

Nath D, Slocombe PM, Stephens PE, Warn A, Hutchinson GR, Yamada KM, Docherty AJ, Murphy G (1999) Interaction of metargidin (ADAM-15) with alphavbeta3 and alpha5beta1 integrins on different haemopoietic cells. J Cell Sci 112 (Pt 4):579–587.

Ohtsuka T, Shiomi T, Shimoda M, Kodama T, Amour A, Murphy G, Ohuchi E, Kobayashi K, Okada Y (2006) ADAM28 is overexpressed in human non-small cell lung carcinomas and correlates with cell proliferation and lymph node metastasis. Int J Cancer 118:263–273.

Ongusaha PP, Kwak JC, Zwible AJ, Macip S, Higashiyama S, Taniguchi N, Fang L, Lee SW (2004) HB-EGF is a potent inducer of tumor growth and angiogenesis. Cancer Res 64:5283–5290.

O'Shea C, McKie N, Buggy Y, Duggan C, Hill AD, McDermott E, O'Higgins N, Duffy MJ (2003) Expression of ADAM-9 mRNA and protein in human breast cancer. Int J Cancer 105:754–761.

Overall CM and Kleifeld O (2006) Tumour microenvironment - opinion: validating matrix metalloproteinases as drug targets and anti-targets for cancer therapy. Nat Rev Cancer 6:227–239.

Overall CM and Lopez-Otin C (2002) Strategies for MMP inhibition in cancer: innovations for the post-trial era. Nat Rev Cancer 2:657–672.

Page-McCaw A, Ewald AJ, Werb Z (2007) Matrix metalloproteinases and the regulation of tissue remodelling. Nat Rev Mol Cell Biol 8:221–233.

Perutelli P (1995) [Disintegrins: potent inhibitors of platelet aggregation]. Recenti Prog Med 86:168–174.

Porter S, Scott SD, Sassoon EM, Williams MR, Jones JL, Girling AC, Ball RY, Edwards DR (2004) Dysregulated expression of adamalysin-thrombospondin genes in human breast carcinoma. Clin Cancer Res 10:2429–2440.

Primakoff P and Myles DG (2000) The ADAM gene family: surface proteins with adhesion and protease activity. Trends in Genetics: 16:83–87.

Qi H, Rand MD, Wu X, Sestan N, Wang W, Rakic P, Xu T, Artavanis-Tsakonas S (1999) Processing of the notch ligand delta by the metalloprotease Kuzbanian. Science 283:91–94.

Rocks N, Paulissen G, Quesada Calvo F, Polette M, Gueders M, Munaut C, Foidart JM, Noel A, Birembaut P, Cataldo D (2006) Expression of a disintegrin and metalloprotease (ADAM and ADAMTS) enzymes in human non-small-cell lung carcinomas (NSCLC). Br J Cancer 94:724–730.

Rocks N, Paulissen G, Quesada-Calvo F, Munaut C, Gonzalez ML, Gueders M, Hacha J, Gilles C, Foidart JM, Noel A, Cataldo DD (2008) ADAMTS-1 metalloproteinase promotes tumor development through the induction of a stromal reaction in vivo. Cancer Res 68: 9541–9550.

Rodriguez-Manzaneque JC, Milchanowski AB, Dufour EK, Leduc R, Iruela-Arispe ML (2000) Characterization of METH-1/ADAMTS1 processing reveals two distinct active forms. J Biol Chem 275:33471–33479.

Rodríiguez-Manzaneque JC, Westling J, Thai SN, Luque A, Knauper V, Murphy G, Sandy JD, Iruela-Arispe ML (2002) ADAMTS1 cleaves aggrecan at multiple sites and is differentially inhibited by metalloproteinase inhibitors. Biochem Biophys Res Commun 293:501–508.

Roemer A, Schwettmann L, Jung M, Roigas J, Kristiansen G, Schnorr D, Loening SA, Jung K, Lichtinghagen R (2004) Increased mRNA expression of ADAMs in renal cell carcinoma and their association with clinical outcome. Oncol Rep 11:529–536.

Roy R, Wewer UM, Zurakowski D, Pories SE, Moses MA (2004) ADAM 12 cleaves extra-cellular matrix proteins and correlates with cancer status and stage. J Biol Chem 279: 51323–51330.

Sagane K, Ohya Y, Hasegawa Y, Tanaka I (1998) Metalloproteinase-like, disintegrin-like, cysteine-rich proteins MDC2 and MDC3: novel human cellular disintegrins highly expressed in the brain. Biochem J 334 (Pt 1):93–98.

Sahin U and Blobel CP (2007) Ectodomain shedding of the EGF-receptor ligand epigen is mediated by ADAM17. FEBS Lett 581:41–44.

Sahin U, Weskamp G, Kelly K, Zhou HM, Higashiyama S, Peschon J, Hartmann D, Saftig P, Blobel CP (2004) Distinct roles for ADAM10 and ADAM17 in ectodomain shedding of six EGFR ligands. J Cell Biol 164:769–779.

Sandy JD, Westling J, Kenagy RD, Iruela-Arispe ML, Verscharen C, Rodriguez-Mazaneque JC, Zimmermann DR, Lemire JM, Fischer JW, Wight TN, Clowes AW (2001) Versican V1 pro-teolysis in human aorta in vivo occurs at the Glu441-Ala442 bond, a site that is cleaved by recombinant ADAMTS-1 and ADAMTS-4. J Biol Chem 276:13372–13378.

Schafer B, Marg B, Gschwind A, Ullrich A (2004) Distinct ADAM metalloproteinases regu-late G protein-coupled receptor-induced cell proliferation and survival. J Biol Chem 279: 47929–47938.

Schulz B, Pruessmeyer J, Maretzky T, Ludwig A, Blobel CP, Saftig P, Reiss K (2008) ADAM10 regulates endothelial permeability and T-Cell transmigration by proteolysis of vascular endothelial cadherin. Circ Res 102:1192–1201.

Schutz A, Hartig W, Wobus M, Grosche J, Wittekind C, Aust G (2005) Expression of ADAM15 in lung carcinomas. Virchows Arch 446:421–429.

Seals DF and Courtneidge SA (2003) The ADAMs family of metalloproteases: multidomain proteins with multiple functions. Genes Dev 17:7–30.

Shigemura K, Sung SY, Kubo H, Arnold RS, Fujisawa M, Gotoh A, Zhau HE, Chung LW (2007) Reactive oxygen species mediate androgen receptor- and serum starvation-elicited downstream signaling of ADAM9 expression in human prostate cancer cells. Prostate 67:722–731.

Shintani Y, Higashiyama S, Ohta M, Hirabayashi H, Yamamoto S, Yoshimasu T, Matsuda H, Matsuura N (2004) Overexpression of ADAM9 in non-small cell lung cancer correlates with brain metastasis. Cancer Res 64:4190–4196.

Shozu M, Minami N, Yokoyama H, Inoue M, Kurihara H, Matsushima K, Kuno K (2005) ADAMTS-1 is involved in normal follicular development, ovulatory process and organization of the medullary vascular network in the ovary. J Mol Endocrinol 35:343–355.

Shtutman M, Zhurinsky J, Simcha I, Albanese C, D'Amico M, Pestell R, Ben-Ze'ev A (1999) The cyclin D1 gene is a target of the beta-catenin/LEF-1 pathway. Proc Natl Acad Sci U S A 96:5522–5527.

Sjöblom T, Jones S, Wood LD, Parsons DW, Lin J, Barber TD, Mandelker D, Leary RJ, Ptak J, Silliman N, Szabo S, Buckhaults P, Farrell C, Meeh P, Markowitz SD, Willis J, Dawson D, Willson JK, Gazdar AF, Hartigan J, Wu L, Liu C, Parmigiani G, Park BH, Bachman KE, Papadopoulos N, Vogelstein B, Kinzler KW, Velculescu VE (2006) The consensus coding sequences of human breast and colorectal cancers. Science 314:268–274.

Somerville RP, Longpre JM, Jungers KA, Engle JM, Ross M, Evanko S, Wight TN, Leduc R, Apte SS (2003) Characterization of ADAMTS-9 and ADAMTS-20 as a distinct ADAMTS subfamily related to Caenorhabditis elegans GON-1. J Biol Chem 278:9503–9513.

Takada H, Imoto I, Tsuda H, Nakanishi Y, Ichikura T, Mochizuki H, Mitsufuji S, Hosoda F, Hirohashi S, Ohki M, Inazawa J (2005) ADAM23, a possible tumor suppressor gene, is frequently silenced in gastric cancers by homozygous deletion or aberrant promoter hypermethylation. Oncogene 24:8051–8060.

Takamune Y, Ikebe T, Nagano O, Nakayama H, Ota K, Obayashi T, Saya H, Shinohara M (2007) ADAM-17 associated with CD44 cleavage and metastasis in oral squamous cell carcinoma. Virchows Arch 450:169–177.

Takeda S, Igarashi T, Mori H, Araki S (2006) Crystal structures of VAP1 reveal ADAMs' MDC domain architecture and its unique C-shaped scaffold. Embo J 25:2388–2396.

Tanaka Y, Miyamoto S, Suzuki SO, Oki E, Yagi H, Sonoda K, Yamazaki A, Mizushima H, Maehara Y, Mekada E, Nakano H (2005) Clinical significance of heparin-binding epidermal growth factor-like growth factor and a disintegrin and metalloprotease 17 expression in human ovarian cancer. Clin Cancer Res 11:4783–4792.

Tang BL (2001) ADAMTS: a novel family of extracellular matrix proteases. Int J Biochem Cell Biol 33:33–44.

Tannapfel A, Anhalt K, Häusermann P, Sommerer F, Benicke M, Uhlmann D, Witzigmann H, Hauss J, Wittekind C (2003) Identification of novel proteins associated with hepatocellular carcinomas using protein microarrays. J Pathol 201:238–249.

Torres-Collado AX, Kisiel W, Iruela-Arispe ML, Rodriguez-Manzaneque JC (2006) ADAMTS1 interacts with, cleaves, and modifies the extracellular location of the matrix inhibitor tissue factor pathway inhibitor-2. J Biol Chem 281:17827–17837.

Tortorella MD, Burn TC, Pratta MA, Abbaszade I, Hollis JM, Liu R, Rosenfeld SA, Copeland RA, Decicco CP, Wynn R, Rockwell A, Yang F, Duke JL, Solomon K, George H, Bruckner R, Nagase H, Itoh Y, Ellis DM, Ross H, Wiswall BH, Murphy K, Hillman MC Jr, Hollis GF, Newton RC, Magolda RL, Trzaskos JM, Arner EC (1999) Purification and cloning of aggrecanase-1: a member of the ADAMTS family of proteins. Science 284: 1664–1666.

Trochon-Joseph V, Martel-Renoir D, Mir LM, Thomaïdis A, Opolon P, Connault E, Li H, Grenet C, Fauvel-Lafève F, Soria J, Legrand C, Soria C, Perricaudet M, Lu H (2004) Evidence of antiangiogenic and antimetastatic activities of the recombinant disintegrin domain of metargidin. Cancer Res 64:2062–2069.

Turk B (2006) Targeting proteases: successes, failures and future prospects. Nat Rev Drug Discov 5:785–799.

Vázquez F, Hastings G, Ortega MA, Lane TF, Oikemus S, Lombardo M, Iruela-Arispe ML (1999) METH-1, a human ortholog of ADAMTS-1, and METH-2 are members of a new family of proteins with angio-inhibitory activity. J Biol Chem 274:23349–23357.

Wildeboer D, Naus S, Amy Sang QX, Bartsch JW, Pagenstecher A (2006) Metalloproteinase dis-integrins ADAM8 and ADAM19 are highly regulated in human primary brain tumors and their expression levels and activities are associated with invasiveness. J Neuropathol Exp Neurol 65:516–527.

Wolfsberg TG, Primakoff P, Myles DG, White JM (1995a) ADAM, a novel family of membrane proteins containing A Disintegrin And Metalloprotease domain: multipotential functions in cell-cell and cell-matrix interactions. J Cell Biol 131:275–278.

Wolfsberg TG, Straight PD, Gerena RL, Huovila AP, Primakoff P, Myles DG, White JM (1995b) ADAM, a widely distributed and developmentally regulated gene family encoding membrane proteins with a disintegrin and metalloprotease domain. Dev Biol 169:378–383.

Yoshimura T, Tomita T, Dixon MF, Axon AT, Robinson PA, Crabtree JE (2002) ADAMs (a dis-integrin and metalloproteinase) messenger RNA expression in Helicobacter pylori-infected, normal, and neoplastic gastric mucosa. J Infect Dis 185:332–340.

Zhang XP, Kamata T, Yokoyama K, Puzon-McLaughlin W, Takada Y (1998) Specific interaction of the recombinant disintegrin-like domain of MDC-15 (metargidin, ADAM-15) with integrin alphavbeta3. J Biol Chem 273:7345–7350.

Zhang Q, Thomas SM, Lui VW, Xi S, Siegfried JM, Fan H, Smithgall TE, Mills GB, Grandis JR (2006) Phosphorylation of TNF-alpha converting enzyme by gastrin-releasing peptide induces amphiregulin release and EGF receptor activation. Proc Natl Acad Sci U S A 103:6901–6906.

Zheng X, Jiang F, Katakowski M, Kalkanis SN, Hong X, Zhang X, Zhang ZG, Yang H, Chopp M (2007) Inhibition of ADAM17 reduces hypoxia-induced brain tumor cell invasiveness. Cancer Sci 98:674–684.

Zigrino P, Mauch C, Fox JW, Nischt R (2005) Adam-9 expression and regulation in human skin melanoma and melanoma cell lines. Int J Cancer 116:853–859.

Chapter 14
Stromal Cells and Tumor Milieu: PDGF et al.

Michele Jacob and Ellen Puré

Cast of Characters

Initiation of the desmoplastic reaction associated with cancer depends on PDGF (Shao et al., 2000). Similarly, PDGF is one of the most potent chemoattractants and activators of fibroblasts, stimulating their differentiation into myofibroblasts, which represent a prominent stromal cell type in carcinomas. Although a translocation resulting in a fusion product between PDGF and COL1A (which encodes type I collagen) is associated with dermatofibrosarcoma protuberans, no mutations in either members of the PDGF family or their receptors have been identified in carcinomas. However, aberrant PDGF signaling has been observed in carcinomas where it promotes desmoplasia and tumor progression (reviewed by Tejada et al., 2006), due to increased secretion of PDGF by tumor cells and/or higher levels of expression of PDGF receptors on stromal fibroblasts (Ebert et al., 1995). In the following chapter, we discuss the fibroblast-to-myofibroblast transition and how stromal cells may impact tumor evolution.

Introduction

The complexity of tumors approximates that of many organs, consisting of tumor cells and a surrounding stroma that is comprised of cellular components such as fibroblasts, inflammatory cells, blood and lymphatic vessels, as well as extracellular matrix (ECM). Over the years, it has become widely accepted that tumor development and progression require crosstalk between tumor cells and stroma. This mutual dependence in carcinomas is not surprising, considering the requirements for bi-directional communication between epithelial and mesenchymal cells to regulate the growth and differentiation of normal tissues during embryogenesis and homeostasis. Oncogenic mutations alter intrinsic signaling pathways of tumor cells. They also

E. Puré (✉)
The Wistar Institute, Philadelphia, PA, USA
e-mail: pure@wistar.org

A. Thomas-Tikhonenko (ed.), *Cancer Genome and Tumor Microenvironment*,
DOI 10.1007/978-1-4419-0711-0_14, © Springer Science+Business Media, LLC 2010

alter the messages communicated by tumor cells to stromal cells, thereby inducing the latter to take on a functional phenotype perhaps unique to the tumor microenvironment (TME). There is even emerging evidence to indicate that stromal cells in the tumor microenvironment may undergo mutations as well and that tumor cells and stromal cells co-evolve. Herein, we focus on the mechanisms by which tumor cells promote the development of tumor-associated fibroblasts (TAFs) (also referred to as cancer-associated fibroblasts, CAFs) and myofibroblasts that are prominent in the process of stromagenesis, and how stromal cells promote tumorigenesis and the evolution of carcinomas.

Much has been learned from panoply of in vitro systems and mouse models used to investigate the role of stromagenesis in cancer. However, although some common themes are emerging, these studies do not point to a single unifying paradigm regarding the impact of stromagenesis on tumor initiation and progression, or the mechanisms involved. This complexity likely reflects differences in the tumor models employed (endogenous tumors, xenografts, ectopic, and orthotopic syngeneic transplant models). Differences between tumor types (breast vs pancreatic, etc.), reminiscent of the selective functions of both epithelial and stromal cells in the organs from which various tumors derive, is another important variable. In addition, the relationship between tumor cells and stroma evolves over the course of tumor progression so that the stage at which these interactions are studied can have a profound impact on outcome. It is thus possible that the stroma initially functions to contain primary tumors. However, as the dialog changes through matrix remodeling, hypoxia, increased intra-tumoral tension and interstitial fluid pressure, changes in secretory patterns, and induction of angiogenesis, stromal fibroblasts/myofibroblasts could become accomplices of tumor cells and shift the balance toward tumor growth and invasiveness. Although many questions remain, it is clear that stromal fibroblasts exert their influence on tumor cells both directly and indirectly, through regulation of ECM remodeling, intra-tumoral inflammatory responses, and angiogenesis. Conversely, it is well established that tumor cells and inflammatory cells can functionally regulate stromal fibroblasts. Interestingly, recent evidence indicates that stromal cells may also be susceptible to genetic mutation and epigenetic regulation in the tumor microenvironment (Hill et al., 2005; Pelham et al., 2006), challenging the notion that in contrast to tumor cells, tumor stromal cells are genetically stable. Stromal cells may thus evolve in response to the genetic evolution and selection of tumor cells, as well as microenvironmental pressures.

Another aspect of tumor progression that we must decipher in order to make significant clinical progress is the role of stromagenesis in metastasis. On the one hand, it is important to determine whether specific mutations in tumor cells translate into changes in stromal cells to facilitate tumor metastasis. On the other hand, we must find out whether stromal fibroblasts promote mutagenic events or confer selective pressure on tumor cells to increase their metastatic potential. Do stromal fibroblasts promote the escape of malignant cells from primary tumors? Do they play a role in site-specific recruitment of tumor cells from the circulation? Are stromal fibroblasts/myofibroblasts critical to establishing microenvironmental niches at distal sites that promote metastatic growth? Do site-specific functions of stromal cells in different organs account for preferential sites of metastasis by specific tumor types? Are myofibroblasts critical to maintaining the self-renewal capacity of putative tumor stem cells? These are all critical questions and a study by Speroni et al. (2009) underscores the importance of the stromal compartment in tumor progression and metastasis development. Using melanoma and fibrosarcoma cell lines injected in the flank or the dorsal region of the foot of mice, they indeed demonstrated that foot tumors grow slow and can metastasize to the lungs, whereas flank tumors grow much faster but do not metastasize. These data thus point to a site-specific role of stromal cells in tumor progression but the underlying mechanisms, the key cell type(s) involved, as well as the relevance for carcinomas remain to be determined. New imaging technologies, the development of more endogenous tumor models in mice, and the use of cell-type-specific transgenic and knockout mice should provide an unprecedented opportunity to address these crucial outstanding questions.

Myofibroblast Phenotype and Function

Myofibroblasts are specialized mesenchymal cells that exhibit characteristics of fibroblasts with smooth muscle cell (SMC)-like features and are enriched in many tumors (Table 14.1). They are characterized by a highly contractile cytoskeletal apparatus and are physically associated with each other through gap junctions, similar to SMC. Unlike SMC, myofibroblasts are smoothelin-negative; smoothelin is thus a reliable marker used to distinguish between myofibroblasts and SMC (Table 14.1). While fibroblasts in vivo do not contain a contractile apparatus and organize their actin filaments mostly into a cortical network, the actin filaments in myofibroblasts associate with non-muscle myosin and/or other contractile proteins to form specialized adhesion complexes – called fibronexi – at the plasma membrane. This high contractile activity allows myofibroblasts to establish the critical tension/force that is necessary to close wounds during the healing process. It is also responsible for the increased tension inherent to most solid tumors and, although the significance remains unclear, it hinders drug delivery and thus favors chemoresistance.

Results from Gabiani's laboratory suggest that there are four different myofibroblast phenotypes in skin wounds (reviewed in Darby and Hewitson, 2007). The classification is based on morphology and the distribution of tissue-specific cytoskeletal markers: type V myofibroblasts express vimentin only; type VA are vimentin and α-smooth muscle actin (αsma)-positive; type VAD express vimentin, αsma, and desmin; and type VD are positive for vimentin and desmin only. On the other hand, Tomasek et al. proposed the existence of two subtypes of myofibroblasts: proto- and differentiated myofibroblasts (Tomasek et al., 2002). Differentiated myofibroblasts exhibit stress fibers and contain αsma. In contrast, proto-myofibroblasts do not express αsma and their stress fibers contain cytoplasmic β-actin. Importantly, incorporation of αsma was reported to strengthen stress fibers compared to β- or γ-actin (Hinz et al., 2001). The biophysical mechanisms conferring such tensile strength on αsma are unknown but in any case, this

Table 14.1 Potential markers for myofibroblasts and other mesenchymal cells

	Fibroblasts	Proto-Mf	Differentiated Mf[a]	SMC	Other cells
Stress fibers	−	+	+	+	−
αsma	−	−	+	+	Pericytes, myoepithelium
Smoothelin	−	−	−	+	−
SM myosin	−	?	Low or −	High	−
S100A4/FSP1	−	?	+	−	T cells, neutrophils, macrophages, tumor cells[b]
Vimentin	+	+	+	+	Mesenchymal[c]
Desmin	−	?	+ (Not in all cases)	+	Endothelial
Calponin	−	?	+	+ (Tumor)	Mesothelial
HMW caldesmon	−	−	−	+	−
cytokeratin	−	−	−	−	Epithelial
Endosialin/Tem1	−	?	+	+	Pericytes, MSC, LEC[d]
FAP	−	+	+	−	Melanocytic
Thy-1/CD90	−	+[e]	+	+ (Culture)	T cells, endothelial
MMP11	−[f]	?	+	−	Perivascular cells, TAM[g]
ED-A FN	−	Low	High		Endothelium

Mf, myofibroblasts; SM myosin, smooth muscle myosin heavy chain; HMW, high molecular weight; MSC, mesenchymal stem cells; LEC, lymphatic endothelial cells; TAM, tumor associated macrophages; ED-A FN, ED-A splice variant of fibronectin. [a]Most investigators identify CAFs as the αsma-positive myofibroblasts, which would be equivalent to the differentiated myofibroblasts described by Tomasek et al. [b]Expression of FSP1 on metastatic tumor cells is thought to precede/accompany EMT (Egeblad et al., 2005). Another group recently reported expression of FSP1 on tumor cells (Maelandsmo et al., 2009). According to them, FSP1 would localize to both the cytoplasm and nucleus of cancer cells but only to the cytoplasm of myofibroblasts. [c]Metastatic tumor cells can also express vimentin, likely as a consequence of undergoing EMT (Hu et al., 2004; Ramaekers et al., 1986). Unpublished data from our laboratory supports this and indicate that the metastatic CT26 colon carcinoma cell line express high levels of vimentin.[d]Whether or not endosialin is expressed on LEC seems controversial (Koyama et al., 2008; Christian et al., 2008; Wicki and Christofori, 2007). [e]Results from our laboratory indicate that fibroblasts grown on plastic (which display characteristics of proto-myofibroblasts) express Thy-1. [f]Since MMP11 is known to be involved in normal and pathological remodeling processes, we do not expect it to be expressed on quiescent fibroblasts (Noel et al., 2008; Matziari et al., 2007). [g]Stojic et al., 2008.

property undoubtedly constitutes an advantage during wound closure. It is also interesting to note that fibroblasts cultured on plastic display the characteristics of proto-myofibroblasts.

Two signals appear to be crucial for the generation of proto-myofibroblasts during embryonic development, wound healing, and tumor growth: mechanical tension and platelet-derived growth factor (PDGF) (Shao et al., 2000) (Fig. 14.1). In such conditions, fibroblasts develop stress fibers and fibronexi and become

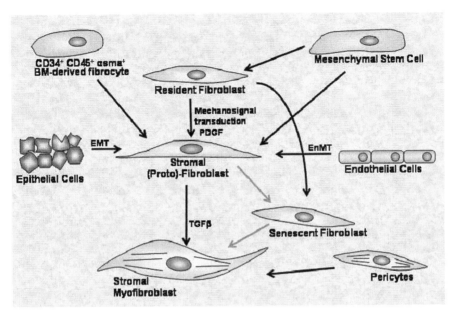

Fig. 14.1 Potential sources and differentiation of tumor stromal fibroblasts/myofibroblasts

proto-myofibroblasts. In addition, proto-myofibroblasts increase their production of fibronectin. More specifically, they start producing the ED-A splice variant of fibronectin, which further promotes differentiation. There are five PDGF isoforms (AA, BB, AB, CC, and DD) and three PDGF receptor dimers (PDGF-R$\alpha\alpha$, -R$\alpha\beta$, and -R$\beta\beta$). All PDGF ligands except PDGF-DD bind to PDGF-R$\alpha\alpha$. Similarly, all PDGF ligands except PDGF-AA bind to PDGF-R$\alpha\beta$ while only PDGF-BB and -DD bind to PDGF-R$\beta\beta$ (reviewed in Pietras et al., 2003; Ostman. 2004). The role of PDGF-AA, -AB, and -BB in wound healing and tumor-associated angiogenesis is well documented. In comparison, the role of PDGF-CC and -DD is poorly understood. Interestingly though, Anderberg et al. (2009) recently showed that PDGF-CC recruits and activates TAFs in a melanoma model. It is also interesting to note that although no mutations have been identified in PDGF or its receptors in carcinomas, the levels of PDGF-R on stromal fibroblasts were seven times higher in samples from pancreatic cancer patients, compared to normal tissues (Ebert et al., 1995). These data clearly emphasize the importance of PDGF-mediated signaling in the tumor stroma and, by extension, in tumor progression.

Sustained mechanical tension is also required for proto-myofibroblasts to acquire the differentiated phenotype. However, mechanical tension, PDGF, and ED-A fibronectin are not sufficient to induce αsma expression. TGFβ1 was shown to be the key to induction of αsma expression and completion of the differentiation process (Fig. 14.1). The underlying mechanisms are not completely understood but a study by Vaahtomeri et al. (2008) showed that Lkb1 (a tumor suppressor also known as STK11) is required. Indeed, they showed that ablation of Lkb1 reduced

TGFβ-dependent transcription of αsma and assembly of stress fibers in embryonic fibroblasts, hence defective myofibroblast differentiation. Importantly, inactivating somatic mutations in Lkb1 have been documented in primary lung adenocarcinomas in humans (Sanchez-Cespedes et al., 2002; Ji et al., 2007). Consistent with these data, a xenograft study by Zhuang et al. (2006) showed that overexpression of Lkb1 in breast cancer cells reduced tumor growth, angiogenesis, and lung metastasis. To the best of our knowledge, whether similar mutations exist in stromal cells has not been addressed. Similarly, various mutations in the TGFβ signaling pathway have been catalogued, including in the TGFβ receptor and Smads but not TGFβ itself. Since this topic is covered in other chapters, we will only make a brief comment on this pathway in a later section.

Derivation and Heterogeneity of Tumor Stromal Fibroblasts

It is interesting to note that, in addition to the type V, VA, VAD, and VD myofibroblasts, some differentiated myofibroblasts (e.g. in granulation tissue) were reported to express αsma but no other smooth muscle-specific proteins whereas others (e.g. in Dupuytren's disease) seem to express smooth muscle myosin and desmin as well. This raises the issue of heterogeneity among myofibroblasts. It has been suggested that myofibroblasts may not represent a distinct cell type from SMC but rather a continuum of intermediate phenotypes between SMC and fibroblasts. Alternatively, myofibroblast heterogeneity can also originate from different mesenchymal precursors under different pathological conditions. For example, in lung fibrosis myofibroblasts derive largely from resident fibroblasts whereas SMC seems to be the main source in atheromatous plaques. Yet in liver fibrosis, hepatic stellate cells (HSC) were identified as the major source. Other progenitors have also been shown to play a role in the generation of myofibroblasts, such as pericytes, CD34+CD45RO+αsma+ bone marrow-derived mesenchymal progenitors referred to as fibrocytes, epithelial cells (through epithelial–mesenchymal transition, or EMT), and endothelial cells (through endothelial–mesenchymal transition, or EnMT) (Larsen et al., 2006; Darby and Hewitson, 2007; Radisky et al., 2007). Recently, a mouse model that allowed direct visualization of both stromal cells and epithelial tumor cells was developed. Using this model of breast cancer, it was demonstrated that EMT occurs in vivo but with a very low incidence (Trimboli et al., 2008). The incidence of metastasis is also very low and might thus be expected to correlate with EMT as previously speculated. However, the same group established that EMT is not a prerequisite for invasion and metastatic progression, at least in this model system.

Whether myofibroblasts represent a continuum of phenotypes between SMC and fibroblasts or derivatives of a variety of cellular sources, the underlying heterogeneity could explain why very few unique markers for myofibroblasts have been identified to date. Regardless, recruitment of fibroblasts from multiple sources by damaged tissues or tumors could be important in meeting the temporarily high demand for cells with high tissue remodeling capacity.

Another point to consider is the functional state of fibroblasts that initially participate in tumorigenesis. Homeostatic fibroblasts, also referred to as resident, interstitial, or quiescent fibroblasts, are not expected to display characteristic features of the activated phenotype. However, once exposed to the tumor microenvironment, resident fibroblasts can be induced to differentiate and exhibit such characteristics. Alternatively, stromal fibroblasts evident at the very early stages of tumorigenesis might undergo prior activation and differentiation, as a consequence of chronic inflammation, fibrosis or senescence, and then contribute to the initiation of tumorigenesis.

A systematic comparison of tumor stromal fibroblasts/myofibroblasts and fibroblasts from sites of chronic inflammation and chronic fibrosis has not been reported. However, considering that chronic inflammation can lead to cancer, and that fibrosis is associated with an increased risk of cancer, it seems probable that fibroblasts activated during inflammation and fibrosis might share many features with tumor-associated fibroblasts. Indeed, a number of genes are differentially expressed in common between these populations, relative to resident fibroblasts under homeostatic conditions. For example, expression of fibroblast activation protein (FAP), which is highly restricted, is a characteristic of tumor-associated fibroblasts, although expression of FAP on TAFs may be heterogenous (Niedermeyer et al., 1997; Park et al., 1999). It is also induced on rheumatoid myofibroblast-like synoviocytes (Bauer et al., 2006), as well as fibroblasts in a number of fibrotic diseases, including liver cirrhosis and idiopathic pulmonary fibrosis (Levy et al., 2002; Acharya et al., 2006). However, the relationship between fibroblasts in the context of inflammation or organ fibrosis and tumor-associated fibroblasts remains to be determined.

Given the link between ageing and the incidence of cancer, as well as between ageing and development of a senescent population of fibroblasts, senescent fibroblasts could be yet another potential source of myofibroblasts. However, very little information is available to either confirm or refute this possibility. Senescent fibroblasts exhibit increased production of growth factors, ECM proteins, and proteinases, similar to myofibroblasts in tumors or injured tissues. Furthermore, senescent fibroblasts were shown to stimulate malignant and premalignant epithelial cells to proliferate in vitro and to form tumors in nude mice (Krtolica et al., 2001). Similarly, radiation-induced senescent fibroblasts were shown to alter the growth characteristics of mammary epithelial cells at different stages of transformation (Tsai et al., 2005). However, it is still unclear whether they promote tumor development or progression in humans. It is also unclear whether they express αsma in vivo and thus truly are equivalent to TAFs/myofibroblasts.

Stromal Fibroblasts: Co-star or Supporting Actor in Tumorigenesis

In cancer patients, desmoplasia – evidenced as an increase in stromal fibroblasts/myofibroblasts, ECM remodeling, and angiogenesis (Fig. 14.2) is often associated with poor prognosis. This observation points to a major role of stromal myofibroblasts in tumor progression.

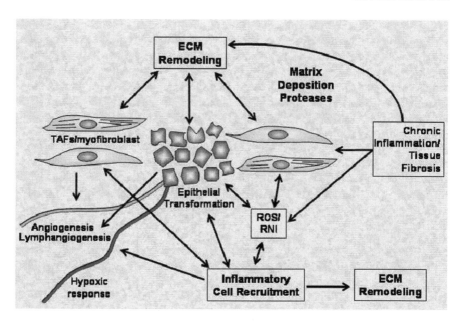

Fig. 14.2 Stromagenesis

Data from Shao et al. (2000) suggest that PDGF secreted by human breast carcinoma cells transplanted in nude mice is solely responsible for initiating fibroblast differentiation and desmoplasia, through a paracrine mechanism. According to these studies, neither PDGF nor any other growth factors produced by host cells were involved. Therefore, it appears that myofibroblasts may not be sufficient to induce epithelial cell-derived tumor development, at least in this particular xenograft model. Several groups used prostate, breast, and pancreatic cancer models to demonstrate that stromal fibroblasts can, however, promote/accelerate tumor development (Hill et al., 2005; Kiaris et al., 2005; Hwang et al., 2008; Cheng et al., 2005b) but those studies did not address the initiation process itself. Recently, Anderberg et al. (2009) suggested that PDGF-CC secreted by tumor cells recruits a subset of PDGF receptor-positive fibroblasts, which then proliferate, differentiate, and secrete osteopontin. Osteopontin, in turn, enhances tumor growth (Pazolli et al., 2009). There is also evidence that tumor-associated fibroblasts isolated from an existing tumor can induce transformation of non-tumorigenic epithelial cells (Tlsty and Hein, 2001). The question remains though: What changes must occur in fibroblasts for them to induce transformation of epithelial cells? Do these changes simply reflect a differentiation program? Do tumor-associated fibroblasts undergo epigenetic regulation or mutation/selection in order to promote malignancy?

Whether or not genetic mutations in fibroblasts are involved, stromal fibroblasts may have the capacity to initiate tumor growth in association with chronic inflammation (Egeblad et al., 2005). Studies have indeed provided evidence for a link between inflammation and stromal initiation of cancer. More specifically, we know that mutagens do not always produce tumors. However, additional tissue insults/injuries long after carcinogen exposure can trigger an inflammatory response that will lead to the generation of a tumor-promoting (reactive) stroma. This, again, may not represent true initiation since prior mutations occurred in epithelial cells. Nevertheless, without inflammation and the subsequent stromal reaction, the transformed or premalignant cells would likely remain dormant. Other prominent examples of association between chronic inflammation and cancer include *Helicobacter pylori* infection and stomach cancer, Crohn's disease and colorectal cancer, chronic pancreatitis and pancreatic cancer, and many more (Radisky and Radisky, 2007).

Activated fibroblasts express and secrete FSP1, also called S100A4. FSP1 has pro-angiogenic properties, which are thought to be mediated by the activation of plasminogen to plasmin, and/or transcriptional upregulation of MMP13 (Egeblad et al., 2005). Both plasmin and MMP13 are thought to play a role in endothelial cell invasion. There is also compelling evidence from mouse models that FSP1 is a crucial factor in the regulation of metastasis. For example, FSP1 expression is increased in metastatic carcinoma cells and this upregulation correlates with EMT, suggesting that EMT is the mechanism by which FSP1 promotes metastasis. Another molecule that could participate in the metastatic process is SDF-1α (also known as CXCL12). SDF-1α is secreted by TAFs and can act directly on carcinoma cells to stimulate their proliferation. It can also lead to the recruitment of endothelial cell precursors, promoting angiogenesis. Furthermore, SDF-1α was proposed to promote metastasis through increased expression in distant organ sites, such as lung and lymph nodes, where it can act as a chemoattractant for tumor cells (Egeblad et al., 2005). These combined results support a role for TAFs in both angiogenesis and metastasis.

Despite the evidence that lymphatic vessels play a critical role in various human cancers, the role of lymphangiogenesis in tumor progression has not been extensively studied. Lymphatic invasion by tumor cells significantly impacts prognosis but we do not know whether pre-existing lymphatic vessels are sufficient for tumor dissemination. One report involving a human study highlighted a correlation between myofibroblast proliferation in the peri-tumoral (but not the intra-tumoral) area and lymphatic microvessel density, as well as between myofibroblast proliferation, lymphatic invasion, and lymph node metastasis (Liang et al., 2005). The underlying mechanisms were not investigated though. Another recent study demonstrated that through their ability to synthesize hyaluronan (HA), TAFs promote lymphangiogenesis and tumor growth (Koyama et al., 2008). Also noteworthy, Webber et al. (2009) reported that through synthesis of TGFβ and an autocrine effect, myofibroblasts maintain an increased HA content in their peri-cellular environment, which correlates with the persistence of the differentiated myofibroblast phenotype. These data further support the evidence presented by Liang et al. (2005).

Mechanisms of Tumor Promotion by TAFs

TAFs can promote tumor progression through several different mechanisms (Mueller and Fusenig, 2004): secretion of pro-migratory ECM components such as tenascin-C, expression of proteases that remodel the ECM, secretion (or release) of growth factors, cytokines and chemokines that act on different cell types to influence tumor growth (Fig. 14.2).

Tenascin-C Affects Various Aspects of Tumorigenesis

Tenascin-C is transiently expressed during embryogenesis and is absent or markedly reduced in most adult tissues. However, both TAFs and transformed epithelial cells produce it. Similarly, its expression is greatly increased during wound healing and inflammation. Potential roles for tenascin-C in cancer include inhibition of immune surveillance (by preventing T cell activation), as well as induction of tumor cell proliferation, angiogenesis, and metastasis (Orend and Chiquet-Ehrismann, 2006). Tenascin-C was also reported to promote migration and interestingly, this effect could be specific to fibroblasts (Trebaul et al., 2007). Furthermore, as is the case for the endogenous anti-angiogenic factors angiostatin, endostatin, and tumstatin, which are derived from plasminogen, collagen XVIII, and collagen IV, respectively (Mueller and Fusenig, 2004), proteolytic degradation of tenascin-C may generate fragments with activities distinct from those of the full-length molecule. Fragments of tenascin-C were indeed shown to induce apoptosis of SMC in vitro whereas the full-length molecule does not (Orend and Chiquet-Ehrismann, 2006).

Serine Proteases and Their Potential Role in Generating a Reservoir of Signaling Molecules

TAFs also express serine proteases such as urokinase-type plasminogen activator (uPA), implicated in the invasion process through its ability to activate plasminogen locally. Once activated, plasmin has very broad substrate specificity; it can degrade fibrin, collagen, laminin, fibronectin, as well as other EMC components (Radisky and Radisky, 2007). Moreover, TAFs express MMPs – in particular MMP1, MMP3, and MMP11 which remodel ECM – and plasmin can activate MMPs. As mentioned above, the remodeling of ECM plays an important role in tumor progression, being a reservoir of latent signaling molecules. Angiostatin (generated from plasminogen by MMP3) is a potent inhibitor of endothelial cell proliferation and angiogenesis. Endostatin (proteolytic fragment of collagen XVIII) inhibits both proliferation and migration of endothelial cells, thereby affecting angiogenesis. Tumstatin (derived from collagen IV) also regulates angiogenesis via its ability to induce apoptosis of endothelial cells. Therefore, the importance of MMPs in tumors is not restricted to its role in ECM remodeling. Their role in processing molecules involved in cell growth, migration, apoptosis, and inflammation is just as critical (Duffy et al., 2008) and MMP11 may be the perfect example of such a case. MMP11 is thought to be expressed mostly in fibroblasts during normal and pathological remodeling processes (Noel et al., 2008; Matziari et al., 2007). Although its role is unknown, it is the only MMP with no known involvement in ECM degradation. It should thus be informative to investigate its substrate specificity. It is also worth noting that unlike other MMPs, MMP11 is secreted in its active form rather than as a proenzyme.

Another protease that recently became the subject of intense investigation is FAP, also known as seprase. FAP is a glycosylated serine protease expressed on the cell surface in conditions of active tissue remodeling, such as embryogenesis, wound healing, cirrhotic liver, fibrotic lungs, and tumors, but not in normal adult tissues (Chen and Kelly, 2003). It is expressed in the majority of carcinomas where its expression is restricted to stromal fibroblasts, as opposed to tumor cells per se, SMC, and other stromal cells. FAP is active as a dimer (homodimer or heterodimer with DPPIV/CD26) and although it was shown to have gelatinase, collagenase, and dipeptidyl peptidase activities in vitro, its in vivo substrate specificity remains undetermined. Similarly, its role in vivo has yet to be defined, being reported as a tumor promoter in some, albeit contrived, tumor models, while in a melanoma model it was reported to act as a tumor suppressor (Cheng et al., 2005a; Cheng et al., 2002; Ramirez-Montagut et al., 2004). Interestingly, FAP was recently shown to have endopeptidase activity in addition to its dipeptidyl peptidase activity, a characteristic not shared by its closest homolog, DPPIV. It will thus be important to develop mouse models that allow to delineate the role of FAP as a dipeptidyl peptidase vs endopeptidase in vivo, so as to understand its role in tumorigenesis.

Interestingly, a recent study revealed that the levels of FAP, MMP11, uPA, various types of collagen, fibronectin, and thrombospondin (see below) mRNA were significantly upregulated in metastasis compared to primary tumors from patients with ovarian serous carcinoma (Bignotti et al., 2007). Although the authors analyzed whole tumor extracts and, therefore, could not determine whether the aforementioned genes were upregulated in TAFs or carcinoma cells, our current knowledge about FAP, MMP11, collagen, and fibronectin leads us to speculate that upregulation of these genes is attributable to TAFs. These observations suggest that TAFs/myofibroblasts contribute greatly to the metastatic process, in agreement with data from Speroni et al. (2009) that we discussed in the introduction.

A Critical Role for Growth Factors, Cytokines, and Other Soluble Factors

TAFs also constitute an important source of growth factors and cytokines that can influence tumor cells, stromal cells, and thus the tumor as a whole (Bhowmick and Moses, 2005). For example, IGF1 and HGF were shown to induce migration and invasion, respectively, in addition to proliferation of epithelial cells. FGF and EGF also stimulate cell proliferation. VEGF and MCP1, on the other hand, were shown to induce angiogenesis and recruitment of inflammatory cells. Wnt-1 seems to promote transformation of epithelial cells without affecting fibroblasts. Finally, TGFβ has been shown to impact many aspects of tumor development/progression. TGFβ can indeed induce EMT, which in many cases enhances tumor dissemination. It can also stimulate collagen synthesis, which may increase the tumor contracture, thereby favoring development of the desmoplastic response and tumor progression. As mentioned earlier, we know that mechanical tension/stress is critical for the conversion of fibroblasts into myofibroblasts (Tomasek et al., 2002). Furthermore,

Wipff et al. recently reported that increasing the Young's modulus (a measure of the stiffness/elasticity of a substrate) of the matrix in which myofibroblasts are grown in vitro, to make it equivalent to that of healing wounds/tissues, can lead to activation of latent TGFβ, suggesting a feedback loop (Wipff et al., 2007). Another way by which TGFβ can promote tumor growth is through immune suppression, preventing an effective immune response against the neoplasm through regulatory T cells (Chen et al., 2005, 2008).

TGFβ is known to inhibit proliferation of normal epithelial cells. However, transformed epithelial cells become non-responsive. The type II TGFβ receptor (TβRII) is frequently inactivated in colon cancers, which explains the desensitization to TGFβ observed in those cases. Whether a similar mechanism operates in other types of tumors remains to be determined. It is otherwise possible that TGFβ resistance results from epigenetic regulation. An additional factor that may be worth considering is the concentration effect. Specifically, there is evidence suggesting that in the femtomolar range, TGFβ acts as a chemotactic molecule for fibroblasts whereas in the picomolar range, it induces their differentiation into myofibroblasts (De Wever and Mareel, 2003). Is it possible then that depending on the concentration of TGFβ (possibly in conjunction with other changes), epithelial cells are responsive or not?

Thrombospondin-1 (TSP1) is a multifunctional matricellular glycoprotein detected at low abundance in normal tissues but strongly expressed in many carcinomas. It regulates the matrix structure by binding directly to fibrillar ECM components such as collagen and fibronectin, and by regulating the activity of extracellular proteases such as MMPs and plasmin. TSP1 also influences the synthesis of matrix proteins through its ability to activate TGFβ. It is expressed mostly by stromal fibroblasts (endothelial and immune stromal cells being minor sources (Lawler and Detmar, 2004) and is known to have immune-regulatory activity (Silzle et al., 2004). In contrast, factors secreted by tumor cells harboring a mutation in H-ras downregulates TSP1 expression. TSP1 also regulates angiogenesis but whether it has pro- or anti-angiogenic properties remains controversial (Silzle et al., 2004; Lawler and Detmar, 2004). Although the majority of data seems to indicate that TSP1 is a potent inhibitor of angiogenesis – via inhibition of endothelial cell migration followed by induction of apoptosis – in the tumor microenvironment, others suggest that it favors angiogenesis (reviewed in Lawler and Detmar, 2004). The different outcomes could again reflect the type of model used. Other effects of TSP1 include modulation of cell adhesion, cytoskeletal reorganization, and apoptosis, all of which are cell-type dependent and probably due to differences in the repertoire of cell surface receptors expressed by the cells in question (Sid et al., 2004).

ROS and RNI: Too Much of a Good Thing is Bad

The production of reactive oxygen species (ROS) and reactive nitrogen intermediates (RNI) is another potentially important factor in the regulation of the tumor microenvironment. ROS can regulate fibroblast, infiltrating inflammatory cell, and tumor cell function, as well as modify ECM. ROS are physiological by-products of normal aerobic metabolism. At low concentrations, ROS act as second messengers in intracellular signaling cascades and affect growth and proliferation. However, excessive production of ROS can overwhelm anti-oxidant mechanisms leading to oxidative stress. ROS are carcinogenic not only by virtue of their ability to increase cell survival, migration, and proliferation, but also their capacity to modify macromolecules and induce DNA damage/genetic lesions inherent to tumor initiation and progression. Many tumor cell lines generate more ROS/RNI than non-transformed epithelial cells. Tumor infiltrating inflammatory cells can also produce ROS/RNI as do quiescent and activated fibroblasts (Nicco et al., 2005), but the role of stromal fibroblast-derived ROS/RNI in tumorigenesis still needs to be determined. Interestingly, ROS can induce cellular senescence, which – as mentioned above – might be a key event in tumor development. However, one should keep in mind that ROS can also induce cell death and could thereby exert anti-tumorigenic activity (Storz, 2005). The role of TAF-derived ROS/RNI in tumor progression warrants further investigation, but the evidence supporting a role for reactive fibroblasts in fibrotic diseases raises the likelihood that production of ROS/RNI may represent yet another mechanism by which stromal fibroblasts contribute to tumorigenesis.

TAFs Pave the Way

In addition to the mechanisms discussed above, Gaggioli et al. (2007) recently demonstrated that through protease– and force-driven ECM remodeling, fibroblasts can pave the way for carcinoma cells that simply move within the same tracks, trailing behind fibroblasts. This provides an additional example of functional interactions between stromal and epithelial cells by which myofibroblasts may promote tumor progression and invasion. However, these results were obtained using an in vitro 3D co-culture model. Therefore, we cannot exclude the possibility that in vivo the desmoplastic reaction – associated with the early stages of cancer represents an attempt of the host to contain the tumor and thereby restrain tumorigenesis. It seems indeed that desmoplasia is less apparent in advanced, highly invasive tumors (Schurch et al., 1981). Accordingly, two studies performed with tumor cell lines that do develop desmoplasia reported an inverse correlation between tumor growth and desmoplasia (reviewed in (Elenbaas and Weinberg, 2001)). Although the underlying mechanisms are unknown, one hypothesis is that expression of lysyl oxidase (by both myofibroblasts and myoepithelial cells) stabilizes the ECM by cross-linking collagen and elastin, thereby increasing its resistance to degradation by MMPs (Elenbaas and Weinberg, 2001). The observation that lysyl oxidase is minimal in invasive tumors is consistent with this hypothesis.

It is thus apparent that stromal fibroblasts play a central role in tumorigenesis both directly as well as indirectly through modification of the tumor microenvironment via multiple autocrine and paracrine mechanisms. Recent data suggests that stromal fibroblasts regulate tumor and stromal cell differentiation/function.

In addition, a new paradigm may be emerging based on recent evidence that the tumor microenvironment can also result in epigenetic and genetic effects on stromal fibroblasts.

Can the Tumor Microenvironment Lead to "Transformation" of Stromal Fibroblasts?

A number of years ago, in reviewing the evidence that stromal contributions may be vital to the growth of tumors, Hanahan and Weinberg (2000) proposed the intriguing possibility that in some tumors both the tumor and stromal cells may exhibit a "departure from normalcy". This suggested that stromal cells may co-evolve with their malignant neighbors. Several subsequent studies provided evidence in favor of this provocative hypothesis. In a mouse model of spontaneous prostate cancer where the epithelial cell cycle was disrupted by cell-specific ablation of pRb function, upregulation of p53 in tumor cells induced upregulation of p53 in stromal fibroblasts through a paracrine loop (Hill et al., 2005). Because an increase in p53 levels leads to growth arrest or apoptosis, a selective pressure was imposed as a result on the stromal fibroblasts, culminating in the preferential expansion of a subpopulation of p53-null fibroblasts (Hill et al., 2005). Preferential expansion of p53-null tumor cells also followed, all of which promoted tumor growth. This model is appealing because of the numerous reports of mutated p53 in the stromal compartment of human carcinomas. Similarly, Maffini et al. (2003) observed that mammary epithelial cells harboring a mutation in the Ha-*ras*-1 gene did not form tumors when injected into cleared fat pads, unless the animals (rats) were pre-exposed to N-nitrosomethylurea (carcinogen) to alter the stroma. Nevertheless, we should be cautious in interpreting these results until it is determined whether the desmoplastic reaction in these models mirrors what is observed in human cancers (Moinfar et al., 2000; Kurose et al., 2001; Wernert et al., 2001; Matsumoto et al., 2003; Paterson et al., 2003; Fukino et al., 2004; Tuhkanen et al., 2004; Bar et al., 2008; Lafkas et al., 2008). Moreover, using cancer-associated fibroblast cultures established from seven primary pancreatic adenocarcinomas, Walter et al. (2008) found no evidence that pancreatic CAFs harbor changes in somatic copy number or immunohistochemical evidence of p53 mutations.

Another recent study also addressed the important question of the genomic integrity of tumor stromal cells. Numerous amplifications and deletions were found in host stromal cells using high-resolution DNA copy number analysis of murine stromal cells from human xenograft tumors in immunodeficient mice (Pelham et al., 2006). In this case, the genetic alterations were widely distributed throughout the genome and they varied between different tumors, but the data suggested that within any one tumor, there was oligoclonal selection of stromal cell variants. Based on these results, the authors put forth that stromal cell components may indeed undergo a co-evolution with tumor cells, at least in the absence of immune pressure. It will be interesting, in future studies, to determine whether such stromal cell variants survive and expand in tumors in immunocompetent hosts.

Conclusion

It is important to keep in mind that – so far – much of the evidence indicating an active role for myofibroblasts in carcinogenesis were obtained using in vitro co-cultures or xenograft tumor models in immunocompromised mice or ectopic syngeneic tumor transplant models. A potential caveat of the xenograft studies pertains to their desmoplastic response. Indeed, the desmoplastic response has been reported to be virtually absent in most human xenograft tumors in nude mice. It is also rare in spontaneous and transplantable animal tumors. In contrast, desmoplasia is common in human cancers (Shao et al., 2000). This paucity of desmoplastic reaction in animal models could be due to the rapid growth of tumor cells, which may overwhelm the host stromal response. Otherwise, it is possible that the tumor cell lines used have lost – through multiple rounds of passage in vitro – their ability to secrete the necessary factor(s) (e.g., PDGF) to induce desmoplasia in the host or that growth at ectopic sites does not replicate the conditions of the tumor microenvironment necessary to promote desmoplasia. Although co-implanting tumor cells with fibroblasts may partially alleviate this problem, it may not circumvent the potential issues raised by the fact that tumor–host interactions likely reflect both tissue– and cancer cell-type-specific functions. Another intriguing alternative comes from a comparative analysis of the effect of O_2 on human and mouse fibroblasts (Parrinello et al., 2003); it suggested that mouse fibroblasts accumulate more DNA damage than human fibroblasts do in standard culture conditions with 20% oxygen. This difference in oxygen sensitivity could thus account for the different rates of proliferation, ageing, and cancer between mouse and humans. Furthermore, such phenotypic divergence might explain why telomere shortening causes human cells to undergo senescence whereas mouse cells eventually senesce despite having long stable telomeres (Parrinello et al., 2003).

The results of ongoing and future studies that increasingly make use of novel models of endogenous tumors in mice to investigate the different aspects of tumor initiation, progression, and metastasis are greatly anticipated. Many such models are being rationally designed based on mechanistic understanding of human tumors. Knowledge on mutations and defects in signaling pathways known to be deregulated in human tumors will become increasingly useful to develop endogenous tumor models that will take into account the aspect of tissue specificity in tumor stromagenesis. Such animals are hoped to provide model systems in which evaluation of therapeutic approaches will be more predictive of clinical efficacy in patients, and will provide the models necessary to obtain proof-of-principle as to whether therapeutically targeting stromal cell function in addition to tumor cells per se, might improve cancer treatments.

References

Acharya PS, Zukas A, Chandan V, Katzenstein AL and Puré E (2006) Fibroblast Activation Protein: a Serine Protease Expressed at the Remodeling Interface in Idiopathic Pulmonary Fibrosis. Hum Pathol 37: 352–360.

Anderberg C, Li H, Fredriksson L, Andrae J, Betsholtz C, Li X, Eriksson U and Pietras K (2009) Paracrine Signaling by Platelet-Derived Growth Factor-CC Promotes Tumor Growth by Recruitment of Cancer-Associated Fibroblasts. Cancer Res 69: 369–378.

Bar J, Feniger-Barish R, Lukashcguk N, Shaham H, Moskovits N, Goldfinger N, Simansky D, Perlman M, Papa M, Yosepovitch A, Rechavi G, Rotter V and Oren M (2008) Cancer cells suppress p53 in adjacent fibroblasts. Oncogene 28: 933–936.

Bauer S, Jendro M, Wadle A, Kleber S, Stenner F, Dinser R, Reich A, Faccin E, Godde S, Dinges H, Muller-Ladner U and Renner C (2006) Fibroblast Activation Protein Is Expressed by Rheumatoid Myofibroblast-Like Synoviocytes. Arthritis Res Ther 8: R171.

Bhowmick NA and Moses HL (2005) Tumor-Stroma Interactions. Curr Opin Genet Dev 15: 97–101.

Bignotti E, Tassi RA, Calza S, Ravaggi A, Bandiera E, Rossi E, Donzelli C, Pasinetti B, Pecorelli S and Santin A D (2007) Gene Expression Profile of Ovarian Serous Papillary Carcinomas: Identification of Metastasis-Associated Genes. Am J Obstet Gynecol 196: 245.

Chen WT and Kelly T (2003) Seprase Complexes in Cellular Invasiveness. Cancer Metastasis Rev 22: 259–269.

Chen ML, Pittet MJ, Gorelik L, Flavell RA, Weissleder R, von Boehmer H and Khazaie K (2005) Regulatory T Cells Suppress Tumor-Specific CD8 T Cell Cytotoxicity Through TGFβ Signals in Vivo. Proc Natl Acad Sci 102: 419–424.

Chen ST, Pan TL, Juan HF, Chen TY, Lin YS and Huang CM (2008) Breast Tumor Microenvironment: Proteomics Highlights the Treatments Targeting Secretome. J Proteome Res 7: 1379–1387.

Cheng JD, Dunbrack RL Jr, Valianou M, Rogatko A, Alpaugh RK and Weiner LM (2002) Promotion of Tumor Growth by Murine Fibroblast Activation Protein, a Serine Protease, in an Animal Model. Cancer Res 62: 4767–4772.

Cheng JD, Valianou M, Canutescu AA, Jaffe EK, Lee HO, Wang H, Lai JH, Bachovchin WW and Weiner LM (2005a) Abrogation of Fibroblast Activation Protein Enzymatic Activity Attenuates Tumor Growth. Mol Cancer Ther 4: 351–360.

Cheng N, Bhowmick NA, Chytil A, Gorksa AE, Brown KA, Muraoka R, Arteaga CL, Neilson EG, Hayward SW and Moses HL (2005b) Loss of TGF-[Beta] Type II Receptor in Fibroblasts Promotes Mammary Carcinoma Growth and Invasion Through Upregulation of TGF-[Alpha]-, MSP- and HGF-Mediated Signaling Networks. Oncogene 24: 5053–5068.

Christian S, Winkler R, Helfrich I, Boos AM, Besemfelder E, Schadendorf D and Augustin HG (2008) Endosialin (Tem1) Is a Marker of Tumor-Associated Myofibroblasts and Tumor Vessel-Associated Mural Cells. Am J Pathol 172: 486–494.

Darby IA and Hewitson TD (2007) Fibroblast Differentiation in Wound Healing and Fibrosis, in International Review of Cytology, A Survey of Cell Biology Kwang WJ ed. Academic Press, pp 143–179.

De Wever O and Mareel M (2003) Role of Tissue Stroma in Cancer Cell Invasion. J Pathol 200: 429–447.

Duffy MJ, McGowan PM and Gallagher WM (2008) Cancer Invasion and Metastasis: Changing Views. J Pathol 214: 283–293.

Ebert M, Yokoyama M, Friess H, Kobrin MS, Buchler MW and Korc M (1995) Induction of Platelet-Derived Growth Factor A and B Chains and Over-expression of Their Receptors in Human Pancreatic Cancers. Int J Cancer 62: 529–535.

Egeblad M, Littlepage LE and Werb Z (2005) The Fibroblastic Coconspirator in Cancer Progression. Cold Spring Harb Symp Quant Biol 70: 383–388.

Elenbaas B and Weinberg RA (2001) Heterotypic Signaling Between Epithelial Tumor Cells and Fibroblasts in Carcinoma Formation. Exp Cell Res 264: 169–184.

Fukino K, Shen L Matsumoto S, Morrison CD, Mutter GL and Eng C (2004) Combined Total Genome Loss of Heterozygosity Scan of Breast Cancer Stroma and Epithelium Reveals Multiplicity of Stromal Targets. Cancer Res 64: 7231–7236.

Gaggioli C, Hooper S, Hidalgo-Carcedo C, Grosse R, Marshall J F, Harrington K and Sahai E (2007) Fibroblast-Led Collective Invasion of Carcinoma Cells with Differing Roles for RhoGTPases in Leading and Following Cells. Nat Cell Biol 9: 1392–1400.

Hanahan D and Weinberg RA (2000) The Hallmarks of Cancer. Cell 100: 57–70.

Hill R, Song Y, Cardiff RD and Van Dyke T (2005) Selective Evolution of Stromal Mesenchyme With P53 Loss in Response to Epithelial Tumorigenesis. Cell 123: 1001–1011.

Hinz B, Celetta G, Tomasek JJ, Gabbiani G and Chaponnier C (2001) Alpha-smooth Muscle Actin Expression Upregulates Fibroblast Contractile Activity. Mol Biol Cell 12: 2730–2741.

Hu L et al. (2004) Association of vimentin overexpression and hepatocellular carcinoma metastasis. Oncogene 23: 298–302.

Hwang RF, Moore T, Arumugam T, Ramachandran V, Amos KD, Rivera A, Ji B, Evans DB and Logsdon CD (2008) Cancer-Associated Stromal Fibroblasts Promote Pancreatic Tumor Progression . Cancer Res 68: 918–926.

Ji H et al. (2007) LKB1 Modulates Lung Cancer Differentiation and Metastasis. Nature 448: 807–811.

Kiaris H, Chatzistamou I, Trimis G, Frangou-Plemmenou M, Pafiti-Kondi A and Kalofoutis A (2005) Evidence for Nonautonomous Effect of P53 Tumor Suppressor in Carcinogenesis. Cancer Res 65: 1627–1630.

Koyama H, Kobayashi N, Harada M, Takeoka M, Kawai Y, Sano K, Fujimori M, Amano J, Ohhashi T, Kannagi R , Kimata K, Taniguchi S and Itano N (2008) Significance of Tumor-Associated Stroma in Promotion of Intratumoral Lymphangiogenesis: Pivotal Role of a Hyaluronan-Rich Tumor Microenvironment. Am J Pathol 172: 179–193.

Krtolica A, Parrinello S, Lockett S, Desprez PY and Campisi J (2001) Senescent Fibroblasts Promote Epithelial Cell Growth and Tumorigenesis: A Link Between Cancer and Aging. Proc Natl Acad Sci 98: 12072–12077.

Kurose K, Hoshaw-Woodard S, Adeyinka A, Lemeshow S, Watson PH and Eng PH (2001) Genetic Model of Multi-step Breast Carcinogenesis Involving the Epithelium and Stroma: Clues to Tumour-Microenvironment Interactions. Hum Mol Genet 10: 1907–1913.

Lafkas D, Trimis G, Papavassiliou AG and Kiaris H (2008) P53 Mutations in Stromal Fibroblasts Sensitize Tumors Against Chemotherapy. Int J Cancer 123: 967–971.

Larsen K, Macleod D, Nihlberg K, Gurcan E, Bjermer L , Marko-Varga G and Westergren-Thorsson G (2006) Specific Haptoglobin Expression in Bronchoalveolar Lavage During Differentiation of Circulating Fibroblast Progenitor Cells in Mild Asthma. J Proteome Res 5: 1479–1483.

Lawler J and Detmar M (2004) Tumor Progression: The Effects of Thrombospondin-1 and -2. Int J Biochem Cell Biol 36: 1038–1045.

Levy ML, McCaughan GW, Abbott CA, Park JE, Cunningham AM, Müller E, Rettig WJ and Gorrell MD (2002) Fibroblast Activation Protein: A Cell Surface Dipeptidyl Peptidase and Gelatinase Expressed by Stellate Cells at the Tissue Remodelling Interface in Human Cirrhosis. Hepatol 29: 1768–1778.

Liang P, Hong JW, Ubukata H, Liu G, Katano M, Motohashi G, Kasuga T, Watanabe Y, Nakada I and Tabuchi T (2005) Myofibroblasts Correlate With Lymphatic Microvessel Density and Lymph Node Metastasis in Early-Stage Invasive Colorectal Carcinoma. Anticancer Res 25: 2705–2712.

Maffini MV, Soto AM, Calabro JM, Ucci AA and Sonnenschein C (2003) The Stroma as a Crucial Target in Rat Mammary gland Carcinogenesis. J Cell Sci 117:1495–1502.

Matsumoto N, Yoshida T, Yamashita K, Numata Y and Okayasu I (2003) Possible Alternative Carcinogenesis Pathway Featuring Microsatellite Instability in Colorectal Cancer Stroma. Br J Cancer 89: 707–712.

Matziari M, Dive V and Yiotakis A (2007) Matrix Metalloproteinase 11 (MMP-11; Stromelysin-3) and Synthetic Inhibitors. Med Res Rev 27: 528–552.

Moinfar F, Man YG, Arnould L, Bratthauer GL, Ratschek M and Tavassoli FA (2000) Concurrent and Independent Genetic Alterations in the Stromal and Epithelial Cells of Mammary Carcinoma: Implications for Tumorigenesis. Cancer Res 60: 2562–2566.

Mueller MM and Fusenig NE (2004) Friends or Foes – Bipolar Effects of the Tumour Stroma in Cancer. Nat Rev Cancer 4: 839–849.

Nicco C, Laurent A, Chereau C, Weill B and Batteux F (2005) Differential Modulation of Normal and Tumor Cell Proliferation by Reactive Oxygen Species. Biomed Pharmacother 59: 169–174.

Niedermeyer J, Scanlan MJ, Garin-Chesa P, Daiber C, Fiebig HH, Old LJ, Rettig WJ and Schnapp A (1997) Mouse Fibroblast Activation Protein: Molecular Cloning, Alternative Splicing and Expression in the Reactive Stroma of Epithelial Cancers. Int J Cancer 71: 383–389.

Noel A, Jost M and Maquoi E (2008) Matrix Metalloproteinases at Cancer Tumor-Host Interface. Semin Cell Dev Biol 19: 52–60.

Orend G and Chiquet-Ehrismann R (2006) Tenascin-C Induced Signaling in Cancer. Cancer Lett 244: 143–163.

Ostman A (2004) PDGF Receptors-Mediators of Autocrine Tumor Growth and Regulators of Tumor Vasculature and Stroma. Cytokine Growth Factor Rev 15: 275–286.

Park JE, Lenter MC, Zimmerman RA, Garin-Chesa P, Old LJ and Rettig WJ (1999) Fibroblast Activation Protein, a Dual Specificity Serine Protease Expressed in Reactive Human Tumor Stromal Fibroblasts. Proc Natl Acad Sci U S A 274: 36505–36512.

Parrinello S, Samper E, Krtolica A, Goldstein J, Melov S and Campisi J (2003) Oxygen Sensitivity Severely Limits the Replicative Lifespan of Murine Fibroblasts. Nat Cell Biol 5: 741–747.

Paterson RF, Ulbright TM, MacLennan GT, Zhang S, Pan CX, Sweeney CJ, Moore CR, Foster RS, Koch MO, Eble JN and Cheng L (2003) Molecular Genetic Alterations in the Laser-Capture-Microdissected Stroma Adjacent to Bladder Carcinoma. Cancer 98: 1830–1836.

Pazzolli E, Luo X, Brehm S, Carbery K, Chung J-J, Prior JL, Doherty J, Demehri S, Salavaggione L, Piwnica-Worms D and Stewart SA (2009) Senescent Stromal-Derived Osteopontin Promotes Preneoplastic Cell Growth. Cancer Res 69: 1230–1239.

Pelham RJ, Rodgers L, Hall I, Lucito R, Nguyen KCQ , Navin N, Hicks J, Mu D, Powers S, Wigler M and Botstein D (2006) Identification of Alterations in DNA Copy Number in Host Stromal Cells During Tumor Progression. Proc Natl Acad Sci 103: 19848–19853.

Pietras K, Sjoblom T, Rubin K, Heldin C-H and Ostman A (2003) PDGF Receptors as Cancer Drug Targets. Cancer Cell 3: 439–443.

Radisky ES and Radisky DC (2007) Stromal Induction of Breast Cancer: Inflammation and Invasion. Rev Endocr Metab Discord 8: 279–287.

Radisky DC, Kenny PA and Bissell MJ (2007) Fibrosis and Cancer: Do Myofibroblasts Come Also From Epithelial Cells Via EMT? J Cell Biochem 101: 830–839.

Ramaekers FC, Haag D, Kant A, Moesker O, Jap PH and Voojis GP (1983) Coexpression of kertain- and vimentin-type intermediate filaments in human metastatic carcinoma cells. Proc. Natl. Acad. Sci. 80: 2618–2622.

Ramirez-Montagut T, Blachere N E, Sviderskaya E V, Bennett D C, Rettig W J, Garin-Chesa P and Houghton AN (2004) FAPalpha, a Surface Peptidase Expressed During Wound Healing, Is a Tumor Suppressor. Oncogene 23: 5435–5446.

Sanchez-Cespedes M, Parrella O, Esteller M, Nomoto S, Trink B, Engles JM, Westra WH, Herman JG and Sidransky D (2002) Inactivation of LKB1/STK11 Is a Common Event in Adenocarcinomas of the Lung. Cancer Res 62: 3659–3662.

Schurch W, Seemayer T A and Legace R (1981) Stromal Myofibroblasts in Primary Invasive and Metastatic Carcinomas. A Combined Immunological, Light and Electron Microscopic Study. Virchows Arch A Pathol Anat Histol 391: 125–139.

Shao ZM, Nguyen M and Barsky SH (2000) Human Breast Carcinoma Desmoplasia Is PDGF Initiated. Oncogene 19: 4337–4345.

Sid B, Sartelet H, Bellon G, El Btaouri H, Rath G, Delorme N, Haye B and Martiny L (2004) Thrombospondin 1: A Multifunctional Protein Implicated in the Regulation of Tumor Growth. Crit Rev Oncol Hematol 49: 245–258.

Silzle T, Randolph GJ, Kreutz M and Kunz-Schughart LA (2004) The Fibroblast: Sentinel Cell and Local Immune Modulator in Tumor Tissue. Int J Cancer 108: 173–180.

Speroni L, de los Angeles Bustuoabad V, Gasparri J, Chiaramoni NS, Taira MC, Ruggiero RA and del Valle Alonso S (2009) Alternative Site of Implantation Affects Tumor Malignancy and Metastatic Potential in Mice. Cancer Biol Ther 8: 1–5.

Stojic J, Hagemann C, Haas S, Herbold C, Kuhnel S, Gerngras S, Roggendorf W, Roosen K and Vince GH (2008) Expression of Matrix Metalloproteinases MMP-1, MMP-11 and MMP-19 Is Correlated With the WHO-Grading of Human Malignant Gliomas. Nerosci Res 60: 40–49.

Storz P (2005) Reactive Oxygen Species in Tumor Progression. Front Biosci 10: 1881–1896.

Tejada ML, Yu L, Dong J, Jung K, Meng G, Peale FV, Frantz GD, Hall L, Liang X, Gerber HP, and Ferrara N (2006) Tumor-Driven Paracrine Platelet-Derived Growth Factor Receptor Alpha Signaling Is a Key Determinant of Stromal Cell Recruitment in a Model of Human Lung Carcinoma. Clin Cancer Res 12:2676–2688.

Tlsty TD and Hein PW (2001) Know Thy Neighbor: Stromal Cells Can Contribute Oncogenic Signals. Curr Opin Genet Dev 11: 54–59.

Tomasek JJ, Gabbiani G, Hinz B, Chaponnier C and Brown RA (2002) Myofibroblasts and Mechano-Regulation of Connective Tissue Remodelling. Nat Rev Mol Cell Biol 3: 349–363.

Trebaul A, Chan EK and Midwood KS (2007) Regulation of Fibroblast Migration by Tenascin-C. Biochem Soc Trans 35: 695–697.

Trimboli AJ, Fukino K, de Bruin A, Wei G, Shen L, Tanner SM, Creasap N, Rosol TJ, Robinson ML, Eng C, Ostrowski MC and Leone G (2008) Direct Evidence for Epithelial-Mesenchymal Transitions in Breast Cancer. Cancer Res 68: 937–945.

Tsai KK, Chuang EY, Little JB and Yuan ZM (2005) Cellular Mechanisms for Low-Dose Ionizing Radiation-Induced Perturbation of the Breast Tissue Microenvironment. Cancer Res 65: 6734–6744.

Tuhkanen H, Anttila M, Kosma VM, Yla-Herttuala S, Heinonen S, Kuronen A, Juhola M, Tammi R and Mannermaa A (2004) Genetic Alterations in the Peritumoral Stromal Cells of Malignant and Borderline Epithelial Ovarian Tumors as Indicated by Allelic Imbalance on Chromosome 3p. Int J Cancer 109: 247–252.

Vaahtomeri K, Bentela E, Laajanen K, Katajisto P, Wipff P-J, Hinz B, Vallenius T, Tiainen M and Makela TP (2008). Lkb1 Is Required for TGFβ-Mediated Myofibroblast Differentiation. J Cell Sci 121: 3531–3540.

Walter K, Omura N, Hong SM, Griffith M and Goggins M (2008) Pancreatic Cancer Associated Fibroblasts Display Normal Allelotypes. Cancer Biol Ther 7: 882–888.

Webber J, Meran S, Steadman R and Phillips A (2009). Hyaluronan Orchestrates TGF-β1 Dependent Maintenance of Myofibroblast Phenotype. J Biol Chem 284: 9083–9092.

Wernert N, Locherbach C, Wellmann A, Behrens P and Hugel A (2001) Presence of Genetic Alterations in Microdissected Stroma of Human Colon and Breast Cancers. Anticancer Res 21: 2259–2264.

Wicki A and Christofori G (2007) The Potential Role of Podoplanin in Tumour Invasion. Br J Cancer 96: 1–5.

Wipff PJ, Rifkin DB, Meister JJ and Hinz B (2007) Myofibroblast Contraction Activates Latent TGF- 1 From the Extracellular Matrix. J Cell Biol 179: 1311–1323.

Zhuang ZG, Di GH, Shen ZZ, Ding J and Shao ZM (2006) Enhanced Expression of LKB1 in Breast Cancer Cells Attenuates Angiogenesis, Invasion, and Metastasic Potential. Mol Cancer Res 4: 843–849.

Chapter 15
TGF-β Signaling Alterations in Neoplastic and Stromal Cells

Qinghua Zeng and Boris Pasche

Cast of Characters

Transforming growth factor beta (TGF-β) plays an central role in cell homeostasis and inherited mutations in the *TGFB1* gene cause Camurati-Engelmann disease, a condition characterized by hyperostosis and sclerosis of the diaphyses of long bones (Janssens et al., 2000; Kinoshita et al., 2000). However, mutations in the TGFB genes do not appear to occur in cancer. In contrast, type I and II TGF-β receptors and their downstream effectors SMADs are often targeted by oncogenic events. For example, loss-of-function mutations in TGFBR1 have been identified in human colorectal cancer cell lines (Ku et al., 2007) and a TGFBR1 polymorphism has been associated with increased cancer risk (Pasche et al., 2004) and is somatically acquired in approximately 2% of primary colon and head and neck tumors. Discovery that Tgfbr1 haploinsufficiency acts as a potent modifier of tumor development in a mouse model of colorectal cancer (Zeng, 2009) prompted validation in humans and led to the identification of two novel haplotypes associated with decreased TGFBR1 allelic expression and markedly increased risk of colorectal cancer (Valle, 2008). Even more frequent event is loss of expression of TGFBR2 owing to frameshift mutations that are found in more than 80% of colorectal cancers with microsatellite instability (Takayama et al., 2006). How these mutations affect tumor progression is described in this chapter.

Introduction

There is a large body of literature that supports a central role for TGF-β in tumor maintenance and progression. TGF-β was initially identified as an oncogene leading to the transformation of mouse fibroblasts (Roberts et al., 1980; Moses and

B. Pasche (✉)
Division of Hematology/Oncology, Department of Medicine and UAB Comprehensive Cancer Center, The University of Alabama at Birmingham, Birmingham, Al, USA
e-mail: boris.pasche@ccc.uab.edu

A. Thomas-Tikhonenko (ed.), *Cancer Genome and Tumor Microenvironment*,
DOI 10.1007/978-1-4419-0711-0_15, © Springer Science+Business Media, LLC 2010

Robinson, 1982). Subsequently, TGF-β has emerged as both a tumor suppressor and a potential inhibitor of cell proliferation (Siegel and Massague, 2003; Roberts et al., 1980; Moses and Robinson, 1982). Paradoxically, TGF-β also modulates processes such as cell invasion, immune regulation, and microenvironment modification. Biological responses to TGF-β are highly contextual throughout development, across different tissues, and also in cancer (Massague, 2008). It is generally accepted that excessive production and or activation of TGF-β by tumor cells can foster cancer progression by mechanisms that include an increase in tumor neoangiogenesis and extracellular matrix production, upregulation of proteases surrounding tumors, and inhibition of immune surveillance in the cancer host (Massague, 2008). In this chapter, we will discuss TGF-β signaling alterations in cancer development.

TGF-β Signaling

TGF-β is a multifunctional cytokine with diverse effects on virtually all cell types and with key roles during embryonic development and tissue homeostasis (Massague et al., 2000). Members of the TGF-β superfamily ligands, such as TGF-β, activin, and BMP, transduce their signals through heterotetrameric complexes comprising two types of serine–threonine kinase receptors, the type 1 and type 2. Upon ligand binding, the type 2 receptor phosphorylates and activates the type 1 receptor, which initiates downstream signaling by phosphorylating the receptor-regulated SMADs (R-SMADs). Each ligand signals through a specific combination of type 2, type 1, and R-Smads (Shi and Massague, 2003). TGF-β binds to the TGF-β type 2 receptor (TGFBR2) and the TGF-β type 1 receptor (TGFBR1, also formerly named TβRI or Alk5 for activin receptor-like kinase 5), although in endothelial cells it can also bind a complex comprising TGFBR2, ACVRL1, and TGFBR1 (Goumans et al., 2003). The type I receptor dictates the specificity for the R-SMADs, TGFBR1, ACVR1B, and ACVR1C phosphorylate SMAD2 and SMAD3 whereas ACVRL1, ACVR1, BMPR1A, and BMPR1B phosphorylate SMAD1, SMAD5, and SMAD8. Once phosphorylated, these R-SMADs transduce the signal to the nucleus in cooperation with the common mediator, SMAD4, to transcriptionally activate or repress different targets genes (Shi and Massague, 2003). The TGF-β superfamily pathways are also negatively regulated. The inhibitory SMADs, SMAD6, and SMAD7 bind the active receptor complexes and also recruit E3 ubiquitin ligase SMURF1/2 to the receptor complexes to degrade them (Imamura et al., 1997; Ebisawa et al., 2001). SMAD7 has also been shown to participate in a complex that dephosphorylates the active TGF-β receptor (Shi et al., 2004).

The TGF-β superfamily signaling pathways are involved in many different biological processes during embryonic development, and in adult organisms they play a role in tissue homeostasis (Massague, 1998). They are also strongly implicated in cancer, since alterations of some specific and some common components of these different pathways have been identified in the majority of human tumors. Cancer is a multistep process resulting from the evolution of a clonal cell population that has escaped from the control of regulatory circuits that normally govern cell proliferation and homeostasis. Two distinct types of genetic alterations have been identified: gain-of-functions in oncogenes that usually result in growth factor-independent cell proliferation, or recessive loss-of-function mutations in tumor suppressors that allow evasion of growth inhibitory signals. The well-characterized growth inhibitory response of TGF-β (Massague et al., 2000) combined with the fact that up to 74% of colon cancer cell lines and 85% of lung cancer cell lines have become resistant to TGF-β antiproliferative effect (Kim et al., 1999; Grady et al., 1999) led several groups to search for evidence of inactivation of components of the TGF-β pathway in human cancer. It has also been found that TGF-β secretion is abundant in many human cancers and the TGF-β-rich microenvironment is associated with poor prognosis, tumor vascularization, and metastasis (Derynck et al., 2001). A dual role for TGF-β in cancer has long been noted, but its mechanistic basis, operating logic, and clinical relevance have remained elusive (Massague, 2008). Understanding the relevance of TGF-β's role in cancer is a prerequisite to fully explore the therapeutic potential of this pathway.

Receptor Alterations in Human Tumors

Changes in TGFBR2 Expression Levels and TGFBR2 Mutations in Cancer

Loss of expression of *TGFBR2* is observed in 44% each of non-small cell lung carcinomas (NSCLC) and bladder cancers, in about 30% of head and neck squamous cell carcinomas (HNSCC) of the esophagus, in 23% of ovarian carcinomas, and in 12.5% of prostate cancers, and also in breast cancers (Fukai et al., 2003; Garrigue-Antar et al., 1996; Gobbi et al., 2000; Kim et al., 1996; Kim et al., 1998; Lynch et al., 1998; Zhang et al., 2004). The *TGFBR2* gene contains an A(10) tract in exon 3 and GT(3) tracts in exon 5 and 7, which are microsatellite sequences prone to replication errors, especially in the presence of MMR gene inactivation. Frameshift mutations of *TGFBR2* are found in more than 80% of microsatellite instability-positive (MSI+) colorectal cancers (Takayama et al., 2006). It is commonly speculated that colorectal cancers acquire partial TGF-β resistance largely because of *TGFBR2* genetic alterations. In fact, the overall incidence of *TGFBR2* mutations is close to 30% in colorectal cancer and is the most common mechanism identified so far that results in TGF-β signaling alterations (Grady et al., 1999; Grady and Markowitz, 2000). Interestingly, some colorectal cancer cell lines, which harbor homozygous mutations of *TGFBR2*, are growth-inhibited by TGF-β, which suggests that under certain circumstance, the cells can bypass *TGFBR2* to maintain growth inhibition (Ilyas et al., 1999).

Whether *TGFBR2* mutations truly contribute to colorectal tumorigenesis or arise as bystander mutations in MSI+ tumors has been a topic of controversy. The fact that *TGFBR2* missense mutations are identified in about 15% of colon cancer cell lines that are microsatellite stable provides some support for the notion that

TGFBR2 serves as a tumor suppressor in colorectal cancer (Grady et al., 1999). To determine the pathogenic relevance of *TGFBR2* inactivation in colorectal cancer, a mouse model that was null for *Tgfbr2* in the colonic epithelium was generated and treated with azoxymethane to induce colorectal cancer formation (Biswas et al., 2004). Mice that lack *Tgfbr2* in the colon epithelium developed more colorectal adenomas and adenocarcinomas and had increased neoplastic proliferation when compared with mice with intact *Tgfbr2* (Biswas et al., 2004). The increased cellular proliferation observed in tissues devoid of *Tgfbr2* is likely due to the failure to inactivate Cdk4 expression as Cdk4 expression is upregulated in MSI+ cancers (Grady et al., 2006). In addition, reconstitution of *TGFBR2* in a MSI+ colorectal cancer cell line resulted in a decrease in Cdk4 expression and activation, accompanied with a decrease in cellular proliferation (Grady et al., 2006). These studies suggest that *TGFBR2* inactivation may be a factor contributing to the transformation of colorectal cancers.

TGFBR1 Mutations and Polymorphisms in Colorectal Cancer

Mutations in *TGFBR1* have been identified in human colorectal cancer cell lines but are uncommon (Ku et al., 2007). However, decreased *TGFBR1* expression levels are frequently observed. In such cells, reconstitution of *TGFBR1* expression has been shown to decrease tumorigenesis. *TGFBR1**6A, a *TGFBR1* polymorphism that consists of a deletion of three alanines within a nine-alanine repeat at the 3' end of exon 1, results in an impairment of TGF-β-mediated antiproliferative response, and has been associated with increased cancer risk (Pasche et al., 2004). Genotyping of germline and tumor DNA has shown that *TGFBR1**6A is somatically acquired in approximately 2% of primary colon and head and neck tumors. Exogenous TGF-β increases thymidine incorporation in breast cancer cells stably transfected with this variant and in colon cancer cells that endogenously harbor this allele (Pasche et al., 2005), suggesting that *TGFBR1**6A has oncogenic properties in established tumor cells.

To determine the role of *TGFBR1**6A in the tumor microenvironment, we microdissected tumors cells, stromal cell, and histologically "normal" epithelial cells adjacent to the tumor from individual with head and neck cancer and evidence of *TGFBR1**6A somatic acquisition within the tumor tissue. In head and neck cancer we found that the *TGFBR1**6A allele was present in the tumor, immediately juxtaposed "normal" squamous epithelium and stroma as well as in adjacent true vocal cord epithelium and stroma. In colon cancer we found that the *TGFBR1**6A allele had been somatically acquired by stromal cells up to 2 cm away from the tumor's edge. Importantly, we found higher *TGFBR1**6A/*TGFBR1* allelic ratios in tumor tissues compared with stromal and epithelial tissues (Bian et al., 2007). Hence, the amount of somatically acquired *TGFBR1**6A allele in normal epithelial and stromal cells surrounding the tumor appears to be inversely proportional to the distance from the primary tumor, suggestive of tumor-centered centrifugal growth (Bian et al., 2007). This provides strong support for the novel concept that *TGFBR1**6A somatic acquisition is a critical event in the early stages of cancer development that is associated with field cancerization (Bian et al., 2007). However, *TGFBR1**6A is not a bona fide oncogene when transfected into NIH 3T3cells. Rather, its decreased TGF-β signaling capabilities result in reduced oncogenesis when compared with wild-type *TGFBR1* (Rosman et al., 2008). To test the hypothesis that decreased *TGFBR1*signaling contributes to colorectal cancer development, we generated a novel mouse model of *TGFBR1* haploinsufficiency (Zeng et al., 2009).

We found that *Tgfbr1* haploinsufficient mice crossed with mice carrying a mutation in the *Apc* tumor suppressor gene, develop two to three times more intestinal tumors than wild-type littermates. Importantly, invasive adenocarcinoma with features of human colon cancer is only identified among $Apc^{Min/+}$; $Tgfbr1^{+/-}$ mice, not among $Apc^{Min/+}$; $Tgfbr1^{+/+}$ mice (Zeng et al., 2009). These findings led us to study whether constitutively decreased *TGFBR1* expression is associated with human cancer. We recently reported that constitutively decreased TGFBR1 expression is an inherited trait associated with significantly increased colorectal cancer risk (Valle et al., 2008).

SMAD Mutation and Isoforms in Colorectal Cancer

TGF-β signaling can also be impaired by deletions or mutations in the *SMAD* genes, which encode for proteins that act downstream of the receptors. *SMAD4*, originally identified as a tumor suppressor gene lost in pancreatic cancers termed *DPC4* (Deleted in Pancreatic Cancer 4) (Hahn et al., 1996), is mutated in 16–25% of colorectal cancer cases, and alterations of *SMAD2* have been identified in about 6% of colorectal cancers (Takayama et al., 2006). In fact, *SMAD2* and *SMAD4* both map to chromosome 18q, a region commonly deleted in colon adenocarcinomas (Grady and Markowitz, 2002). *SMAD4* mutations occur in more than half of pancreatic carcinomas and are close in prevalence to mutations in *KRAS*, *TP53*, and *CDKN2A* (formerly named *p16INK4A*) (Jaffee et al., 2002). *SMAD4* mutations are found in more than half of sporadic colorectal tumors without microsatellite instability (but not in tumors with microsatellite instability), in a high proportion of esophageal tumors, and with less frequency in other cancers (Sjoblom et al., 2006).

Germline mutations of *SMAD4* cause juvenile polyposis (Howe et al., 1998) as well as hamartomatous polyposis (Sweet et al., 2005). While both *Smad2*-null and *Smad4*-null mice die in utero, mice with heterozygous deletion of *Smad4* are predisposed to gastrointestinal polyps that can eventually develop into tumors (Mishra et al., 2005), which suggests that *Smad4* functions as a tumor suppressor in colorectal cancer progression. In agreement with these findings, it has recently been shown that TGF-β-induced epithelial–mesenchymal transition is not dependent on *SMAD4*, and *SMAD4* mainly mediates the antiproliferative response to TGF-β (Levy and Hill, 2005). A recent study showed that mice with selective loss of *Smad4*-dependent signaling in T cell develop spontaneous epithelial cancers throughout the gastrointestinal tract, including colon and rectum, where tumors are heavily infiltrated with plasma cells. Importantly, mice with epithelial-specific deletion of the *Smad4* gene do not have the same phenotype (Kim et al., 2006). These results suggest that SMAD4 mediates crosstalk between stromal and epithelial cells, and interference with this process may eventually lead to cancer.

Until recently *SMAD3*mutations in human colorectal cancer were thought to be rare (Ku et al., 2007) and their true pathogenic role has yet to be defined. However, a recent report suggests that SMAD3 mutations are among the most common mutations observed in this disease (Sjoblom et al., 2006). Interestingly, mice with loss of *Smad3* develop a high frequency of metastatic colon carcinoma by 6 months of age (Zhu et al., 1998). It was also reported that skin wounds heal faster, with a rapid rate of keratinocyte proliferation and migration in *Smad3* null mice (Ashcroft et al., 1999). However, two additional lines of *Smad3*-deficient mice do not develop colonic adenocarcinoma (Datto et al., 1995; Yang et al., 1999). Recently, it has been reported that Helicobacter-induced chronic inflammation may explain this discrepancy (Maggio-Price et al., 2006). *Smad3*-null mice maintained in a bacteria-free environment did not develop colon cancer for up to 9 months, while infection of these mice with the gram-negative enterohepatic bacteria Helicobacter triggered colon cancer in more than half of the animals. This suggests that bacterial infection plays an important role in triggering colorectal cancer in the context of gene mutations in the TGF-β signaling pathway(Maggio-Price et al., 2006).

In acute myelogenous leukemia (AML), transcriptional repressors encoded by the chimeric genes *AML1/EVI-1* from a 3:21 translocation and *AML1/ETO* from an 8:21 translocation interact with SMAD3 and suppress TGF-β signaling (Letterio, 2005). SMAD3 has two phosphoisoforms: one phosphorylated at the C-terminal region (pSMAD3C) by TGFBR1, and the other phosphorylated at the linker region (pSMAD3L) by JNK (Yamagata et al., 2005). While SMAD3C is expressed in normal colorectal epithelial cells and inhibits their growth, pSMAD3L is highly expressed in late-stage sporadic colorectal tumors and mediates mesenchymal cell invasion (Yamagata et al., 2005). It has been suggested that during sporadic colorectal carcinogenesis, tumor cells gain growth advantage through a shift from TGFBR1/pSMAD3C-mediated to JNK/pSMAD3L-mediated signaling (Matsuzaki et al., 2006; Matsuzaki, 2006).

SMAD Antagonists

SMAD6 and SMAD7 are inhibitory SMADs that negatively control TGF-β signaling in response to feedback loops and antagonistic signals (Massague et al., 2005). SMAD6 competes with SMAD4 for binding to receptor-activated

SMAD1 and SMAD7 recruits SMURF to TGF-β and BMP receptors for inactivation. Overexpression of SMAD7 and suppression of TGF-β signaling has been reported in endometrial carcinomas and thyroid follicular tumors (Cerutti et al., 2003; Dowdy et al., 2005). Interestingly, a recent genome-wide association study has shown that common alleles of *SMAD7* that lead to decreased SMAD7 mRNA expression are associated with colorectal cancer risk (Broderick et al., 2007). SMAD function is also directly inhibited by transcriptional repressors such as SKI and SNON (SKI-like). Deletions as well as amplification of *SKI* and *SKIL* have been reported in colorectal and esophageal cancers, raising the possibility that these genes act as oncogenes or tumor suppressor genes depending on the context (Zhu et al., 2007).

TGF-β Signaling Alterations Within the Stromal Compartment

Next, we will discuss the role of altered TGF-β signaling in the stromal compartment and tumor microenvironment. The tumor microenvironment is defined as the non-epithelial components of the area immediately surrounding tumor cells including fibroblasts, immune cells, extracellular matrix (ECM), and blood vessels. The TGF-β signaling pathway is a critical regulator of cancer initiation, development, progression through tumor cell autonomous signaling, and interactions within tumor microenvironment. The complex role that TGF-β plays in cancer via cell autonomous mechanisms has been extensively investigated (Roberts and Wakefield, 2003).

TGF-β Signaling in Stromal Fibroblasts

A study investigating the loss of TGF-β signaling in fibroblasts during mammary gland development demonstrated that fibroblasts can regulate adjacent epithelial cell morphogenesis. Zinc-inducible overexpression of a dominant negative TGFBR2 transgene resulted in attenuation of TGF-β signaling in the stroma adjacent to mammary epithelia (Joseph et al., 1999). The loss of TGF-β signaling in fibroblasts increased lateral ductal branching and correlated with an increased level of HGF mRNA expression. These results suggested that TGF-β signaling could contribute to the regulation of stromal–epithelial interactions in vivo.

A subsequent report of conditional inactivation of the *Tgfbr2* gene in mouse fibroblasts provided the first unequivocal proof of principle that abrogation of TGF-β signaling within the stroma leads to cancer development. Indeed, these mice had evidence of stromal hyperplasia with accompanying nuclear atypia and hyperplasia of adjacent epithelial cells resulting in prostatic intraepithelial neoplasia (PIN) (Bhowmick et al., 2004). The forestomach of these mice had increased abundance of fibroblasts, but the stromal expansion was accompanied by invasive squamous cell carcinoma. Similarly, abrogation of TGF-β signaling in mammary fibroblasts resulted in an increased rate of fibroblast proliferation (Cheng et al., 2005). When engrafted under the kidney capsule with mammary carcinoma cells, *Tgfbr2*-null fibroblasts were able to promote adjacent carcinoma growth and invasion through upregulation of paracrine factors including TGF-α, macrophage-stimulating protein (MSP), and HGF (Cheng et al., 2005). These secreted factors induced phosphorylation and activation of their cognate receptors ErbB1 and ErbB2, RON, and c-Met, respectively. Inhibition of downstream signaling from the cognate receptors through administration of pharmacologic inhibitiors (TGF-α) or neutralizing antibodies (MSP, HGF, c-Met) limited proliferation and invasion (Cheng et al., 2005).

TGF-β *Signaling in the Immune System*

It has long been known that chronic inflammation can promote tumor progression (Coussens and Werb, 2002). Mice with *Smad4*-null T cells exhibit an expansion of the gastrointestinal stromal compartment with a significant plasma cell infiltrate that is associated with increased levels of IgA locally and in the serum. The loss of *Smad4* expression results in skewed maturation toward a *Th2* phenotype, with increased levels of cytokines including IL-4,-5,-6, and -13 in vivo and in vitro. Knock-out mice produced through expression of Cre under control of the designed promoter went on to spontaneously develop carcinoma in the gastrointestinal tract. In addition, these mice also exhibit a high rate of oral squamous cell carcinoma. This study illustrates a concept and mechanism wherein the loss of TGF-β signaling from a stromal component, independent of an epithelial cell autonomous defect, can initiate and promote carcinoma in vivo.

Whether alterations of stromal TGFBR1 signaling account for the significant increase in colorectal cancer susceptibility incurred by *Tgfbr1* haploinsufficient mice (Zeng et al., 2009) and individuals with constitutively decreased TGFBR1 expression (Valle et al., 2008) will need to be further studied. Also relevant to cancer development are the effects of TGF-β on stromal lymphocytes. TGF-β is a key enforcer of immune tolerance and tumors that produce high levels of this cytokine may be shielded from immune surveillance. On the other hand, defective TGF-β responsiveness in immune cells can lead to chronic inflammation, which creates a protumorigenic environment. Tumor-derived TGF-β may recruit other stromal cell types such as myofibroblasts (at the invading tumor front) and osteoclasts (in bone metastases), thus furthering tumor spread (Massague, 2008).

The TGF-β signaling pathway is a potent regulator of the immune system (Kirkbride and Blobe, 2003), and its immunosuppressive effects are predominantly mediated by its effects on T cells and antigen-presenting cells (APCs). TGF-β inhibits IL-2-dependent proliferation of T cells, and prevents naive T cells from acquiring effector functions (Gorelik and Flavell, 2002). TGF-β may also mediates its immunosuppressive effects on T cells through $CD4^+CD25^+$ regulator T cells, which secrete TGF-β1 and express cell surface-bound TGF-β1 (Nakamura et al., 2001). TGF-β also has potent effects on APCs, with autocrine TGF-β inhibiting tissue macrophage activation (Bogdan et al., 1992) and promoting differentiation of dendritic cells from precursors (Riedl et al., 1997).

TGF-β Signaling and EMT

Another tumorigenic effect of TGF-β signaling is the induction of epithelial–mesenchymal transition (EMT) in human cancer (Shipitsin et al., 2007). EMT is a well-coordinated process during embryonic development and a pathological feature in neoplasia and fibrosis (Thiery, 2003). Cells undergoing EMT lose expression of E-cadherin and other components of epithelial junctions. Instead, they produce a mesenchymal cell cytoskeleton and acquire motility and invasive properties. It was first reported in mouse heart formation and palate fusion, in some mammary cell lines and in mouse models of skin carcinogenesis that TGF-β is a potent inducer of EMT (Derynck and Akhurst, 2007; Thiery, 2003). TGF-β-induced EMT is observed in transformed epithelial progenitor cells with tumor propagating ability (Mani et al., 2008). EMT-like processes contribute to tumor invasion and dissemination owing to the cell junction free, motile phenotype they confer. Carcinoma cells with mesenchymal traits have been observed in the invasion front of carcinomas and may reflect a series of interconnected features that: carcinomas are propagated by transformed progenitor cells, progenitor cells are competent to undergo EMT, EMT is triggered at the invasion front, which ultimately augments the disseminative capacity of these cells (Mani et al., 2008; Massague, 2008).

TGF-β promotes EMT by a combination of SMAD-dependent transcriptional events and SMAD-independent effects on cell junction complexes. SMAD-mediated expression of HMGA2 (high mobility group A2) induces expression of SNAIL, SLUG, and TWIST (Thuault et al., 2006; Thuault et al., 2008). Independent of SMAD activity, TGFBR2-mediated phosphorylation of PAR6 promotes the dissolution of cell junction complexes (Ozdamar et al., 2005). In mouse tumors and cell lines, TGF-β-induced EMT is Smad-dependent and enhanced by Ras signaling (Derynck and Akhurst, 2007). TGF-β also enhances cell motility by cooperating with HER2 signals, as observed in breast cancer cells overexpressing HER2 (Seton-Rogers et al., 2004).

Conclusions

Recently a systematic, genome-wide scans of several types of cancer (breast cancer, colorectal cancer, pancreatic cancer, and glioblastoma) have revealed important novel information on the genetic underpinnings of these diseases. Sequencing the protein-coding regions of more than 13,000 genes in breast and colon cancer, 189 genes were identified, with an average of 11 per tumor that were clearly mutated in breast and colon tumors. The vast majority of these genes such as *SMAD3* were not known to be genetically altered in tumors and are predicted to affect a wide range of cellular functions, including transcription, adhesion, and invasion (Sjoblom et al., 2006). The results are limited to the genome-wide sequencing of only 11 breast and 11 colon tumors, but they provide the first proof of concept that this comprehensive approach holds great promise with respect to the genetic understanding of cancer.

In summary, both pathway-specific and global genomic approaches highlight the central role of TGF-β alterations in cancer development and progression. TGF-β pathway alterations in cancer illustrate the complex but crucial role of stromal cells with respect to cancer development and progression.

Acknowledgments Supported by grants from CA112520, CA108741 from the NCI and AR048098-070007 from the NIH.

References

Ashcroft GS, Yang X, Glick AB, Weinstein M, Letterio JJ, Mizel DE, Anzano M, Greenwell-Wild T, Wahl SM, Deng CX, Roberts AB. 1999. Mice lacking Smad3 show accelerated wound healing and an impaired local inflammatory response. Nat Cell Biol 1:260–266.

Bhowmick NA, Chytil A, Plieth D, Gorska AE, Dumont N, Shappell S, Washington MK, Neilson EG, Moses HL. 2004. TGF-{beta} Signaling in fibroblasts modulates the oncogenic potential of adjacent epithelia. Science 303:848–851.

Bian Y, Knobloch TJ, Sadim M, Kaklamani V, Raji A, Yang GY, Weghorst CM, Pasche B. 2007. Somatic acquisition of TGFBR1*6A by epithelial and stromal cells during head and neck and colon cancer development. Hum Mol Genet 16:3128–3135.

Biswas S, Chytil A, Washington K, Romero-Gallo J, Gorska AE, Wirth PS, Gautam S, Moses HL, Grady WM. 2004. Transforming growth factor {beta} receptor Type II Inactivation promotes the establishment and progression of colon cancer. Cancer Res 64:4687–4692.

Bogdan C, Paik J, Vodovotz Y, Nathan C. 1992. Contrasting mechanisms for suppression of macrophage cytokine release by transforming growth factor-beta and interleukin-10. J Biol Chem 267:23301–23308.

Broderick P, Carvajal-Carmona L, Pittman AM, Webb E, Howarth K, Rowan A, Lubbe S, Spain S, Sullivan K, Fielding S, Jaeger E, Vijayakrishnan J, Kemp Z, Gorman M, Chandler I, Papaemmanuil E, Penegar S, Wood W, Sellick G, Qureshi M, Teixeira A, Domingo E, Barclay E, Martin L, Sieber O, Kerr D, Gray R, Peto J, Cazier JB, Tomlinson I, Houlston RS. 2007. A genome-wide association study shows that common alleles of SMAD7 influence colorectal cancer risk. Nat Genet 39:1315–1317.

Cerutti JM, Ebina KN, Matsuo SE, Martins L, Maciel RM, Kimura ET. 2003. Expression of Smad4 and Smad7 in human thyroid follicular carcinoma cell lines. J Endocrinol Invest 26:516–521

Cheng N, Bhowmick NA, Chytil A, Gorksa AE, Brown KA, Muraoka R, Arteaga CL, Neilson EG, Hayward SW, Moses HL. 2005. Loss of TGF-beta type II receptor in fibroblasts promotes mammary carcinoma growth and invasion through upregulation of TGF-alpha-, MSP- and HGF-mediated signaling networks. Oncogene 24:5053–5068.

Coussens LM and Werb Z. 2002. Inflammation and cancer. Nature 420:860–867.

Datto MB, Li Y, Panus JF, Howe DJ, Xiong Y, Wang XF. 1995. Transforming growth factor beta induces the cyclin-dependent kinase inhibitor p21 through a p53-independent mechanism. Proc Natl Acad Sci U S A 92:5545–5549.

Derynck R and Akhurst RJ. 2007. Differentiation plasticity regulated by TGF-[beta] family proteins in development and disease. Nat Cell Biol 9:1000–1004.

Derynck R, Akhurst RJ, Balmain A. 2001. TGF-beta signaling in tumor suppression and cancer progression. Nat Genet 29:117–129.

Dowdy SC, Mariani A, Reinholz MM, Keeney GL, Spelsberg TC, Podratz KC, Janknecht R. 2005. Overexpression of the TGF-beta antagonist Smad7 in endometrial cancer. Gynecol Oncol 96:368–373.

Ebisawa T, Fukuchi M, Murakami G, Chiba T, Tanaka K, Imamura T, Miyazono K. 2001. Smurf1 interacts with transforming growth factor-beta type I receptor through Smad7 and induces receptor degradation. J Biol Chem 276:12477–12480.

Fukai Y, Fukuchi M, Masuda N, Osawa H, Kato H, Nakajima T, Kuwano H. 2003. Reduced expression of transforming growth factor-beta receptors is an unfavorable prognostic factor in human esophageal squamous cell carcinoma. Int J Cancer 104:161–166.

Garrigue-Antar L, Souza RF, Vellucci VF, Meltzer SJ, Reiss M. 1996. Loss of transforming growth factor-beta type II receptor gene expression in primary human esophageal cancer. Lab Invest 75:263–272.

Gobbi H, Arteaga CL, Jensen RA, Simpson JF, Dupont WD, Olson SJ, Schuyler PA, Plummer WD, Page DL, david.page@mcmail.vanderbilt.edu, Benign bd, Ductal carcinoma is, Immunohistochemistry, Invasive mc, Transforming growth factor beta receptors. 2000. Loss of expression of transforming growth factor beta type II receptor correlates with high tumour grade in human breast in-situ and invasive carcinomas. Histopathology 36:168–177.

Gorelik L, Flavell RA. 2002. Transforming growth factor-beta in T-cell biology. Nat Rev Immunol 2:46–53.

Goumans MJ, Valdimarsdottir G, Itoh S, Lebrin F, Larsson J, Mummery C, Karlsson S, ten Dijke P. 2003. Activin receptor-like kinase (ALK)1 is an antagonistic mediator of lateral TGF[beta]/ALK5 signaling. Mol Cell 12:817–828.

Grady WM and Markowitz S. 2000. Genomic instability and colorectal cancer. Current Opinion in Gastroenterology 16:62–67.

Grady WM and Markowitz SD. 2002. Genetic and epigenetic alterations in colon cancer. Annu Rev Genom Hum Genet 3:101–128.

Grady WM, Myeroff LL, Swinler SE, Rajput A, Thiagalingam S, Lutterbaugh JD, Neumann A, Brattain MG, Chang J, Kim SJ, Kinzler KW, Vogelstein B, Willson JK, Markowitz S. 1999. Mutational inactivation of transforming growth factor beta receptor type II in microsatellite stable colon cancers. Cancer Res 59:320–324.

Grady WM, Willis JE, Trobridge P, Romero-Gallo J, Munoz N, Olechnowicz J, Ferguson K, Gautam S, Markowitz SD. 2006. Proliferation and Cdk4 expression in microsatellite unstable colon cancers with TGFBR2 mutations. Int J Cancer 118:600–608.

Hahn SA, Schutte M, Hoque AT, Moskaluk CA, da Costa LT, Rozenblum E, Weinstein CL, Fischer A, Yeo CJ, Hruban RH, Kern SE. 1996. Dpc4, a candidate tumor suppressor gene at human chromosome 18q21.1. [see comments]. Science 271:350–353.

Howe JR, Roth S, Ringold JC, Summers RW, Jarvinen HJ, Sistonen P, Tomlinson IP, Houlston RS, Bevan S, Mitros FA, Stone EM, Aaltonen LA. 1998. Mutations in the SMAD4/DPC4 gene in juvenile polyposis. Science 280:1086–1088.

Ilyas M, Efstathiou JA, Straub J, Kim HC, Bodmer WF. 1999. Transforming growth factor beta stimulation of colorectal cancer cell lines: Type II receptor bypass and changes in adhesion molecule expression. Proc 96:3087–3091.

Imamura T, Takase M, Nishihara A, Oeda E, Hanai J, Kawabata M, Miyazono K. 1997. Smad6 inhibits signalling by the tgf-beta superfamily. Nature 389:622–626.

Jaffee EM, Hruban RH, Canto M, Kern SE. 2002. Focus on pancreas cancer. Cancer Cell 2: 25–28.

Janssens K, Gershoni-Baruch R, Guanabens N, Migone N, Ralston S, Bonduelle M, Lissens W, Van ML, Vanhoenacker F, Verbruggen L, Van HW. 2000. Mutations in the gene encoding the latency-associated peptide of TGF-beta 1 cause Camurati-Engelmann disease. Nat Genet 26:273–275.

Joseph H, Gorska AE, Sohn P, Moses HL, Serra R. 1999. Overexpression of a kinase-deficient transforming growth factor-beta type II receptor in mouse mammary stroma results in increased epithelial branching. Molecular Biology of the Cell 10:1221–1234.

Kim IY, Ahn HJ, Zelner DJ, Shaw JW, Lang S, Kato R, Oefelein MG, Miyazono K, Nemeth JA, Kozlowski JM, Lee C. 1996. Loss of expression of transforming growth factor beta type i and type ii receptors correlates with tumor grade in human prostate cancer. Clin Cancer Res 2:1255–1261.

Kim IY, Ahn HJ, Lang S, Oefelein MG, Oyasu R, Kozlowski JM, Lee C. 1998. Loss of expression of transforming growth factor-beta receptors is associated with poor prognosis in prostate cancer patients. Clini Cancer Res 4:1625–1630.

Kim WS, Park C, Jung YS, Kim HS, Han JH, Park CH, Kim K, Kim J, Shim YM, Park K. 1999. Reduced transforming growth factor-beta type II receptor (TGF-beta RII) expression in adenocarcinoma of the lung. Anticancer Res 19:301–306.

Kim BG, Li C, Qiao W, Mamura M, Kasperczak B, Anver M, Wolfraim L, Hong S, Mushinski E, Potter M, Kim SJ, Fu XY, Deng C, Letterio JJ. 2006. Smad4 signalling in T cells is required for suppression of gastrointestinal cancer. Nature 441:1015–1019.

Kinoshita A, Saito T, Tomita H, Makita Y, Yoshida K, Ghadami M, Yamada K, Kondo S, Ikegawa S, Nishimura G, Fukushima Y, Nakagomi T, Saito H, Sugimoto T, Kamegaya M, Hisa K, Murray JC, Taniguchi N, Niikawa N, Yoshiura K. 2000. Domain-specific mutations in TGFB1 result in Camurati-Engelmann disease. Nat Genet 26:19–20.

Kirkbride KC, Blobe GC. 2003. Inhibiting the TGF-beta signalling pathway as a means of cancer immunotherapy. Expert Opin Biol Ther 3:251–261.

Ku JL, Park SH, Yoon KA, Shin YK, Kim KH, Choi JS, Kang HC, Kim IJ, Han IO, Park JG. 2007. Genetic alterations of the TGF-beta signaling pathway in colorectal cancer cell lines: A novel mutation in Smad3 associated with the inactivation of TGF-beta-induced transcriptional activation. Cancer Lett 247:283–292.

Letterio JJ. 2005. TGF-beta signaling in T cells: Roles in lymphoid and epithelial neoplasia. Oncog 24:5701–5712.

Levy L, Hill CS. 2005. Smad4 dependency defines two classes of transforming growth factor {beta} (TGF-{beta}) target genes and distinguishes TGF-{beta}-induced epithelial-mesenchymal transition from its antiproliferative and migratory responses. Mol Cell Biol 25:8108–8125.

Lynch MA, Nakashima R, Song H, Degroff VL, Wang D, Enomoto T, Weghorst CM. 1998. Mutational analysis of the transforming growth factor beta receptor type II gene in human ovarian carcinoma. Cancer Res 58:4227–4232.

Maggio-Price L, Treuting P, Zeng W, Tsang M, Bielefeldt-Ohmann H, Iritani BM. 2006. Helicobacter Infection Is Required for Inflammation and Colon Cancer in Smad3-Deficient Mice. Cancer Res 66:828–838.

Mani SA, Guo W, Liao MJ, Eaton EN, Ayyanan A, Zhou AY, Brooks M, Reinhard F, Zhang CC, Shipitsin M, Campbell LL, Polyak K, Brisken C, Yang J, Weinberg RA. 2008. The epithelial-mesenchymal transition generates cells with properties of stem cells. Cell 133:704–715.

Massague J. 1998. TGF-beta signal transduction. Annu Rev Biochem 67:753–791.

Massague J. 2008. TGF-beta in Cancer. Cell 134:215–230.

Massague J, Blain SW, Lo RS. 2000. TGFbeta signaling in growth control, cancer, and heritable disorders. Cell 103:295–309.

Massague J, Seoane J, Wotton D. 2005. Smad transcription factors. Genes Dev 19:2783–2810.

Matsuzaki K. 2006. Smad3 phosphoisoform-mediated signaling during sporadic human colorectal carcinogenesis. Histol Histopathol 21:645–662.

Matsuzaki K, Seki T, Okazaki K. 2006. TGF-beta during human colorectal carcinogenesis: The shift from epithelial to mesenchymal signaling. Inflammopharmacology 14:198–203.

Mishra L, Shetty K, Tang Y, Stuart A, Byers SW. 2005. The role of TGF-beta and Wnt signaling in gastrointestinal stem cells and cancer. Oncog 24:5775–5789.

Moses HL, Robinson RA. 1982. Growth factors, growth factor receptors, and cell cycle control mechanisms in chemically transformed cells. Fed Proc 41:3008–3011.

Nakamura K, Kitani A, Strober W. 2001. Cell contact-dependent immunosuppression by CD4(+)CD25(+) regulatory T cells is mediated by cell surface-bound transforming growth factor beta. J Exp Med 194:629–644.

Ozdamar B, Bose R, Barrios-Rodiles M, Wang HR, Zhang Y, Wrana JL. 2005. Regulation of the polarity protein Par6 by TGFbeta receptors controls epithelial cell plasticity. Science 307: 1603–1609.

Pasche B, Kaklamani VG, Hou N, Young T, Rademaker A, Peterlongo P, Ellis N, Offit K, Caldes T, Reiss M, Zheng T. 2004. TGFBR1*6A and cancer: A meta-analysis of 12 case-control studies. J Clin Oncol 22:756–758.

Pasche B, Knobloch TJ, Bian Y, Liu J, Phukan S, Rosman D, Kaklamani V, Baddi L, Siddiqui FS, Frankel W, Prior TW, Schuller DE, Agrawal A, Lang J, Dolan ME, Vokes EE, Lane WS, Huang CC, Caldes T, Di Cristofano A, Hampel H, Nilsson I, von Heijne G, Fodde R, Murty VVVS, de la Chapelle A, Weghorst CM. 2005. Somatic acquisition and signaling of TGFBR1*6A in cancer. JAMA 294:1634–1646.

Riedl E, Strobl H, Majdic O, Knapp W. 1997. Tgf-beta-1 promotes in vitro generation of dendritic cells by protecting progenitor cells from apoptosis. J Immunol 158:1591–1597.

Roberts AB and Wakefield LM. 2003. The two faces of transforming growth factor {beta} in carcinogenesis. PNAS 100:8621.

Roberts AB, Lamb LC, Newton DL, Sporn MB, De Larco JE, Todaro GJ. 1980. Transforming growth factors: isolation of polypeptides from virally and chemically transformed cells by acid/ethanol extraction. Proc Natl Acad Sci U S A 77:3494–3498.

Rosman DS, Phukan S, Huang CC, Pasche B. 2008. TGFBR1*6A enhances the migration and invasion of MCF-7 breast cancer cells through RhoA activation. Cancer Res 68:1319–1328.

Seton-Rogers SE, Lu Y, Hines LM, Koundinya M, LaBaer J, Muthuswamy SK, Brugge JS. 2004. Cooperation of the ErbB2 receptor and transforming growth factor beta in induction of migration and invasion in mammary epithelial cells. Proc Natl Acad Sci U S A 101: 1257–1262.

Shi Y and Massague J. 2003. Mechanisms of TGF-beta signaling from cell membrane to the nucleus. Cell 113:685–700.

Shi W, Sun C, He B, Xiong W, Shi X, Yao D, Cao X. 2004. GADD34-PP1c recruited by Smad7 dephosphorylates TGFbeta type I receptor. J Cell Biol 164:291–300.

Shipitsin M, Campbell LL, Argani P, Weremowicz S, Bloushtain-Qimron N, Yao J, Nikolskaya T, Serebryiskaya T, Beroukhim R, Hu M, Halushka MK, Sukumar S, Parker LM, Anderson KS, Harris LN, Garber JE, Richardson AL, Schnitt SJ, Nikolsky Y, Gelman RS, Polyak K. 2007. Molecular definition of breast tumor heterogeneity. Cancer Cell 11:259–273.

Siegel PM and Massague J. 2003. Cytostatic and apoptotic actions of TGF-beta in homeostasis and cancer. Nat Rev Cancer 3:807–820.

Sjoblom T, Jones S, Wood LD, Parsons DW, Lin J, Barber TD, Mandelker D, Leary RJ, Ptak J, Silliman N, Szabo S, Buckhaults P, Farrell C, Meeh P, Markowitz SD, Willis J, Dawson D, Willson JKV, Gazdar AF, Hartigan J, Wu L, Liu C, Parmigiani G, Park BH, Bachman KE, Papadopoulos N, Vogelstein B, Kinzler KW, Velculescu VE. 2006. The consensus coding sequences of human breast and colorectal cancers. Science 314:268–274.

Sweet K, Willis J, Zhou XP, Gallione C, Sawada T, Alhopuro P, Khoo SK, Patocs A, Martin C, Bridgeman S, Heinz J, Pilarski R, Lehtonen R, Prior TW, Frebourg T, Teh BT, Marchuk DA, Aaltonen LA, Eng C. 2005. Molecular classification of patients with unexplained hamartomatous and hyperplastic polyposis. JAMA 294:2465–2473.

Takayama T, Miyanishi K, Hayashi T, Sato Y, Niitsu Y. 2006. Colorectal cancer: Genetics of development and metastasis. J Gastroenterol 41:185–192.

Thiery JP. 2003. Epithelial-mesenchymal transitions in development and pathologies. Curr Opin Cell Biol 15:740–746.

Thuault S, Valcourt U, Petersen M, Manfioletti G, Heldin CH, Moustakas A. 2006. Transforming growth factor-{beta} employs HMGA2 to elicit epithelial-mesenchymal transition. J Cell Biol 174:175–183.

Thuault S, Tan EJ, Peinado H, Cano A, Heldin CH, Moustakas A. 2008. HMGA2 and Smads co-regulate SNAIL1 expression during induction of epithelial-to-mesenchymal transition. J Biol Chem 283:33437–33446.

Valle L, Serena-Acedo T, Liyanarachchi S, Hampel H, Comeras I, Li Z, Zeng Q, Zhang HT, Pennison MJ, Sadim M, Pasche B, Tanner SM, de la Chapelle A. 2008. Germline allele-specific expression of TGFBR1 confers an increased risk of colorectal cancer. Science 115 9397.

Yamagata H, Matsuzaki K, Mori S, Yoshida K, Tahashi Y, Furukawa F, Sekimoto G, Watanabe T, Uemura Y, Sakaida N, Yoshioka K, Kamiyama Y, Seki T, Okazaki K. 2005. Acceleration of Smad2 and Smad3 phosphorylation via c-Jun NH2-terminal kinase during human colorectal carcinogenesis. Cancer Res 65:157–165.

Yang X, Letterio JJ, Lechleider RJ, Chen L, Hayman R, Gu H, Roberts AB, Deng CX. 1999. Targeted disruption of SMAD3 results in impaired mucosal immunity and diminished T cell responsiveness to TGF-beta. EMBO Journal 18:1280–1291.

Zeng Q, Phukan S, Xu Y, Sadim M, Rosman DS, Pennison M, Liao J, Yang GY, Huang CC, Valle L, Di Cristofano A, de la Chapelle A, Pasche B. 2009. Tgfbr1 haploinsufficiency is a potent modifier of colorectal cancer development. Cancer Res 69:678–686.

Zhang HT, Chen XF, Wang MH, Wang JC, Qi QY, Zhang RM, Xu WQ, Fei QY, Wang F, Cheng QQ, Chen F, Zhu CS, Tao SH, Luo Z. 2004. Defective expression of transforming growth factor {beta} receptor type II is associated with CpG methylated promoter in primary non-small cell lung cancer. Clin Cancer Res 10:2359–2367.

Zhu YA, Richardson JA, Parada LF, Graff JM. 1998. Smad3 mutant mice develop metastatic colorectal cancer. Cell 94:703–714.

Zhu Q, Krakowski AR, Dunham EE, Wang L, Bandyopadhyay A, Berdeaux R, Martin GS, Sun L, Luo K. 2007. Dual role of SnoN in mammalian tumorigenesis. Mol Cell Biol 27:324–339.

Part V
Getting Attention:
Immune Recognition and Inflammation

Chapter 16
Genetic Instability and Chronic Inflammation in Gastrointestinal Cancers

Antonia R. Sepulveda and John P. Lynch

Cast of Characters

Genetic instability and inflammation are closely intertwined processes. While the induction of genetic instability in the setting of inflammation is easy to conceptualize, the reverse occurs as well. It has been appreciated for some time now that colon cancers that arise in the setting of DNA mismatch repair (MMR) deficiencies have a significant lymphocyte infiltration, suggesting an inflammatory response. This characteristic is being used clinically by pathologists to identify the approximately 15% of human colon cancers that develop with microsatellite instability (MSI) rather than the more common chromosomal instability. Inactivating mutations or gene silencing of hMLH1 or hMSH2, which are essential for normal MMR, are frequently observed in these cancers and account for the vast majority of hereditary non-polyposis colorectal cancer (HNPCC, or Lynch syndrome I) (Ionov et al. 1993; Thibodeau et al. 1993; Fishel et al. 1993; Leach et al. 1993). How the induction of MSI leads to the increased inflammatory response remains unknown. What is better understood is how chronic inflammatory processes provoke genetic instabilities that lead to the development of cancer.

Introduction

Inflammation, both acute and chronic, is a common medical disorder that places a significant burden upon health-care systems worldwide. Chronic inflammatory conditions are especially burdensome. Not only must the pain and disability directly associated with these disorders be managed, but patients and health-care providers must be vigilant for the long-term consequences often associated with these diseases. Cancer is one such sequela, with many different types of neoplasia associated with chronic inflammatory diseases. In fact, it has been estimated that as many as

J.P. Lynch (✉)
Division of Gastroenterology/650 CRB, 415 Curie Blvd., Philadelphia, PA, USA
e-mail: lynchj@mail.med.upenn.edu

A. Thomas-Tikhonenko (ed.), *Cancer Genome and Tumor Microenvironment*,
DOI 10.1007/978-1-4419-0711-0_16, © Springer Science+Business Media, LLC 2010

one-third to one-half of all cancers are associated in some manner with inflammatory conditions (Nam and Murthy 2004). It is therefore a problem of great clinical importance.

The association between inflammation and cancer is not a new one. It was first suggested more than a century ago when Virchow noted an inflammatory infiltration in some tumors (Nam and Murthy 2004). However, definitive proof of a connection became apparent only in the last 20 years. Careful clinical-observational studies demonstrating the correlation with statistical certainty and a better molecular understanding of carcinogenesis and the toxic microenvironment produced by inflammation all helped convince investigators and clinicians alike of the validity of this association. In the remainder of this chapter, we will discuss the association between inflammation and cancer, with an emphasis on the multiple mechanisms by which inflammatory conditions alter the cellular microenvironment to promote carcinogenesis.

Role of Inflammation in GI Cancer Development

Chronic inflammatory conditions have been associated with carcinogenesis in a number of tissues and organ systems (Table 16.1). It appears that gastrointestinal (GI) organs may in fact be particularly susceptible to this process, though the reasons for this are unclear. Every major organ of the GI tract is subject to one or more disease processes that can result in a chronic inflammatory condition. While the etiologies for these processes can vary considerably, all are known to increase the risk

Table 16.1 Association between chronic inflammatory conditions and cancer in humans

Tissue	Type of inflammation or etiologic agent	Associated cancer
Lung	Asbestos fibers, silica particles, smoking	Mesothelioma and lung cancer
Salivary gland	Sialadenitis	Salivary gland carcinoma
Bladder	1. Chronic cystitis (indwelling catheter) 2. *Shistosoma haematobium* infection	Bladder carcinoma
Esophagus	Gastric and bile acid reflux	Esophageal adenocarcinoma
Stomach	1. *Helicobacter pylori* infections 2. Autoimmune gastritis	1. Intestinal-type adenocarcinoma 2. MALT lymphoma
Bile ducts	1. Liver fluke infections (*Clonorchis sinensis* and *Opisthorchis* species) 2. Primary sclerosing cholangitis	Cholangiocarcinoma
Pancreas	Chronic pancreatitis from any cause including hereditary, alcoholic	Pancreatic adenocarcinoma
Liver	1. Hepatitis B 2. Cirrhosis from any cause including Hepatitis C, alcohol, and autoimmune	Hepatocellular carcinoma
Small intestine	1. Celiac disease 2. Crohn's disease	1. Malt lymphoma 2. Adenocarcinoma
Colon	Ulcerative colitis, Crohn's colitis	Colon adenocarcinoma

for cancer. These findings have prompted the ongoing mechanistic studies into how inflammatory conditions promote carcinogenesis and have suggested interventions that have begun to reduce the frequency of some GI cancers.

Helicobacter pylori *Gastritis and Gastric Cancer*

Infectious causes for gastritis and peptic ulcer disease were unknown until the seminal studies of Barry Marshall and Robin Warren established a role for the bacterium *Helicobacter pylori* (Marshall and Warren 1984). Subsequently, human observational studies established an association between *H. pylori* infection and gastric cancer. Prospective case–control (Forman et al. 1991; Parsonnet et al. 1991a) and meta-analyses (Huang et al. 1998; Sepulveda and Graham 2002) supported this conclusion. Moreover, a number of studies also linked *H. pylori* infection to gastric lymphomas, also known as MALT-type lymphomas (mucosa-associated lymphoid tissue tumor) (Wotherspoon et al. 1991; Parsonnet et al. 1994; Eck et al. 1999). Perhaps the clearest demonstration that *H. pylori* infection and the resultant chronic gastritis cause gastric cancer and lymphoma is that eradication of the infection diminishes the risk for cancer. Nearly half of the localized, early MALT lymphomas will completely regress with *H. pylori* eradication (Wotherspoon et al. 1993; Fischbach et al. 2004; Kim et al. 2007). Moreover, *H. pylori* eradication reduced the risk for gastric carcinogenesis in one randomized, placebo-controlled trial, but only in those patients with no atrophy or intestinal metaplasia (Wong et al. 2004).

Hereditary Pancreatitis and Pancreatic Cancer

An equally compelling demonstration of the association between chronic inflammatory conditions and cancer is observed in patients with hereditary pancreatitis. Hereditary pancreatitis (HP) is an autosomally inherited predisposition to recurrent episodes of acute pancreatitis. Symptoms are often first manifest in childhood, as early as 5 years of age, with the majority becoming symptomatic by age 20 (Sossenheimer et al. 1997; Keim et al. 2003). HP is caused primarily by inherited mutations in the gene encoding cationic trypsinogen (*PRSS1*) (Whitcomb et al. 1996; Teich et al. 2006). Typically, these mutations either enhance trypsin stability, preventing its normal inactivation, or augment trypsinogen autoactivation (Teich et al. 2006). Soon after the recognition of this inherited disorder, it was noted that several family kindreds also experienced high rates of pancreatic cancer (Whitcomb and Pogue-Geile 2002). Typically, pancreatic cancers occur in HP patients only after 20 or more years of pancreatitis (Howes et al. 2004). This fact suggests that it is the chronic inflammation that causes the cancer, not the *PRSS1* mutation. This pattern thus supports the hypothesis that chronic inflammation can promote carcinogenesis in the pancreas.

Ulcerative Colitis and Colon Cancer Risk

Ulcerative colitis (UC) is a chronic, relapsing inflammatory condition of the colon (Stenson 1995). The pathogenesis of UC is presently unclear. Currently, it is believed that UC patients have a genetically based predisposition for the disease. They must also then be exposed to certain environmental factors that serve to trigger the maladaptive chronic inflammatory response. UC has been associated with colon cancer for more than 80 years (Bargen 1928; Loftus 2006). An increased risk for colon cancer in UC patients was established by the 1970s with reports suggesting a cumulative probability of developing colon cancer as high as 60% after 40 years of disease (Devroede et al. 1971). Subsequent studies have better defined that risk, and the picture that emerges is that increasing the extent, duration, and degree of inflammation all increase the risk for the subsequent development of colon cancer (Loftus 2006). Disease duration is perhaps the best-established risk factor for colon cancer in UC. The average patient with UC and colon cancer has had their colitis for a decade and a half (Delaunoit et al. 2006; Loftus 2006). In a meta-analysis of 19 separate studies, both the annual and cumulative colorectal cancer incidences increased with UC disease duration. The annual and cumulative incidences increased from 0.2 and 1.6%, respectively, after 10 years of disease to 0.7 and 8.3%, respectively, after 20 years, then to 1.2 and 18.4 %, respectively, after 30 years of UC (Eaden et al. 2001).

The extent of the colon involved with inflammation is also a well-established risk factor for cancer in UC patients. Patients with pan colitis had a colorectal cancer (CRC) risk that was 20 times greater than those with disease limited to the rectum (Ekbom et al. 1990; Eaden et al. 2001). A more recent study has confirmed this risk gradient based on disease extent (Jess et al. 2006). Lastly, disease severity has been recently established as an important risk factor for colon cancer in UC patients (Rutter et al. 2004a,b). While symptomatic measures of severity have never correlated with a colon cancer risk, histologic and endoscopic findings diagnostic of more severe disease were associated with increased rates of colon cancer. Together, the correlation of UC disease extent, severity, and duration with the risk for colon cancer supports the conclusion that the chronic inflammatory process promotes colon carcinogenesis.

Aspirin, NSAIDs, and Cancer Prevention

The evidence presented thus far supports an association between chronic inflammatory conditions and cancer. Studies of cancer chemoprevention provide a different perspective on this question. A number of groups have explored the potential use of aspirin, non-steroidal anti-inflammatory (NSAIDs) drugs, and COX-2 inhibitors for primary and secondary cancer chemoprevention. All of these agents are potent anti-inflammatory agents. Their primary clinical use is to treat both acute and chronic inflammatory conditions. All are presently thought to exert their anti-cancer effects in part as inhibitors of prostaglandin biosynthesis (Lynch and Lichtenstein 2004).

Levels of Evidence Implicating Chronic Inflammation in Human Carcinogenesis

* **Human epidemiologic studies**
  o Cancers arise in chronic inflammatory conditions with different etiologies including genetic, infectious, and environmental exposures
  o Disease duration, extent, and intensity predicts cancer risk
* **Pathology findings and associations**
  o Finding DNA mutations associated with cancer in non-cancerous, chronically-inflamed tissues
  o Demonstration of ROS and RNS mediated DNA damage in chronically-inflamed human tissues
  o The expression patterns of cytokines, chemokines, and eicosanoids in human cancers and their association with disease progression
* **Pharmacologic**
  o Medical therapies that control inflammation reduce cancer risk
* **Animal models**
  o Induction of chronic inflammatory conditions in animals causes cancer
  o Modulation of cytokine or eicosanoid expression levels can enhance or hinder carcinogenesis and cancer progression
* **Cell culture and in vitro models**
  o identification of the DNA mutations associated with ROS and RNS
  o Demonstration of the pro-proliferative, antiapoptotic, pro-angiogenic and metastasis-promoting effects of immune-modulators like cytokines, chemokines, and eicosanoids.

Fig. 16.1 Evidence implicating chronic inflammation in human carcinogenesis

Multiple studies from the United States and Europe have generally confirmed that frequent users of aspirin or other NSAIDS have reduced rates of esophageal, gastric, and colon cancers (Kune et al. 1988; Langman et al. 2000; Akre et al. 2001; Gonzalez-Perez et al. 2003). Moreover, meta-analyses have further concluded that regular aspirin or NSAID use may be chemoprotective for gastric and esophageal cancers (Gonzalez-Perez et al. 2003). These drugs may be particularly beneficial in patients with familial adenomatosis polyposis (FAP), an inherited predisposition to colon cancer (Giardiello et al. 2002; Phillips et al. 2002). However, the benefits of these drugs as cancer chemopreventive agents for average-risk individuals remain unclear, as the protective effects are most apparent at doses which are associated with drug side effects (Ulrich et al. 2006).

In summary, there is substantial epidemiologic and pharmacologic evidence implicating the inflammatory environment as a causative factor for human carcinogenesis (Fig. 16.1). Not only discussed but also supporting this conclusion is a large body of experimental animal and cell-culture data. In the remainder of this chapter, we will consider which components of the inflammatory environment might be contributing to carcinogenesis. We will also utilize research regarding two human chronic inflammatory diseases, *H. pylori* gastritis and ulcerative colitis, to model how the inflammatory microenvironment promotes carcinogenesis in humans.

Mechanisms by Which Inflammation Promotes Carcinogenesis

The current models suggest that the chronic inflammatory process creates a microenvironment that favors neoplastic transformation (Coussens and Werb 2002). The inflammatory microenvironment differs from the normal environment primarily in the presence of activated immune cells and an excess production of inflammatory mediators including eicosanoids, cytokines, chemokines, and toxic-free radicals derived from reactive oxygen and nitrogen species (ROS and RNS). These inflammatory mediators not only regulate the immune response, they also stimulate mesenchymal and epithelial cells to foster repair and tissue regeneration. Epithelial cell proliferation and migration are stimulated, and programmed cell death (apoptosis) is inhibited. Moreover, angiogenesis is induced, and the oxidative stresses in the inflammatory microenvironment overwhelm normal protective mechanisms and cause severe damage to cellular proteins, lipid membranes, and nuclear DNA. Together, this creates an environment in which the emergence of a transformed, neoplastic cell is more likely to occur.

The Role of Cytokines and Chemokines in Human Carcinogenesis

Cytokines and chemokines are small extracellular signaling proteins. They were initially thought to be exclusively secreted by and signal to the immune system, but are now known to be synthesized by many cell types (Balkwill 2004). Moreover, cytokine and chemokine receptors are expressed quite broadly, thus they appear to target a greater variety of cells than was originally anticipated. Adding to this complexity is the observation that cytokine signaling can have many seemingly opposing effects. Depending on which cytokines are secreted and which cell types express receptors, cytokines can induce immune activation or suppression, be proinflammatory or anti-inflammatory, and enhance cell survival or stimulate apoptosis (Balkwill 2004). Cytokines also can stimulate cell proliferation and enhance cell trafficking (Fig. 16.2). The latter effect is primarily directed toward fostering wound repair and angiogenesis. Thus, in the chronic inflammatory microenvironment, the increased secretion of cytokines and chemokines by both immune and stromal cells supports tumorigenesis (Lin and Karin 2007).

Interleukin-6 (IL-6) is a potent inflammatory cytokine that has been associated with the initiation and progression of many different cancers largely due to its effects on proliferation and programmed cell death (Lin and Karin 2007). Recent studies have implicated IL-6 in the pathogenesis of Kaposi's sarcoma (Osborne et al. 1999), multiple myeloma (Bommert et al. 2006), and colon cancer (Rose-John et al. 2006). Moreover, a polymorphism in the promoter region of IL-6, which has been linked to higher expression levels of this cytokine, is associated with a poor prognosis in breast cancer (Berger 2004). Tumor necrosis factor alpha (TNF-α) is another important cytokine with prominent roles in chronic inflammatory conditions. It is typically produced by inflammatory cells in the tumor microenvironment or the tumor cells themselves. While, as its name might suggest, it can induce apoptosis in some normal and cancer cells, TNF-α is also required by many cancers to promote cell proliferation and survival (Lin and Karin 2007). Human polymorphisms that lead to increased TNF-α production are associated with increased rates of several cancers including multiple myeloma, bladder, breast, gastric, and hepatocellular

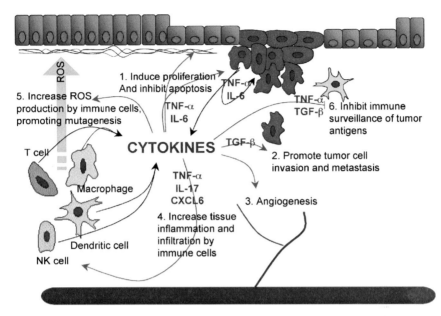

Fig. 16.2 Cytokines promote carcinogenesis through several mechanisms.Cytokines expressed by both tumor cells and inflammatory cells contribute to carcinogenesis in a number of ways. 1. Induce cell proliferation and inhibit the tumor-suppressor apoptosis pathways in target cells. 2. Promote cell migration, thereby enhancing tumor cell metastasis. 3. Cytokines signal to endothelial cells and stimulate angiogenesis. 4. Cytokines and chemokines are chemotactic and provoke inflammatory cell migration into the involved tissue. Moreover, cytokines influence the differentiation and activity of dendritic, macrophage, lymphocytic, and NK cells. 5. Pro-inflammatory cytokines stimulate ROS production by phagocytic and non-phagocytic cells, increasing oxidative stresses and DNA mutagenesis. 6. Anti-inflammatory cytokines can promote tumor growth by inhibiting normal cancer surveillance mechanisms, such as blocking dendritic cell activation, suppressing anti-tumor T-cell responses, blocking macrophage, NK cell, and neutrophil activity, and enhance the function of regulatory T cells

carcinomas (HCC) (Mocellin et al. 2005). TNF-α also stimulates the production of reactive oxygen species (ROS) by macrophages and NK cells (Hussain et al. 2003). These genotoxic molecules can cause DNA mutations and, if not corrected by DNA repair mechanisms, can induce carcinogenesis.

Chemokines are cytokines known to regulate the directed migration of leukocytes during the inflammatory response (Koizumi et al. 2007). However, chemokine receptors are now known to be expressed in many different cancer types and are thought to contribute to the metastatic behavior of cancer cells (Murakami et al. 2004; Koizumi et al. 2007). Some cancers may metastasize to certain tissues based on which chemokines are being expressed (Koizumi et al. 2007). For example, the chemokine CXCL12 can attract migrating breast cancer cells to the lymph node and lung (Muller et al. 2001). CXCL12 signaling has other tumorigenic effects as well. In ovarian, melanoma, and neuroblastoma cancers, CXCL12 inhibits apoptosis and induces matrix metalloproteinase expression which enhances tumor cell migration and invasion (Scotton et al. 2001, 2002). Lastly, tumor-derived cytokines and chemokines can modulate the immune response to inhibit normal surveillance mechanisms that target neoplastic cells. They also promote leukocyte infiltration, which leads to degradation of stromal elements, thereby further enhancing neoplastic cell migration and metastasis (Mocellin et al. 2001; Balkwill 2002; Coussens and Werb 2002; Farrow and Evers 2002; White et al. 2002).

Eicosanoids in Inflammation and Cancer

Eicosanoids are oxygenated lipids with important signaling functions. They are produced by metabolizing arachidonic acid in response to growth factors, hormones, or inflammatory cytokines (Crofford 2001; Pidgeon et al. 2007; Wang et al. 2007). Eicosanoids include the prostanoids (prostaglandins and thromboxane) and leukotrienes. Prostanoids are important modulators of immune, renal, platelet, and reproductive functions, and serve as critical trophic factors that maintain epithelial integrity in the GI tract (Wang et al. 2007). Leukotrienes also regulate immune function, but they have other important roles including the regulation of platelet and endothelial cell function, smooth-muscle cell contractility, and epithelial cell secretory behavior (Pidgeon et al. 2007).

The first step in eicosanoid biosynthesis involves the release of arachidonic acid from phospholipid membranes catalyzed primarily by phospholipase A_2 (PLA$_2$) or phospholipase C (PLC) (Fig. 16.3) (Crofford 2001; Pidgeon et al. 2007; Wang

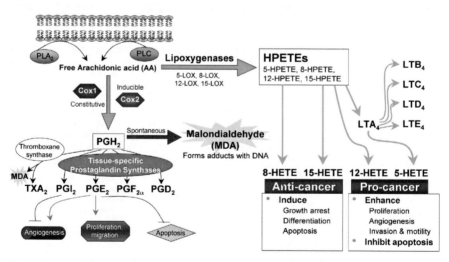

Fig. 16.3 Eicosanoid synthetic pathways. The pathway for prostaglandin and leukotriene biosynthesis from arachidonic acid is illustrated. Phospholipases A_2 and C (PLA$_2$ and PLC) release arachidonic acid from cell membranes, which is then converted by the cyclooxygenases and lipoxygenases into PGH$_2$ and HPETEs, respectively. The generation of the genotoxic bifunctional electrophile malondialdehyde (MDA) is indicated. The effects of eicosanoids on the inflammatory microenvironment that support tumorigenesis are indicated

et al. 2007). The free arachidonic acid is then shunted either toward prostanoid or leukotriene production by the actions of the cyclooxygenase or lipoxygenase enzymes, respectively (Fig. 16.3) (Crofford 2001; Pidgeon et al. 2007; Wang et al. 2007). Cyclooxygenases (Cox-1 and Cox-2) catalyze the rate-limiting step in prostaglandin biosynthesis, the production of prostaglandin H_2 (PGH_2) from arachidonic acid. PGH_2 is then converted to the final prostanoid product by the actions of tissue-specific isomerases. Similarly, lipoxygenases (5-LOX, 8-LOX, 12-LOX, and 15-LOX) catalyze the conversion of arachidonic acid into cyclic hydroperoxyeicosatetraenoic acids (HPETEs) which are then enzymatically converted to hydroxyeicosatetraenoic acids (HETEs) and leukotriene A_4 (Fig. 16.3) (Pidgeon et al. 2007).

In the setting of inflammation, eicosanoids activate responses that enhance the repair of an injury (Crofford 2001; Pidgeon et al. 2007; Wang et al. 2007). Eicosanoid activity induces vasodilation and increases vessel permeability promoting tissue swelling. This effect, in conjunction with the chemotactic properties of eicosanoids, induces an influx of macrophages, lymphocytes, and neutrophils. Eicosanoids also stimulate epithelial cell proliferation and inhibit programmed cell death. This is a useful property when dealing with an acute insult or in its role as a trophic factor for gastrointestinal epithelium (Cohn et al. 1997). However, these properties can also support cancer initiation and promotion (Fig. 16.3).

Eicosanoids have been associated with promoting colonic neoplasia due to their ability to enhance cell proliferation, inhibit apoptosis (Husain et al. 2002; Lynch and Lichtenstein 2004; Pai et al. 2002), induce angiogenesis (Fosslien 2001; Leahy et al. 2002), promote extracellular matrix remodeling, and suppress normal immune surveillance mechanisms (Kambayashi et al. 1995; Kucharzik et al. 1997; Wendum et al. 2004; Yang and Carbone 2004; Chell et al. 2006). These effects are seen in other non-GI cancers as well (Pidgeon et al. 2007; Wang et al. 2007). Due to these many beneficial effects on tumor growth and survival, increased eicosanoid biosynthesis can be seen in cancers that do not arise in the setting of chronic inflammation (Lynch and Lichtenstein 2004). Therefore, targeting eicosanoid biosynthetic pathways remains an area of active interest and is a focus in human cancer prevention and cancer therapy trials (Pidgeon et al. 2007; Wang et al. 2007).

DNA Damage Associated with Chronic Inflammation

While cytokine and eicosanoid signals serve to initiate and maintain the inflammatory process, highly reactive free-radical species like ROS and RNS serve as key effectors of inflammation. These reactive oxygen and nitrogen species are typically generated in mitochondria and the peroxisome (Federico et al. 2007). Protecting cells from these reactive species are a broad array of antioxidant defenders, including superoxide dismutase, catalase, glutathione peroxidase, and glutathione-S-transferase, among other cellular and dietary products (Valko et al. 2007). Oxidative stress occurs when the ROS, RNS, and active intermediates are in excess to the antioxidant defenders. Oxidative stress is a normal byproduct of the inflammatory process. Pro-inflammatory cytokines and chemokines can induce ROS and RNS production in both phagocytic and nonphagocytic cells (Federico et al. 2007). These reactive species in the inflammatory microenvironment help kill bacteria and viruses, fight infection, and enhance wound repair.

DNA nucleotide bases are fairly stable chemically in the normal cellular environment. Despite this stability, free-radical species can chemically react with the double-stranded DNA to alter it in many ways (Fig. 16.4). ROS species can induce single- and double-stranded DNA breaks; modify the purine, pyrimidine, or deoxyribose subunits; produce DNA intrastrand adducts and chemically crosslink DNA and associated proteins (Valko et al. 2005, 2006). If not recognized prior to DNA replication, the modified purine and pyrimidine bases may mispair, causing transition or transversion point mutations (G -> A or G -> T, respectively). Similarly, the potent vasoactive signaling gas NO that is actively produced during an inflammatory response can react with superoxide to form peroxynitrite, another highly reactive species. Peroxynitrite can then react with guanine to yield 8-nitroguanine. 8-Nitroguanine is mutagenic and mispairs with adenosine to produce a G -> T transversion mutation. This transversion mutation is frequently observed in *RAS* and *p53* genes and directly contributes to carcinogenesis in a number of tissues (Yermilov et al. 1995; Suzuki et al. 2005).

Lipid hydroperoxides are another product of inflammation and free-radical reactions. They are formed either from the action of a ROS on polyunsaturated fatty acids or as specific products of eicosanoid biosynthesis (Fig. 16.3) (Blair 2001; Federico et al. 2007). Homolytic decomposition of these products can give rise

The free radicals ROS and RNS promote DNA damage and carcinogenesis

* **ROS-induced single and double-stranded DNA breaks**
  o Requires functioning checkpoint genes and p53 activity
  o can cause programmed cell death (apoptosis)
  o Repaired by non-homologous end-joining and/or homologous recombination
* **Modification of purine, pyrimidine, or deoxyribose subunits by ROS**
  o Modifications can alter DNA base pairing
  o If not corrected, can cause transition and transversion point mutations
  o Repaired by BER and MMR
* **DNA intrastrand adducts and DNA-protein crosslinking**
  o Can induce apoptosis or cell senescence
  o Repaired by homologous recombination
* **Formation of peroxynitrite by reaction of NO with superoxide (O_2^-)**
  o Peroxynitrite reacts with guanine to yield 8-oxo-7,8-dihydro-2′-deoxyguanosine and 8-nitroguanine
  o This is a cause of G>T transversions if not corrected
  o Repaired by BER and MMR
* **Reaction with proteins impairs function**
  o Oxidative stress impairs MMR function and increases MSI
* **Eicosanoid biosynthesis is a source of lipid hydroperoxides**
  o These decompose into DNA-reactive bifunctional electrophiles like 4-hydroxynonal (HNE)
  o Repaired by BER and MMR

Fig. 16.4 Contributions of reactive oxygen and nitrogen species to DNA damage and carcinogenesis

to a number of genotoxic bifunctional electrophiles including malondialdehyde (MDA), 4-hydroxy-2(E)-nonenal (HNE), and 4-oxo-2(E)-nonenal (ONE), among others (Prescott and White 1996; Blair 2001, 2008). MDA is formed from the natural breakdown of PGH2 and during thromboxane biosynthesis. It is a potent mutagen forming adducts with DNA nucleosides (Prescott and White 1996; Wendum et al. 2004). HNE is the most abundant of these bifunctional aldehydes produced during periods of oxidative stress (Federico et al. 2007). At low levels it stimulates cell proliferation, but at higher levels it forms adducts with DNA and can induce apoptosis. In addition to the electrophiles produced by eicosanoid biosynthesis, the cyclooxygenase and lipoxygenase enzymes can convert linoleic acid, another abundant polyunsaturated fatty acid, into several related hydroperoxyoctadecadenoic acids (HPODEs) (Blair 2001, 2008). These HPODEs also decompose and give rise to the genotoxic electrophiles HNE and ONE. Thus, genotoxic bifunctional aldehydes are produced by several mechanisms during the inflammatory response, further contributing to the oxidative stress of the cell.

Oxidative stress from a chronic inflammatory process can thus irreversibly damage DNA. If the ROS- and RNS-mediated DNA damage is not extensive, repair mechanisms like non-homologous end-joining (NHEJ), homologous recombination (HR), DNA mismatch repair (MMR), and base excision repair (BER) can identify the mutations and often affect a complete repair (Lynch and Rustgi 2005). These repair processes, along with programmed cell death (apoptosis) and cell senescence, are the primary means by which cells prevent neoplastic transformation in the setting of oxidative stress from a chronic inflammatory process.

Genetic Instability and DNA Repair Mechanisms

Genetic instability is a common trait of human cancers (Lengauer et al. 1997; Cahill et al. 1999). There are a number of different genetic alterations that can be observed commonly in human cancers including point mutations; altered DNA methylation patterns; and gene rearrangements, amplifications, and deletions. Several distinct forms of genetic instability have been identified that give rise to these mutations, including chromosomal instability (CIN), microsatellite instability (MSI), epigenetic instability, and the instabilities associated with inactivation of the nucleotide excision repair (NER) or base excision repair (BER) pathways (Lynch and Rustgi 2005). Of these five mechanisms, four are commonly involved in the pathogenesis of gastrointestinal cancers (Lengauer et al. 1998; Breivik and Gaudernack 1999; Jiricny and Marra 2003; Sancar et al. 2004).

Chromosomal Instability in Gastrointestinal Cancers

Aneuploidy is a complex trait of cancer cells marked primarily by gains or losses of whole chromosomes. In addition, other common features include smaller chromosomal rearrangements, such as non-reciprocal translocations that can cause segmental gene amplifications and/or losses. This complex set of features gives rise to the cancer phenotype described as chromosomal instability or CIN (Lengauer et al. 1998). A common feature of CIN cancers is the loss of heterozygosity (LOH) that frequently targets and thereby inactivates tumor-suppressor genes. Common genes inactivated by LOH in GI cancers include the *APC* gene (chromosome 5q), *p53*(17p), and *DPC4/SMAD4* (18p). Growth-promoting cellular proto-oncogenes such as the *EGF receptor* or *cyclin D1* are conversely frequently amplified by the chromosomal rearrangements in many human malignancies (Hollstein et al. 1988; Ormandy et al. 2003; Sunpaweravong et al. 2005). These genetic changes obviously promote cell transformation and tumor growth. The degree of CIN increases as cells progress toward cancer, worsening as the degree of dysplasia advances. These complex traits associated with CIN and aneuploidy have been rather difficult to replicate in the laboratory until relatively recently.

The causes of CIN remain unknown, but significant advances have been made recently. Most certainly, DNA damage, cell cycle, and spindle checkpoints play a role in this process, as does telomere maintenence (Lengauer et al. 1997; Cahill et al. 1998; Bharadwaj and Yu 2004; Sharpless and DePinho 2004). The breast cancer-related *BRCA1* and *BRCA2* genes, *ATM*, and *p53* genes play critical roles in the DNA damage checkpoints and are known to play important roles in human tumorigenesis (Lengauer et al. 1997; Nagy et al. 2004). Inactivation of the DNA damage checkpoint controls yields cells more tolerant of severe DNA damage and permissive of neoplastic transformation and CIN events, as evidenced by the increased risk for cancer in families carrying germline mutations of these genes (Motoyama and Naka 2004; Sancar et al. 2004).

Cell cycle and spindle checkpoint genes have also been implicated in CIN (Cahill et al. 1998; Shibata et al. 2002; Corn et al. 2003; Toyota et al. 2003; Honda et al. 2004). Recent work investigating the role of telomere maintenance in both normal and neoplastic cells has provided novel insights into the generation of non-reciprocal translocations and gene amplifications (Sharpless and DePinho 2004). Telomeres are structures that serve to indicate the natural ends of chromosomes and distinguish them from true DNA double-stranded breaks. However, telomeres erode with each DNA replication cycle unless maintained by the enzyme telomerase. Telomerase is normally expressed only in stem cells. Once telomere protection is eroded, cells recognize chromosomal ends as double-stranded DNA breaks and cells initiate repairs, including non-homologous end-joining (NHEJ) and homologous recombination (HR). Dicentric chromosomes are frequently formed by the fusion of two chromosome ends. If these dicentric chromosomes are pulled in opposite directions during mitosis, they break at random points, resulting in non-reciprocal translocations. The broken ends reactivate NHEJ and are fused again, possibly with another chromosome. This process is repeated with each cell division, resulting in massive genomic instability, a state called telomere crisis (Sharpless and DePinho 2004). This model is supported by many observations, both in vitro and in vivo. (Engelhardt et al. 1997; Artandi et al. 2000; Gisselsson et al. 2001; Hermsen et al. 2002; Plentz et al. 2003). Together these findings suggest telomere erosion, along with loss of DNA damage, cell cycle, and mitotic spindle checkpoints contribute greatly to the CIN genetic instability observed in many human cancers.

Microsatellite Instability and DNA Mismatch Repair

Microsatellite instability (MSI) is perhaps the best understood of the genetic instabilities (Kolodner and Marsischky 1999; Peltomaki 2001; Jiricny and Marra 2003; Nagy et al. 2004). The DNA mismatch repair (MMR) system is a multiprotein complex of MutS homologues hMSH2, hMSH3 and hMSH6, and the MutL homologues hMLH1, hPMS1, hPMS2, and hMLH3 (Peltomaki 2001; Heinen et al. 2002; Jiricny and Marra 2003; Nagy et al. 2004). This multiprotein complex recognizes and repairs the base–base mismatches and short insertion/deletion mispairings which spontaneously occur with DNA replication. Short repetitive DNA segments, known as microsatellites, are especially vulnerable to this type of error (Lengauer et al. 1998; Peltomaki 2001; Jiricny and Marra 2003; Nagy et al. 2004). DNA mismatch repair deficiency leads to frameshift mutations which can alter the coding regions of genes. Current guidelines for the identification of MSI in colon cancers utilize a consensus panel of five mononucleotide and dinucleotide markers (Boland et al. 1998; Vasen et al. 1999; Umar et al. 2004). Instability in two or more markers is designated as microsatellite-high (MSI-H). Instability in one marker is termed as microsatellite-low (MSI-L), and absence of instability is termed as microsatellite-stable (MSS).

MSI cancers tend to be diploid or near diploid rather than aneuploid. They also tend to be resistant to DNA-damaging chemotherapeutic agents and have a better prognosis (Lengauer et al. 1998; Peltomaki 2001). MSI instability can arise in either familial (hereditary non-polyposis colon cancer – HNPCC) or sporadic GI cancers, although the mechanisms responsible for each are different. MSI is seen in a portion of colonic (approximately 15%), pancreatic (13%), and gastric cancers (10 to 27%). In these cancers the MMR system is inactivated, either by germline disruption (HNPCC) or by epigenetic silencing of the *hMLH1* gene (sporadic cancers).

Nearly all mutations selected for in MSI cancers tend to lead to inactivation of target genes. Genes targeted by MSI may differ between tissues. Best understood are the genes targeted in colon cancer. In the colon, approximately 70% of HNPCC cancers acquire frameshift mutations in APC (Huang et al. 1996; Miyaki et al. 1999). The TGF-βRII and insulin-like growth factor-II receptors (IGFIIR) are also frequently inactivated by mutations in MSI neoplasms (Parsons et al. 1995; Souza et al. 1996; Grady et al. 1998). BAX, an important p53 pro-apoptotic effector, is inactivated in 55% of MSI colon cancers, yet p53 itself is not (Rampino et al. 1997; Yagi et al. 1998; Losi et al. 1997; Samowitz et al. 2001). Other genes frequently mutated in MSI colon cancers include MED1 (Riccio et al. 1999), ATM (Ejima et al. 2000), the DNA helicase BLM (Calin et al. 2000), and the transcription factor E2F-4 (Yoshitaka et al. 1996). In summary, inhibition of MMR promotes the accumulation of frameshift mutations that inactivate tumor suppressors, promote growth, and accelerate malignant transformation of epithelial cells.

Base Excision Repair (BER)

As has been discussed previously, DNA can be chemically altered by reactive species such as ROS or activated methyl- and alkyl radicals, or by spontaneous nucleotide deaminations, particularly in stressed cells. These changes can alter the non-covalent interactions between nucleotides and lead to base mispairing during DNA replication if not corrected (Jiricny and Marra 2003). The mispairings lead to point mutations, described as transition or transversion mutations (G -> A or G -> T, respectively). Point mutations can cause missense (change in an amino acid) and nonsense (insertion of a stop codon) mutations if they occur in protein coding sequences of genes. The base excision repair (BER) pathway identifies the modified bases and initiates their repair.

Unlike CIN and MSI, which appear to be mutually exclusive (Lengauer et al. 1998), BER defects can be observed in both CIN and MSI colon cancers, as well as a subgroup that are CIN and MSI stable (Jass et al. 2002; Jiricny and Marra 2003; Jass 2004). Two components of the BER pathway have been implicated in GI cancer pathogenesis, MED1(MBD4) and hMYH (Riccio et al. 1999; Petronzelli et al. 2000; Jones et al. 2002; Jiricny and Marra 2003; Sampson et al. 2003; Sieber et al. 2003; Kambara et al. 2004). MED1(MBD4) is a glycosylase that repairs spontaneous deaminations of methylcytosines. It is frequently mutated by microsatellite instability in MSI tumors, and its inactivation is associated with an increase in C -> T transition mutations (Bader et al. 1999; Riccio et al. 1999).

Germline mutations in the *hMYH* gene are reportedly the cause of the familial colon cancer syndrome MYH adenomatous polyposis (MAP) (Jones et al. 2002; Sampson et al. 2003; Sieber et al. 2003). MAP-associated colon cancers are diploid and are somewhat stable genetically (CIN-/MSI-). Fundamentally, they are characterized by high rates of G -> T transversion mutations. *hMYH*, together with *OGG1* and *MTH1*, identify and excise the 8-hydroxydeoxyguanosine (8-OHdG) formed from ROS damage to DNA. If not corrected, the 8-OHdG can mispair with adenine, leading to the G -> T transversions characteristic of MAP. The *APC* gene is frequently inactivated by premature nonsense codons in 50% of the MAP cancers, due to G -> T transversions. G -> T mutations also cause activating missense mutations in codon 12 of *Ki-RAS*, leading to inappropriate activation of this potent oncogene (Jones et al. 2002; Lipton et al. 2003; Sampson et al. 2003; Sieber et al. 2003). However, inactivation of the tumor-suppressors *p53, SMAD4*, and *TGF-βII receptor* genes do not frequently occur in MAP colon cancers.

The *methylguanine methyl transferase* gene (*MGMT*) is not a member of the BER pathway but it performs a related function. Agents that methylate DNA preferentially target the N7 position of guanine. This adduct is repaired by the BER system. Less frequently, these agents attack the O6 position of guanine or the O4 position of thymine. MGMT recognizes these modifications and removes the alkyl adduct through a "suicide reaction" in which the adduct is irreversibly transferred to the reactive site of the MGMT protein (Gerson 2004). Failure to remove these alkyl groups prior to DNA replication results in G -> A transition mutations due to mispairing. For this reason, the *MGMT* gene has been hypothesized to play a significant role in gastrointestinal malignancies (Jass et al. 2002; Gerson 2004; Jass 2004). Supporting this contention, the *MGMT* gene is frequently silenced by promoter hypermethylation in cancers of the colon, stomach, esophagus, prostate, and CNS (Bello et al. 2004; Gerson 2004; Lind et al. 2004; Yang et al. 2005). In summary, repair of chemically modified DNA bases is a critical function that can be an important source of genetic instability in cells in which these pathways are disrupted.

DNA Methylation and Epigenetic Instability in GI Cancers

Epigenetic mechanisms refer to the interrelated processes of DNA methylation, gene imprinting, and histone acetylation (Yoder et al. 1997; Walsh et al. 1998). They are based on regulated methylation of the cytosine bases in CpG dinucleotides. CpG methylation is believed to determine whether chromatin is in an open, transcriptionally active conformation (unmethylated CpG) or in compacted state closed-off from transcriptional regulators (highly methylated CpG). The patterns of CpG methylation are conserved with cell division and are typically transmitted to daughter cells. For this reason, it is a useful mechanism for permanent gene silencing utilized by both normal and cancer cells (Baylin and Herman 2000). Disordered CpG island methylation is now recognized to be involved in the pathogenesis of many gastrointestinal cancers (Cunningham et al. 1998; Veigl et al. 1998; Cui et al. 2002; Nie et al. 2002; Strathdee 2002; Cruz-Correa et al. 2004; Lund and van Lohuizen 2004).

While epigenetic instability can be seen in both CIN and MSI cancers, the selection of certain gene targets can influence whether the cancer is MSI or CIN or has BER-associated defects. For instance, the mitotic checkpoint gene *checkpoint with forkhead associated and ring-finger* (*Chfr*) is frequently silenced by promoter hypermethylation in colon, esophageal, and gastric cancers (Shibata et al. 2002; Corn et al. 2003; Toyota et al. 2003; Honda et al. 2004), which may foster CIN development. In contrast, the *hMLH1* gene promoter is silenced in 80% of sporadic colon cancers with MSI (Kuismanen et al. 2000). Lastly, the frequency of G -> A transition mutations is increased in many cancers by the epigenetic silencing of the *MGMT* gene (Bello et al. 2004; Lind et al. 2004; Yang et al. 2005).

Other genes targeted by promoter hypermethylation frequently play important roles regulating cell proliferation, apoptosis, cell migration, and angiogenesis. The *secreted frizzled-related protein (SFRP)*, *E-cadherin*, and *p16* genes are preferentially silenced in colorectal, gastric, and pancreatic cancers, respectively (Ueki et al. 2000; Strathdee 2002; Suzuki et al. 2004). CpG island hypermethylation of the MDM2 inhibitor *p14^{ARF}* reduces p53's response to oncogene activation and DNA damage (Esteller et al. 2000, 2001a,b). The *VHL* and *thrombospondin-1* genes are frequently silenced by promoter hypermethylation in gastrointestinal cancers, which stimulates angiogenesis and fosters tumor growth (Ahuja et al. 1997; Kuroki et al. 2003; Oue et al. 2003; Xu et al. 2004). Lastly, tumor cell metastasis is enhanced by disruption of the extracellular matrix or loss of cell–cell adhesion, as occurs with epigenetic silencing of *TIMP3* and *E-cadherin* genes, respectively (Ueki et al. 2000; Iguchi et al. 2001; Kang et al. 2001; Lind et al. 2004).

In summary, genetic instability is a complex phenotype frequently manifest in human cancers. These instabilities arise from defects in DNA repair mechanisms or inactivation of critical cell cycle, DNA damage, and mitotic checkpoints. Cancers that progress due to chronic inflammation are no different, frequently expressing CIN, MSI, BER, and epigenetic defects and inactivating these same critical checkpoints. We will explore this further using *H. pylori*-induced gastric cancer and ulcerative colitis-associated colon cancer to illustrate these concepts further.

H. pylori Infection Induces an Inflammatory Microenvironment that Promotes Gastric Carcinogenesis

H. pylori *and Gastric Cancer*

The development of gastric cancer is usually a multistep process which leads to increasing deregulation of gastric epithelial cells at the molecular level, resulting in characteristic histologic changes of the gastric mucosa. These molecular and morphologic changes of the epithelium of the stomach result from the effects of a combination of factors including the diet, genetic susceptibility, and chronic inflammation of the stomach, most commonly due to *Helicobacter pylori*-associated gastritis (Parsonnet et al. 1991a,b; Correa 1992; Palli et al. 1997; El-Omar et al. 2000).

The association of *Helicobacter pylori* infection and gastric adenocarcinomas has led to the classification of *H. pylori* as a definite human carcinogen by a World Health Organization panel in 1994 (Anonymous 1994). Over the last two decades, since the first reports by Warren and Marshal implicating *H. pylori* as the causal agent of gastritis and ulcers (Warren and Marshall 1983; Marshall 1995), research has focused on the association of *H. pylori* gastritis and gastric cancer and has led to significant advances in our understanding. *H. pylori* infection appears to play a predominant role during the initiating steps of gastric cancer, provoking an inflammatory response to the infection that ultimately promotes neoplastic progression.

H. pylori *Strains, Bacterial Virulence Factors, and Gastric Cancer*

It has been widely recognized that certain *H. pylori* bacterial strains have specific human disease associations. This association is in part due to virulence factors that play a role in *H. pylori* pathogenesis. The best known and most significant of the virulence factors are the vacuolating cytotoxin (VacA) and the cytotoxin-associated antigen A (CagA) proteins (Cover and Blanke 2005; Handa et al. 2007).

VacA is a secreted 88-kDa protein which causes vacuolization and induces apoptosis of epithelial cells (Cover and Blanke 2005). VacA has been shown to have

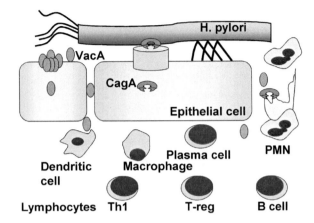

Fig. 16.5 Gastric mucosa inflammatory response to *H. pylori* and bacterial virulence factors

immunomodulatory effects upon B-lymphocyte antigen presentation, the regulation of T-cell-mediated cytokine responses, the inhibition of T-lymphocyte activation and proliferation, and the inhibition of T-lymphocyte-induced B-cell proliferation (Fig. 16.5) (Gebert et al. 2003, 2004; Fischer et al. 2004 Torres et al. 2007). These studies suggested that the immunomodulatory actions of VacA toxin on T and B lymphocytes contributes to the ability of *H. pylori* to establish a persistent chronic infection (Torres et al. 2007).

The *cagA* gene encodes a 125–145-kDa protein and is one of the genes that constitute the *Cag* pathogenicity island (Censini et al. 1996; Handa et al. 2007). Recent studies have characterized the functional domains of the CagA protein, further elucidated their roles in *H. pylori* pathogenesis. The *Cag* pathogenicity island encodes a type IV secretion system, which is used by the bacterium to inject the CagA protein into gastric epithelial cells (Fig. 16.5). Once intracellular, CagA interacts with several signaling pathways in both tyrosine phosphorylation-dependent and tyrosine phosphorylation-independent manners. The injected CagA undergoes tyrosine phosphorylation by the epithelial cell Src kinase at the EPIYA sites. This phosphorylation allows it to then bind the Src homology 2 domain-containing tyrosine phosphatase (SHP2), deregulating the activity of this phosphatase (Handa et al. 2007).

There is considerable evidence that the CagA protein plays an important role in gastric carcinogenesis. *H. pylori* strains that produce the CagA protein are associated with an increased risk of gastric carcinoma, at least in part because these strains cause a greater inflammatory response and mucosal damage. CagA-positive strains have been shown to induce higher levels of interleukin-8 (IL-8) as compared to CagA-negative strains, resulting in greater gastric mucosa inflammation (Crabtree et al. 1994, 1995). Moreover, it was recently reported that transgenic mice expressing the CagA protein developed gastric epithelial hyperplasia, gastric polyps, and adenocarcinomas of the stomach and small intestine (Ohnishi et al. 2008).

It is now well established that different *H. pylori* strains produce variants of the CagA protein. Some structural variants of CagA have a stronger association with gastric cancer. The CagA type C strains have been associated with more severe degrees of atrophic gastritis and gastric cancer (Yamaoka et al. 1998). In addition, strain differences regarding EPYIA phosphorylation may alter the risk for gastric carcinogenesis. *H. pylori* strains with an East-Asian pattern of EPYIA phosphorylation are associated with an increased incidence of gastric cancer (Hatakeyama and Higashi 2005; Handa et al. 2007). In summary, the VacA and CagA proteins are important bacterial virulence factors that contribute to *H. pylori*-associated gastric carcinogenesis.

Histologic Changes Associated with *H.* pylori *Gastritis*

H. pylori infection of the stomach elicits an inflammatory response with infiltration of the gastric mucosa by neutrophils, macrophages, and T- and B lymphocytes (Robinson et al. 2007; Wilson and Crabtree 2007). At the tissue level, progression from *H. pylori* chronic gastritis to gastric cancer consists of a sequence of mucosal changes. Long-lasting chronic gastritis, beginning in childhood and lasting into to adulthood, often produces gastric epithelial atrophy. This atrophy is almost

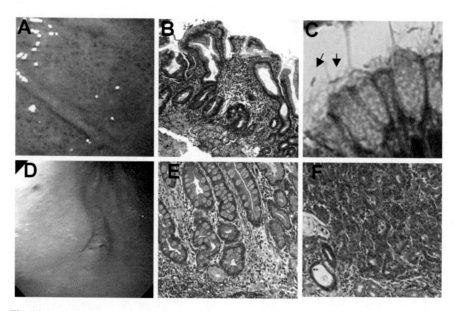

Fig. 16.6 *H. pylori* gastritis and gastric adenocarcinoma. (**A**) Endoscopic image of gastric antrum demonstrates erythematous mucosa associated with chronic gastritis. (**B**) Histology of gastric antrum demonstrating *H. pylori* associated with chronic gastritis. (**C**) *H. pylori* organisms indicated by the arrows are located on the mucus layer and in close contact with epithelial cells on the surface of the gastric mucosa. (**D**) Endoscopic image of gastric adenocarcinoma. (**E**) Gastric mucosa with extensive intestinal metaplasia present in the background stomach of the same patient with adenocarcinoma (**F**). Hematoxylin and eosin stain's original magnification 100X (**B, C, E**) and 400X (**F**). Endoscopic images contributed by Dr. Gregory Ginsberg, University of Pennsylvania

always accompanied by the replacement of the normal gastric glands with an intestinal metaplasia (Fig. 16.6). As these changes occur there is an increased risk for the development of gastric epithelial dysplasia and adenocarcinoma (Nomura et al. 1991; Parsonnet et al. 1991a,b; Anonymous 1994; Correa 1995; Dixon 1995).

H. pylori-associated gastric cancers characteristically arise with chronic active and atrophic gastritis in the background mucosa. These gastric cancers are most frequently of the so-called intestinal type, and they are predominantly well to moderately differentiated adenocarcinomas (Fig. 16.6). However, poorly differentiated carcinomas, classified as diffuse type, may also occur in these patients (Huang et al. 1998; Sepulveda et al. 2000).

Patients who are at higher risk of progression to cancer often have the most extensive forms of atrophic gastritis with intestinal metaplasia involving large areas of the stomach, including the gastric body and fundus. This pattern of gastritis has been described as pangastritis or multifocal atrophic gastritis (Correa 1992; Dixon et al. 1996; Cassaro et al. 2000; Kimura 2000; Sipponen and Marshall 2000). Extensive gastritis involving the parietal compartment of the gastric body and fundus leads to hypochlorhydria, allowing for bacterial overgrowth and increased carcinogenic activity in the stomach through the conversion of nitrites to carcinogenic nitroso-N compounds (Recavarren-Arce et al. 1991; Kodama et al. 2003). This pattern of pangastritis is also seen in the family relatives of patients of gastric cancer, suggesting host susceptibility factors may be contributing to this disease pattern and the associated increase risk for gastric cancer (Sepulveda et al. 2002).

Host Susceptibility and the Inflammatory Microenvironment Caused by H. pylori Infection

Genetic susceptibility factors that increase the risk of gastric cancer development in *H. pylori*-infected patients have been identified. Among the best understood are pro-inflammatory gene polymorphisms. Pro-inflammatory IL-1 gene polymorphisms have been shown to increase the risk of gastric cancer and cancer precursors in the setting of an *H. pylori* infection. Individuals with polymorphisms in the IL-1beta (IL-1B-31*C or -511*T) or the IL-1RN (receptor antagonist) genes (IL-1RN*2/*2 genotypes) are at increased risk of hypochlorhydria, gastric atrophy, and gastric cancer in response to *H. pylori* colonization (El-Omar et al. 2000; El-Omar et al. 2003; Machado et al. 2003; El-Omar 2006).

Recent studies in mice have suggested a role for bone marrow-derived stem cells as an alternative model for the origin of gastric cancer in chronic *H. pylori* gastritis. *H. pylori*-associated inflammation and atrophy creates an abnormal microenvironment favoring engraftment of bone marrow-derived stem cells into the chronically inflamed gastric epithelium. It is suggested that these cells do not enter in the pathway of complete differentiation, but rather follow a program of uncontrolled replication, progressive loss of differentiation, and neoplastic invasive behavior (Houghton et al. 2004; Correa and Houghton 2007; Katoh 2007; Giannakis et al. 2008). However, data from human studies supporting a similar role for bone

370 A.R. Sepulveda and J.P. Lynch

Fig. 16.7
Inflammation-associated
mutagenesis and pathways of
DNA repair in gastric
carcinogenesis

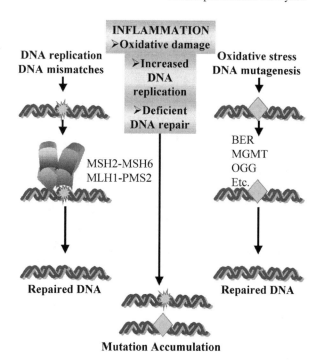

Mutation Accumulation

marrow-derived stem cells in human gastric carcinogenesis have not yet been reported.

Chronic *H. pylori* infections induce profound changes in the gastric epithelium by the combined actions that the bacterial products and the inflammatory mediators have on cell survival, proliferation, differentiation, and DNA integrity (Fig. 16.7). These factors together contribute to a sustained inflammatory response in the infected gastric mucosa. This chronic and continuously active immunologic response is in part responsible for damage to the epithelium, through the release of oxygen radicals (Shimada et al. 1999) and production of chemokines that can bind receptors on epithelial cells to alter cellular responses. Moreover, these bacterial products, including the well-characterized virulence factors (CagA and VacA), directly affect the gastric epithelial cells and inflammatory cells, resulting in increased rates of cell apoptosis, proliferation, and mutagenesis (Moss et al. 1996; Peek et al. 1997; Farinati et al. 1998; Shirin et al. 2000; Yao et al. 2006; Handa et al. 2007).

H. pylori infection of the stomach elicits a host inflammatory response that includes both humoral and cellular immune responses, as well as activation of the innate and acquired immune systems (Robinson et al. 2007; Wilson and Crabtree 2007). Once *H. pylori* colonizes and infects the stomach, the disease persists as chronic gastritis, unless appropriate treatment to eradicate the microorganisms is provided (Malfertheiner et al. 2007). The long-term chronic infection by *H. pylori* requires its evasion from the immune system surveillance. The mechanisms that lead to *H. pylori* immune evasion and chronic gastritis are currently being unraveled. We know it depends in part upon the direct action of *H. pylori* bacterial products on macrophages, dendritic cells, and gastric epithelial cells. These mechanisms are illustrated in Fig. 16.5 (Cover and Blanke 2005; Robinson et al. 2007; Wilson and Crabtree 2007). Several steps are represented, with several occurring simultaneously:

(1) *H. pylori* organisms contact the apical aspect of epithelial cells located on the gastric mucosal surface and in the gastric foveolae, where the organisms may contact stem cells. This contact prompts an intracellular signaling cascade within the epithelial cells that alters gene expression patterns and induces the basal secretion of cytokines like IL-8. These cytokines can activate macrophages, dendritic cells, and other inflammatory cells present within the lamina propria (Fig. 16.5)

(2) Some *H. pylori* organisms enter the lamina propria after damage is inflicted to the surface epithelial layer, permitting *H. pylori* to directly interact with immune response cells.

(3) Once they are stimulated by the bacterial products, mucosal macrophages, dendritic cells, and epithelial cells in turn activate T lymphocytes (with a predominant Th1 response), regulatory T lymphocytes (T-Regs), B lymphocytes (which mature into mucosal plasma cells), and neutrophils (which actively phagocytize *H. pylori* organisms). This effect is mediated both by direct contact from dendritic cells or the secretion of pro-inflammatory cytokines by the macrophages, dendritic cells, and gastric epithelial cells.

Genetic Instability in Gastric Epithelium Is Induced by **H. pylori** *Infection*

This inflammatory microenvironment, over many years, can serve as both an inducer and a promoter of gastric carcinogenesis. ROS are generated by the inflammatory and epithelial cells after activation by cytokines and the *H. pylori* bacterial products. In addition, *H. pylori*-associated gastritis is reported to have increased levels of inducible nitric oxide synthase (iNOS) and cyclooxygenase (COX2) enzymes, which can enhance the production of nitric oxide (NO) and prostaglandins, respectively. These products and their biosynthetic pathways further increase the oxidative stresses and resulting damage (Plummer et al. 1995; Fu et al. 1999; Grisham et al. 2000; Li et al. 2000). Moreover, the reduced level of oxygen radical scavengers, such as glutathione and glutathione-S-transferase, during *H. pylori* gastritis also contributes to the higher levels of oxygen radicals observed in the mucosa of *H. pylori*-infected patients (Verhulst et al. 2000).

The genetic changes associated with inflammation and increased oxidative stress, including epigenetic modifications, point mutations, and larger DNA insertions and deletions, can precede the onset of dysplasia and cancer in *H. pylori* gastritis (Gologan et al. 2005). Increased oxidative stress can also directly inhibit DNA repair functions, further accelerating gastric epithelial mutagenesis (Gologan et al. 2005). Finally, it has been hypothesized that the hypochlorhydria and atrophic mucosa produce a microenvironment that increases the genotoxicity of ingested environmental carcinogens. Together, these combined processes can accelerated the onset of gastric cancer.

DNA Repair Mechanisms Protecting the Gastric Epithelium from **H. pylori-***Associated Cancer*

Several DNA repair systems are required for correction of DNA damage associated with *H. pylori* gastritis. They include the DNA MMR system and the BER pathway. Other related mechanisms are also important, including the enzymes MGMT and polymorphic glycosylase (OGG1). Inactivation of these repair pathways are often an early event in the pathway to gastric cancer.

A number of investigators have looked for evidence that the MMR repair pathway was inactivated in the early stages of gastritis and gastric cancer. In pre-neoplastic tissues, only a small subset of cells may carry the MSI phenotype and, therefore, the MSI status may be underestimated. Despite this limitation, several studies have reported a role of DNA mismatch repair deficiency in the mutations that accumulate during *H. pylori* infection (Leung et al. 2000; Kim et al. 2002a; Yao et al. 2006). Microsatellite instability can be detected in the intestinal metaplasia from patients with gastric cancer, indicating that MSI can occur in the pre-cancerous mucosa (Semba et al. 1996; Hamamoto et al. 1997; Ottini et al. 1997; Fang et al. 1999; Kobayashi et al. 2000; Leung et al. 2000). Microsatellite instability was reported in 13% of chronic gastritis cases, 20% intestinal metaplasias, 25% of intestinal metaplasia with dysplasia, and 38% of gastric cancers examined, indicating a stepwise acquisition or clonal selection of MSI in gastric carcinogenesis (Ling et al. 2004). Supporting a role for MSI in the progression from *H. pylori* chronic gastritis to gastric cancer, several studies reported that patients with MSI-positive tumors showed a significantly higher frequency of active *H. pylori* infection (Wu et al. 1998; Leung et al. 2000; Wu et al. 2000). Using a co-culture in vitro system, studies from our laboratory have shown that gastric cancer cell lines exposed to *H. pylori* had diminished levels of DNA mismatch repair proteins hMLH1 and hMSH2 (Kim et al. 2002a). These changes were functionally significant as they were associated with increased mutagenesis of an MSI-type frameshift reporter vector (Yao et al. 2006).

The BER pathway also appears to be inactivated during the development of *H. pylori*-associated gastritis and cancer. Increased levels of 8-OhdG have been detected in the DNA isolated from the gastric mucosa of *H. pylori*-infected patients. These increased levels were detected in the early gastritis stage as well as the later intestinal metaplasia and gastric atrophy stages. It is interesting to note that the levels of 8-OHdG in the gastric mucosa significantly decreased after eradication of *H. pylori* infection, directly linking the bacterial infection to the increased oxidative DNA damage (Hahm et al. 1997; Farinati et al. 1998). Repair of the mutant base 8-OHdG is by the actions of the BER pathway including the glycosylase (OGG1). A gene polymorphism that may affect OGG1 function was reported frequently in patients with intestinal metaplasia and gastric cancer, suggesting that deficient OGG1 function may increase mutagenesis and thereby promote gastric carcinogenesis (Farinati et al. 2008).

O-(6)-Alkylguanine DNA adducts can also arise with ROS-mediated DNA damage. This modified base can mispair with thymidine during DNA replication and cause G -> A point mutations if not corrected. These types of point mutations occur with oxidative DNA damage and are frequently observed in the *p53* gene, as well as other genes involved in gastric carcinogenesis (Shiao et al. 1994). The O-(6)-methylguanine DNA methyltransferase (MGMT) enzyme removes the O-(6)-alkyl adducts, restoring normal base pairing. MGMT enzyme activity is frequently lost early in the development of gastric carcinogenesis, suggesting a role for this DNA repair protein in gastric cancer development (Park et al. 2001).

Patterns of Gene Mutations and Epigenetic Alterations Associated with the Progression from Gastric Intestinal Metaplasia to Cancer

Epigenetic gene modifications and DNA mutagenesis both precede neoplastic progression during gastric carcinogenesis. Both of these types of genetic changes have been observed in *H. pylori* gastritis and the subsequent pre-neoplastic and neoplastic mucosal lesions (Fig. 16.8) (Gologan et al. 2005). These changes can be difficult to detect during early gastritis because the mutations are present in only a small subset of the mucosal cell population. However, during the intestinal metaplasia stage, there is an expansion of cell clones with mutations that provide survival advantages. This clonal expansion increases the detectable signal and can often facilitate the identification of these mutational events in vivo (Leung et al. 2000; Mihara et al. 2006).

Epigenetic DNA changes and gene silencing, MSI type DNA mutations, LOH associated with chromosomal instability, as well as point mutations have all been described in early gastric cancer. Similar to colon cancer, CIN and MSI are the two main pathways that underlie gastric cancer progression. However, many of the molecular changes observed in cancer tissues are not specific to either pathway, resulting in considerable overlap in gastric cancer subtypes. MSI was reported in 17–35% of gastric adenomas (Kashiwagi et al. 2000; Kim et al. 2002b; Abraham et al. 2003) and in 17–59% gastric carcinomas (Strickler et al. 1994; Hayden et al. 1998; Sepulveda et al. 1999; Kashiwagi et al. 2000; Leung et al. 2000; Kim et al. 2002b; Lee et al. 2002b; Abraham et al. 2003). High level of MSI in gastric adenomas and cancer, determined by MSI at greater than 30% tested loci (Umar et al. 2004), has been associated with the epigenetic silencing of the MMR gene *hMLH1*

Gastric Carcinogenesis

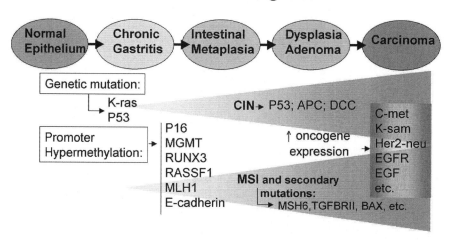

Fig. 16.8 Molecular events in the development and progression of gastric neoplasia. Gastric cancers are characterized by complex patterns of genomic changes related to histology and stage of progression. The two main pathways of gastric cancer progression include CIN and MSI. Many of the molecular changes that occur are not specific to either pathway and there is thus considerable overlap of molecular mechanisms of gastric cancer progression

(Edmonston et al. 2000; Baek et al. 2001; Fleisher et al. 2001; Umar et al. 2004). Gastric tumors with MSI-H also typically harbor frameshift mutations in the coding regions of other cancer-related genes, including *BAX, IGFRII, TGFβRII, hMSH3*, and *hMSH6* (Myeroff et al. 1995; Chung et al. 1997; Ottini et al. 1997; Yamamoto et al. 1997; Shinmura et al. 1998). In MSI-H gastric adenomas, frameshift mutations of *TGFbetaRII* were detected in 38–88% of the cases, *BAX* in 13%, *hMSH3* in 13%, and *E2F-4* in 50% of the specimens tested (Kim et al. 1999, 2000).

Point mutations and loss of heterozygosity at multiple gene loci have been detected in intestinal metaplasia, preceding the development of adenomas and gastric carcinomas (Kobayashi et al. 2000). Mutations of the *p53* and *APC* tumor-suppressor genes have been reported in both intestinal metaplasia and gastric dysplasia (Nakatsuru et al. 1993; Correa and Shiao 1994; Shiao et al. 1994; Imatani et al. 1996). *APC* gene mutations, including stop-codon and frameshift mutations, were reported in 46% and 5q allelic loss in 33% of informative cases of gastric adenoma (Abraham et al. 2003) and in 45% carcinomas (Lee et al. 2002a). Activating *Ki-RAS* mutations at codon 12 were less commonly observed, being present in only 14% of biopsies with atrophic gastritis, and in less than 10% of adenomas and carcinomas (Hunt et al. 2001; Lee et al. 2002b).

Gene silencing by epigenetic DNA modifications occurs throughout the progression from gastritis to gastric cancer (Gologan et al. 2005). Genes that play a role in cell cycle progression, DNA repair, and cell adhesion as well as several tumor-suppressor genes are reportedly regulated by epigenetic mechanisms. In gastric carcinogenesis, CpG island methylation and gene silencing are seen with many genes including *hMLH1, p14, p15, p16, E-cadherin, RUNX3, thromobospondin-1 (THBS1), tissue inhibitor of metalloproteinase 3 (TIMP-3), COX-2,* and *MGMT* (Toyota et al. 1999; Kang et al. 2001; To et al. 2002; Kang et al. 2003; Waki et al. 2003; Lee et al. 2004). The mechanisms that regulate CpG methylation and gene silencing during *H. pylori*-associated gastritis and progression to cancer are not currently known. Recent studies have suggested that polymorphisms in the pro-inflammatory *Interleukin-1β* gene were associated with CpG island methylation of target genes (Chan et al. 2007). Moreover, CpG methylation of the E-cadherin promoter was induced in cells treated with IL-1β (Qian et al. 2008). These data suggest that components of the inflammatory cascade induced by *H. pylori* may contribute to orchestration of the epigenetic response in *H. pylori*-associated carcinogenesis.

In summary, the spectrum of gene expression changes, mutations, and epigenetic alterations in gastric intestinal metaplasia, dysplasia, and cancer reflect the combined effects of chronic inflammation and *Helicobacter* bacterium products. The integration of these components will improve our ability to determine the likelihood of progression to cancer and may provide novel targets for early detection and therapy of gastric cancer.

Ulcerative Colitis as a Paradigm for Inflammation-Associated Carcinogenesis

Clinical Manifestations of Ulcerative Colitis

Ulcerative colitis is a chronic relapsing inflammatory condition of the colonic mucosa. It is manifest in most patients by the presence of diarrhea, abdominal pain, tenesmus, and rectal bleeding (Stenson 1995). The intensity of these symptoms can vary significantly, from mild to severe. The mucosa is typically more friable, with frequent petechiae, exudates, and frank hemorrhages (Fig. 16.9). In severe cases bleeding can be very intense, mucosal ulcerations become evident, and inflammatory pseudopolyps often develop (Stenson 1995). The inflammation can involve the whole colon or be limited to a lesser portion, but it almost always involves the rectum and is contiguous (no "skip" or uninvolved normal regions within the involved areas of the colon).

At the microscopic level, UC is marked by an intense infiltration of neutrophils that are limited to the mucosa and submucosa (Fig. 16.9) (Stenson 1995). Common findings include the presence of crypt abscesses, mucosal ulcerations, regenerative crypt fissuring, and goblet cell depletion (Fig. 16.9). These findings are often present even in those whose symptoms have resolved. The condition can wax and wane over the course of decades, with recurrent bouts of severe colitis interspersed with periods of relative disease quiescence. Often, however, even within these quiescent periods, there is endoscopic and microscopic evidence of ongoing mucosal inflammation. The molecular basis for UC remains elusive despite many years of research.

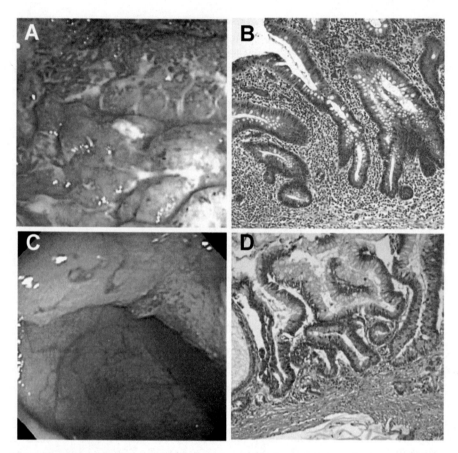

Fig. 16.9 Ulcerative colitis and adenocarcinoma. (**A**) Endoscopic image of colon demonstrates irregular erythematous mucosa in a patient with active ulcerative colitis. (**B**) Histology of chronic active ulcerative colitis depicting crypt architecture distortion, increased mucosal chronic inflammation, and acute cryptitis. (**C**) Endoscopic image and (**D**) histology of colonic adenocarcinoma arising from a dysplastic lesion in a patient with ulcerative colitis. Hematoxylin and eosin stains original magnification 100X (**B, C**). Endoscopic images contributed by Drs. Gregory Ginsberg and Anil Rustgi, University of Pennsylvania

Currently, it is believed that UC arises through an interaction of genetic factors with environmental exposures (Baumgart and Carding 2007).

Epidemiological studies have demonstrated an aggregation of UC in families, as well as a disease concordance in monozygotic twins. Indeed, several susceptibility genes have been described (Baumgart and Carding 2007). These findings suggest a genetic basis to UC. However, the inheritance pattern is complex, with disease concordance in monozygotic twins only 10%, suggesting the genetic contribution is not dominant. Rather, it appears that genetics may determine susceptibility, but environmental exposures, including exposure to normal bacterial flora, may serve as the critical disease trigger (Baumgart and Carding 2007).

The Inflammatory Microenvironment in Ulcerative Colitis

Despite the tremendous variety in bacterial colonizers in the colon, the normal mucosal immune system is not in a constant state of activation. This tolerance for the colonic flora is acquired within the first 2 years of life (Baumgart and Carding 2007). It depends on the production of regulatory immune cells by the adaptive immune system to inhibit immune activation or to suppress immune effectors once they have become active. With normal tolerance present, there is a balance between effector and regulatory immune subpopulations. This balance is actively maintained by the antigen-presenting dendritic cells through the secretion of suppressor cytokines like interleukin-10 (Banchereau and Steinman 1998; Hart et al. 2004).

It remains unclear what the inciting event is that causes UC. Several possibilities include an incomplete or "leaky" epithelial barrier permitting influx of bacterial antigens, atypical innate immune system activity, abnormal antigen-presenting cells that incorrectly recognize commensal bacteria and activate effector T cells, or alternatively the absence of normal regulatory dendritic and T-cell function that suppress an active immune response (Stenson 1995; Baumgart and Carding 2007). All of these abnormalities are present in ulcerative colitis and contribute to the persistence of the inflammatory response.

Once professional and non-professional antigen-presenting cells are activated, they release potent chemokines like interleukin-8, macrophage inflammatory protein 1 (α and β), monocyte chemoattractant proteins 1, 2, and 3, among others, to intensify the inflammatory response (Charo and Ransohoff 2006; Baumgart and Carding 2007). Neutrophils, macrophages, and lymphocytes actively migrate to the colonic mucosa in response. Pro-inflammatory cytokines like Il-1, Il-5, Il-6, Il-13, and TNF-α are also released, prompting the maturation of immune effectors including natural killer T cells and activated macrophages and granulocytes. These activated effectors then begin the production of antimicrobial metabolites including the genotoxic superoxide (O^{2-}), hydroxy radical ($\cdot OH$), and hydrogen peroxide (H_2O_2). Eicosanoid and NO biosynthesis are also induced in response to cytokine signaling, resulting in the production of additional mutagenic metabolites like lipid hydroperoxides, ROS, and RNS (Valko et al. 2005; Federico et al. 2007). This inflammatory response is meant to persist for only brief periods until the infection has resolved. However, in ulcerative colitis patients, this genotoxic microenvironment can persist for years, thereby promoting carcinogenesis.

Molecular Pathways for the Induction of Carcinogenesis in UC

The chronic inflammatory environment in UC applies unique stresses upon colonic epithelial cells. Oxidative injury and the actions of cytotoxic immune cells can induce colonocyte apoptosis and mucosal ulcerations. The continuously renewing epithelium must expand its proliferative capacity in order to respond to this ongoing injury and promote mucosal restitution (Boland et al. 2005; Itzkowitz 2006). This is made more difficult by the ROS and RNS species released by activated immune cells, which damage DNA (Fig. 16.10) (Valko et al. 2005; Federico et al. 2007). This appears to be the fundamental factor driving carcinogenesis in UC. Cells normally have many ways to respond to DNA damage. DNA repair mechanisms like non-homologous end-joining (NHEJ) and homologous recombination (HR), MMR, and BER are very effective and can often complete the necessary repairs. However, they can be overwhelmed if the injury is too great. Moreover, enzymes involved in MMR are sensitive to ROS and RNS species and can be inactivated by oxidation, diminishing MMR activity (Chang et al. 2002). Therefore in active UC, normal DNA repair mechanisms may be inadequate. Other tumor-suppressor mechanisms may then be employed to prevent the survival and replication of cells with DNA damage including apoptosis or cell senescence.

These important tumor-suppressor mechanisms are abrogated early in the progression to cancer in ulcerative colitis (Fig. 16.10). Intracellular signals initiated by cytokines and prostaglandins promote intestinal cell proliferation and inhibit apoptosis. In UC and other inflammatory conditions, cytokines like IL-6 bind with receptors to initiate intracellular signaling, which includes activation of the serine–threonine kinase Akt (Rose-John et al. 2006). Akt promotes cell survival by inhibiting the pro-apoptotic factors p53, BAD, and FoxO1 (Vivanco and Sawyers 2002). Prostaglandins have similar effects on intestinal epithelial cells, also largely mediated by activation of the Akt pathway (Stenson 2007).

Another important response to inflammation that enhances carcinogenesis is the activation of the transcription factor NFκB (Boland et al. 2005). NFκB proteins play a central role in the inflammatory response for many cells. NfκB is activated in response to a variety of stimuli including cytokines, bacteria, and bacterial products (via the innate immune system); DNA damage; and growth factors (Karrasch and Jobin 2008). In the intestinal epithelium, NFκB induces the expression of COX2 and of pro-inflammatory cytokines IL-1, TNF-α, IL-12p40, and IL-23p19 (Karrasch and Jobin 2008). This serves to amplify and maintain the inflammatory response. NFκB activity in intestinal epithelial cells also promotes the expression of the anti-apoptotic factor inhibitor of apoptosis protein (IAP) and B-cell leukemia/lymphoma (Bcl-XL). Together, the cytokines, prostaglandins, and NFκB act to promote the survival and proliferation of epithelial cells in UC that may have significant DNA damage which would otherwise induce apoptosis or senescence. Some of these cells may acquire a mutation that yields a survival advantage, a process that if repeated can ultimately lead to the emergence of colon cancer (Fig. 16.10).

Genetic Instability and Molecular Alterations in Colitis-Associated Cancers

Colon cancers that develop in the setting of UC are genetically unstable, much as are sporadic colon cancers. Despite the significant differences in their underlying pathogenesis, the patterns of instability are quite similar (Itzkowitz 2006).

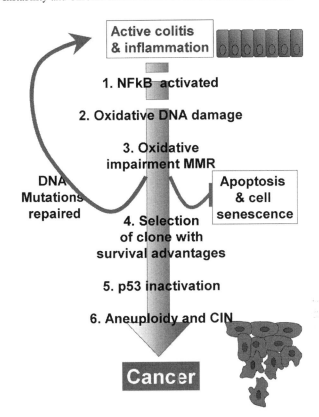

Fig. 16.10 Current model describing the emergence of colon cancer in the setting of ulcerative colitis. Chronic inflammation produces a microenvironment that stimulates NFκB activation in epithelial cells. NFκB promotes cell proliferation and inhibits apoptosis of damaged epithelial cells. Oxidative stress is increased in the inflammatory microenvironment, causing damage to epithelial cell lipid membranes, proteins, and DNA. Cellular repairs are initiated, however, some repair mechanisms like MMR may be diminished by the oxidative stress. Cells that complete repairs are able to replicate their DNA and progress through the cell cycle to help reconstitute the injured colonic epithelial barrier. Cells that cannot complete repairs either undergo apoptosis and die or irreversibly exit the cell cycle and undergo cell senescence. Rarely a cell acquires a mutation that allows it to avoid apoptosis or senescence. This clone gives rise to daughter cells that acquire additional mutations, with inactivation of the tumor-suppressor p53 frequently being acquired early in this process. Once p53 has been inactivated, genetic instability increases, aneuploidy and CIN develop, and a fully transformed cancer cell is selected and a tumor forms

The rates of chromosomal (CIN) and microsatellite instabilities (MSI) in colitis-associated cancers are identical to those seen in sporadic colon cancers (85 and 15%, respectively). Despite these similarities, significant differences exist regarding the molecular events that precede the onset of these cancers.

In a subset of UC colon cancers, the cause of MSI-H is the silencing of the MMR gene hMLH1 by promoter hypermethylation, much as it is in sporadic cancers (Fleisher et al. 2000). However, MSI-L is observed in non-cancerous and cancerous UC epithelium at a much greater frequency than that seen in sporadic cancers (Boland et al. 2005). There have been several explanations proposed for this observation. MMR enzymes are known to be inactivated by free radicals directly (Chang et al. 2002). This would diminish repair activity and possibly cause an MSI-L phenotype. It has also been hypothesized that massive oxidative DNA damage can overwhelm the ability of the MMR pathway to correct the damage. While this has never been directly proven, it was indirectly established (Hofseth et al. 2003). BER activity, which is increased in response to oxidative DNA damage, requires MMR enzymes to complete the repair. This leads to an adaptive imbalance in MMR enzymes caused by the increased BER demands. This imbalance has been observed in vivo in MSI-L UC cancers and can be demonstrated in vitro using several experimental systems (Hofseth et al. 2003). Therefore, MSI likely plays an important role in the genetic instability of most UC-associated colon cancers.

Other important differences between colitis-associated and sporadic colon cancers exist. This includes the significance and/or timing of certain genetic alterations. In sporadic and familial MSI-H colon cancers, mutational inactivation of the TGFβ receptor II gene by MSI occurs in 80% of tested cancers, and is frequently a late event, coming with the transition from late adenoma to cancer (Lynch and Hoops 2002; Lynch and Rustgi 2005). In UC-associated colon cancers with MSI, TGFβRII mutations are much less common, observed in only 17% of these cancers (Fig. 16.11) (Itzkowitz 2006). The pattern of genes inactivated by MSI in colitis-associated cancers is not well established; it is therefore unknown if other significant differences exist between sporadic and colitis-associated MSI cancers.

Another important difference is the *adenomatous polyposis coli* (APC) gene, which is mutated in the majority (80%) of all sporadic colon cancers (Lynch and Hoops 2002). In sporadic and familial cancers, this gene is typically inactivated by the early adenoma stage (Fig. 16.11). This leads to unopposed Wnt/β-catenin activity, which enhances carcinogenesis by promoting cell proliferation, migration, angiogenesis, and inhibiting apoptosis (Lynch and Rustgi 2005). However, in UC-associated colon cancers, *APC* mutations or LOH are seen in only 14 to 33% of cancers, based on several studies (Greenwald et al. 1992; Redston et al. 1995; Tomlinson et al. 1998; Aust et al. 2002). Moreover, the *APC* mutations occur much later in UC cancers, associated with the transition from high-grade dysplasia to carcinoma (Itzkowitz 2006). This significant genetic variance from sporadic colon cancer is likely due to the inflammatory environment in UC. The activation of NFκB in colon epithelial cells by cytokine signaling promotes cell proliferation and inhibits apoptosis. These effects may make APC inactivation unnecessary as a prerequisite for colitis-associated carcinogenesis(Boland et al. 2005).

The tumor-suppressor p53 is another study in contrasts (Fig. 16.11). While the tumor-suppressor p53 is mutated at a high rate in both sporadic and UC colon cancers, p53 mutations tend to occur much earlier in the colitis-associated cancers (Burmer et al. 1992; Yin et al. 1993; Brentnall et al. 1994; Hussain et al. 2000). p53 mutations and LOH are late events in sporadic CRC, typically associated with the progression from late adenoma to cancer (Lynch and Hoops 2002). However, in UC carcinogenesis, p53 mutations can be detected early, often preceding the onset

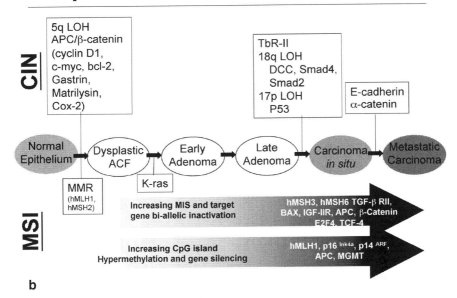

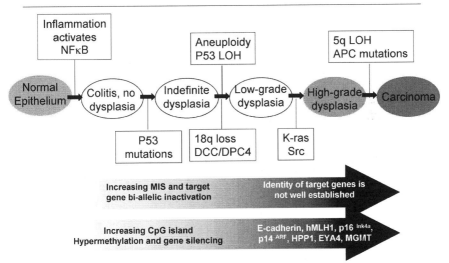

Fig. 16.11 Molecular events common in the development of sporadic and colitis-associated colon cancer–based on the model proposed by Fearon and Vogelstein in 1990. (**a**) Genetic events associated with both CIN and MSI forms of sporadic colon cancer in humans. (**b**) Molecular changes reported in the pathway to UC-associated colon cancer

of dysplasia and aneuploidy (Brentnall et al. 1994; Hussain et al. 2000). Mutations in p53 were detected in 19% of biopsies without dysplasia, with the frequency increasing as the degree of dysplasia advanced (Holzmann et al. 1998).

As the "guardian of the genome," p53 is critically important in the response to DNA damage (Meek 2004). In the setting of mild DNA damage, p53 will induce p21 gene expression and halt cell cycle progression in S-phase until the damage is repaired. When DNA damage is more extensive, p53 can induce apoptosis or cell senescence, thereby preventing DNA replication and the passage of the mutational events on to daughter cells. The early inactivation of p53 seen in UC-associated cancers contributes to the rapid progression to colon cancer that is seen in these patients. Cells lacking adequate p53 function have a survival advantage over other epithelial cells in the inflammatory UC microenvironment. Absent p53 activity, genetic instability, and aneuploidy does not induce cell death. Mutations accumulate, and ultimately a cell clone emerges that possesses the required features of a cancer cell (Lynch and Rustgi 2005).

In summary, the chronic inflammatory environment of UC provides a milieu that is supportive for the emergence of colon cancer cells. While from a genetic and clinical perspective there are many similarities between sporadic and CACs, we now know there to be substantial differences with respect to the genes targeted and the timing of these mutations. It has been speculated that these differences constitute a separate "pathway" for the transformation of colonocytes into cancer cells. There remains much that we still do not know regarding the molecular basis for these human pathologies. Research ongoing now and in the future will yield new insights into this important clinical and scientific question.

Conclusions

The inflammatory process is an important biological mechanism by which multicellular organisms respond to injury and infection. As such it is critically important for the health and well-being of the organism. However, if unchecked, or in the setting of a chronic infectious process, the immune response can be deleterious. One important sequela of a chronic inflammatory process is the development of cancer. This relationship has been well documented in humans and animals both epidemiologically and experimentally. We now know the inflammatory microenvironment to be carcinogenic. Inflammation causes the expression of genotoxins like ROS, RNS, and lipid hydroperoxides, which constantly bombard and damage the cell's membranes, proteins, and DNA. Cells are also constantly stimulated by cytokines and eicosanoids, enhancing their proliferation and protecting them from death in this stressed setting. Robust DNA repair mechanisms like NHEJ, HR, BER, and MMR collaborate to maintain the fidelity of the original DNA sequence. Moreover, when repairs cannot be completed, other mechanisms exist to prevent cell replication and the transmission of this damage as mutations to daughter cells, including cellular apoptosis and senescence. The fact that cancers typically do not emerge from chronically inflamed tissues for several decades testifies to the vigorousness of these pathways. However, ultimately a rare cell clone emerges that has derived survival advantages from this mutagenic environment, and a cancer develops. Our improved understanding of this process is yielding novel therapeutic approaches to treat and ultimately prevent this devastating complication of chronic inflammatory conditions.

References

Abraham SC, Park SJ, Lee JH, Mugartegui L, Wu TT (2003) Genetic alterations in gastric adenomas of intestinal and foveolar phenotypes. Mod Pathol 16:786–795.

Ahuja N, Mohan AL, Li Q, Stolker JM, Herman JG, Hamilton SR, Baylin SB, Issa JP (1997) Association between CpG island methylation and microsatellite instability in colorectal cancer. Cancer Res 57:3370–3374.

Akre K, Ekstrom AM, Signorello LB, Hansson LE, Nyren O (2001) Aspirin and risk for gastric cancer: a population-based case-control study in Sweden. Br J Cancer 84:965–968.

Anonymous (1994) Live flukes and *Helicobacter pylori*. IARC Working group on the Evaluation of Carcinogenic Risks to Humans. Lyon. 7–14 June 1994. IARC Monogr Eval Carcinog Risks Hum 61:1–241.

Artandi SE, Chang S, Lee SL, Alson S, Gottlieb GJ, Chin L, DePinho RA (2000) Telomere dysfunction promotes non-reciprocal translocations and epithelial cancers in mice. Nature 406:641–645.

Aust DE, Terdiman JP, Willenbucher RF, Chang CG, Molinaro-Clark A, Baretton GB, Loehrs U, Waldman FM (2002) The APC/beta-catenin pathway in ulcerative colitis-related colorectal carcinomas: a mutational analysis. Cancer 94:1421–1427.

Bader S, Walker M, Hendrich B, Bird A, Bird C, Hooper M, Wyllie A (1999) Somatic frameshift mutations in the MBD4 gene of sporadic colon cancers with mismatch repair deficiency. Oncogene 18:8044–8047.

Baek MJ, Kang H, Kim SE, Park JH, Lee JS, Paik YK, Kim H (2001) Expression of hMLH1 is inactivated in the gastric adenomas with enhanced microsatellite instability. Br J Cancer 85:1147–1152.

Balkwill F (2002) Tumor necrosis factor or tumor promoting factor? Cytokine Growth Factor Rev 13:135–141.

Balkwill FR (2004) Inflammatory cytokines: their role in tumor growth and progression. In: Cancer and Inflammation. Birkhauser Verlag Basel, Basel.

Banchereau J and Steinman RM (1998) Dendritic cells and the control of immunity. Nature 392:245–252.

Bargen JA (1928) Chronic ulcerative colitis associated with malignant disease. Arch Surg 17:561–576.

Baumgart DC and Carding SR (2007) Inflammatory bowel disease: cause and immunobiology. Lancet 369:1627–1640.

Baylin SB and Herman JG (2000) DNA hypermethylation in tumorigenesis: epigenetics joins genetics. Trends Genet 16:168–174.

Bello MJ, Alonso ME, Aminoso C, Anselmo NP, Arjona D, Gonzalez-Gomez P, Lopez-Marin I, de Campos JM, Gutierrez M, Isla A, Kusak ME, Lassaletta L, Sarasa JL, Vaquero J, Casartelli C, Rey JA (2004) Hypermethylation of the DNA repair gene MGMT: association with TP53 G:C to A:T transitions in a series of 469 nervous system tumors. Mutat Res 554:23–32.

Berger FG (2004) The interleukin-6 gene: a susceptibility factor that may contribute to racial and ethnic disparities in breast cancer mortality. Breast Cancer Res Treat 88:281–285.

Bharadwaj R and Yu H (2004) The spindle checkpoint, aneuploidy, and cancer. Oncogene 23:2016–2027.

Blair IA (2001) Lipid hydroperoxide-mediated DNA damage. Exp Gerontol 36:1473–1481.

Blair IA (2008) DNA adducts with lipid peroxidation products. J Biol Chem 283:15545–15549.

Boland CR, Thibodeau SN, Hamilton SR, Sidransky D, Eshleman JR, Burt RW, Meltzer SJ, Rodriguez-Bigas MA, Fodde R, Ranzani GN, Srivastava S (1998) A National Cancer Institute Workshop on Microsatellite Instability for cancer detection and familial predisposition: development of international criteria for the determination of microsatellite instability in colorectal cancer. Cancer Res 58:5248–5257.

Boland CR, Luciani MG, Gasche C, Goel A (2005) Infection, inflammation, and gastrointestinal cancer. Gut 54:1321–1331.

Bommert K, Bargou RC, Stuhmer T (2006) Signalling and survival pathways in multiple myeloma. Eur J Cancer 42:1574–1580.

Breivik J and Gaudernack G (1999) Genomic instability, DNA methylation, and natural selection in colorectal carcinogenesis. Semin Cancer Biol 9:245–254.

Brentnall TA, Crispin DA, Rabinovitch PS, Haggitt RC, Rubin CE, Stevens AC, Burmer GC (1994) Mutations in the p53 gene: an early marker of neoplastic progression in ulcerative colitis. Gastroenterology 107:369–378.

Burmer GC, Rabinovitch PS, Haggitt RC, Crispin DA, Brentnall TA, Kolli VR, Stevens AC, Rubin CE (1992) Neoplastic progression in ulcerative colitis: histology, DNA content, and loss of a p53 allele. Gastroenterology 103:1602–1610.

Cahill DP, Lengauer C, Yu J, Riggins GJ, Willson JK, Markowitz SD, Kinzler KW, Vogelstein B (1998) Mutations of mitotic checkpoint genes in human cancers. Nature 392:300–303.

Cahill DP, Kinzler KW, Vogelstein B, Lengauer C (1999) Genetic instability and darwinian selection in tumours. Trends Cell Biol 9:M57–60.

Calin GA, Gafa R, Tibiletti MG, Herlea V, Becheanu G, Cavazzini L, Barbanti-Brodano G, Nenci I, Negrini M, Lanza G (2000) Genetic progression in microsatellite instability high (MSI-H) colon cancers correlates with clinico-pathological parameters: A study of the TGRbetaRII, BAX, hMSH3, hMSH6, IGFIIR and BLM genes. Int J Cancer 89:230–235.

Cassaro M, Rugge M, Gutierrez O, Leandro G, Graham DY, Genta RM (2000) Topographic patterns of intestinal metaplasia and gastric cancer. Am J Gastroenterol 95:1431–1438.

Censini S, Lange C, Xiang Z, Crabtree JE, Ghiara P, Borodovsky M, Rappuoli R, Covacci A (1996) cag, a pathogenicity island of Helicobacter pylori, encodes type I-specific and disease-associated virulence factors. Proc Natl Acad Sci U S A 93:14648–14653.

Chan AO, Chu KM, Huang C, Lam KF, Leung SY, Sun YW, Ko S, Xia HH, Cho CH, Hui WM, Lam SK, Rashid A (2007) Association between Helicobacter pylori infection and interleukin 1beta polymorphism predispose to CpG island methylation in gastric cancer. Gut 56:595–597.

Chang CL, Marra G, Chauhan DP, Ha HT, Chang DK, Ricciardiello L, Randolph A, Carethers JM, Boland CR (2002) Oxidative stress inactivates the human DNA mismatch repair system. Am J Physiol Cell Physiol 283:C148–154.

Charo IF and Ransohoff RM (2006) The many roles of chemokines and chemokine receptors in inflammation. N Engl J Med 354:610–621.

Chell SD, Witherden IR, Dobson RR, Moorghen M, Herman AA, Qualtrough D, Williams AC, Paraskeva C (2006) Increased EP4 receptor expression in colorectal cancer progression promotes cell growth and anchorage independence. Cancer Res 66:3106–3113.

Chung YJ, Park SW, Song JM, Lee KY, Seo EJ, Choi SW, Rhyu MG (1997) Evidence of genetic progression in human gastric carcinomas with microsatellite instability. Oncogene 15:1719–1726.

Cohn SM, Schloemann S, Tessner T, Seibert K, Stenson WF (1997) Crypt stem cell survival in the mouse intestinal epithelium is regulated by prostaglandins synthesized through cyclooxygenase-1. J Clin Invest 99:1367–1379.

Corn PG, Summers MK, Fogt F, Virmani AK, Gazdar AF, Halazonetis TD, El-Deiry WS (2003) Frequent hypermethylation of the 5′ CpG island of the mitotic stress checkpoint gene Chfr in colorectal and non-small cell lung cancer. Carcinogenesis 24:47–51.

Correa P (1992) Human gastric carcinogenesis: a multistep and multifactorial process– First American Cancer Society Award Lecture on Cancer Epidemiology and Prevention. Cancer Res 52:6735–6740.

Correa P (1995) Helicobacter pylori and gastric carcinogenesis. Am J Surg Pathol 19:S37–S43.

Correa P and Houghton J (2007) Carcinogenesis of Helicobacter pylori. Gastroenterology 133:659–672.

Correa P and Shiao Y-H (1994) Phenotypic and genotypic events in gastric carcinogenesis. Cancer Res 54 (Supplement):1941–1943.

Coussens LM and Werb Z (2002) Inflammation and cancer. Nature 420:860–867.

Cover TL and Blanke SR (2005) Helicobacter pylori VacA, a paradigm for toxin multifunctionality. Nat Rev Microbiol 3:320–332.

Crabtree JE, Covacci A, Farmery SM, Xiang Z, Tompkins DS, Perry S, Lindley IJ, Rappuoli R (1995) Helicobacter pylori induced interleukin-8 expression in gastric epithelial cells is associated with CagA positive phenotype. J Clin Pathol 48:41–45.

Crabtree JE, Wyatt JI, Trejdosiewicz LK, Peichl P, Nichols PH, Ramsay N, Primrose JN, Lindley IJ (1994) Interleukin-8 expression in Helicobacter pylori infected, normal, and neoplastic gastroduodenal mucosa. J Clin Pathol 47:61–66.

Crofford LJ (2001) Prostaglandin biology. Gastroenterol Clin North Am 30:863–876.

Cruz-Correa M, Cui H, Giardiello FM, Powe NR, Hylind L, Robinson A, Hutcheon DF, Kafonek DR, Brandenburg S, Wu Y, He X, Feinberg AP (2004) Loss of imprinting of insulin growth factor II gene: a potential heritable biomarker for colon neoplasia predisposition. Gastroenterology 126:964–970.

Cui H, Onyango P, Brandenburg S, Wu Y, Hsieh CL, Feinberg AP (2002) Loss of imprinting in colorectal cancer linked to hypomethylation of H19 and IGF2. Cancer Res 62:6442–6446.

Cunningham JM, Christensen ER, Tester DJ, Kim CY, Roche PC, Burgart LJ, Thibodeau SN (1998) Hypermethylation of the hMLH1 promoter in colon cancer with microsatellite instability. Cancer Res 58:3455–3460.

Delaunoit T, Limburg PJ, Goldberg RM, Lymp JF, Loftus EV, Jr. (2006) Colorectal cancer prognosis among patients with inflammatory bowel disease. Clin Gastroenterol Hepatol 4:335–342.

Devroede GJ, Taylor WF, Sauer WG, Jackman RJ, Stickler GB (1971) Cancer risk and life expectancy of children with ulcerative colitis. N Engl J Med 285:17–21.

Dixon MF (1995) Histological responses to Helicobacter pylori infection: gastritis, atrophy and preneoplasia. Baillieres Clin Gastroenterol 9:467–486.

Dixon MF, Genta RM, Yardley JH, Correa P (1996) Classification and grading of gastritis. The updated Sydney system. International workshop on the histopathology of gastritis, Houston 1994. Am J Surg Pathol 20:1161–1181.

Eaden JA, Abrams KR, Mayberry JF (2001) The risk of colorectal cancer in ulcerative colitis: a meta-analysis. Gut 48:526–535.

Eck M, Greiner A, Schmausser B, Eck H, Kolve M, Fischbach W, Strecker P, Muller-Hermelink HK (1999) Evaluation of Helicobacter pylori in gastric MALT-type lymphoma: differences between histologic and serologic diagnosis. Mod Pathol 12:1148–1151.

Edmonston TB, Cuesta KH, Burkholder S, Barusevicius A, Rose D, Kovatich AJ, Boman B, Fry R, Fishel R, Palazzo JP (2000) Colorectal carcinomas with high microsatellite instability: defining a distinct immunologic and molecular entity with respect to prognostic markers. Hum Pathol 31:1506–1514.

Ejima Y, Yang L, Sasaki MS (2000) Aberrant splicing of the ATM gene associated with shortening of the intronic mononucleotide tract in human colon tumor cell lines: a novel mutation target of microsatellite instability. Int J Cancer 86:262–268.

Ekbom A, Helmick C, Zack M, Adami HO (1990) Ulcerative colitis and colorectal cancer. A population-based study. N Engl J Med 323:1228–1233.

El-Omar EM (2006) Role of host genes in sporadic gastric cancer. Best Pract Res Clin Gastroenterol 20:675–686.

El-Omar EM, Carrington M, Chow WH, McColl KE, Bream JH, Young HA, Herrera J, Lissowska J, Yuan CC, Rothman N, Lanyon G, Martin M, Fraumeni JF, Jr., Rabkin CS (2000) Interleukin-1 polymorphisms associated with increased risk of gastric cancer. Nature 404:398–402.

El-Omar EM, Rabkin CS, Gammon MD, Vaughan TL, Risch HA, Schoenberg JB, Stanford JL, Mayne ST, Goedert J, Blot WJ, Fraumeni JF, Jr., Chow WH (2003) Increased risk of noncardia gastric cancer associated with proinflammatory cytokine gene polymorphisms. Gastroenterology 124:1193–1201.

Engelhardt M, Drullinsky P, Guillem J, Moore MA (1997) Telomerase and telomere length in the development and progression of premalignant lesions to colorectal cancer. Clin Cancer Res 3:1931–1941.

Esteller M, Tortola S, Toyota M, Capella G, Peinado MA, Baylin SB, Herman JG (2000) Hypermethylation-associated inactivation of p14(ARF) is independent of p16(INK4a) methylation and p53 mutational status. Cancer Res 60:129–133.

Esteller M, Cordon-Cardo C, Corn PG, Meltzer SJ, Pohar KS, Watkins DN, Capella G, Peinado MA, Matias-Guiu X, Prat J, Baylin SB, Herman JG (2001a) p14ARF silencing by promoter hypermethylation mediates abnormal intracellular localization of MDM2. Cancer Res 61:2816–2821.

Esteller M, Corn PG, Baylin SB, Herman JG (2001b) A gene hypermethylation profile of human cancer. Cancer Res 61:3225–3229.

Fang DC, Jass JR, Wang DX, Zhou XD, Luo YH, Young J (1999) Infrequent loss of heterozygosity of APC/MCC and DCC genes in gastric cancer showing DNA microsatellite instability. J Clin Pathol 52:504–508.

Farinati F, Cardin R, Degan P, Rugge M, Mario FD, Bonvicini P, Naccarato R (1998) Oxidative DNA damage accumulation in gastric carcinogenesis. Gut 42:351–356.

Farinati F, Cardin R, Bortolami M, Nitti D, Basso D, de Bernard M, Cassaro M, Sergio A, Rugge M (2008) Oxidative DNA damage in gastric cancer: CagA status and OGG1 gene polymorphism. Int J Cancer 123:51–55.

Farrow B and Evers BM (2002) Inflammation and the development of pancreatic cancer. Surg Oncol 10:153–169.

Federico A, Morgillo F, Tuccillo C, Ciardiello F, Loguercio C (2007) Chronic inflammation and oxidative stress in human carcinogenesis. Int J Cancer 121:2381–2386.

Fischbach W, Goebeler-Kolve ME, Dragosics B, Greiner A, Stolte M (2004) Long term outcome of patients with gastric marginal zone B cell lymphoma of mucosa associated lymphoid tissue (MALT) following exclusive Helicobacter pylori eradication therapy: experience from a large prospective series. Gut 53:34–37.

Fischer W, Gebert B, Haas R (2004) Novel activities of the Helicobacter pylori vacuolating cytotoxin: from epithelial cells towards the immune system. Int J Med Microbiol 293:539–547.

Fishel R, Lescoe MK, Rao MR, Copeland NG, Jenkins NA, Garber J, Kane M, Kolodner R (1993) The human mutator gene homolog MSH2 and its association with hereditary nonpolyposis colon cancer. Cell 75:1027–1038.

Fleisher AS, Esteller M, Harpaz N, Leytin A, Rashid A, Xu Y, Liang J, Stine OC, Yin J, Zou TT, Abraham JM, Kong D, Wilson KT, James SP, Herman JG, Meltzer SJ (2000) Microsatellite instability in inflammatory bowel disease-associated neoplastic lesions is associated with hypermethylation and diminished expression of the DNA mismatch repair gene, hMLH1. Cancer Res 60:4864–4868.

Fleisher AS, Esteller M, Tamura G, Rashid A, Stine OC, Yin J, Zou TT, Abraham JM, Kong D, Nishizuka S, James SP, Wilson KT, Herman JG, Meltzer SJ (2001) Hypermethylation of the hMLH1 gene promoter is associated with microsatellite instability in early human gastric neoplasia. Oncogene 20:329–335.

Forman D, Newell DG, Fullerton F, Yarnell JW, Stacey AR, Wald N, Sitas F (1991) Association between infection with Helicobacter pylori and risk of gastric cancer: evidence from a prospective investigation. BMJ 302:1302–1305.

Fosslien E (2001) Review: molecular pathology of cyclooxygenase-2 in cancer-induced angiogenesis. Ann Clin Lab Sci 31:325–348.

Fu S, Ramanujam KS, Wong A, Fantry GT, Drachenberg CB, James SP, Meltzer SJ, Wilson KT (1999) Increased expression and cellular localization of inducible nitric oxide synthase and cyclooxygenase 2 in Helicobacter pylori gastritis. Gastroenterology 116:1319–1329.

Gebert B, Fischer W, Haas R (2004) The Helicobacter pylori vacuolating cytotoxin: from cellular vacuolation to immunosuppressive activities. Rev Physiol Biochem Pharmacol 152: 205–220.

Gebert B, Fischer W, Weiss E, Hoffmann R, Haas R (2003) Helicobacter pylori vacuolating cytotoxin inhibits T lymphocyte activation. Science 301:1099–1102.

Gerson SL (2004) MGMT: its role in cancer aetiology and cancer therapeutics. Nat Rev Cancer 4:296–307.

Giannakis M, Chen SL, Karam SM, Engstrand L, Gordon JI (2008) Helicobacter pylori evolution during progression from chronic atrophic gastritis to gastric cancer and its impact on gastric stem cells. Proc Natl Acad Sci U S A 105:4358–4363.

Giardiello FM, Yang VW, Hylind LM, Krush AJ, Petersen GM, Trimbath JD, Piantadosi S, Garrett E, Geiman DE, Hubbard W, Offerhaus GJ, Hamilton SR (2002) Primary chemoprevention of familial adenomatous polyposis with sulindac. N Engl J Med 346:1054–1059.

Gisselsson D, Jonson T, Petersen A, Strombeck B, Dal Cin P, Hoglund M, Mitelman F, Mertens F, Mandahl N (2001) Telomere dysfunction triggers extensive DNA fragmentation and evolution of complex chromosome abnormalities in human malignant tumors. Proc Natl Acad Sci U S A 98:12683–12688.

Gologan A, Graham DY, Sepulveda AR (2005) Molecular Markers in Helicobacter pylori-Associated Gastric Carcinogenesis. Clin Lab Med 25:197–222.

Gonzalez-Perez A, Garcia Rodriguez LA, Lopez-Ridaura R (2003) Effects of non-steroidal anti-inflammatory drugs on cancer sites other than the colon and rectum: a meta-analysis. BMC Cancer 3:28.

Grady WM, Rajput A, Myeroff L, Liu DF, Kwon K, Willis J, Markowitz S (1998) Mutation of the type II transforming growth factor-beta receptor is coincident with the transformation of human colon adenomas to malignant carcinomas. Cancer Res 58:3101–3104.

Greenwald BD, Harpaz N, Yin J, Huang Y, Tong Y, Brown VL, McDaniel T, Newkirk C, Resau JH, Meltzer SJ (1992) Loss of heterozygosity affecting the p53, Rb, and mcc/apc tumor suppressor gene loci in dysplastic and cancerous ulcerative colitis. Cancer Res 52:741–745.

Grisham MB, Jourd'heuil D, Wink DA (2000) Review article: chronic inflammation and reactive oxygen and nitrogen metabolism–implications in DNA damage and mutagenesis. Aliment Pharmacol Ther 14 Suppl 1:3–9.

Hahm KB, Lee KJ, Choi SY, Kim JH, Cho SW, Yim H, Park SJ, Chung MH (1997) Possibility of chemoprevention by the eradication of Helicobacter pylori: oxidative DNA damage and apoptosis in H. pylori infection. Am J Gastroenterol 92:1853–1857.

Hamamoto T, Yokozaki H, Semba S, Yasui W, Yunotani S, Miyazaki K, Tahara E (1997) Altered microsatellites in incomplete-type intestinal metaplasia adjacent to primary gastric cancers. J Clin Pathol 50:841–846.

Handa O, Naito Y, Yoshikawa T (2007) CagA protein of Helicobacter pylori: a hijacker of gastric epithelial cell signaling. Biochem Pharmacol 73:1697–1702.

Hart AL, Lammers K, Brigidi P, Vitali B, Rizzello F, Gionchetti P, Campieri M, Kamm MA, Knight SC, Stagg AJ (2004) Modulation of human dendritic cell phenotype and function by probiotic bacteria. Gut 53:1602–1609.

Hatakeyama M and Higashi H (2005) Helicobacter pylori CagA: a new paradigm for bacterial carcinogenesis. Cancer Sci 96:835–843.

Hayden JD, Martin IG, Cawkwell L, Quirke P (1998) The role of microsatellite instability in gastric carcinoma. Gut 42:300–303.

Heinen CD, Schmutte C, Fishel R (2002) DNA repair and tumorigenesis: lessons from hereditary cancer syndromes. Cancer Biol Ther 1:477–485.

388 A.R. Sepulveda and J.P. Lynch

Hermsen M, Postma C, Baak J, Weiss M, Rapallo A, Sciutto A, Roemen G, Arends JW, Williams R, Giaretti W, De Goeij A, Meijer G (2002) Colorectal adenoma to carcinoma progression follows multiple pathways of chromosomal instability. Gastroenterology 123:1109–1119.

Hofseth LJ, Khan MA, Ambrose M, Nikolayeva O, Xu-Welliver M, Kartalou M, Hussain SP, Roth RB, Zhou X, Mechanic LE, Zurer I, Rotter V, Samson LD, Harris CC (2003) The adaptive imbalance in base excision-repair enzymes generates microsatellite instability in chronic inflammation. J Clin Invest 112:1887–1894.

Hollstein MC, Smits AM, Galiana C, Yamasaki H, Bos JL, Mandard A, Partensky C, Montesano R (1988) Amplification of epidermal growth factor receptor gene but no evidence of ras mutations in primary human esophageal cancers. Cancer Res 48:5119–5123.

Holzmann K, Klump B, Borchard F, Hsieh CJ, Kuhn A, Gaco V, Gregor M, Porschen R (1998) Comparative analysis of histology, DNA content, p53 and Ki-ras mutations in colectomy specimens with long-standing ulcerative colitis. Int J Cancer 76:1–6.

Honda T, Tamura G, Waki T, Kawata S, Nishizuka S, Motoyama T (2004) Promoter hypermethylation of the Chfr gene in neoplastic and non-neoplastic gastric epithelia. Br J Cancer 90:2013–2016.

Houghton J, Stoicov C, Nomura S, Rogers AB, Carlson J, Li H, Cai X, Fox JG, Goldenring JR, Wang TC (2004) Gastric cancer originating from bone marrow-derived cells. Science 306:1568–1571.

Howes N, Lerch MM, Greenhalf W, Stocken DD, Ellis I, Simon P, Truninger K, Ammann R, Cavallini G, Charnley RM, Uomo G, Delhaye M, Spicak J, Drumm B, Jansen J, Mountford R, Whitcomb DC, Neoptolemos JP (2004) Clinical and genetic characteristics of hereditary pancreatitis in Europe. Clin Gastroenterol Hepatol 2:252–261.

Huang J, Papadopoulos N, McKinley AJ, Farrington SM, Curtis LJ, Wyllie AH, Zheng S, Willson JK, Markowitz SD, Morin P, Kinzler KW, Vogelstein B, Dunlop MG (1996) APC mutations in colorectal tumors with mismatch repair deficiency. Proc Natl Acad Sci U S A 93:9049–9054.

Huang JQ, Sridhar S, Chen Y, Hunt RH (1998) Meta-analysis of the relationship between Helicobacter pylori seropositivity and gastric cancer. Gastroenterology 114:1169–1179.

Hunt JD, Mera R, Strimas A, Gillespie AT, Ruiz B, Correa P, Fontham ET (2001) KRAS mutations are not predictive for progression of preneoplastic gastric lesions. Cancer Epidemiol Biomarkers Prev 10:79–80.

Husain SS, Szabo IL, Tamawski AS (2002) NSAID inhibition of GI cancer growth: clinical implications and molecular mechanisms of action. Am J Gastroenterol 97:542–553.

Hussain SP, Amstad P, Raja K, Ambs S, Nagashima M, Bennett WP, Shields PG, Ham AJ, Swenberg JA, Marrogi AJ, Harris CC (2000) Increased p53 mutation load in noncancerous colon tissue from ulcerative colitis: a cancer-prone chronic inflammatory disease. Cancer Res 60:3333–3337.

Hussain SP, Hofseth LJ, Harris CC (2003) Radical causes of cancer. Nat Rev Cancer 3:276–285.

Iguchi C, Nio Y, Takeda H, Yamasawa K, Hirahara N, Toga T, Itakura M, Tamura K (2001) Plant polysaccharide PSK: cytostatic effects on growth and invasion; modulating effect on the expression of HLA and adhesion molecules on human gastric and colonic tumor cell surface. Anticancer Res 21:1007–1013.

Imatani A, Sasano H, Asaki S, Toyota T, Saito M, Masuda T, Nagura H (1996) Analysis of p53 abnormalities in endoscopic gastric biopsies. Anticancer Res 16:2049–2056.

Ionov Y, Peinado MA, Malkhosyan S, Shibata D, Perucho M (1993) Ubiquitous somatic mutations in simple repeated sequences reveal a new mechanism for colonic carcinogenesis. Nature 363:558–561.

Itzkowitz SH (2006) Molecular biology of dysplasia and cancer in inflammatory bowel disease. Gastroenterol Clin North Am 35:553–571.

Jass JR (2004) Hyperplastic polyps and colorectal cancer: is there a link? Clin Gastroenterol Hepatol 2:1–8.

Jass JR, Whitehall VL, Young J, Leggett BA (2002) Emerging concepts in colorectal neoplasia. Gastroenterology 123:862–876.

Jess T, Loftus EV, Jr., Velayos FS, Harmsen WS, Zinsmeister AR, Smyrk TC, Schleck CD, Tremaine WJ, Melton LJ, 3rd, Munkholm P, Sandborn WJ (2006) Risk of intestinal cancer in inflammatory bowel disease: a population-based study from olmsted county, Minnesota. Gastroenterology 130:1039–1046.

Jiricny J and Marra G (2003) DNA repair defects in colon cancer. Curr Opin Genet Dev 13:61–69.

Jones S, Emmerson P, Maynard J, Best JM, Jordan S, Williams GT, Sampson JR, Cheadle JP (2002) Biallelic germline mutations in MYH predispose to multiple colorectal adenoma and somatic G:C -> T:A mutations. Hum Mol Genet 11:2961–2967.

Kambara T, Whitehall VL, Spring KJ, Barker MA, Arnold S, Wynter CV, Matsubara N, Tanaka N, Young JP, Leggett BA, Jass JR (2004) Role of inherited defects of MYH in the development of sporadic colorectal cancer. Genes Chromosomes Cancer 40:1–9.

Kambayashi T, Alexander HR, Fong M, Strassmann G (1995) Potential involvement of IL-10 in suppressing tumor-associated macrophages. Colon-26-derived prostaglandin E2 inhibits TNF-alpha release via a mechanism involving IL-10. J Immunol 154:3383–3390.

Kang GH, Shim YH, Jung HY, Kim WH, Ro JY, Rhyu MG (2001) CpG island methylation in premalignant stages of gastric carcinoma. Cancer Res 61:2847–2851.

Kang GH, Lee S, Kim JS, Jung HY (2003) Profile of aberrant CpG island methylation along the multistep pathway of gastric carcinogenesis. Lab Invest 83:635–641.

Karrasch T and Jobin C (2008) NF-kappaB and the intestine: friend or foe? Inflamm Bowel Dis 14:114–124.

Kashiwagi K, Watanabe M, Ezaki T, Kanai T, Ishii H, Mukai M, Hibi T (2000) Clinical usefulness of microsatellite instability for the prediction of gastric adenoma or adenocarcinoma in patients with chronic gastritis. Br J Cancer 82:1814–1818.

Katoh M (2007) Dysregulation of stem cell signaling network due to germline mutation, SNP, Helicobacter pylori infection, epigenetic change and genetic alteration in gastric cancer. Cancer Biol Ther 6:832–839.

Keim V, Witt H, Bauer N, Bodeker H, Rosendahl J, Teich N, Mossner J (2003) The course of genetically determined chronic pancreatitis. JOP 4:146–154.

Kim JJ, Baek MJ, Kim L, Kim NG, Lee YC, Song SY, Noh SH, Kim H (1999) Accumulated frameshift mutations at coding nucleotide repeats during the progression of gastric carcinoma with microsatellite instability. Lab Invest 79:1113–1120.

Kim HS, Woo DK, Bae SI, Kim YI, Kim WH (2000) Microsatellite instability in the adenoma-carcinoma sequence of the stomach. Lab Invest 80:57–64.

Kim JJ, Tao H, Carloni E, Leung WK, Graham DY, Sepulveda AR (2002a) Helicobacter pylori impairs DNA mismatch repair in gastric epithelial cells. Gastroenterology 123:542–553.

Kim JS, Chung SJ, Choi YS, Cheon JH, Kim CW, Kim SG, Jung HC, Song IS (2007) Helicobacter pylori eradication for low-grade gastric mucosa-associated lymphoid tissue lymphoma is more successful in inducing remission in distal compared to proximal disease. Br J Cancer 96:1324–1328.

Kim SS, Bhang CS, Min KO, Chae HS, Choi SW, Lee CD, Lim KW, Chung IS, Park DH (2002b) p53 mutations and microsatellite instabilities in the subtype of intestinal metaplasia of the stomach. J Korean Med Sci 17:490–496.

Kimura K (2000) Gastritis and gastric cancer. Asia. Gastroenterol Clin North Am 29:609–621.

Kobayashi K, Okamoto T, Takayama S, Akiyama M, Ohno T, Yamada H (2000) Genetic instability in intestinal metaplasia is a frequent event leading to well-differentiated early adenocarcinoma of the stomach. Eur J Cancer 36:1113–1119.

Kodama K, Sumii K, Kawano M, Kido T, Nojima K, Sumii M, Haruma K, Yoshihara M, Chayama K (2003) Gastric juice nitrite and vitamin C in patients with gastric cancer and atrophic gastritis: is low acidity solely responsible for cancer risk? Eur J Gastroenterol Hepatol 15:987–993.

Koizumi K, Hojo S, Akashi T, Yasumoto K, Saiki I (2007) Chemokine receptors in cancer metastasis and cancer cell-derived chemokines in host immune response. Cancer Sci 98:1652–1658.

Kolodner RD and Marsischky GT (1999) Eukaryotic DNA mismatch repair. Curr Opin Genet Dev 9:89–96.

Kucharzik T, Lugering N, Winde G, Domschke W, Stoll R (1997) Colon carcinoma cell lines stimulate monocytes and lamina propria mononuclear cells to produce IL-10. Clin Exp Immunol 110:296–302.

Kuismanen SA, Holmberg MT, Salovaara R, de la Chapelle A, Peltomaki P (2000) Genetic and epigenetic modification of MLH1 accounts for a major share of microsatellite-unstable colorectal cancers. Am J Pathol 156:1773–1779.

Kune GA, Kune S, Watson LF (1988) Colorectal cancer risk, chronic illnesses, operations, and medications: case control results from the Melbourne Colorectal Cancer Study. Cancer Res 48:4399–4404.

Kuroki T, Trapasso F, Yendamuri S, Matsuyama A, Alder H, Mori M, Croce CM (2003) Allele loss and promoter hypermethylation of VHL, RAR-beta, RASSF1A, and FHIT tumor suppressor genes on chromosome 3p in esophageal squamous cell carcinoma. Cancer Res 63:3724–3728.

Langman MJ, Cheng KK, Gilman EA, Lancashire RJ (2000) Effect of anti-inflammatory drugs on overall risk of common cancer: case-control study in general practice research database. BMJ 320:1642–1646.

Leach FS, Nicolaides NC, Papadopoulos N, Liu B, Jen J, Parsons R, Peltomaki P, Sistonen P, Aaltonen LA, Nystrom-Lahti M, Guan XY, Zhang J, Meltzer PS, Yu JW, Kao FT, Chen DJ, Cerosaletti KM, Fournier RE, Todd S, Lewis T, Leach RJ, Naylor SL, Weissenbach J, Mecklin JP, Järvinen H, Petersen GM, Hamilton SR, Trent JM, de la Chapelle A, Kinzler KW, Vogelstein B (1993) Mutations of a mutS homolog in hereditary nonpolyposis colorectal cancer. Cell 75:1215–1225.

Leahy KM, Ornberg RL, Wang Y, Zweifel BS, Koki AT, Masferrer JL (2002) Cyclooxygenase-2 inhibition by celecoxib reduces proliferation and induces apoptosis in angiogenic endothelial cells in vivo. Cancer Res 62:625–631.

Lee HS, Choi SI, Lee HK, Kim HS, Yang HK, Kang GH, Kim YI, Lee BL, Kim WH (2002a) Distinct clinical features and outcomes of gastric cancers with microsatellite instability. Mod Pathol 15:632–640.

Lee JH, Abraham SC, Kim HS, Nam JH, Choi C, Lee MC, Park CS, Juhng SW, Rashid A, Hamilton SR, Wu TT (2002b) Inverse relationship between APC gene mutation in gastric adenomas and development of adenocarcinoma. Am J Pathol 161:611–618.

Lee JH, Park SJ, Abraham SC, Seo JS, Nam JH, Choi C, Juhng SW, Rashid A, Hamilton SR, Wu TT (2004) Frequent CpG island methylation in precursor lesions and early gastric adenocarcinomas. Oncogene 23:4646–4654.

Lengauer C, Kinzler KW, Vogelstein B (1997) Genetic instability in colorectal cancers. Nature 386:623–627.

Lengauer C, Kinzler KW, Vogelstein B (1998) Genetic instabilities in human cancers. Nature 396:643–649.

Leung WK, Kim JJ, Kim JG, Graham DY, Sepulveda AR (2000) Microsatellite instability in gastric intestinal metaplasia in patients with and without gastric cancer. Am J Pathol 156:537–543.

Li CQ, Pignatelli B, Ohshima H (2000) Coexpression of interleukin-8 and inducible nitric oxide synthase in gastric mucosa infected with cagA+ Helicobacter pylori. Dig Dis Sci 45:55–62.

Lin WW and Karin M (2007) A cytokine-mediated link between innate immunity, inflammation, and cancer. J Clin Invest 117:1175–1183.

Lind GE, Thorstensen L, Lovig T, Meling GI, Hamelin R, Rognum TO, Esteller M, Lothe RA (2004) A CpG island hypermethylation profile of primary colorectal carcinomas and colon cancer cell lines. Mol Cancer 3:28.

Ling XL, Fang DC, Wang RQ, Yang SM, Fang L (2004) Mitochondrial microsatellite instability in gastric cancer and its precancerous lesions. World J Gastroenterol 10:800–803.

Lipton L, Halford SE, Johnson V, Novelli MR, Jones A, Cummings C, Barclay E, Sieber O, Sadat A, Bisgaard ML, Hodgson SV, Aaltonen LA, Thomas HJ, Tomlinson IP (2003) Carcinogenesis in MYH-associated polyposis follows a distinct genetic pathway. Cancer Res 63:7595–7599.

Loftus EV, Jr. (2006) Epidemiology and risk factors for colorectal dysplasia and cancer in ulcerative colitis. Gastroenterol Clin North Am 35:517–531.

Losi L, Ponz de Leon M, Jiricny J, Di Gregorio C, Benatti P, Percesepe A, Fante R, Roncucci L, Pedroni M, Benhatter J (1997) K-ras and p53 mutations in hereditary non-polyposis colorectal cancers. Int J Cancer 74(1):94–96.

Lund AH and van Lohuizen M (2004) Epigenetics and cancer. Genes Dev 18:2315–2335.

Lynch JP and Hoops TC (2002) The genetic pathogenesis of colorectal cancer. Hematol Oncol Clin North Am 16:1–36.

Lynch JP and Lichtenstein GR (2004) Cyclooxygenase Activity in Gastrointestinal Cancer Development and Progression – Prospects as a Therapeutic Target. In: Morgan D, Fossman U, Nakaqda M (eds) Cancer and Inflammation. Birkhauser Verlag Basel, Basel, pp. 147–176.

Lynch JP and Rustgi AK (2005) Mechanisms of GI Malignancies. In: Johnson LR, Barret KE, Gishan FK, Merchant JL, Said HM, Wood JD (eds) Physiology of the Gastrointestinal Tract, Fourth edn. Elsevier, San Diego, CA, pp. 477–498.

Machado JC, Figueiredo C, Canedo P, Pharoah P, Carvalho R, Nabais S, Castro Alves C, Campos ML, Van Doorn LJ, Caldas C, Seruca R, Carneiro F, Sobrinho-Simoes M (2003) A proinflammatory genetic profile increases the risk for chronic atrophic gastritis and gastric carcinoma. Gastroenterology 125:364–371.

Malfertheiner P, Megraud F, O'Morain C, Bazzoli F, El-Omar E, Graham D, Hunt R, Rokkas T, Vakil N, Kuipers EJ (2007) Current concepts in the management of Helicobacter pylori infection: the Maastricht III Consensus Report. Gut 56:772–781.

Marshall BJ (1995) *Helicobacter pylori*: the etiologic agent for peptic ulcer. JAMA 274: 1064–1066.

Marshall BJ and Warren JR (1984) Unidentified curved bacilli in the stomach of patients with gastritis and peptic ulceration. Lancet 1:1311–1315.

Meek DW (2004) The p53 response to DNA damage. DNA Repair (Amst) 3:1049–1056.

Mihara M, Yoshida Y, Tsukamoto T, Inada K, Nakanishi Y, Yagi Y, Imai K, Sugimura T, Tatematsu M, Ushijima T (2006) Methylation of multiple genes in gastric glands with intestinal metaplasia: A disorder with polyclonal origins. Am J Pathol 169:1643–1651.

Miyaki M, Iijima T, Kimura J, Yasuno M, Mori T, Hayashi Y, Koike M, Shitara N, Iwama T, Kuroki T (1999) Frequent mutation of beta-catenin and APC genes in primary colorectal tumors from patients with hereditary nonpolyposis colorectal cancer. Cancer Res 59:4506–4509.

Mocellin S, Wang E, Marincola FM (2001) Cytokines and immune response in the tumor microenvironment. J Immunother 24:392–407.

Mocellin S, Rossi CR, Pilati P, Nitti D (2005) Tumor necrosis factor, cancer and anticancer therapy. Cytokine Growth Factor Rev 16:35–53.

Moss SF, Calam J, Agarwal B, Wang S, Holt PR (1996) Induction of gastric epithelial apoptosis by Helicobacter pylori. Gut 38:498–501.

Motoyama N and Naka K (2004) DNA damage tumor suppressor genes and genomic instability. Curr Opin Genet Dev 14:11–16.

Muller A, Homey B, Soto H, Ge N, Catron D, Buchanan ME, McClanahan T, Murphy E, Yuan W, Wagner SN, Barrera JL, Mohar A, Verastegui E, Zlotnik A (2001) Involvement of chemokine receptors in breast cancer metastasis. Nature 410:50–56.

Murakami T, Cardones AR, Hwang ST (2004) Chemokine receptors and melanoma metastasis. J Dermatol Sci 36:71–78.

Myeroff LL, Parsons R, Kim SJ, Hedrick L, Cho KR, Orth K, Mathis M, Kinzler KW, Lutterbaugh J, Park K, Bang Y-J, Lee HY, Park J-G, Lynch HT, Roberts AB, Vogeistein B, and Markowitz SD (1995) A transforming growth factor beta receptor type II gene mutation common in colon and gastric but rare in endometrial cancers with microsatellite instability. Cancer Res 55: 5545–5547.

Nagy R, Sweet K, Eng C (2004) Highly penetrant hereditary cancer syndromes. Oncogene 23:6445–6470.

Nakatsuru S, Yanagisawa A, Furukawa Y, Ichii S, Kato Y, Nakamura Y, Horii A (1993) Somatic mutations of the APC gene in precancerous lesion of the stomach. Hum Mol Genet 2: 1463–1465.

Nam JH and Murthy S (2004) Chronic inflammation and cancer in various organ systems. In: Cancer and Inflammation. Birkhauser Verlag Basel, Basel

Nie Y, Liao J, Zhao X, Song Y, Yang GY, Wang LD, Yang CS (2002) Detection of multiple gene hypermethylation in the development of esophageal squamous cell carcinoma. Carcinogenesis 23:1713–1720.

Nomura A, Stemmermann GN, Chyou PH, Kato I, Perez GI, Blaser MJ (1991) Helicobacter pylori infection and gastric carcinoma among Japanese Americans in Hawaii. N Engl J Med 325:1132–1136.

Ohnishi N, Yuasa H, Tanaka S, Sawa H, Miura M, Matsui A, Higashi H, Musashi M, Iwabuchi K, Suzuki M, Yamada G, Azuma T, Hatakeyama M (2008) Transgenic expression of Helicobacter pylori CagA induces gastrointestinal and hematopoietic neoplasms in mouse. Proc Natl Acad Sci U S A 105:1003–1008.

Ormandy CJ, Musgrove EA, Hui R, Daly RJ, Sutherland RL (2003) Cyclin D1, EMS1 and 11q13 amplification in breast cancer. Breast Cancer Res Treat 78:323–335.

Osborne J, Moore PS, Chang Y (1999) KSHV-encoded viral IL-6 activates multiple human IL-6 signaling pathways. Hum Immunol 60:921–927.

Ottini L, Palli D, Falchetti M, D'Amico C, Amorosi A, Saieva C, Calzolari A, Cimoli F, Tatarelli C, De Marchis L, Masala G, Mariani-Costantini R, Cama A (1997) Microsatellite instability in gastric cancer is associated with tumor location and family history in a high-risk population from Tuscany. Cancer Res 57:4523–4529.

Oue N, Matsumura S, Nakayama H, Kitadai Y, Taniyama K, Matsusaki K, Yasui W (2003) Reduced expression of the TSP1 gene and its association with promoter hypermethylation in gastric carcinoma. Oncology 64:423–429.

Pai R, Soreghan B, Szabo IL, Pavelka M, Baatar D, Tarnawski AS (2002) Prostaglandin E2 transactivates EGF receptor: a novel mechanism for promoting colon cancer growth and gastrointestinal hypertrophy. Nat Med 8:289–293.

Palli D, Caporaso NE, Shiao YH, Saieva C, Amorosi A, Masala G, Rice JM, Fraumeni JF, Jr. (1997) Diet, Helicobacter pylori, and p53 mutations in gastric cancer: a molecular epidemiology study in Italy. Cancer Epidemiol Biomarkers Prev 6:1065–1069.

Park TJ, Han SU, Cho YK, Paik WK, Kim YB, Lim IK (2001) Methylation of O(6)-methylguanine-DNA methyltransferase gene is associated significantly with K-ras mutation, lymph node invasion, tumor staging, and disease free survival in patients with gastric carcinoma. Cancer 92:2760–2768.

Parsonnet J, Friedman GD, Vandersteen DP, Chang Y, Vogelman JH, Orentreich N, Sibley RK (1991b) Helicobacter pylori infection and the risk of gastric carcinoma. N Engl J Med 325:1127–1131.

Parsonnet J, Vandersteen D, Goates J, Sibley RK, Pritikin J, Chang Y (1991b) Helicobacter pylori infection in intestinal- and diffuse-type gastric adenocarcinomas. J Natl Cancer Inst 83: 640–643.

Parsonnet J, Hansen S, Rodriguez L, Gelb AB, Warnke RA, Jellum E, Orentreich N, Vogelman JH, Friedman GD (1994) Helicobacter pylori infection and gastric lymphoma. N Engl J Med 330:1267–1271.

Parsons R, Myeroff LL, Liu B, Willson JK, Markowitz SD, Kinzler KW, Vogelstein B (1995) Microsatellite instability and mutations of the transforming growth factor beta type II receptor gene in colorectal cancer. Cancer Res 55:5548–5550.

Peek RM, Jr., Moss SF, Tham KT, Perez-Perez GI, Wang S, Miller GG, Atherton JC, Holt PR, Blaser MJ (1997) Helicobacter pylori cagA+ strains and dissociation of gastric epithelial cell proliferation from apoptosis [see comments]. J Natl Cancer Inst 89:863–868.

Peltomaki P (2001) Deficient DNA mismatch repair: a common etiologic factor for colon cancer. Hum Mol Genet 10:735–740.

Petronzelli F, Riccio A, Markham GD, Seeholzer SH, Stoerker J, Genuardi M, Yeung AT, Matsumoto Y, Bellacosa A (2000) Biphasic kinetics of the human DNA repair protein MED1 (MBD4), a mismatch-specific DNA N-glycosylase. J Biol Chem 275:32422–32429.

Phillips RK, Wallace MH, Lynch PM, Hawk E, Gordon GB, Saunders BP, Wakabayashi N, Shen Y, Zimmerman S, Godio L, Rodrigues-Bigas M, Su LK, Sherman J, Kelloff G, Levin B, Steinbach G (2002) A randomised, double blind, placebo controlled study of celecoxib, a selective cyclooxygenase 2 inhibitor, on duodenal polyposis in familial adenomatous polyposis. Gut 50:857–860.

Pidgeon GP, Lysaght J, Krishnamoorthy S, Reynolds JV, O'Byrne K, Nie D, Honn KV (2007) Lipoxygenase metabolism: roles in tumor progression and survival. Cancer Metastasis Rev 26:503–524.

Plentz RR, Wiemann SU, Flemming P, Meier PN, Kubicka S, Kreipe H, Manns MP, Rudolph KL (2003) Telomere shortening of epithelial cells characterises the adenoma-carcinoma transition of human colorectal cancer. Gut 52:1304–1307.

Plummer SM, Hall M, Faux SP (1995) Oxidation and genotoxicity of fecapentaene-12 are potentiated by prostaglandin H synthase. Carcinogenesis 16:1023–1028.

Prescott SM and White RL (1996) Self-promotion? Intimate connections between APC and prostaglandin H synthase-2. Cell 87:783–786.

Qian X, Huang C, Cho CH, Hui WM, Rashid A, Chan AO (2008) E-cadherin promoter hypermethylation induced by interleukin-1beta treatment or H. pylori infection in human gastric cancer cell lines. Cancer Lett 263:107–113.

Rampino N, Yamamoto H, Ionov Y, Li Y, Sawai H, Reed JC, Perucho M (1997) Somatic frameshift mutations in the BAX gene in colon cancers of the microsatellite mutator phenotype. Science 275:967–969.

Recavarren-Arce S, Leon-Barua R, Cok J, Berendson R, Gilman RH, Ramirez-Ramos A, Rodriguez C, Spira WM (1991) Helicobacter pylori and progressive gastric pathology that predisposes to gastric cancer. Scand J Gastroenterol Suppl 181:51–57.

Redston MS, Papadopoulos N, Caldas C, Kinzler KW, Kern SE (1995) Common occurrence of APC and K-ras gene mutations in the spectrum of colitis-associated neoplasias. Gastroenterology 108:383–392.

Riccio A, Aaltonen LA, Godwin AK, Loukola A, Percesepe A, Salovaara R, Masciullo V, Genuardi M, Paravatou-Petsotas M, Bassi DE, Ruggeri BA, Klein-Szanto AJ, Testa JR, Neri G, Bellacosa A (1999) The DNA repair gene MBD4 (MED1) is mutated in human carcinomas with microsatellite instability. Nat Genet 23:266–268.

Robinson K, Argent RH, Atherton JC (2007) The inflammatory and immune response to Helicobacter pylori infection. Best Pract Res Clin Gastroenterol 21:237–259.

Rose-John S, Scheller J, Elson G, Jones SA (2006) Interleukin-6 biology is coordinated by membrane-bound and soluble receptors: role in inflammation and cancer. J Leukoc Biol 80:227–236.

Rutter M, Saunders B, Wilkinson K, Rumbles S, Schofield G, Kamm M, Williams C, Price A, Talbot I, Forbes A (2004a) Severity of inflammation is a risk factor for colorectal neoplasia in ulcerative colitis. Gastroenterology 126:451–459.

Rutter MD, Saunders BP, Wilkinson KH, Rumbles S, Schofield G, Kamm MA, Williams CB, Price AB, Talbot IC, Forbes A (2004b) Cancer surveillance in longstanding ulcerative colitis: endoscopic appearances help predict cancer risk. Gut 53:1813–1816.

Samowitz WS, Holden JA, Curtin K, Edwards SL, Walker AR, Lin HA, Robertson MA, Nichols MF, Gruenthal KM, Lynch BJ, Leppert MF, Slattery ML (2001) Inverse relationship between microsatellite instability and K-ras and p53 gene alterations in colon cancer. Am J Pathol 158(4):1517–1524.

Sampson JR, Dolwani S, Jones S, Eccles D, Ellis A, Evans DG, Frayling I, Jordan S, Maher ER, Mak T, Maynard J, Pigatto F, Shaw J, Cheadle JP (2003) Autosomal recessive colorectal adenomatous polyposis due to inherited mutations of MYH. Lancet 362:39–41.

Sancar A, Lindsey-Boltz LA, Unsal-Kacmaz K, Linn S (2004) Molecular mechanisms of mammalian DNA repair and the DNA damage checkpoints. Annu Rev Biochem 73:39–85.

Scotton CJ, Wilson JL, Milliken D, Stamp G, Balkwill FR (2001) Epithelial cancer cell migration: a role for chemokine receptors? Cancer Res 61:4961–4965.

Scotton CJ, Wilson JL, Scott K, Stamp G, Wilbanks GD, Fricker S, Bridger G, Balkwill FR (2002) Multiple actions of the chemokine CXCL12 on epithelial tumor cells in human ovarian cancer. Cancer Res 62:5930–5938.

Semba S, Yokozaki H, Yamamoto S, Yasui W, Tahara E (1996) Microsatellite instability in precancerous lesions and adenocarcinomas of the stomach. Cancer 77:1620–1627.

Sepulveda AR and Graham DY (2002) Role of Helicobacter pylori in gastric carcinogenesis. Gastroenterol Clin North Am 31:517–535, x.

Sepulveda AR, Santos AC, Yamaoka Y, Wu L, Gutierrez O, Kim JG, Graham DY (1999) Marked differences in the frequency of microsatellite instability in gastric cancer from different countries. Am J Gastroenterol 94:3034–3038.

Sepulveda AR, Wu L, Ota H, Gutierrez O, Kim JG, Genta RM, Graham DY (2000) Molecular identification of main cellular lineages as a tool for the classification of gastric cancer. Hum Pathol 31:566–574.

Sepulveda A, Peterson LE, Shelton J, Gutierrez O, Graham DY (2002) Histological patterns of gastritis in H. pylori-infected individuals with a family history of gastric cancer. Am J Gastroenterol 97:1365–1370.

Sharpless NE and DePinho RA (2004) Telomeres, stem cells, senescence, and cancer. J Clin Invest 113:160–168.

Shiao YH, Rugge M, Correa P, Lehmann HP, Scheer WD (1994) p53 alteration in gastric precancerous lesions. Am J Pathol 144:511–517.

Shibata Y, Haruki N, Kuwabara Y, Ishiguro H, Shinoda N, Sato A, Kimura M, Koyama H, Toyama T, Nishiwaki T, Kudo J, Terashita Y, Konishi S, Sugiura H, Fujii Y (2002) Chfr expression is downregulated by CpG island hypermethylation in esophageal cancer. Carcinogenesis 23:1695–1699.

Shimada T, Watanabe N, Hiraishi H, Terano A (1999) Redox regulation of interleukin-8 expression in MKN28 cells. Dig Dis Sci 44:266–273.

Shinmura K, Tani M, Isogaki J, Wang Y, Sugimura H, Yokota J (1998) RER phenotype and its associated mutations in familial gastric cancer. Carcinogenesis 19:247–251.

Shirin H, Sordillo EM, Kolevska TK, Hibshoosh H, Kawabata Y, Oh SH, Kuebler JF, Delohery T, Weghorst CM, Weinstein IB, Moss SF (2000) Chronic helicobacter pylori infection induces an apoptosis-resistant phenotype associated with decreased expression of p27(kip1). Infect Immun 68:5321–5328.

Sieber OM, Lipton L, Crabtree M, Heinimann K, Fidalgo P, Phillips RK, Bisgaard ML, Orntoft TF, Aaltonen LA, Hodgson SV, Thomas HJ, Tomlinson IP (2003) Multiple colorectal adenomas, classic adenomatous polyposis, and germ-line mutations in MYH. N Engl J Med 348:791–799.

Sipponen P and Marshall BJ (2000) Gastritis and gastric cancer. Western countries. Gastroenterol Clin North Am 29:579–592, v–vi.

Sossenheimer MJ, Aston CE, Preston RA, Gates LK, Jr., Ulrich CD, Martin SP, Zhang Y, Gorry MC, Ehrlich GD, Whitcomb DC (1997) Clinical characteristics of hereditary pancreatitis in a large family, based on high-risk haplotype. The Midwest Multicenter Pancreatic Study Group (MMPSG). Am J Gastroenterol 92:1113–1116.

Souza RF, Appel R, Yin J, Wang S, Smolinski KN, Abraham JM, Zou TT, Shi YQ, Lei J, Cottrell J, Cymes K, Biden K, Simms L, Leggett B, Lynch PM, Frazier M, Powell SM, Harpaz N, Sugimura H, Young J, Meltzer SJ (1996) Microsatellite instability in the insulin-like growth factor II receptor gene in gastrointestinal tumours. Nat Genet 14:255–257.

Stenson WF (1995) Inflammatory Bowel Disease. In: Yamada T (ed) Textbook of Gastroenterology, Second edn. J.B. Lippincott Company, Philadelphia, pp. 1748–1805.

Stenson WF (2007) Prostaglandins and epithelial response to injury. Curr Opin Gastroenterol 23:107–110.

Strathdee G (2002) Epigenetic versus genetic alterations in the inactivation of E-cadherin. Semin Cancer Biol 12:373–379.

Strickler JG, Zheng J, Shu Q, Burgart LJ, Alberts SR, Shibata D (1994) p53 mutations and microsatellite instability in sporadic gastric cancer: when guardians fail. Cancer Res 54: 4750–4755.

Sunpaweravong P, Sunpaweravong S, Puttawibul P, Mitarnun W, Zeng C, Baron AE, Franklin W, Said S, Varella-Garcia M (2005) Epidermal growth factor receptor and cyclin D1 are independently amplified and overexpressed in esophageal squamous cell carcinoma. J Cancer Res Clin Oncol 131:111–119.

Suzuki H, Watkins DN, Jair KW, Schuebel KE, Markowitz SD, Dong Chen W, Pretlow TP, Yang B, Akiyama Y, Van Engeland M, Toyota M, Tokino T, Hinoda Y, Imai K, Herman JG, Baylin SB (2004) Epigenetic inactivation of SFRP genes allows constitutive WNT signaling in colorectal cancer. Nat Genet 36:417–422.

Suzuki N, Yasui M, Geacintov NE, Shafirovich V, Shibutani S (2005) Miscoding events during DNA synthesis past the nitration-damaged base 8-nitroguanine. Biochemistry 44:9238–9245.

Teich N, Rosendahl J, Toth M, Mossner J, Sahin-Toth M (2006) Mutations of human cationic trypsinogen (PRSS1) and chronic pancreatitis. Hum Mutat 27:721–730.

Thibodeau SN, Bren G, Schaid D (1993) Microsatellite instability in cancer of the proximal colon. Science 260:816–819.

To KF, Leung WK, Lee TL, Yu J, Tong JH, Chan MW, Ng EK, Chung SC, Sung JJ (2002) Promoter hypermethylation of tumor-related genes in gastric intestinal metaplasia of patients with and without gastric cancer. Int J Cancer 102:623–628.

Tomlinson I, Ilyas M, Johnson V, Davies A, Clark G, Talbot I, Bodmer W (1998) A comparison of the genetic pathways involved in the pathogenesis of three types of colorectal cancer. J Pathol 184:148–152.

Torres VJ, VanCompernolle SE, Sundrud MS, Unutmaz D, Cover TL (2007) Helicobacter pylori vacuolating cytotoxin inhibits activation-induced proliferation of human T and B lymphocyte subsets. J Immunol 179:5433–5440.

Toyota M, Ahuja N, Suzuki H, Itoh F, Ohe-Toyota M, Imai K, Baylin SB, Issa JP (1999) Aberrant methylation in gastric cancer associated with the CpG island methylator phenotype. Cancer Res 59:5438–5442.

Toyota M, Sasaki Y, Satoh A, Ogi K, Kikuchi T, Suzuki H, Mita H, Tanaka N, Itoh F, Issa JP, Jair KW, Schuebel KE, Imai K, Tokino T (2003) Epigenetic inactivation of CHFR in human tumors. Proc Natl Acad Sci U S A 100:7818–7823.

Ueki T, Toyota M, Sohn T, Yeo CJ, Issa JP, Hruban RH, Goggins M (2000) Hypermethylation of multiple genes in pancreatic adenocarcinoma. Cancer Res 60:1835–1839.

Ulrich CM, Bigler J, Potter JD (2006) Non-steroidal anti-inflammatory drugs for cancer prevention: promise, perils and pharmacogenetics. Nat Rev Cancer 6:130–140.

Umar A, Boland CR, Terdiman JP, Syngal S, de la Chapelle A, Ruschoff J, Fishel R, Lindor NM, Burgart LJ, Hamelin R, Hamilton SR, Hiatt RA, Jass J, Lindblom A, Lynch HT, Peltomaki P, Ramsey SD, Rodriguez-Bigas MA, Vasen HF, Hawk ET, Barrett JC, Freedman AN, Srivastava S (2004) Revised Bethesda Guidelines for hereditary nonpolyposis colorectal cancer (Lynch syndrome) and microsatellite instability. J Natl Cancer Inst 96:261–268.

Valko M, Morris H, Cronin MT (2005) Metals, toxicity and oxidative stress. Curr Med Chem 12:1161–1208.

Valko M, Rhodes CJ, Moncol J, Izakovic M, Mazur M (2006) Free radicals, metals and antioxidants in oxidative stress-induced cancer. Chem Biol Interact 160:1–40.

Valko M, Leibfritz D, Moncol J, Cronin MT, Mazur M, Telser J (2007) Free radicals and antioxidants in normal physiological functions and human disease. Int J Biochem Cell Biol 39:44–84.

Vasen HF, Watson P, Mecklin JP, Lynch HT (1999) New clinical criteria for hereditary nonpolyposis colorectal cancer (HNPCC, Lynch syndrome) proposed by the International Collaborative group on HNPCC. Gastroenterology 116:1453–1456.

Veigl ML, Kasturi L, Olechnowicz J, Ma AH, Lutterbaugh JD, Periyasamy S, Li GM, Drummond J, Modrich PL, Sedwick WD, Markowitz SD (1998) Biallelic inactivation of hMLH1 by epigenetic gene silencing, a novel mechanism causing human MSI cancers. Proc Natl Acad Sci U S A 95:8698–8702.

Verhulst ML, van Oijen AH, Roelofs HM, Peters WH, Jansen JB (2000) Antral glutathione concentration and glutathione S-transferase activity in patients with and without Helicobacter pylori. Dig Dis Sci 45:629–632.

Vivanco I and Sawyers CL (2002) The phosphatidylinositol 3-Kinase AKT pathway in human cancer. Nat Rev Cancer 2:489–501.

Waki T, Tamura G, Sato M, Terashima M, Nishizuka S, Motoyama T (2003) Promoter methylation status of DAP-kinase and RUNX3 genes in neoplastic and non-neoplastic gastric epithelia. Cancer Sci 94:360–364.

Walsh CP, Chaillet JR, Bestor TH (1998) Transcription of IAP endogenous retroviruses is constrained by cytosine methylation. Nat Genet 20:116–117.

Wang MT, Honn KV, Nie D (2007) Cyclooxygenases, prostanoids, and tumor progression. Cancer Metastasis Rev 26:525–534.

Warren JR and Marshall B (1983) Unidentified curved bacilli on gastric epithelium in active chronic gastritis. Lancet 1:1273–1275.

Wendum D, Masliah J, Trugnan G, Flejou JF (2004) Cyclooxygenase-2 and its role in colorectal cancer development. Virchows Arch 445:327–333.

Whitcomb DC and Pogue-Geile K (2002) Pancreatitis as a risk for pancreatic cancer. Gastroenterol Clin North Am 31:663–678.

Whitcomb DC, Gorry MC, Preston RA, Furey W, Sossenheimer MJ, Ulrich CD, Martin SP, Gates LK, Jr., Amann ST, Toskes PP, Liddle R, McGrath K, Uomo G, Post JC, Ehrlich GD (1996) Hereditary pancreatitis is caused by a mutation in the cationic trypsinogen gene. Nat Genet 14:141–145.

White ES, Strieter RM, Arenberg DA (2002) Chemokines as therapeutic targets in non-small cell lung cancer. Curr Med Chem Anti-Canc Agents 2:403–417.

Wilson KT and Crabtree JE (2007) Immunology of Helicobacter pylori: insights into the failure of the immune response and perspectives on vaccine studies. Gastroenterology 133:288–308.

Wong BC, Lam SK, Wong WM, Chen JS, Zheng TT, Feng RE, Lai KC, Hu WH, Yuen ST, Leung SY, Fong DY, Ho J, Ching CK (2004) Helicobacter pylori eradication to prevent gastric cancer in a high-risk region of China: a randomized controlled trial. JAMA 291:187–194.

Wotherspoon AC, Ortiz-Hidalgo C, Falzon MR, Isaacson PG (1991) Helicobacter pylori-associated gastritis and primary B-cell gastric lymphoma. Lancet 338:1175–1176.

Wotherspoon AC, Doglioni C, Diss TC, Pan L, Moschini A, de Boni M, Isaacson PG (1993) Regression of primary low-grade B-cell gastric lymphoma of mucosa-associated lymphoid tissue type after eradication of Helicobacter pylori. Lancet 342:575–577.

Wu MS, Lee CW, Shun CT, Wang HP, Lee WJ, Sheu JC, Lin JT (1998) Clinicopathological significance of altered loci of replication error and microsatellite instability-associated mutations in gastric cancer. Cancer Res 58:1494–1497.

Wu MS, Lee CW, Shun CT, Wang HP, Lee WJ, Chang MC, Sheu JC, Lin JT (2000) Distinct clinicopathologic and genetic profiles in sporadic gastric cancer with different mutator phenotypes. Genes Chromosomes Cancer 27:403–411.

Xu XL, Yu J, Zhang HY, Sun MH, Gu J, Du X, Shi DR, Wang P, Yang ZH, Zhu JD (2004) Methylation profile of the promoter CpG islands of 31 genes that may contribute to colorectal carcinogenesis. World J Gastroenterol 10:3441–3454.

Yagi OK, Akiyama Y, Nomizu T, Iwama T, Endo M, Yuasa Y (1998) Proapoptotic gene BAX is frequently mutated in hereditary nonpolyposis colorectal cancers but not in adenomas. Gastroenterology 114:268–274.

Yamamoto H, Sawai H, Perucho M (1997) Frameshift somatic mutations in gastrointestinal cancer of the microsatellite mutator phenotype. Cancer Res 57:4420–4426.

Yamaoka Y, Kodama T, Kashima K, Graham DY, Sepulveda AR (1998) Variants of the 3′ region of the cagA gene in Helicobacter pylori isolates from patients with different H. pylori-associated diseases. J Clin Microbiol 36:2258–2263.

Yang B, House MG, Guo M, Herman JG, Clark DP (2005) Promoter methylation profiles of tumor suppressor genes in intrahepatic and extrahepatic cholangiocarcinoma. Mod Pathol 18(3):412–420.

Yang L and Carbone DP (2004) Tumor-host immune interactions and dendritic cell dysfunction. Adv Cancer Res 92:13–27.

Yao Y, Tao H, Park DI, Sepulveda JL, Sepulveda AR (2006) Demonstration and characterization of mutations induced by Helicobacter pylori organisms in gastric epithelial cells. Helicobacter 11:272–286.

Yermilov V, Rubio J, Becchi M, Friesen MD, Pignatelli B, Ohshima H (1995) Formation of 8-nitroguanine by the reaction of guanine with peroxynitrite in vitro. Carcinogenesis 16:2045–2050.

Yin J, Harpaz N, Tong Y, Huang Y, Laurin J, Greenwald BD, Hontanosas M, Newkirk C, Meltzer SJ (1993) p53 point mutations in dysplastic and cancerous ulcerative colitis lesions. Gastroenterology 104:1633–1639.

Yoder JA, Walsh CP, Bestor TH (1997) Cytosine methylation and the ecology of intragenomic parasites. Trends Genet 13:335–340.

Yoshitaka T, Matsubara N, Ikeda M, Tanino M, Hanafusa H, Tanaka N, Shimizu K (1996) Mutations of E2F-4 trinucleotide repeats in colorectal cancer with microsatellite instability. Biochem Biophys Res Commun 227:553–557.

Chapter 17
Immunoglobulin Gene Rearrangements, Oncogenic Translocations, B-Cell Receptor Signaling, and B Lymphomagenesis

Murali Gururajan and Subbarao Bondada

Cast of Characters

Reciprocal chromosomal translocations involving one of the immunoglobulin (Ig) loci and a proto-oncogene are a hallmark of many types of B-cell lymphoma (Vanasse et al. 1999). As a consequence of such translocations, the oncogene comes under the control of the active Ig locus, causing a deregulated, constitutive expression of the oncogene. Examples of such translocations include Bcl-2-IgH translocation associated with follicular lymphoma, Bcl-6-IgH associated with diffuse large B-cell lymphoma, c-Myc translocation associated with Burkitt's lymphoma, and Pax-5 translocation associated with marginal zone and large cell lymphomas. Dysregulated expression of oncogenes often affects lymphoma growth by altering the expression of key genes that lie downstream of BCR – for example, the ability of Pax-5 to promote lymphomagenesis correlated with expression of components of BCR signaling pathway, including upregulation of Igα and CD19 antigens and downregulation of BCR-negative regulators, such as CD22 and PIR-B (Cozma et al. 2007). Despite translocations involving Ig locus, majority of the B-cell lymphomas retain functional B-cell receptor (Kuppers and Dalla-Favera 2001; Kuppers 2005) and disruption of the B-cell receptor expression inhibited their growth (Gururajan et al. 2006). In addition, somatic hypermutation, a process involving random mutations in the Ig variable regions, unique to B cells, generates B-cell receptors of higher affinity even as lymphoma cells continue to divide. The mutated BCRs seem to retain their function as evidenced by hyperactive signaling molecules downstream of the BCR, including constitutive phosphorylation of several key tyrosine kinases and MAP kinases (Gururajan et al. 2005, 2006, 2007). The importance of BCR signaling in B-cell lymphomas in the context of IgH translocations is described below.

S. Bondada (✉)
Department of Microbiology, Immunology and Molecular Genetics, Markey Cancer Center, University of Kentucky, 800 Rose St., Lexington, KY, USA
e-mail: bondada@email.uky.edu

A. Thomas-Tikhonenko (ed.), *Cancer Genome and Tumor Microenvironment*,
DOI 10.1007/978-1-4419-0711-0_17, © Springer Science+Business Media, LLC 2010

Introduction

B lymphocytes are critical components of humoral immunity, and T lymphocytes are essential for cell-mediated immunity. Upon encountering an antigen, B cells proliferate and differentiate into plasma cells, which secrete antibodies. The function of antibodies is to neutralize the antigen and clear the infection. B cells originate from the bone marrow and migrate to secondary lymphoid organs such as spleen and lymph nodes where they complete their maturation. Mature B cells reside in the follicles and are the major players in humoral immunity. B cell recognizes the antigen through its surface B-cell receptor (BCR), which is a membrane-bound form of IgM or IgD for naïve B cells and may be of other isotypes for memory B cells. Signaling through the B-cell receptor is critical for B cells to differentiate into fully mature cells and also to become plasma cells. Several transcription factors regulate B-cell development in the bone marrow, and some of them act downstream of BCR (Singh et al. 2005b). Some of these transcription factors (PU.1, Ikaros, E2A, EBF, Pax-5, Bcl-11) determine commitment of bone marrow stem cells to the B-cell lineage. By knocking out specific transcription factors in mouse models, the molecular circuitry responsible for B-cell development has been defined (Smith and Sigvardsson 2004; Singh et al. 2005b). In addition to their role in B-cell maturation, transcription factors (BLIMP-1, XBP-1) also regulate B-cell differentiation into plasma cells (Calame 2001). These studies on transcription factors are important as they enable us to understand the ontogeny of B cells, a leading arm of the humoral immune response in the context of an infection. In addition to combating the infection, dysregulation of normal B cells due to alterations in B-cell subsets, transcription factors, apoptosis, and signaling pathways also contributes to the pathological condition called "autoimmunity" (Mandik-Nayak et al. 1999; Hardy et al. 2000; Peng 2007). Thus, B cells represent two edges of the sword: a normal B cell producing antibodies to counteract the infection and an abnormal B cell producing pathological antibodies that destroy body's own cells (breakdown of tolerance).

In contrast to normal B cells, which are in a resting state, B lymphomas are composed of transformed B cells. The mechanisms underlying B-lymphoma development (termed lymphomagenesis) are not fully understood. The most common mechanism that promotes normal B-cell transformation into a cancer cell is the chromosomal translocation of specific oncogenes (often transcription factors) next to the immunoglobulin gene loci (Kuppers et al. 1999; Kuppers 2005). However, mouse models developed to mimic the disease process by incorporating oncogenes into these hotspots fail to fully recapitulate human disease (Kuppers et al. 1999; Kuppers 2005). Either this is due to a poorly understood delay in tumor formation or the oncogene is not sufficient to drive the process. These findings suggest that some other signals may be required in addition to dysregulated expression of specific oncogenes.

B lymphomas comprise the fifth most common cancer types in the world. It is estimated that approximately 95% of the lymphomas are of B-cell type and are classified depending upon their stage of differentiation (Kuppers 2005). The current

World Health Organization lymphoma classification and the Revised European–American Lymphoma classification list 15 types of B lymphomas (Kuppers 2005). The different types of lymphomas have implications in terms of pathogenesis, treatment, and outcome.

The cellular origin of human B-cell lymphomas and the identification of key transforming events including chromosomal translocations in lymphoma pathogenesis is becoming increasingly known (Kuppers et al. 1999). However, it is clear that B-cell lymphomas are not as autonomous as previously thought – key factors that are critical for normal B-cell survival, proliferation, and differentiation are also required for the B-lymphoma pathogenesis (Kuppers 2005). The cell types that give rise to B-cell lymphomas, the transforming events, the role of antigen, and the microenvironment in the B-lymphoma pathogenesis will be addressed in detail in this chapter.

B-cell Development and B Lymphomagenesis

B-cell development occurs as distinct steps in the bone marrow and concludes when a B-cell precursor successfully rearranges immunoglobulin (Ig) heavy- and light-chain genes expressing a functional surface antigen receptor. Cells that express a functional BCR differentiate into immature naïve B cells and leave the bone marrow, after undergoing negative selection to remove self-reactive B cells, whereas B-cell precursors that fail to express a BCR undergo apoptosis (Reth et al. 1991; Flaswinkel and Reth 1994; Rajewsky 1996; Torres et al. 1996; Smith and Reth 2004). BCR cross-linking leads to activation of protein tyrosine kinases (PTKs), the Src family kinase (SFK) Lyn, the Syk kinase, and the Tec-family kinase Btk (Bruton's tyrosine kinase). The upstream activated Src and non-Src family kinases in turn activate downstream kinases including ERK, JNK, p38, PI-3K, Akt, PLC-γ, and others (Niiro and Clark 2002). Many of these intermediate targets regulate several downstream transcription factors including NF-κB, AP-1, and Egr-1. The recognition of antigen by BCR leads to B-cell activation, and in the presence of additional signals (T-helper cell-derived cytokines) leads to B-cell proliferation and differentiation into antibody-secreting plasma cells.

Reciprocal chromosomal translocations involving one of the immunoglobulin loci and a proto-oncogene are a hallmark of many types of B-cell lymphoma (Vanasse et al. 1999). As a consequence of such translocations, the oncogene comes under the control of the active Ig locus, causing a deregulated, constitutive expression of the oncogene. Examples of such translocations include Bcl-2-IgH translocation associated with follicular lymphoma, Bcl-6-IgH associated with diffuse large B-cell lymphoma, and c-Myc translocation associated with Burkitt's lymphoma (Kuppers et al. 1999; Janz 2006).

The causes for the DNA strand breaks in the oncogenes involved in translocation are not well understood. Defects in the repair of DNA strand breaks may have a role in the translocation of oncogenes (Beecham et al. 1994). The process of class switch recombination and somatic hypermutation contribute to lymphoma pathogenesis not only by causing chromosomal translocations but probably also by targeting non-Ig genes (Vanasse et al. 1999). Translocations and exon 1 mutations of Bcl-6 are found in 50% of DLBCL cases (Cattoretti et al. 2005). Such mutations might promote the development of lymphomas by disrupting the negative autoregulatory circuit that normally controls Bcl-6 expression (Wang et al. 2002; Pasqualucci et al. 2003). Mutations of the Bcl-6 proto-oncogene disrupt its negative autoregulation in diffuse large B-cell lymphoma (Pasqualucci et al. 2003). This possibility was supported by the finding that the chromosomal breakpoints are frequently found at the sites that are hypermutated (Cattoretti et al. 2005). Activation-induced cytidine deaminase (AID), an enzyme essential for class switch recombination and somatic mutation, enhances B-cell lymphomagenesis in Eμ-myc transgenic mice and is required for Bcl-6-dependent lymphoma development, strongly supporting the notion that DNA strand breaks initiated during CSR and SHM may facilitate oncogene transloca- tions (Cattoretti et al. 2005; Pasqualucci et al. 2006; Kotani et al. 2007; Pasqualucci et al. 2008).

Role of the BCR in Normal B-Cell Development and B-Cell Lymphomas

BCR-Induced Normal B-Cell Survival

B cells undergo selection process in the bone marrow and spleen to express a func- tional B-cell receptor (Kitamura et al. 1991; Rajewsky 1992; Ehlich et al. 1993). Pre-B cells express a functional pre-BCR consisting of μ-heavy chain and a surro- gate light chain, which is replaced by kappa or lambda light chains in the immature B cells. Membrane-bound BCR on pre-B, immature and mature B cells, is asso- ciated with two co-receptors, Ig-α and Ig-β. These co-receptors are expressed on B-cell surface throughout B-cell development except in plasma cells, which do not express any cell surface BCR. They are important for signal transduction in B cells, since the μ-heavy chains that anchor BCR on cell membrane have only a three amino acid long cytoplasmic domain, which is insufficient to assemble a signalosome complex (Niiro and Clark 2002). The co-receptors, Ig-α and Ig-β, have a small extracellular domain and a long cytoplasmic domain that transmits activation signals to B cells. The cytoplasmic domain of the co-receptors contains two immune-receptor tyrosine-based activation motifs (ITAM) that are substrates for the SFK and Syk protein tyrosine kinase. Although antigen specificity of the pre-BCR is much debated, its expression is essential for B-cell development. This appears to be related to its ability to transmit tonic signals, since expression of the ITAM domains of Ig-α and Ig-β is sufficient to drive B-cell development in the bone marrow (Bannish et al. 2001).

In immature B cells BCR is important for selection against autoreactive B cells (Chen et al. 1994; Nemazee and Weigert 2000; Wardemann et al. 2003). In the periphery, B cells derived from the germinal centers undergo somatic mutation and those that express high-affinity BCR survive and differentiate into memory or plasma cells (Gu et al. 1991; Chen et al. 1994; Su et al. 2004). It has been shown recently that deletion of surface BCR in mature B cells results in death of such cells (Kraus et al. 2004). Thus, using a conditional transgenic mouse model, Kraus and colleagues demonstrated that removal of surface BCR in resting mature B cells results in apoptosis and loss of such cells in the periphery (Lam et al. 1997; Kraus et al. 2004). Moreover, introduction of mutations in the Igα cytoplasmic ITAM motifs in an inducible and cell-stage restricted manner led to loss of mature B cells (Kraus et al. 2004). These seminal studies laid foundation to the concept that basal or tonic signaling by the BCR is required for the survival of naïve B cells.

Requirement of BCR for B-Lymphoma Development

A role for BCR in lymphoma development was proposed almost 50 years ago and has been addressed in experimental models from time to time (Dameshek and Schwartz 1959). The basic hypothesis has been that antigen-dependent stimulation of B cells provides both multiple opportunities for cell division, and a random chance for mutagenic events that lead to transformation of an antigen-specific B cell. Consistent with this model several autoimmune diseases have been associated with lymphoma development (Guyomard et al. 2003; Jonsson et al. 2007). Similarly, chronic stimulation associated with infectious agents, such as EBV, hepatitis C virus, and *Helicobactor pylori*, have all been shown to promote B-lymphoma development. Often, but not always, MALT lymphoma-derived BCRs are specific to *H. pylori*-derived antigens (Isaacson and Du 2004). Chronic stimulation can be from the B-cell receptor-derived signaling, as well as from T cells that may activate B cells. Follicular and diffuse large B-cell lymphomas are often infiltrated with T cells (Dave et al. 2004). Very recently the role of T cells in B-lymphoma development was tested elegantly in an animal model by Zangani et al., who developed T-helper cells specific for a B-cell idiotype (Id) expressed in an Ig transgenic mouse. Repeated injection of these T-helper cells into Id⁺, but not Id⁻ mice, resulted in B-cell tumor development in 100% of the mice (Zangani et al. 2007). Moreover, expression of ITAM motifs critical for B-cell receptor signaling led to the transformation of fibroblasts and mammary epithelial cells *in vitro* (Grande et al. 2006), providing direct support to the concept that BCR-mediated signaling can lead to oncogenic transformation.

Most of the B-cell lymphomas of the non-Hodgkin's type (widely prevalent type) express surface BCR. Interestingly, follicular lymphoma, a subtype of non-Hodgkin's lymphoma responds to treatment with antibodies specific to the idiotype expressed by the B-cell receptor of the lymphoma cells. However, patients progressively develop resistance to the anti-idiotype antibody treatment. Notably, the resistance to anti-idiotype treatment does not result from the complete loss of the BCR but only a loss of the idiotype (Bahler and Levy 1992). The preservation of BCR expression in the variants may be due to a requirement for BCR-derived signals for the lymphoma growth. (Brown et al. 1989; Bahler and Levy 1992; Maloney et al. 1992). These findings suggest that BCR expression might be important for survival of B lymphomas (Kuppers 2005). Consistent with this notion is the finding that most chromosomal translocations involving oncogenes occur in the non-productively rearranged Ig loci with a few exceptions (Kuppers 2005). The expression of stereotyped Ig molecules with minimal or no somatic mutation but with common V regions that share CDR3 regions by several CLL patients has been used to that a significant fraction of small cell lymphoma may be antigen selected (Messmer et al. 2004). As noted above, a role for antigen-induced signaling is suggested by the strong association between *H. pylori* infection and B lymphoma (Isaacson and Du 2004). The rare appearance of BCR-negative variants in many lymphomas with ongoing somatic mutation such as follicular lymphoma, Burkitt's lymphoma, diffuse large B-cell lymphoma, and MALT lymphoma support the notion that B-cell lymphomas undergo selection process like normal B cells.

The influence of BCR expression on B-lymphoma development was demonstrated in an elegant mouse model by Refaeli et al. (2008). This system made use of the E_μ-Myc transgenic mouse model that develops B lymphomas as mice age. Breeding of the E_μ-Myc mice to the transgenic mice that express the B-cell receptor specific to lysozyme allowed a direct test of the role of antigen and BCR signals in B-lymphoma development. The presence of antigen promoted the development of large B-cell lymphomas like DLBCL that are specific to the antigen (lysozyme), whereas in the absence of antigen the B-cell malignancy was similar to chronic B-lymphocytic leukemia. Presence of antigen accelerated the development of B lymphoma significantly in E_μ-Myc-HEL-BCR mice compared to E_μ-Myc mice alone (Refaeli et al. 2008).

Constitutive or Tonic BCR Signaling in B-Lymphoma Maintenance

Previous observations on the importance of BCR expression for B lymphoma could be interpreted as BCR having a role in B-lymphoma development but not maintenance. Also these studies did not distinguish if BCR signals are triggered by antigen binding or by its mere presence. We discovered that Burkitt's lymphoma cells, that have the c-myc oncogenes translocated into the Ig locus, required JNK-mediated signals for c-myc expression and survival (Gururajan et al. 2005). Since JNK can be activated by BCR cross-linking in naïve B cells, we hypothesized that JNK activation in these lymphomas may be BCR dependent (Wu et al. 2001; Gururajan et al. 2005). We propose the hypothesis that BCR-derived signals, that contribute to the survival of normal resting B cells, are also important for the continued growth of B-cell lymphomas. In support of such a hypothesis, we demonstrated that several components of BCR signaling pathway (Syk, JNK, Egr-1) are constitutively activated in B-lymphoma cells and that such constitutive activation of signaling pathways was BCR dependent (Gururajan et al. 2005; Gururajan et al. 2007). Thus, down-modulation of BCR expression in B-lymphoma cells is accompanied by a reduction in activation of several critical signaling intermediates such as c-Jun N-terminal kinase (JNK) and Akt, and a decrease in cellular levels of growth and survival-related factors such as EGR-1, Bcl-xL, and Cyclin D2. These results predict a critical role for BCR-derived trophic (Akt, Egr-1, and Bcl-xL) and proliferation (Cyclin D2) signals in the continued expansion and survival of B-lymphoma cells (Gururajan et al. 2006). These findings have clinical implications, as targeting machinery that are part of BCR complex will aid in the design of novel therapeutics for treating B lymphoma. Recent evidence in support of a role for constitutive or tonic BCR signaling in B-lymphoma maintenance is summarized below.

Role of Syk in BCR Signaling and B-Cell Development

Igα and Igβ molecules in the BCR complex are critical for signaling via the immunoreceptor tyrosine-based activation (ITAM) motifs present in their cytoplasmic domains. ITAM motifs transmit signals that lead to activation of several tyrosine kinases upon BCR cross-linking. Syk is a non-receptor tyrosine kinase expressed by all hematopoietic cells, including B, T, and NK cells (Turner et al. 2000). In the absence of Syk, immature B cells can be detected in the T-cell zones of the spleen but fail to undergo maturation into recirculating B cells (Turner et al. 1995, 1997). These results suggest that Syk is an essential transducer of BCR signals required for the transition of immature into mature recirculating B cells. Using reverse genetics approach to reconstitute proximal BCR components in the Drosophila cell system, Rolli and colleagues demonstrated that Syk phosphorylates both the tyrosines of the ITAM motifs of the BCR co-receptors Ig-α and Ig-β (Rolli et al. 2002). Syk becomes activated upon phosphorylation of Tyr 525 and Tyr 526 (Hutchcroft et al. 1991) and induces multiple signaling pathways including PI3K, NF-κB, PLC-γ, and JNK (Cornall et al. 2000; Arndt et al. 2004; Takada and Aggarwal 2004). NF-κB, a potent anti-apoptotic factor, is activated in a Syk and JNK-dependent manner in response to TNF stimulation and oxidative stress (Craxton et al. 1999; Gold et al. 1999; Ozes et al. 1999; Romashkova and Makarov 1999; Ding et al. 2000; Pogue et al. 2000; Takano et al. 2002). Loss of Syk expression in breast tumors as a result of DNA hypermethylation promotes tumor cell proliferation and invasion and predicts shorter survival of breast cancer patients (Yuan et al. 2001; Toyama et al. 2003; Gatalica and Bing 2005; Wang et al. 2005). Unlike breast cancer cells, where Syk is shown to be a tumor suppressor, Syk has a pro-survival role in normal B-cell development suggesting multiple roles for Syk depending on the cellular context. An oncogenic role for Syk in pre-B cells was shown by overexpressing Syk in bone marrow pre-B cells, which gave rise to leukemias (Wossning et al. 2006).

Syk is Constitutively Activated in B Lymphomas and Is Critical for B-Lymphoma Survival and Proliferation

A variety of B-lymphoma cells (cell lines and primary tumors from mouse and tumor samples from human patients) expressed constitutively active Syk with little or no active Syk in normal splenic and peripheral blood B cells (Gururajan et al. 2007). Using two different approaches to inhibit Syk activation, it was shown that Syk is critical for B-lymphoma survival and proliferation (Gururajan et al. 2007). Curcumin, a natural compound present in *Curcuma longa*, has anti-cancer and anti-inflammatory properties (Shishodia et al. 2007). We have shown that curcumin is a potent inhibitor of B-lymphoma growth (Han et al. 1999). Many previous experiments demonstrated that curcumin targets critical cellular substrates, including NF-κB, Akt, and JNK. The proximal signaling pathways that are targeted by curcumin are poorly understood. Although curcumin-induced apoptosis is Akt dependent, surprisingly curcumin does not directly inhibit Akt (in vitro kinase assay) or its recently identified key regulator mTOR/rictor complex (Sarbassov et al. 2005; Gururajan et al. 2007). For the first time, we demonstrated that under *in vitro* conditions, curcumin can directly inhibit phosphorylation of Syk and thus identified Syk as a novel target for curcumin in B-lymphoma cells. Consistent with the concept that Syk is a direct target of curcumin, Lyn activity and Igα phosphorylation, which are upstream of Syk activation, are not affected by curcumin in B-lymphoma cells (Gururajan et al. 2007). It appears that curcumin-mediated targeting of these pathways is Syk dependent. Thus, by targeting Syk, all downstream components are downregulated, which is a potential way to modulate pathways that are diversified from the proximal components. Using a Syk selective inhibitor (Piceatannol) and by small interfering RNA that targets Syk, it was demonstrated that constitutive Syk activity is critical for B-lymphoma growth (Gururajan et al. 2007).

In follicular lymphomas Syk was more rapidly activated in tumor B cells than in tumor infiltrating normal B cells (Irish et al. 2006). It was demonstrated that diffuse large B-cell lymphoma cell lines that express surface BCR were highly-sensitive to the ATP-competitive Syk inhibitor, R406, which blocked SYK525/526 autophosphorylation and downstream signaling (Chen et al. 2008). Blocking Syk led to apoptosis of such cells. These DLBCL cell lines with an intact BCR signaling pathway and sensitivity to the SYK inhibitor were designated as "BCR" tumors on the basis of their transcriptional profiles. A majority of DLBCL cell lines exhibited tonic BCR signaling and Syk-dependent survival, but a subset of lines had no detectable BCR. The BCR-negative B cells were insensitive to Syk inhibition and were designated "non-BCR" DLBCLs (Chen et al. 2008). Since inhibition of Syk by selective inhibitors seems to be promising, oral Syk inhibitors are currently being explored for early-stage clinical trials in human lymphoma patients (Chen et al. 2008).

Role of BCR-Induced Mitogen-Activated Protein Kinases (MAPK) in B Lymphoma

MAPKs are a group of serine/threonine protein kinases activated by a wide variety of extracellular signals including BCR ligation. MAPKs include ERK1/2 (extra-cellular signal-regulated kinase), JNK1/2 (c-jun amino-terminal kinase) and p38 MAPK. Extensive work by several groups has established that Map kinase pathways play critical roles in the pathogenesis of various hematologic malignancies, providing new molecular targets for future therapeutic approaches (James et al. 2003; Kerr et al. 2003; Platanias 2003; Staber et al. 2004). Thus, inhibition of JNK activation with the pharmacological JNK inhibitor, SP600125, induces growth arrest in myeloma cell lines (Hideshima et al. 2003). Certain follicular lymphomas upon transformation into diffuse large B-cell lymphomas express constitutively active form of p38 MAPK and its inhibition with SB203580, the pharmacological inhibitor, induces growth arrest and apoptosis (Elenitoba-Johnson et al. 2003). There is also evidence implicating abnormal expression of c-Jun, which is a downstream effectorof JNK pathway, in the proliferation of malignant Hodgkin's lymphoma cells (Mathas et al. 2002).

JNK MAPK and Its Role in Cell Survival, Proliferation, and Apoptosis

JNK is activated in response to certain growth factors or stresses like UV radiation. Stress-induced JNK activation often leads to cell death through activation of the mitochondrial apoptotic pathway in many cell types including neuronal cells, prostate cancer cells, and fibroblasts (Le-Niculescu et al. 1999; Mielke and Herdegen 2000; Deng et al. 2003; Shimada et al. 2003). On the contrary, JNK can promote survival of BCR/ABL transformed leukemic cells (Hess et al. 2002). Triggering the JNK pathway in vitro with a BCR-ABL tyrosine kinase leads to a dramatic increase in B-cell transformation. Moreover, JNK is required for IL-3-mediated cell survival through its ability to phosphorylate and inactivate the proapoptotic Bcl-2 family protein BAD (Yu et al. 2004). JNK protein kinases are coded for by three genes, *Jnk1*, *Jnk2*, and *Jnk3*. *Jnk1* and *Jnk2* are the more widely expressed isoforms of JNK. *Jnk3* is limited in expression, being restricted primarily to the brain, heart, and testis. JNK is activated by upstream MAPK kinases, MKK7, and MKK4 (Davis 2000; Tournier et al. 2001; Weston and Davis 2002). Activated JNK phosphorylates and activates its major substrate c-jun, as well as several other transcription factors and proteins, required for cell survival, proliferation, transformation, and cell death (Shaulian and Karin 2002).

The dual role of JNK in both apoptotic and survival signaling pathways indicates that the functional role of JNK is complex. Cells lacking both JNK isoforms exhibit a defect in proliferation similar to c-Jun-deficient cells (Schreiber et al. 1999; Sabapathy et al. 2004). Indicating an isoform specific role, absence of JNK2 enhances proliferation, whereas JNK1 deletion delays G1-S progression. This appears to be related to the ability of JNK2 in unstimulated cells to promote degradation of c-Jun, whereas JNK1 enhances phosphorylation of c-Jun (Sabapathy et al. 2004). The biological outcome of JNK activation depends on the cellular context, time course of activation, and the balance between the ability of JNK to signal both apoptosis and cell survival. The complexity of the cellular response to JNK activation can be illustrated by the diverse actions of the pro-inflammatory cytokine TNF-α. Sustained activation of JNK correlates with TNF-induced apoptosis of rat mesangial cells (Guo et al. 1998). On the other hand, JNK1 and JNK2 double knockout fibroblasts are more sensitive to TNF-induced apoptosis compared to wild-type fibroblasts suggesting a pro-survival role for JNK signaling in these cells (Lamb et al. 2003). Using a dominant-negative mutant of TRAF2 (TNF Receptor-Associated Factor-2), it is seen that TRAF2 provides anti-apoptotic signals by activating JNK following cross-linking of TNF receptor superfamily members in lymphocytes (Lee et al. 1997). Recent findings that MKK7 (an upstream activator of JNK) knockout hepatocytes fail to proliferate and mouse embryo fibroblasts that lack MKK7 undergo cellular senescence and G_2/M growth arrest further support a role for JNK in cell cycle progression (Wada and Penninger 2004).

Signaling through CD72, CD40, or B-cell receptor (BCR) ligation induces activation of MAP kinases, like JNK, in primary splenic B cells (Sakata et al. 1995; Wu et al. 2001; Xie et al. 2004). However, no defect in BCR- or CD72-induced proliferation is observed in B cells from JNK1$^{-/-}$ or JNK2$^{-/-}$ mice (Wu et al. 2001). This is probably due to a redundancy of function between the two isoforms as JNK1 and JNK2 double knockouts exhibit embryonic lethality (Kuan et al. 1999). In T cells, JNK2 is required for the differentiation of CD4+ T cells to Th1 cells and impaired IFN-γ production is observed in T cells from JNK2$^{-/-}$ mice (Yang et al. 1998). Moreover, JNK2 but not JNK1 was regulated by the Carma1-Bcl-10 complex, which is downstream of both BCR and TCR signaling pathways (Blonska et al. 2007).

JNK, the MAPK Which Regulates Several Downstream Effectors, Is Constitutively Activated in B Lymphomas and Is Critical for B-Lymphoma Growth

Using a pharmacological inhibitor, it was shown that JNK activity is essential for BCR-induced proliferation of both normal murine splenic B cells and peripheral blood human B cells (Wu et al. 2001; Gururajan et al. 2005). Many B lymphoma cell lines, as well as primary tumor samples of both human and murine origin, constitutively express an activated form of JNK (pJNK) and its major substrate c-jun (phospho-c-jun), whereas naïve B cells exhibit very little activation of JNK in the absence of mitogenic stimulation (Gururajan et al. 2005). This basal JNK activity is required for B-lymphoma proliferation. Inhibition of JNK activation with SP600125 or inhibition of JNK expression by siRNA resulted in reduced basal proliferation of several murine B-lymphoma cell lines, human Burkitt B-lymphoma cells as well as human diffuse large B-cell lymphoma cell lines. These findings for the first time demonstrated that JNK activity is critical for B-lymphoma proliferation. Recently, it was shown that NPM-ALK, a tyrosine kinase associated with anaplastic large cell lymphoma, induced lymphoma cell proliferation in a JNK and c-jun-dependent manner (Leventaki et al. 2007). This study suggested that the constitutive JNK activity is not only critical for lymphoma maintenance but also for lymphomagenesis. Moreover, a role for JNK and c-Jun induction in the survival and metastasis of *Theileria*-transformed B cells was demonstrated by Langsley and colleagues. Blocking JNK and c-jun by inhibitors and siRNA led to failure of transformation of B cells by *Theileria* parasite (Lizundia et al. 2006). Constitutive JNK activation is not limited to B lymphomas, since it was also found in HTLV-1 associated adult

T cell leukemia patients (Xu et al. 1996). An examination of gene expression profiling data on diffuse large B-cell lymphoma reveals an enhanced expression of JNK mRNA in at least 60% of the samples although this was not noted by these authors (Alizadeh et al. 2000).

Many B lymphomas overexpress c-Myc due to chromosomal translocations, and this overexpression is important for their proliferation and cell cycle progression (Fischer et al. 1994; Lovec et al. 1994; Wu et al. 1996; Baudino et al. 2003; Sanchez-Beato et al. 2003). JNK is known to upregulate c-Myc expression in response to growth factors like PDGF (Iavarone et al. 2003). Moreover, it has been shown that WEHI-231 B-lymphoma cells stably transfected with c-Myc are resistant to anti-IgM-induced growth arrest (Wu et al. 1996). There was a significant reduction in c-Myc protein in both SP600125 and JNK-specific siRNA treated WEHI-231 B lymphoma suggesting that inhibition of JNK may cause growth arrest by inhibiting c-Myc expression. c-Myc translocation is common in Burkitt's B-lymphoma cells which leads to its overexpression (Kuppers 2005). However, in Burkitt's lymphomas, often c-Myc gene is translocated to the IgH locus, whose expression may still be regulated by the MAPK pathway. This may account for the growth inhibition of these cells by the JNK inhibitor.

c-Myc expression has been shown to be cell cycle dependent. Elevated c-Myc levels are observed during G_1 and G_2/M phases of cell cycle with moderate levels at the S phase and c-Myc is shown to co-operate with Ras to induce cdc2, a kinase required for G_2/M progression (Seth et al. 1993). Moreover, drug-induced G2/M arrest of Jurkat T cells is correlated with c-Myc downregulation (Villamarin et al. 2002). It is possible that JNK regulates c-Myc during G_2/M phase of cell cycle progression, since MKK7 knockout fibroblasts, in which JNK activation is compromised, undergo G_2/M arrest and cellular senescence (Wada and Penninger 2004). Downregulated c-Myc might account for the G_2/M arrest observed in SP600125-treated cells. This is consistent with the protective effect of CD40, as CD40 signaling restored c-Myc levels (Merino et al. 1995). Moreover, ectopic expression of c-Myc in WEHI-231 cells overcomes the G_2/M arrest induced by the JNK inhibitor. The pro-survival role for JNK in B-lymphoma growth is further substantiated by in vivo studies in a mouse model of B lymphoma (Gururajan et al 2005). In summary, these data demonstrate that the proliferation of primary B cells and B-lymphoma cells is dependent on JNK activation. These findings suggest that targeting JNK may have some important therapeutic implications in the treatment of B lymphomas (Manning and Davis 2003).

The significance of two other MAPK family members, including ERK and p38, in B-lymphoma growth regulation was tested. Although these B lymphomas express activated forms of ERK constitutively, inhibition of its activity by two different inhibitors PD98059 and UO126 affected basal proliferation of some but not all lymphoma cell lines studied (Gururajan et al. 2005; Ke et al. 2006). Moreover, the p38 inhibitor SB203580 did not inhibit the proliferation of two B-lymphoma cell lines tested. However, p38 MAP kinase has recently been shown to be activated during progression of follicular lymphoma into diffuse large B-cell lymphoma

(Elenitoba-Johnson et al. 2003). Hence more B lymphomas have to be examined for the relative importance of different MAPK enzymes for lymphoma growth.

Transcription Factors Including Egr-1 and Pax-5 Sustain BCR Signaling in B Lymphoma

In this section, we focus on two transcription factors that have a role in BCR signaling and may have implications for B-cell development and transformation. Egr-1 is a zinc finger-containing transcription factor that is a member of a family with three other members, Egr-2, Egr-3, and Egr-4. Egr-1 is a widely expressed immediate early gene, with diverse consequences on cell growth, apoptosis, as well as production of pro-inflammatory cytokines (Liu et al. 1998). In naïve B cells BCR cross-linking enhances Egr-1 expression rapidly in Ras-dependent manner (McMahon and Monroe 1995). Egr-1 is required for expression of CD44 and ICAM-1 molecules in B cells (McMahon and Monroe 1996). Early studies suggested that Egr-1 deficiency does not have profound effects on immune cell development and function (Lee et al. 1995). Recently we discovered that Egr-1 deficiency enhances B lymphopoiesis in the bone marrow but specifically diminished marginal zone B cell development in the periphery (Gururajan et al 2008).

Pax-5, also known as B-cell specific activator protein or BSAP, is involved in the commitment of early B-cell precursors to B lineage by its ability to promote transcription of Rag-2 required for VDJ recombination and several B-cell specific genes such as CD19, *Mb-1*, and *BLNK*. Pax-5 deletion arrests B-cell development at the pro-B-cell stage (Smith and Sigvardsson 2004; Singh et al. 2007). The Pax-5 deficient B cells can, however, be differentiated into cells of other lineages such as macrophages, dendritic cells, osteocytes, granulocytes, etc., in the presence of suitable signals, suggesting that Pax-5 acts as a repressor as well. Recently several Pax-5 targets whose expression is enhanced or repressed by Pax-5 have been described (Pridans et al. 2008). The BCR co-receptor, Igα, is one of the genes upregulated by Pax-5 expression. Notch-1 is an early lineage commitment factor that is suppressed by Pax-5. Pax-5 expression continues throughout B-cell development but is extinguished upon differentiation into plasma cells (Calame 2001).

Egr-1 Is Critical for B-Lymphoma Growth

Egr-1 is upregulated in normal B cells when the BCR is cross-linked (Seyfert et al. 1989; Ke et al. 2006). Unlike normal B cells, the murine B-lymphoma, BKS-2 constitutively expressed Egr-1 and BCR cross-linking led to a reduction in Egr-1 mRNA accompanied by strong growth inhibition (Muthukkumar et al. 1997). In addition, anti-sense nucleotides specific for Egr-1 significantly diminished the growth of BKS-2 B lymphoma (Muthukkumar et al. 1997; Ke et al. 2006). LPS-mediated rescue of WEHI-231 B lymphoma from anti-IgM-induced growth arrest involved upregulation of Egr-1 gene (Seyfert et al. 1989). This pro-growth induc-ing property of Egr-1 in B lymphoma is in contrast to its role in suppressing tumor transformation in several human tumor cell lines, including fibrosarcoma cells, breast carcinoma, glioblastoma, and its role in ionizing radiation-induced growth inhibition in human melanoma cells (Huang et al. 1995, 1997; Ahmed et al. 1996). In one report, there was a lack of correlation between Egr-1 expres-sion and anti-Ig-mediated growth inhibition in the WEHI-231 lymphoma cells (Gottschalk et al. 1993). The relevance of constitutive expression of Egr-1 for lym-phoma growth was addressed by blocking Egr-1 activity using WT-*Egr* construct, a repressor of Egr-1 (Madden et al. 1991). Consistent with the idea that Egr-1 is a growth promoting transcription factor, it was found that blocking Egr-1 with a retroviral-mediated introduction of WT-*Egr* significantly reduced the growth of two different B-lymphoma cell lines (Ke et al. 2006). It was proposed that constitu-tive Egr-1 expression promotes induction of some of the previously characterized target genes including *cyclin D2*, *c-Myc*, and inhibition of *p19INK4d*, a cell cycle inhibitor. A role for Egr-1 in B-lymphoma growth is further supported by consti-tutive expression of Egr-1 in body cavity lymphoma isolated from AIDS patients and its decrease in expression upon growth inhibition (Sun et al. 2001). EBV-mediated B-cell transformation was also accompanied by a rapid upregulation of Egr-1 expression (Calogero et al. 1996). Examination of the published microarray analysis of gene expression in diffuse large B-cell lymphomas revealed that 35% of the patient samples exhibit constitutive expression of Egr-1, which is probably an underestimate since this study uses several transformed cells to normalize the data (Alizadeh et al. 2000).

Pax-5 Is Critical for B-Lymphoma Growth

Pax-5 is found to be translocated into the Ig locus in marginal zone lymphoma (Morrison et al. 1998). The chromosomal translocation t(9:14) is associated with 50% of large cell lymphoma cases. Cloning of the breakpoint region by Iida et al. (1996) revealed the presence of Pax-5 gene fused to the Ig heavy chain region and a significant increase in Pax-5 expression. Recently, it was demonstrated that Pax-5 expression promoted lymphoma growth *in vivo* in mouse models (Cozma et al. 2007). The ability of Pax-5 to promote lymphomagenesis correlated with expression of components of BCR signaling pathway including upregulation of Igα and CD19 antigens, B-cell linker (Blnk), Bruton's agammaglobulinemia tyrosine kinase (Btk), PKCβ1, and phospholipase C-γ and downregulation of BCR-negative regulators such as CD22 and PIR-B (Cozma et al. 2007). This ability of Pax-5 is reversed by the interruption of the chain of signaling events downstream of Igα. On the other hand, a constitutively active ITAM construct recapitulated the tumor-promoting effects of Pax-5, suggesting that Pax-5 expression may upregulate BCR signals (Cozma et al. 2007). These findings not only demonstrate the molec-ular mechanisms by which Pax-5 promotes lymphoma growth, but also directly established the role of BCR signaling in lymphomagenesis.

Model for Constitutive BCR Signaling and Its Implications for Basal B-Lymphoma Growth

The importance of constitutive or tonic BCR signaling for naïve B-cell survival is now well established (Lam et al. 1997; Kraus et al. 2004). In B-lymphoma cells, this constitutive BCR signaling is further enhanced when compared to the naïve B cells as revealed by increased tyrosine phosphorylation of Igα and Igβ BCR co-receptors (Gururajan et al. 2006). Recently we observed that Src family kinases (SFK) like Lyn are also constitutively active in B-lymphoma cells (Ke et al manuscript in preparation), which could explain the increased phosphorylation of BCR co-receptors, as SFKs are thought to be key initiators of BCR signaling (Niiro and Clark 2002). We propose that the elevated levels of tonic BCR signaling are required for continued growth of B-lymphoma cells. The BCR activation leads to constitutive Syk activation in B-lymphoma cells (Fig. 17.1). Constitutive Syk activation leads to activation of several downstream kinases including Akt and MAP kinases like JNK. Akt promotes cell survival by phosphorylation of Bad and key cell

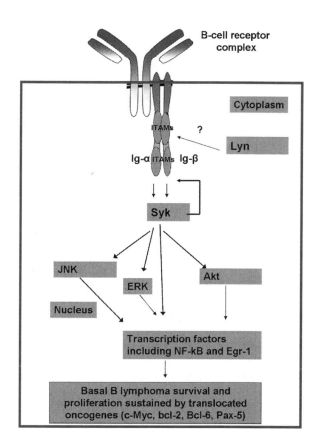

Fig. 17.1 Key intermediates in tonic BCR signaling pathway which contribute to B-lymphoma growth

cycle-related genes. JNK promotes cell survival through Egr-1 and cell cycle pro-gression through c-Myc. The critical and most compelling evidence for this model comes from the data pointing to the fact that when BCR expression is inhibited by siRNA that targets Igα or Igβ expression, activation of all the above-mentioned signaling molecules is downregulated, accompanied by a decrease in cell viability and cell cycle progression of B-lymphoma cells (Gururajan et al. 2006). The other compelling evidence for this model comes from the observations that when each component of this module is targeted using specific siRNA or pharmacological inhibitors, there was a decrease in cell survival and cell cycle progression of B-lymphoma cells *in vitro*. Pharmacological inhibitors of Syk and JNK also decreased lymphoma burden *in vivo*. Thus BCR and its signaling machinery are critical for basal survival and proliferation of B lymphoma (Fig. 17.1). The precise mechanism for initiating and regulating tonic BCR signaling remains unknown. Several lines of evidence suggest that this process could be ligand dependent or independent.

Ligand-Dependent BCR Signaling in Lymphomagenesis

The proposed model does not address the origin of the constitutive BCR signaling in B lymphomas. One source of BCR signaling can be the availability of antigen in the form of an autoantigen or an infectious agent. Indeed, autoantibodies have been demonstrated frequently in lymphoma patients (Guyomard et al. 2003). This is very prevalent in small cell lymphoma (Chiorazzi and Ferrarini 2003). Role of ligand-dependent BCR signaling for lymphoma growth and development is best illustrated by the lymphomas associated with *H. pylori* and hepatitis C virus infections.

Infection and Lymphoma

The epidemiological evidence of an association between *H. pylori* infection and mucosa-associated lymphoid tissue (MALT) lymphoma came from the study of Parsonnet et al., who showed that *H. pylori* infection precedes the development of MALT lymphoma (Parsonnet et al. 1994; Parsonnet and Isaacson 2004). The first direct evidence for a link between *H. pylori* gastritis and MALT lymphoma came from Isaacson et al.,who observed lymphoma regression in five of six patients after cure of *H. pylori* infection and from other groups (Isaacson 1999). It was demonstrated that there is regression of MALT lymphoma in 70% of patients treated with an antibacterial agent against *H. pylori* (Bayerdorffer et al. 1995; Cammarota et al. 1995; Isaacson 1999; Thiede et al. 2000). Analysis of D region rearrange-ments suggested that MALT B-lymphoma clones have undergone antigen selection indicating that antigen stimulation may have a role in B-lymphoma development (Bertoni et al. 1997). This is further supported by the observations that the Ig sequences in low-grade MALT lymphomas exhibit somatic mutation and the B cells appear to be of germinal center origin (Du et al. 1996). The regression of MALT lymphoma brought about by eradication of *H. pylori* infection provides one of the best evidences for ligand-dependent BCR signaling in lymphomagenesis. The specificity of lymphoma-derived immunoglobulins to *H. pylori*-derived antigens has been questioned by a recent study, although others have found common idiotypes and autoantigen reactivity (Lenze et al. 2006). Antigen-specific T cells also appear to have a critical role in MALT lymphoma.

The histological, clinical, and biological studies have focused on the association between *H. pylori* infection and low-grade gastric MALT lymphoma. However, clinical and morphological data suggested that some low-grade lymphomas may develop into high-grade MALT lymphomas. Cure of *H. pylori* infection associated with an early-stage tumor resulted in complete tumor regression in more than 80% of patients (Bayerdorffer et al. 1995, 1997). It has been observed that tumors with transition to high-grade malignancy did not respond to cure of the *H. pylori* infection suggesting that other factors might play a role in addition to *H. pylori* infection (Morgner et al. 2001). Factors including T cell help may play a role either through direct interaction with *H. pylori*-specific B cells or bystander activation. Cytokines from T cells and/or innate immune cells including macrophages and dendritic cells could play an important role in sustaining BCR signals in B-lymphoma growth in vivo in MALT lymphomas. Elucidating such factors in detail will help understand the disease process and design of therapies for better treatment of patients with advanced stages of tumors.

Epidemiological studies have shown association between hepatitis C virus (HCV) infection and non-Hodgkin's lymphoma (Landau et al. 2007; Suarez et al. 2007; Zignego et al. 2007). There is evidence for antigen-driven clonal expansion leading from oligoclonal to monoclonal proliferation and frank malignancy. Similar to MALT lymphomas in *H. pylori* infection, antiviral treatment with interferon and ribavirin dramatically reduces the growth of HCV-associated splenic lymphoma (Hermine et al. 2002). HCV infection of B cells in vitro leads to somatic mutation of oncogenes such as *Bcl-6*. One report describes direct infection of malignant B cells in a patient with HCV, but this is not essential since HCV-encoded E2 protein can bind to CD81 on B cells and induce somatic mutation (Machida et al. 2005). Nevertheless, these studies clearly point to the role of antigen or microenvironment in B lymphomagenesis.

Microenvironmental Regulation of B-Lymphoma Growth

Recent studies highlight the contributions of microenvironment in B-lymphoma pathogenesis. Rituxan (Rituximab) is an anti-CD20 monoclonal antibody which depletes all the B cells, including lymphoma cells from the body of lymphoma patients (Martin and Chan 2006). Studies in mouse models revealed that there are mechanistic differences in the Rituximab-mediated depletion of circulating and non-circulating types of malignancies. The circulating but not non-circulating B cells are efficiently depleted with anti-CD20 monoclonal antibody therapy (Gong et al. 2005). These differences highlight the potential involvement of other factors in the tissues for lymphoma cell survival. The presence of infiltrating T cells in lymphoma tissue has been well documented. In animal models, idiotype-specific T cells induced vigorous proliferation of B cells bearing the idiotype which led to their subsequent transformation (Zangani et al. 2007). Together, these data indicate that microenvironment likely plays an important role in clinical response. One key factor that was shown to play a role in B-lymphoma growth is BAFF (Gong et al. 2005). The interrelationship of BAFF and depleting ability of anti-hCD20 mAbs was demonstrated in a mouse model. In a transgenic mouse that expresses human CD20 in B cells, efficient B-cell depletion was obtained when anti-CD20 therapy was combined with TACI-Fc, a fusion protein that scavenges BAFF (Gong et al. 2005). This study provided a mechanistic basis for the potential combinatorial therapy of anti-hCD20 mAb with antagonists of BAFF to enhance the efficacy of B-cell immunotherapy in the treatment of lymphomas. This study also highlighted the role of microenvironment in B lymphomagenesis, as BAFF is secreted by marginal zone macrophages in the marginal sinus of the spleen.

It has been known for a long time that primary lymphoma cells from patients are very difficult to adapt to *in vitro* culture. In addition to genetic changes, the majority of human non-Hodgkin's lymphoma remain dependent on their microenvironment during disease progression and therefore long-term cultures of lymphoma cells without stromal support is not possible *in vitro*. It was demonstrated recently that lymphoma cells are dependent on hedgehog ligands secreted by stromal cells in lymphoid organs (Dierks et al. 2007). Overexpression of activated Smo^{W535L} (ligand for hedgehog) in mouse model of lymphoma induced highly proliferative lymphomas in the skin. Moreover, it was demonstrated that Indian (Ihh) and sonic (Shh) hedgehog proteins are ligands produced by stromal cells in the bone marrow, the spleen, and the lymph nodes that allow survival and expansion of lymphoma cells *in vitro* and *in vivo* (Dierks et al. 2007). These experiments indicate that hedgehog pathway activation is critical for lymphoma growth *in vivo* and that hedgehog ligands might be one of the limiting factors that determine the localization of lymphoma. Pharmacological intervention of hedgehog signaling could represent a new therapeutic approach for NHL.

Ligand-Independent BCR Signaling in Lymphomagenesis

Unlike MALT lymphomas, where *H. pylori* infection correlated with disease outcome and treatment, and some non-Hodgkin's lymphomas that are associated with HCV infection, majority of the non-Hodgkin's lymphomas lack such correlation (Kuppers 2005). Hence the BCR signaling may derive from autoantigen stimulation or is ligand independent. The concept of ligand-independent BCR signaling in B cells is supported by the observations that in B cells, inactivation of PTPs with pervanadate or H_2O_2 resulted in ligand-independent BCR signaling and phosphorylation of downstream substrates including Syk (Rolli et al. 2002).

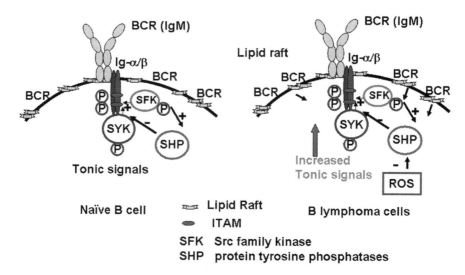

Fig. 17.2 Tonic BCR signaling is elevated in B lymphoma

A ligand-independent signaling role for BCR is strongly supported by the observations of Bannish et al. (2001) who showed that ITAM domains of Ig-α and Ig-β when linked to a myristoylation domain can signal B-cell development in the absence of B-cell receptor. Both viral and Ig-derived ITAMs were sufficient to induce in vitro transformation of epithelial cells and fibroblasts (Grande et al. 2006, 2007). Monroe and colleagues have proposed a model in which the tonic signaling is regulated by the steady-state activity of BCR-associated PTKs and PTPs (Monroe 2006). According to this model, a transient ligand-independent signal is generated by the assembly of positive regulators within the BCR complex and this assembly leads to activation of BCR-associated PTKs, ITAM phosphorylation of Ig-α/β signaling complexes, and Syk phosphorylation. Thereafter, the transient signaling at individual BCR complexes is rapidly terminated by multiple negative regulators including PTPs such as PTPROt. This balance can be disrupted by reactive oxygen species since PTPs that regulate BCR signals are reversibly inactivated by free radicals (Singh et al. 2005a). In B-lymphoma cells, inhibition of such negative regulators by oxidative stress and other factors, leads to a stabilized PTK activation, thereby sustaining BCR-derived signals (Bannish et al. 2001; Fuentes-Panana et al. 2004; Monroe 2006) (Fig. 17.2).

Another possibility is that the BCR in B lymphomas is constitutively associated with lipid rafts, which are cholesterol-containing microdomains that have been shown to be critical for receptor signaling in immune cells and non-immune cells (Dykstra et al. 2003; Gupta et al. 2006; Zeyda and Stulnig 2006) (Fig. 17.2). In B cells, BCR cross-linking induces association of the BCR with lipid rafts where it may have access to SFK-like lyn for initial ITAM tyrosine phosphorylation, which can be further amplified by the Syk kinase (Tolar et al. 2005). CD19, a positive regulator of BCR signaling is also associated with lipid rafts and prolongs BCR association with lipid rafts (Cherukuri et al. 2001). Such BCR–lipid raft association is defective in anergic B cells (Blery et al. 2006). The two models, reactive oxygen species to inactivate phosphatases that regulate BCR signaling and the lipid raft hypothesis may not be mutually exclusive of each other, since oxidative stress has been shown to promote lipid raft formation in T cells (Lu et al. 2007).

Conclusions

Non-Hodgkin's lymphoma (NHL) is the fifth most common cancer in the United States; however, only around 30 to 60% of these cases can be cured through modern therapies such as radiation therapy, chemotherapy, or biological therapy (Lymphoma Research Foundation, USA). Rituximab, an anti-CD20 antibody, is the most recent addition to lymphoma therapy but is not effective for late-stage B lymphomas (Ng 2007). So, there is a need to identify novel therapeutic targets. In this context, BCR signaling gains importance. In terms of B-lymphoma pathogenesis, targeting machinery unique to BCR complex will open up a whole new approach for treating B lymphoma. Targeting molecules (e.g., Syk and JNK) downstream of BCR in B lymphoma will lead to the disruption of signals generated by the microenvironment (BCR induced) as well as the oncogenic translocations, which may enable a better block in B-lymphoma growth.

References

Ahmed MM, Venkatasubbarao K, Fruitwala SM, Muthukkumar S, Wood DP Jr, Sells SF, Mohiuddin M, Rangnekar VM. 1996. EGR-1 induction is required for maximal radiosensitivity in A375-C6 melanoma cells. J Biol Chem 271:29231–29237.

Alizadeh AA, Eisen MB, Davis RE, Ma C, Lossos IS, Rosenwald A, Boldrick JC, Sabet H, Tran T, Yu X, Powell JI, Yang L, Marti GE, Moore T, Hudson J Jr, Lu L, Lewis DB, Tibshirani R, Sherlock G, Chan WC, Greiner TC, Weisenburger DD, Armitage JO, Warnke R, Levy R, Wilson W, Grever MR, Byrd JC, Botstein D, Brown PO, Staudt LM. 2000. Distinct types of diffuse large B-cell lymphoma identified by gene expression profiling. Nature 403:503–511.

Arndt PG, Suzuki N, Avdi NJ, Malcolm KC, Worthen GS. 2004. Lipopolysaccharide-induced c-Jun NH2-terminal kinase activation in human neutrophils: role of phosphatidylinositol 3-Kinase and Syk-mediated pathways. J Biol Chem 279:10883–10891.

Bahler DW and Levy R. 1992. Clonal evolution of a follicular lymphoma: Evidence for antigen selection. Proc Natl Acad Sci U S A 89:6770–6774.

Bannish G, Fuentes-Panana EM, Cambier JC, Pear WS, Monroe JG. 2001. Ligand-independent signaling functions for the B lymphocyte antigen receptor and their role in positive selection during B Lymphopoiesis. J Exp Med 194:1583–1596.

Baudino TA, Maclean KH, Brennan J, Parganas E, Yang C, Aslanian A, Lees JA, Sherr CJ, Roussel MF, Cleveland JL. 2003. Myc-mediated proliferation and lymphomagenesis, but not apoptosis, are compromised by E2f1 loss. Mol Cell 11:905–914.

Bayerdörffer E, Neubauer A, Rudolph B, Thiede C, Lehn N, Eidt S, Stolte M. 1995. Regression of primary gastric lymphoma of mucosa-associated lymphoid tissue type after cure of Helicobacter pylori infection. MALT Lymphoma Study Group. Lancet 345:1591–1594.

Bayerdorffer E, Miehlke S, Neubauer A, Stolte M. 1997. Gastric MALT-lymphoma and Helicobacter pylori infection. Aliment Pharmacol Ther 11 Suppl 1:89–94.

Beecham EJ, Jones GM, Link C, Huppi K, Potter M, Mushinski JF, Bohr VA. 1994. DNA repair defects associated with chromosomal translocation breaksite regions. Mol Cell Biol 14: 1204–1212.

Bertoni F, Cazzaniga G, Bosshard G, Roggero E, Barbazza R, De Boni M, Capella C, Pedrinis E, Cavalli F, Biondi A, Zucca E. 1997. Immunoglobulin heavy chain diversity genes rearrangement pattern indicates that MALT-type gastric lymphoma B cells have undergone an antigen selection process. Br J Haematol 97:830–836.

Blery M, Tze L, Miosge LA, Jun JE, Goodnow CC. 2006. Essential role of membrane cholesterol in accelerated BCR internalization and uncoupling from NF-{kappa}B in B cell clonal anergy. J Exp Med 203:1773–1783.

Blonska M, Pappu BP, Matsumoto R, Li H, Su B, Wang D, Lin X. 2007. The CARMA1-Bcl10 signaling complex selectively regulates JNK2 kinase in the T cell receptor-signaling pathway. Immunity 26:55–66.

Brown SL, Miller RA, Horning SJ, Czerwinski D, Hart SM, McElderry R, Basham T, Warnke RA, Merigan TC, Levy R. 1989. Treatment of B-cell lymphomas with anti-idiotype antibodies alone and in combination with alpha interferon. Blood 73:651–661.

Calame KL. 2001. Plasma cells: Finding new light at the end of B cell development. Nat Immunol 2:1103–1108.

Calogero A, Cuomo L, D'Onofrio M, de Grazia U, Spinsanti P, Mercola D, Faggioni A, Frati L, Adamson ED, Ragona G. 1996. Expression of Egr-1 correlates with the transformed phenotype and the type of viral latency in EBV genome positive lymphoid cell lines. Oncogene. 13: 2105–2112.

Cammarota G, Tursi A, Montalto M, Papa A, Branca G, Vecchio FM, Renzi C, Verzí A, Armuzzi A, Pretolani S, et al. 1995. Prevention and treatment of low-grade B-cell primary gastric lymphoma by anti-H. pylori therapy. J Clin Gastroenterol 21:118–122.

Cattoretti G, Pasqualucci L, Ballon G, Tam W, Nandula SV, Shen Q, Mo T, Murty VV, Dalla-Favera R. 2005. Deregulated BCL6 expression recapitulates the pathogenesis of human diffuse large B cell lymphomas in mice. Cancer Cell 7:445.

Chen C, Radic MZ, Erikson J, Camper SA, Litwin S, Hardy RR, Weigert M. 1994. Deletion and editing of B cells that express antibodies to DNA. J Immunol. 152:1970–1982.

Chen L, Monti S, Juszczynski P, Daley J, Chen W, Witzig TE, Habermann TM, Kutok JL, Shipp MA. 2008. SYK-dependent tonic B-cell receptor signaling is a rational treatment target in diffuse large B-cell lymphoma. Blood 111:2230–2237.

Cherukuri A, Cheng PC, Sohn HW, Pierce SK. 2001. The CD19/CD21 complex functions to prolong B cell antigen receptor signaling from lipid rafts. Immunity 14:169–179.

Chiorazzi N and Ferrarini M. 2003. B cell chronic lymphocytic leukemia: lessons learned from studies of the B cell antigen receptor. Annu Rev Immunol 21:841–894.

Cornall RJ, Cheng AM, Pawson T, Goodnow CC. 2000. Role of Syk in B-cell development and antigen-receptor signaling. Proc Natl Acad Sci U S A 97:1713–1718.

Cozma D, Yu D, Hodawadekar S, Azvolinsky A, Grande S, Tobias JW, Metzgar MH, Paterson J, Erikson J, Marafioti T, Monroe JG, Atchison ML, Thomas-Tikhonenko A. 2007. B cell activator PAX5 promotes lymphomagenesis through stimulation of B cell receptor signaling. J Clin Invest 117:2602–2610.

Craxton A, Jiang A, Kurosaki T, Clark EA. 1999. Syk and Bruton's tyrosine kinase are required for B cell antigen receptor-mediated activation of the kinase Akt. J Biol Chem 274: 30644–30650.

Dameshek W and Schwartz RS. 1959. Editorial: Leukemia and auto-immunization – Some possible relationships. Blood 14:1151–1158.

Dave SS, Wright G, Tan B, Rosenwald A, Gascoyne RD, Chan WC, Fisher RI, Braziel RM, Rimsza LM, Grogan TM, Miller TP, LeBlanc M, Greiner TC, Weisenburger DD, Lynch JC, Vose J, Armitage JO, Smeland EB, Kvaloy S, Holte H, Delabie J, Connors JM, Lansdorp PM, Ouyang Q, Lister TA, Davies AJ, Norton AJ, Muller-Hermelink HK, Ott G, Campo E, Montserrat E, Wilson WH, Jaffe ES, Simon R, Yang L, Powell J, Zhao H, Goldschmidt N, Chiorazzi M,

Staudt LM. 2004. Prediction of survival in follicular lymphoma based on molecular features of tumor-infiltrating immune cells. N Engl J Med 351:2159–2169.

Davis RJ. 2000. Signal transduction by the JNK group of MAP kinases. Cell 103:239–252.

Deng Y, Ren X, Yang L, Lin Y, Wu X. 2003. A JNK-dependent pathway is required for TNFalpha-induced apoptosis. Cell 115:61–70.

Dierks C, Grbic J, Zirlik K, Beigi R, Englund NP, Guo GR, Veelken H, Engelhardt M, Mertelsmann R, Kelleher JF, Schultz P, Warmuth M. 2007. Essential role of stromally induced hedgehog signaling in B-cell malignancies. Nat Med 13:944–951.

Ding J, Takano T, Gao S, Han W, Noda C, Yanagi S, Yamamura H. 2000. Syk is required for the activation of Akt survival pathway in B cells exposed to oxidative stress. J Biol Chem 275:30873–30877.

Du M, Diss TC, Xu C, Peng H, Isaacson PG, Pan L. 1996. Ongoing mutation in MALT lymphoma immunoglobulin gene suggests that antigen stimulation plays a role in the clonal expansion. Leukemia 10:1190–1197.

Dykstra M, Cherukuri A, Sohn HW, Tzeng SJ, Pierce SK. 2003. Location is everything: lipid rafts and immune cell signaling. Annu Rev Immunol 21:457–481.

Ehlich A, Schaal S, Gu H, Kitamura D, Muller W, Rajewsky K. 1993. Immunoglobulin heavy and light chain genes rearrange independently at early stages of B cell development. Cell 72: 695–704.

Elenitoba-Johnson KS, Jenson SD, Abbott RT, Palais RA, Bohling SD, Lin Z, Tripp S, Shami PJ, Wang LY, Coupland RW, Buckstein R, Perez-Ordonez B, Perkins SL, Dube ID, Lim MS. 2003. Involvement of multiple signaling pathways in follicular lymphoma transformation: p38-mitogen-activated protein kinase as a target for therapy. PNAS 100:7259–7264.

Fischer G, Kent SC, Joseph L, Green DR, Scott DW. 1994. Lymphoma models for B cell activation and tolerance. X. Anti-mu-mediated growth arrest and apoptosis of murine B cell lymphomas is prevented by the stabilization of myc. J Exp Med 179:221–228.

Flaswinkel H, Reth M. 1994. Dual role of the tyrosine activation motif of the Ig-alpha protein during signal transduction via the B cell antigen receptor. Embo J 13:83–89.

Fuentes-Panana EM, Bannish G, Monroe JG. 2004. Basal B-cell receptor signaling in B lymphocytes: Mechanisms of regulation and role in positive selection, differentiation, and peripheral survival. Immunol Rev 197:26–40.

Gatalica Z and Bing Z. 2005. Syk tyrosine kinase expression during multistep mammary carcinogenesis. Croat Med J 46:372–376.

Gold MR, Scheid MP, Santos L, Dang-Lawson M, Roth RA, Matsuuchi L, Duronio V, Krebs DL. 1999. The B cell antigen receptor activates the Akt (protein kinase B)/glycogen synthase kinase-3 signaling pathway via phosphatidylinositol 3-kinase. J Immunol 163: 1894–1905.

Gong Q, Ou Q, Ye S, Lee WP, Cornelius J, Diehl L, Lin WY, Hu Z, Lu Y, Chen Y, Wu Y, Meng YG, Gribling P, Lin Z, Nguyen K, Tran T, Zhang Y, Rosen H, Martin F, Chan AC. 2005. Importance of cellular microenvironment and circulatory dynamics in B cell immunotherapy. J Immunol 174:817–826.

Gottschalk AR, Joseph LJ, Quintans J. 1993. Differential induction of Egr-1 expression in WEHI-231 sublines does not correlate with apoptosis. Eur J Immunol 23:2011–2015.

Grande SM, Katz E, Crowley JE, Bernardini MS, Ross SR, Monroe JG. 2006. Cellular ITAM-containing proteins are oncoproteins in nonhematopoietic cells. Oncogene 25:2748–2757.

Grande SM, Bannish G, Fuentes-Panana EM, Katz E, Monroe JG. 2007. Tonic B-cell and viral ITAM signaling: Context is everything. Immunol Rev 218:214–234.

Gu H, Tarlinton D, Muller W, Rajewsky K, Forster I. 1991. Most peripheral B cells in mice are ligand selected. J Exp Med 173:1357–1371.

Guo YL, Baysal K, Kang B, Yang LJ, Williamson JR. 1998. Correlation between sustained c-Jun N-terminal protein kinase activation and apoptosis induced by tumor necrosis factor-alpha in rat mesangial cells. J Biol Chem 273:4027–4034.

Gupta N, Wollscheid B, Watts JD, Scheer B, Aebersold R, DeFranco AL. 2006. Quantitative proteomic analysis of B cell lipid rafts reveals that ezrin regulates antigen receptor-mediated lipid raft dynamics. Nat Immunol 7:625–633.

Gururajan M, Chui R, Karuppannan AK, Ke J, Jennings CD, Bondada S. 2005. c-Jun N-terminal kinase (JNK) is required for survival and proliferation of B-lymphoma cells. Blood 106: 1382–1391.

Gururajan M, Jennings CD, Bondada S. 2006. Cutting edge: constitutive B cell receptor signaling is critical for basal growth of B lymphoma. J Immunol 176:5715–5719.

Gururajan M, Dasu T, Shahidain S, Jennings CD, Robertson DA, Rangnekar VM, Bondada S. 2007. Spleen tyrosine kinase (Syk), a novel target of curcumin, is required for B lymphoma growth. J Immunol 178:111–121.

Gururajan M, Simmons A, Dasu T, Spear BT, Calulot C, Robertson DA, Wiest DL, Monroe JG, Bondada S. 2008. Early growth response gene-1 (Egr-1) is required for B cell development, proliferation and immune response. J Immunol 181:4590–4602.

Guyomard S, Salles G, Coudurier M, Rousset H, Coiffier B, Bienvenu J, Fabien N. 2003. Prevalence and pattern of antinuclear autoantibodies in 347 patients with non-Hodgkin's lymphoma. Br J Haematol 123:90–99.

Han SS, Chung ST, Robertson DA, Ranjan D, Bondada S. 1999. Curcumin causes the growth arrest and apoptosis of B cell lymphoma by downregulation of egr-1, c-myc, bcl-XL, NF-kappa B, and p53. Clin Immunol 93:152–161.

Hardy RR, Li YS, Allman D, Asano M, Gui M, Hayakawa K. 2000. B-cell commitment, development and selection. Immunol Rev 175:23–32.

Hermine O, Lefrère F, Bronowicki JP, Mariette X, Jondeau K, Eclache-Saudreau V, Delmas B, Valensi F, Cacoub P, Brechot C, Varet B, Troussard X. 2002. Regression of splenic lymphoma with villous lymphocytes after treatment of hepatitis C virus infection. N Engl J Med 347: 89–94.

Hess P, Pihan G, Sawyers CL, Flavell RA, Davis RJ. 2002. Survival signaling mediated by c-Jun NH(2)-terminal kinase in transformed B lymphoblasts. Nat Genet 32:201–205.

Hideshima T, Hayashi T, Chauhan D, Akiyama M, Richardson P, Anderson K. 2003. Biologic sequelae of c-Jun NH(2)-terminal kinase (JNK) activation in multiple myeloma cell lines. Oncogene 22:8797–8801.

Huang RP, Liu C, Fan Y, Mercola D, Adamson ED. 1995. Egr-1 negatively regulates human tumor cell growth via the DNA-binding domain. Cancer Res. 55:5054–5062.

Huang RP, Fan Y, de Belle I, Niemeyer C, Gottardis MM, Mercola D, Adamson ED. 1997. Decreased Egr-1 expression in human, mouse and rat mammary cells and tissue correlates with tumor formation. Int J Cancer 72:102–109.

Hutchcroft JE, Harrsion ML, Geahlen RL. 1991. B lymphocyte activation is accompanied by phosphorylation of a 72-kDa protein-tyrosine kinase. J Biol Chem 266:14846–14849.

Iavarone C, Catania A, Marinissen MJ, Visconti R, Acunzo M, Tarantino C, Carlomagno MS, Bruni CB, Gutkind JS, Chiariello M. 2003. The platelet-derived growth factor controls c-myc expression through a JNK- and AP-1-dependent signaling pathway. J Biol Chem 278: 50024–50030.

Iida S, Rao PH, Nallasivam P, Hibshoosh H, Butler M, Louie DC, Dyomin V, Ohno H, Chaganti RS, Dalla-Favera R. 1996. The t(9;14)(p13;q32) chromosomal translocation associated with lymphoplasmacytoid lymphoma involves the PAX-5 gene. Blood 88:4110–4117.

Irish JM, Czerwinski DK, Nolan GP, Levy R. 2006. Altered B cell receptor signaling kinetics distinguish human follicular lymphoma B cells from tumor infiltrating non-malignant B cells. Blood 108:3135–3142.

Isaacson PG. 1999. Mucosa-associated lymphoid tissue lymphoma. Semin Hematol 36:139–147.

Isaacson PG and Du M-Q. 2004. MALT lymphoma: From morphology to molecules. Nat Rev Cancer 4:644–653.

James JA, Smith MA, Court EL, Yip C, Ching Y, Willson C, Smith JG. 2003. An investigation of the effects of the MEK inhibitor U0126 on apoptosis in acute leukemia. Hematol J 4:427–432.

Janz S. 2006. Myc translocations in B cell and plasma cell neoplasms. DNA Repair 5:1213–1224.

Jonsson R, Nginamau E, Szyszko E, Brokstad KA. 2007. Role of B cells in Sjogren's syndrome– from benign lymphoproliferation to overt malignancy. Front Biosci 12:2159–2170.

Ke J, Gururajan M, Kumar A, Simmons A, Turcios L, Chelvarajan RL, Cohen DM, Wiest DL, Monroe JG, Bondada S. 2006. The role of MAP kinases in BCR induced down-regulation of Egr-1 in immature B lymphoma cells. J Biol Chem 281:39806–39818.

Kerr AH, James JA, Smith MA, Willson C, Court EL, Smith JG. 2003. An investigation of the MEK/ERK inhibitor U0126 in acute myeloid leukemia. Ann N Y Acad Sci 1010:86–89.

Kitamura D, Roes J, Kuhn R, Rajewsky K. 1991. A B cell-deficient mouse by targeted disruption of the membrane exon of the immunoglobulin mu chain gene. Nature 350:423–426.

Kotani A, Kakazu N, Tsuruyama T, Okazaki IM, Muramatsu M, Kinoshita K, Nagaoka H, Yabe D, Honjo T. 2007. Activation-induced cytidine deaminase (AID) promotes B cell lymphomagenesis in Emu-cmyc transgenic mice. PNAS 104:1616–1620.

Kraus M, Alimzhanov MB, Rajewsky N, Rajewsky K.. 2004. Survival of resting mature B lymphocytes depends on BCR signaling via the Igalpha/beta heterodimer. Cell 117:787–800.

Kuan CY, Yang DD, Samanta Roy DR, Davis RJ, Rakic P, Flavell RA. 1999. The Jnk1 and Jnk2 protein kinases are required for regional specific apoptosis during early brain development. Neuron 22:667–676.

Kuppers R. 2005. Mechanisms of B-cell lymphoma pathogenesis. Nat Rev Cancer 5:251–262.

Kuppers R and Dalla-Favera R. 2001. Mechanisms of chromosomal translocations in B cell lymphomas. Oncogene 20:5580–5594.

Kuppers R, Klein U, Hansmann M-L, Rajewsky K. 1999. Cellular origin of human B-cell lymphomas. N Engl J Med 341:1520–1529.

Lam KP, Kuhn R, Rajewsky K. 1997. In vivo ablation of surface immunoglobulin on mature B cells by inducible gene targeting results in rapid cell death. Cell 90:1073–1083.

Lamb JA, Ventura JJ, Hess P, Flavell RA, Davis RJ. 2003. JunD mediates survival signaling by the JNK signal transduction pathway. Mol Cell 11:1479–1489.

Landau D-A, Saadoun D, Calabrese LH, Cacoub P. 2007. The pathophysiology of HCV induced B-cell clonal disorders. Autoimmun Rev 6:581–587.

Le-Niculescu H, Bonfoco E, Kasuya Y, Claret FX, Green DR, Karin M. 1999. Withdrawal of survival factors results in activation of the JNK pathway in neuronal cells leading to Fas ligand induction and cell death. Mol Cell Biol 19:751–763.

Lee SL, Tourtellotte LC, Wesselschmidt RL, Milbrandt J. 1995. Growth and differentiation proceeds normally in cells deficient in the immediate early gene NGFI-A. J Biol Chem 270:9971–9977.

Lee SY, Reichlin A, Santana A, Sokol KA, Nussenzweig MC, Choi Y. 1997. TRAF2 is essential for JNK but not NF-kappaB activation and regulates lymphocyte proliferation and survival. Immunity 7:703–713.

Lenze D, Berg E, Volkmer-Engert R, Weiser AA, Greiner A, Knörr-Wittmann C, Anagnostopoulos I, Stein H, Hummel M. 2006. Influence of antigen on the development of MALT lymphoma. Blood 107:1141–1148.

Leventaki V, Drakos E, Medeiros LJ, Lim MS, Elenitoba-Johnson KS, Claret FX, Rassidakis GZ. 2007. NPM-ALK oncogenic kinase promotes cell-cycle progression through activation of JNK/cJun signaling in anaplastic large-cell lymphoma. Blood 110:1621–1630.

Liu C, Rangnekar VM, Adamson E, Mercola D. 1998. Suppression of growth and transformation and induction of apoptosis by EGR-1. Cancer Gene Ther. 5:3–28.

Lizundia R, Chaussepied M, Huerre M, Werling D, Di Santo JP, Langsley G. 2006. c-Jun NH2-terminal kinase/c-Jun signaling promotes survival and metastasis of B lymphocytes transformed by Theileria. Cancer Res 66:6105–6110.

Lovec H, Grzeschiczek A, Kowalski MB, Moroy T. 1994. Cyclin D1/bcl-1 cooperates with myc genes in the generation of B-cell lymphoma in transgenic mice. Embo J 13:3487–3495.

Lu S-P, Lin Feng M-H, Huang H-L, Huang Y-C, Tsou W-I, Lai M-Z. 2007. Reactive oxygen species promote raft formation in T lymphocytes. Free Radic Biol Med 42:936–944.

Machida K, Cheng KTH, Pavio N, Sung VMH, Lai MMC. 2005. Hepatitis C Virus E2-CD81 Interaction induces hypermutation of the immunoglobulin gene in B cells. J Virol 79: 8079–8089.

Madden SL, Cook DM, Morris JF, Gashler A, Sukhatme VP, Rauscher FJ, III. 1991. Transcriptional repression mediated by the WT1 Wilms tumor gene product. Science 253:1550–1553.

Maloney DG, Brown S, Czerwinski DK, Liles TM, Hart SM, Miller RA, Levy R. 1992. Monoclonal anti-idiotype antibody therapy of B-cell lymphoma: The addition of a short course of chemotherapy does not interfere with the antitumor effect nor prevent the emergence of idiotype-negative variant cells. Blood 80:1502–1510.

Mandik-Nayak L, Seo SJ, Sokol C, Potts KM, Bui A, Erikson J. 1999. MRL-lpr/lpr mice exhibit a defect in maintaining developmental arrest and follicular exclusion of anti-double-stranded DNA B cells. J Exp Med 189:1799–1814.

Manning AM and Davis RJ. 2003. Targeting JNK for therapeutic benefit: from junk to gold? Nat Rev Drug Discov 2:554–565.

Martin F and Chan AC. 2006. B cell immunobiology in disease: evolving concepts from the clinic. Annu Rev Immunol 24:467–496.

Mathas S, Hinz M, Anagnostopoulos I, Krappmann D, Lietz A, Jundt F, Bommert K, Mechta-Grigoriou F, Stein H, Dörken B, Scheidereit C. 2002. Aberrantly expressed c-Jun and JunB are a hallmark of Hodgkin lymphoma cells, stimulate proliferation and synergize with NF-kappa B. Embo J 21:4104–4113.

McMahon SB and Monroe JG. 1995. Activation of the p21ras pathway couples antigen receptor stimulation to induction of the primary response gene egr-1 in B lymphocytes. J Exp Med 181:417–422.

McMahon SB and Monroe JG. 1996. The role of early growth response gene 1 (egr-1) in regulation of the immune response. J Leukoc Biol 60:159–166.

Merino R, Grillot DA, Simonian PL, Muthukkumar S, Fanslow WC, Bondada S, Núñez G. 1995. Modulation of anti-IgM-induced B cell apoptosis by Bcl-xL and CD40 in WEHI-231 cells. Dissociation from cell cycle arrest and dependence on the avidity of the antibody-IgM receptor interaction. J Immunol 155:3830–3838.

Messmer BT, Albesiano E, Efremov DG, Ghiotto F, Allen SL, Kolitz J, Foa R, Damle RN, Fais F, Messmer D, Rai KR, Ferrarini M, Chiorazzi N. 2004. Multiple distinct sets of stereotyped antigen receptors Indicate a role for antigen in promoting chronic lymphocytic leukemia. J Exp Med 200:519–525.

Mielke K and Herdegen T. 2000. JNK and p38 stress kinases – degenerative effectors of signal-transduction-cascades in the nervous system. Prog Neurobiol 61:45–60.

Monroe JG. 2006. ITAM-mediated tonic signalling through pre-BCR and BCR complexes. Nat Rev Immunol 6:283–294.

Morgner A, Thiede C, Bayerdörffer E, Alpen B, Wündisch T, Neubauer A, Stolte M. 2001. Long-term follow-up of gastric MALT lymphoma after H. pylori eradication. Curr Gastroenterol Rep 3:516–522.

Morrison AM, Jager U, Chott A, Schebesta M, Haas OA, Busslinger M. 1998. Deregulated PAX-5 transcription from a translocated IgH promoter in marginal zone lymphoma. Blood 92: 3865–3878.

Muthukkumar S, Han SS, Rangnekar VM, Bondada S. 1997. Role of Egr-1 gene expression in B cell receptor-induced apoptosis in an immature B cell lymphoma. J Biol Chem 272: 27987–27993.

Nemazee D and Weigert M. 2000. Revising B cell receptors. J Exp Med 191:1813–1818.

Ng AK. 2007. Diffuse large B-cell lymphoma. Semin Radiat Oncol 17:169–175.

Niiro H and Clark EA. 2002. Regulation of B-cell fate by antigen-receptor signals. Nat Rev Immunol 2:945–956.

Ozes ON, Mayo LD, Gustin JA, Pfeffer SR, Pfeffer LM, Donner DB. 1999. NF-kappaB activation by tumour necrosis factor requires the Akt serine-threonine kinase. Nature 401: 82–85.

Parsonnet J and Isaacson PG. 2004. Bacterial infection and MALT lymphoma. N Engl J Med 350:213–215.

Parsonnet J, Hansen S, Rodriguez L, Gelb AB, Warnke RA, Jellum E, Orentreich N, Vogelman JH, Friedman GD. 1994. Helicobacter pylori infection and gastric lymphoma. N Engl J Med 330:1267–1271.

Pasqualucci L, Kitaura Y, Gu H, Dalla-Favera R. 2006. PKA-mediated phosphorylation regulates the function of activation-induced deaminase (AID) in B cells. PNAS 103:395–400.

Pasqualucci L, Migliazza A, Basso K, Houldsworth J, Chaganti RS, Dalla-Favera R. 2003. Mutations of the BCL6 proto-oncogene disrupt its negative autoregulation in diffuse large B-cell lymphoma. Blood 101:2914–2923.

Pasqualucci L, Bhagat G, Jankovic M, Compagno M, Smith P, Muramatsu M, Honjo T, Morse HC 3rd, Nussenzweig MC, Dalla-Favera R. 2008. AID is required for germinal center-derived lymphomagenesis. Nat Genet 40:108–112.

Peng SL. 2007. Immune regulation by Foxo transcription factors. Autoimmunity 40:462–469.

Platanias LC. 2003. Map kinase signaling pathways and hematologic malignancies. Blood 101:4667–4679.

Pogue SL, Kurosaki T, Bolen J, Herbst R. 2000. B cell antigen receptor-induced activation of Akt promotes B cell survival and is dependent on Syk kinase. J Immunol 165:1300–1306.

Pridans C, Holmes ML, Polli M, Wettenhall JM, Dakic A, Corcoran LM, Smyth GK, Nutt SL. 2008. Identification of Pax5 target genes in early B cell differentiation. J Immunol 180:1719–1728.

Rajewsky K. 1992. Early and late B-cell development in the mouse. Curr Opin Immunol 4:171–176.

Rajewsky K. 1996. Clonal selection and learning in the antibody system. Nature 381:751–758.

Refaeli Y, Young RM, Turner BC, Duda J, Field KA, Bishop JM. 2008. The B cell antigen receptor and overexpression of MYC can cooperate in the genesis of B cell lymphomas. PLoS Biol 6:e152.

Reth M, Hombach J, Wienands J, Campbell KS, Chien N, Justement LB, Cambier JC. 1991. The B-cell antigen receptor complex. Immunol Today 12:196–201.

Rolli V, Gallwitz M, Wossning T, Flemming A, Schamel WW, Zürn C, Reth M. 2002. Amplification of B cell antigen receptor signaling by a Syk/ITAM positive feedback loop. Mol Cell 10:1057–1069.

Romashkova JA and Makarov SS. 1999. NF-kappaB is a target of AKT in anti-apoptotic PDGF signalling. Nature 401:86–90.

Sabapathy K, Hochedlinger K, Nam SY, Bauer A, Karin M, Wagner EF. 2004. Distinct roles for JNK1 and JNK2 in regulating JNK activity and c-Jun-dependent cell proliferation. Molecular Cell 15:713–725.

Sakata N, Patel HR, Terada N, Aruffo A, Johnson GL, Gelfand EW. 1995. Selective activation of c-Jun kinase mitogen-activated protein kinase by CD40 on human B cells. J Biol Chem 270:30823–30828.

Sanchez-Beato M, Sanchez-Aguilera A, Piris MA. 2003. Cell cycle deregulation in B-cell lymphomas. Blood 101:1220–1235.

Sarbassov DD, Guertin DA, Ali SM, Sabatini DM. 2005. Phosphorylation and regulation of Akt/PKB by the rictor-mTOR complex. Science 307:1098–1101.

Schreiber M, Kolbus A, Piu F, Szabowski A, Möhle-Steinlein U, Tian J, Karin M, Angel P, Wagner EF. 1999. Control of cell cycle progression by c-Jun is p53 dependent. Genes Dev 13:607–619.

Seth A, Gupta S, Davis RJ. 1993. Cell cycle regulation of the c-Myc transcriptional activation domain. Mol Cell Biol 13:4125–4136.

Seyfert VL, Sukhatme VP, Monroe JG. 1989. Differential expression of a zinc finger-encoding gene in response to positive versus negative signaling through receptor immunoglobulin in murine B lymphocytes. Mol Cell Biol 9:2083–2088.

Shaulian E and Karin M. 2002. AP-1 as a regulator of cell life and death. Nat Cell Biol 4:E131–136.

Shimada K, Nakamura M, Ishida E, Kishi M, Yonehara S, Konishi N. 2003. c-Jun NH2-terminal kinase-dependent Fas activation contributes to etoposide-induced apoptosis in p53-mutated prostate cancer cells. Prostate 55:265–280.

Shishodia S, Chaturvedi MM, Aggarwal BB. 2007. Role of curcumin in cancer therapy. Curr Probl Cancer 31:243–305.

Singh DK, Kumar D, Siddiqui Z, Basu SK, Kumar V, Rao KVS. 2005a. The strength of receptor signaling is centrally controlled through a cooperative loop between Ca2+ and an oxidant signal. Cell 121:281.

Singh H, Medina KL, Pongubala JMR. 2005b. Gene regulatory networks special feature: Contingent gene regulatory networks and B cell fate specification. PNAS 102:4949–4953.

Singh H, Pongubala JM, Medina KL. 2007. Gene regulatory networks that orchestrate the development of B lymphocyte precursors. Adv Exp Med Biol 596:57–62.

Smith SH and Reth M. 2004. Perspectives on the nature of BCR-mediated survival signals. Mol Cell 14:696–697.

Smith E and Sigvardsson M. 2004. The roles of transcription factors in B lymphocyte commitment, development, and transformation. J Leukoc Biol 75:973–981.

Staber PB, Linkesch W, Zauner D, Beham-Schmid C, Guelly C, Schauer S, Sill H, Hoefler G. 2004. Common alterations in gene expression and increased proliferation in recurrent acute myeloid leukemia. Oncogene 23:894–904.

Su TT, Guo B, Wei B, Braun J, Rawlings DJ. 2004. Signaling in transitional type 2 B cells is critical for peripheral B-cell development. Immunol Rev 197:161–178.

Suarez F, Lefrere F, Besson C, Hermine O. 2007. Splenic lymphoma with villous lymphocytes, mixed cryoglobulinemia and HCV infection: Deciphering the role of HCV in B-cell lymphomagenesis. Dig Liver Dis 39 Suppl 1:S32–37.

Sun Y, Huang PL, Li JJ, Huang YQ, Zhang L, Lee-Huang S. 2001. Anti-HIV agent MAP30 modulates the expression profile of viral and cellular genes for proliferation and apoptosis in AIDS-related lymphoma cells infected with Kaposi's sarcoma-associated virus. Biochem Biophys Res Commun 287:983–994.

Takada Y and Aggarwal BB. 2004. TNF activates Syk protein tyrosine kinase leading to TNF-induced MAPK activation, NF-kappaB activation, and apoptosis. J Immunol 173: 1066–1077.

Takano T, Sada K, Yamamura H. 2002. Role of protein-tyrosine kinase syk in oxidative stress signaling in B cells. Antioxid Redox Signal 4:533–541.

Thiede C, Wündisch T, Neubauer B, Alpen B, Morgner A, Ritter M, Ehninger G, Stolte M, Bayerdörffer E, Neubauer A. 2000. Eradication of Helicobacter pylori and stability of remissions in low-grade gastric B-cell lymphomas of the mucosa-associated lymphoid tissue: results of an ongoing multicenter trial. Recent Results Cancer Res 156:125–133.

Tolar P, Sohn HW, Pierce SK. 2005. The initiation of antigen-induced B cell antigen receptor signaling viewed in living cells by fluorescence resonance energy transfer. Nat Immunol 6:1168–1176.

Torres RM, Flaswinkel H, Reth M, Rajewsky K. 1996. Aberrant B cell development and immune response in mice with a compromised BCR complex. Science 272:1804–1808.

Tournier C, Dong C, Turner TK, Jones SN, Flavell RA, Davis RJ. 2001. MKK7 is an essential component of the JNK signal transduction pathway activated by proinflammatory cytokines. Genes Dev 15:1419–1426.

Toyama T, Iwase H, Yamashita H, Hara Y, Omoto Y, Sugiura H, Zhang Z, Fujii Y. 2003. Reduced expression of the Syk gene is correlated with poor prognosis in human breast cancer. Cancer Lett 189:97–102.

Turner M, Mee PJ, Costello PS, Williams O, Price AA, Duddy LP, Furlong MT, Geahlen RL, Tybulewicz VL. 1995. Perinatal lethality and blocked B-cell development in mice lacking the tyrosine kinase Syk. Nature 378:298–302.

Turner M, Gulbranson-Judge A, Quinn ME, Walters AE, MacLennan IC, Tybulewicz VL. 1997. Syk tyrosine kinase is required for the positive selection of immature B cells into the recirculating B cell pool. J Exp Med 186:2013–2021.

Turner M, Schweighoffer E, Colucci F, Di Santo JP, Tybulewicz VL. 2000. Tyrosine kinase SYK: essential functions for immunoreceptor signalling. Immunol Today 21:148–154.

Vanasse GJ, Concannon P, Willerford DM. 1999. Regulated genomic instability and neoplasia in the lymphoid lineage. Blood 94:3997–4010.

Villamarin S, Ferrer-Miralles N, Mansilla S, Priebe W, Portugal J. 2002. Induction of G(2)/M arrest and inhibition of c-myc and p53 transcription by WP631 in Jurkat T lymphocytes. Biochem Pharmacol 63:1251–1258.

Wada T and Penninger JM. 2004. Stress kinase MKK7: Savior of cell cycle arrest and cellular senescence. Cell Cycle 3:577–579.

Wang X, Li Z, Naganuma A, Ye BH. 2002. Negative autoregulation of BCL-6 is bypassed by genetic alterations in diffuse large B cell lymphomas. Proc Natl Acad Sci U S A 99: 15018–15023.

Wang L, Devarajan E, He J, Reddy SP, Dai JL. 2005. Transcription repressor activity of spleen tyrosine kinase mediates breast tumor suppression. Cancer Res 65:10289–10297.

Wardemann H, Yurasov S, Schaefer A, Young JW, Meffre E, Nussenzweig MC. 2003. Predominant autoantibody production by early human B cell precursors. Science 301:1374–1377.

Weston CR and Davis RJ. 2002. The JNK signal transduction pathway. Curr Opin Genet Dev 12:14–21.

Wossning T, Herzog S, Köhler F, Meixlsperger S, Kulathu Y, Mittler G, Abe A, Fuchs U, Borkhardt A, Jumaa H. 2006. Deregulated Syk inhibits differentiation and induces growth factor-independent proliferation of pre-B cells. J Exp Med 203:2829–2840.

Wu M, Arsura M, Bellas RE, FitzGerald MJ, Lee H, Schauer SL, Sherr DH, Sonenshein GE. 1996. Inhibition of c-myc expression induces apoptosis of WEHI 231 murine B cells. Mol Cell Biol 16:5015–5025.

Wu HJ, Venkataraman C, Estus S, Dong C, Davis RJ, Flavell RA, Bondada S. 2001. Positive signaling through CD72 induces mitogen-activated protein kinase activation and synergizes with B cell receptor signals to induce X-linked immunodeficiency B cell proliferation. J Immunol 167:1263–1273.

Xie P, Hostager BS, Bishop GA. 2004. Requirement for TRAF3 in Signaling by LMP1 But Not CD40 in B Lymphocytes. J Exp Med 199:661–671.

Xu X, Heidenreich O, Kitajima I, McGuire K, Li Q, Su B, Nerenberg M. 1996. Constitutively activated JNK is associated with HTLV-1 mediated tumorigenesis. Oncogene 13:135–142.

Yang DD, Conze D, Whitmarsh AJ, Barrett T, Davis RJ, Rincón M, Flavell RA. 1998. Differentiation of CD4+ T cells to Th1 cells requires MAP kinase JNK2. Immunity 9:575–585.

Yu C, Minemoto Y, Zhang J, Liu J, Tang F, Bui TN, Xiang J, Lin A. 2004. JNK suppresses apoptosis via phosphorylation of the proapoptotic Bcl-2 family protein BAD. Mol Cell 13:329–340.

Yuan Y, Mendez R, Sahin A, Dai JL. 2001. Hypermethylation leads to silencing of the SYK gene in human breast cancer. Cancer Res 61:5558–5561.

Zangani MM, Frøyland M, Qiu GY, Meza-Zepeda LA, Kutok JL, Thompson KM, Munthe LA, Bogen B. 2007. Lymphomas can develop from B cells chronically helped by idiotype-specific T cells. J Exp Med 204:1181–1191.

Zeyda M and Stulnig TM. 2006. Lipid Rafts & Co.: An integrated model of membrane organization in T cell activation. Prog Lipid Res 45:187–202.

Zignego AL, Giannini C, Ferri C. 2007. Hepatitis C virus-related lymphoproliferative disorders: An overview. World J Gastroenterol 13:2467–2478.

Chapter 18
Modulation of Philadelphia Chromosome-Positive Hematological Malignancies by the Bone Marrow Microenvironment

Lin Wang, Heather O'Leary, and Laura F. Gibson

Cast of Characters

Hematological malignancies often have cytogenetically distinct chromosomal translocations, resulting in fusion proteins that lead to dysregulation of specific signaling pathways and distinct phenotypic outcomes. The constitutively active Bcr-Abl kinase defines the underlying cause for several forms of leukemia in humans. Due to different breakpoints in the *Bcr* gene, the reciprocal translocation between chromosomes 9 and 22 (the Philadelphia chromosome; (Ph+) (Nowell, 2007; Koretzky, 2007)) generates proto-oncoproteins of variable size. The p210 Bcr-Abl fusion protein is predominantly associated with CML during the chronic phase, but can also be detected in acute lymphoblastic leukemia (ALL) during blast transformation. In contrast, the p185 Bcr-Abl fusion protein is most often associated with the generation of de novo B-lineage ALL, but also has been shown to be expressed in rare cases of T-cell ALL, mast cell ALL, as well as in endothelial cells derived from patients with CML. While high, constitutive Abl kinase activity is thought to be the driving force in initiation and progression of leukemic disease, the bone marrow microenvironment also plays a pivotal role in maintaining Ph+ leukemic stem cells. In the following chapter we discuss the interplay between expression of the Bcr-Abl fusion protein and bone marrow microenvironment-derived cues and their collective influence on leukemogenesis.

Introduction

For almost all patients with chronic myelogenous leukemia (CML), generation of the constitutively active, non-receptor tyrosine kinase Bcr-Abl (Ph+) fusion protein is the hallmark event that targets leukemic transformation of a primitive hematopoietic cell (Nowell, 2007; Koretzky, 2007). As such, CML provides a reasonable

L.F. Gibson (✉)
Mary Babb Randolph Cancer Center, West Virginia University Health Sciences Center, Morgantown WV
e-mail: lgibson@hsc.wvu.edu

A. Thomas-Tikhonenko (ed.), *Cancer Genome and Tumor Microenvironment*,
DOI 10.1007/978-1-4419-0711-0_18, © Springer Science+Business Media, LLC 2010

context in which to consider the mechanisms by which changes inherent to a tumor cell converge with signals from its surrounding microenvironment to collectively define the nature of the disease. CML is characterized by the presence of a t(9;22) chromosomal translocation by which dysregulated Bcr-Abl kinase activity is conferred via oligomerization of the truncated Bcr protein (Tauchi et al., 1997; Fan et al., 2003; Hantschel and Superti-Furga, 2004). Dependent upon the specific breakpoint in the *Bcr* and *Abl* genes two forms of the fusion product are generated, indicated as p210 or p185/p190. Subsequently, Abl kinase activity plays a pivotal role in initiating and maintaining the disease throughout its chronic phase to blast crisis (He et al., 2002). While the molecular basis for Bcr–Abl promotion of the transition of CML chronic phase to blast crisis is still under investigation, this specific aspect of the disease serves as an elegant paradigm for understanding how hematopoietic cells with specific "hard-wired" mutations evolve to acquire the capacity for self-renewal (Melo and Barnes, 2007; Savona and Talpaz, 2008). In particular, this chapter discusses how the marrow microenvironment may modulate the leukemic stem cell properties of unique tumors that result from inherent genetic alterations.

Alterations of Adhesion Molecule Expression Are Functionally Distinct in CML Chronic Phase and Blast Crisis

Bone marrow stromal cells express diverse adhesion molecules, cytokines, and chemokines that position them to interact with both normal hematopoietic cells as well as leukemic cells that share receptor expression (Fig. 18.1). Additionally, components of the extracellular matrix (ECM) in the marrow microenvironment provide signaling cues to healthy and transformed hematopoietic stem and progenitor cells. Consequently, increased expression or activity of integrins, chemokine receptors, or receptors for ECM that occur downstream of Bcr-Abl expression increases the magnitude of response to the microenvironment. This response can be manifested as increased tumor stem cell survival or proliferation, or maintenance of a tumor stem cell phenotype.

As compared to the well-documented roles of Bcr-Abl oncoprotein in leukemic cell proliferation and survival, its impact on Ph+ leukemic-stromal cell interactions, leukemic cell migration, and cytoskeletal remodeling are less well defined. There are several observations relevant to the anti-apoptotic effects of the Bcr-Abl fusion protein (Stoklosa et al., 2008; Deininger et al., 2000a), and the regulatory effects on mitotic/cell cycle progression in Bcr-Abl-expressing leukemic cells (Dierov et al., 2004; Gordon et al., 1987). Importantly, the influence of the Bcr-Abl oncoprotein on leukemic cell adhesive and migratory behaviors is distinct during the chronic phase and blast crisis. Many adhesion molecules previously characterized as being expressed on non-hematopoietic tissues, or uniquely expressed during embryogenesis, are also expressed on Bcr-Abl positive leukemic cells. This suggests a potential role of this oncoprotein in leukemic transformation of Ph+ CML to acute myeloid

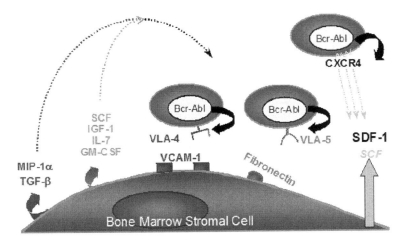

Fig. 18.1 Bone marrow microenvironment interaction with tumor cells is mediated by both physical and soluble factors. Tumor cells that either metastasize to, or initiate, in bone marrow microenvironment niches express diverse cytokine and chemokine receptors that position them to respond to stromal cell-derived cues. Expression of the Bcr-Abl fusion gene has been associated with alterations of expression and/or activity of VLA-4, VLA-5, CXCR4, and integrin 6 (not shown) as one means by which constitutive kinase activity alters the capacity of Ph+ hematopoietic tumors to respond to microenvironment signals

or lymphoblastic leukemias, reflected in part by a "stem cell like" phenotype. Based on their unique qualities, cells in chronic or blast crisis will be considered separately when appropriate.

Diminished Adhesion Molecule Expression and Increased Migratory Capacity During the Indolent, Chronic Phase of CML (CML-CP)

Dysregulated Bcr-Abl kinase, and the subsequent perturbation of a variety of cell signaling pathways, dramatically alters the molecules that physically anchor hematopoietic cells to the marrow microenvironment. A large body of literature indicates decreased adhesion molecule expression, increased migratory capacity, and dysregulated matrix protease expression during the early phase of the disease (Gordon et al., 1987; Renshaw et al., 1995; Zhao et al., 2001; Ramaraj et al., 2004; Jongen-Lavrencic et al., 2005; Kronenwett et al., 2005; Wertheim et al., 2002b). Although the mechanisms underlying increased detachment of leukemic cells from the marrow matrix remain elusive, these observations are consistent with the heavy tumor burden manifested as hyperleukocytosis and splenic enlargement during the chronic phase of CML. Egress of Ph+ leukemic cells from marrow niches in CML-CP has been reported to result from decreased α4/β1 (VLA-4) or α5/β1 integrin

(VLA-5) expression and affinity (Lundell et al., 1996; Bhatia and Verfaillie, 1998; Bhatia et al., 1995; Bhatia et al., 1996), enhanced MMP expression (Kronenwett et al., 2005; Sun et al., 2008), increased cell motility, or interruption of the CXCL12 (SDF-1)/CXCR4 signaling axis (Salgia et al., 1997; Ptasznik et al., 2002). In addition, diminished expression of ICAM-1, P-Selectin, L-Selectin, Plakoglobulin, and CCL-7 have also been reported (Jongen-Lavrencic et al., 2005; Kronenwett et al., 2005; Pelletier et al., 2004). Of note, the previously mentioned observations were largely drawn from experiments utilizing either samples collected from patients with CML-CP, or during prolonged latency of CML-like myeloproliferative diseases.

Additional data have been derived from cells induced to a transformed phenotype by retroviral-mediated Bcr-Abl transduction or Bcr-Abl transgene expression. In general, the role of Bcr-Abl in cellular functions including adhesion and migration during CML-CP is opposite to its normal counterpart c-Abl (including the Drosophila Abl or D-Abl and the Abl-related gene product, Arg). Genetic ablation of c-Abl and Arg, or chemical inhibition of their activities with Imatinib mesylate (referred to throughout as Imatinib), results in decreased cell adhesion and increased cell migration (Kain and Klemke, 2001; Frasca et al., 2001), and enforced expression of Abl or Arg abrogate the inhibitory effects on cell migration (Kain and Klemke, 2001). These reports suggest an essential role of the Abl family of non-receptor tyrosine kinases in mediating anchorage of cells to the stromal matrix (Hernandez et al., 2004). The opposing role of Bcr-Abl to its normal counterparts, in terms of cell adhesion and migration, raises the possibility that formation of the chimeric Bcr-Abl protein may serve as a dominant-negative form of Abl, competitively acting on normal Abl partner proteins during the initiation of CML at its early, indolent phase. These opposing functions of Abl and Bcr-Abl are consistent with the complexity of understanding oncoprotein function in general. Further, they prompt us to consider how these genetic alterations may position Ph+ leukemic cells to respond uniquely to the microenvironment cues in the context of adhesion.

Enhanced Adhesion and Decreased Migratory Molecule Expression During the Aggressive, Blast Crisis Phase of CML (CML-BC)

Enhanced adhesion and firm binding of Ph+ leukemic cells to the marrow stroma are thought to occur during CML-BC, coincident with an acute transformation of the indolent to a more aggressive leukemic stem cell (LSC) state. Early reports indicate that Bcr-Abl enhances VLA-4 and VLA-5 integrin function (Bazzoni et al., 1996), with introduction of Bcr-Abl into Mo7e, 32D, or BaF/3 hematopoietic cells promoting leukemic cell binding to immobilized fibronectin and VCAM-1 (Bazzoni et al., 1996). Although these observations were not directly attributed to increased expression of integrins on leukemic cells, this observation is consistent with a functional alteration, correlated with Bcr-Abl kinase, that drives abnormal cytoskeletal remodeling, integrin clustering, and enhanced cell adhesion in cells with sustained expression of the Bcr-Abl chimeric protein (Li et al., 2007c). Heightened integrin α6 activity is observed in BV173, an acute lymphoblast leukemia derived from blast crisis of CML (Deininger et al., 2000b). Increased α6 integrin expression associated with Bcr-Abl kinase activity is reduced nearly 20-fold when BV173 cells are exposed to the tyrosine kinase inhibitor STI-571(Imatinib) connecting Bcr-Abl activity to downstream integrin expression (Deininger et al., 2000b). In the 32D/Bcr-Abl model, increased integrin β1 expression is present on the surface of transformed cells and contributes to increased binding to fibronectin, collagen type I, and bone marrow stromal cells (Fierro et al., 2008). Collectively, the work from several outstanding groups suggests diverse consequences of sustained Bcr-Abl expression on integrin expression and function. These changes provide the potential for Ph+ tumor cells to have amplified capacity to respond to stromal cell signals that are initiated by physical interaction.

Enhanced attachment of leukemic progenitors to marrow matrix at CML-BC is also associated with a decreased expression of CXCR4, or CCL9 (Geay et al., 2005; Iotti et al., 2007). Reduced response to CXCL12 is also demonstrated by cells subsequent to ECM attachment (Salgia et al., 1999). Imatinib treatment of CD34+ cells from patients in blast crisis markedly reverses the inhibitory effect of Bcr-Abl on CXCR4 mRNA and protein expression (Geay et al., 2005). A functional connection between increased integrin expression and diminished CXCL12/CXCR4 signaling has also been recently revealed (Chen et al., 2008). In CD34+ cells collected from CML-BC patients, Bcr-Abl increased expression of the β2 integrin LFA-1 (Chen et al., 2008), and this increase correlated with a complete loss of responsiveness to CXCL12, characterized by diminished inside-out signaling involving CXCR4 and the Src family kinase Lyn (Chen et al., 2008).

Dysregulated cell adhesion and migration during CML-BC are also associated with modified cytoskeletal actin re-organization in leukemic blasts. Increased adhesion of α5/β1 integrin to fibronectin is facilitated by the physical interaction between the Bcr-Abl C-terminal actin-binding domain and F-actin (Wertheim et al., 2003). The importance of this interaction was emphasized by the observation that p190 Bcr-Abl transgenic mice demonstrate latency that was markedly prolonged, with development of myeloproliferative disease significantly decreased, when the C-terminal F-actin-binding domain is deleted (Heisterkamp et al., 2000). Intriguingly, Bcr-Abl-induced immobilization and anchoring of leukemic blasts to the marrow substratum are not directly correlated to its kinase activity (Wertheim et al., 2002a). Expression of an inactive p210 mutant in leukemic blasts, or Imatinib treatment of Meg-01 cells that express functional p210, does not result in abrogation of adhesion (Wertheim et al., 2002a). These observations support the notion that additional mechanism(s), independent of Bcr-Abl kinase activity, modulate adhesion. Alternatively, sustained Bcr-Abl kinase activity may result in stable modifications that promote altered interaction with elements of the marrow microenvironment, even when Bcr-Abl kinase activity is blunted. The potential role of cadherin family proteins as mediators of cell–cell interactions, with specific emphasis on Ph+ hematological malignancies, is considered in the following section.

Expression of the Cadherin Family of Proteins by Diverse Cell Types

VE-cadherin expression in non-endothelial cells has been previously identified and characterized in cytotrophoblast stem cells and was shown to be required for successful endovascular invasion and normal placentation (Zhou et al., 1997; Hendrix et al., 2001; Hendrix et al., 2003; Hess et al., 2006). Subsequently, Mary Hendrix et al. (Hendrix et al., 2001) reported that VE-cadherin was expressed in highly aggressive melanoma and contributed to vascular mimicry. Notable are the observations that gestational trophoblastic neoplasia and aggressive melanoma are highly metastatic with frequent central nervous system involvement (Rustin et al., 1989; Khuntia et al., 2006). High-risk refractory gestational trophoblastic neoplasia was reported to have a approximately 45–54% brain invasion (Rustin et al., 1989; Khuntia et al., 2006; Pesce et al., 1999; Soper, 1990) and highly aggressive melanoma accounts for 10–15% of multifocal metastases in the central nervous system (CNS) (Khuntia et al., 2006). It is also widely recognized that, as compared to acute non-lymphoblastic leukemia (ANLL), non-Hodgkin's lymphoma or Hodgkin's lymphoma, acute lymphoblastic leukemia (ALL) is clinically manifested with a much higher frequency of CNS involvement. Because non-endothelial cells with VE-cadherin expression identified so far share a common clinical feature, CNS involvement, it is tempting to speculate that VE-cadherin expression plays an important role in mediating invasion of the CNS microenvironment. As such, Bcr-Abl induction of signals that stabilize VE-cadherin may be relevant in several microenvironment contexts, with discussion of the bone marrow as our primary site of focus.

In the marrow microenvironment, endosteal osteoblasts and sinusoidal vascular endothelial cells constitute two types of specialized niches for the maintenance of primitive hematopoietic stem cells (HSCs) (Zhang et al., 2003; Calvi et al., 2003; Kiel et al., 2005). Accordingly, the N-cadherin+ osteoblast niche and VE-cadherin+ vascular niche retain N-cadherin+ or VE-cadherin+ HSCs through homotypic interactions (Haug et al., 2008). While N-cadherin and VE-cadherin may be simultaneously expressed on vascular endothelial cells (Navarro et al., 1998; Luo and Radice, 2005), expression of both types of cadherin molecules was previously thought to be only on restricted tissue types including osteoblasts, endothelial cells, and neural tissues. However, p190 (referred to by some investigators as p185) Bcr-Abl transgenic lymphoblastic leukemic cells unexpectedly express N-cadherin molecules (Zhang et al., 2007). The N-cadherin-positive leukemic subpopulation demonstrated a growth advantage and resistance to farnesyltransferase inhibitors in the presence of bone marrow stromal cells (Zhang et al., 2007). We have recently reported that Ph+ ALL cells also express VE-cadherin, which confers enhanced self-renewal properties via accumulation and activation of β-catenin (Wang et al., 2007). These cells also co-express N-cadherin (unpublished data from our laboratory). Expression of N-cadherin or VE-cadherin appears to be downstream of Bcr-Abl kinase activity, since treatment of endothelial cells with Imatinib markedly reduces the expression of VE-cadherin (Vrekoussis et al., 2006). The isolation of Bcr-Abl-expressing endothelial cells from patients with CML is intriguing, and supports the notion that Bcr-Abl alone is sufficient to drive VE-cadherin expression at the hemangioblast stage from which both tumor and endothelial populations may be derived (Gunsilius et al., 2000; Fang et al., 2005).

Two "categories" of cell adhesion require consideration when evaluating how the adhesive qualities of Ph+ tumor cells respond to microenvironment signals. The first is "conditional adhesion", which involves ligand/receptor engagement such as integrin/fibronectin or CXCL12/CXCR4 interactions as mentioned previously. Constitutive adhesion encompasses homotypic interactions between the homologous cadherin family of proteins such as N-cadherin and VE-cadherin expressed on the bone marrow niche and leukemic cells. The concept of "constitutive adhesion" differs from "conditional adhesion" as the dissociation of homotypic interactions between cadherin family of molecules may require active interruption. This can be accomplished by several proteases including MMP9/ADAM10/15-mediated cleavage of the ectodomain of E-cadherin (Najy et al., 2008; Symowicz et al., 2007; Gavert et al., 2007), ADAM10/γ-secretase driven N-cadherin cleavage (Shoval et al., 2007; Reiss et al., 2005), ADAM10-facilitated protocadherin cleavage (Reiss et al., 2006) or ADAM10-dependent cleavage of VE-cadherin (Schulz et al., 2008). In contrast, "conditional adhesion" involves the modulation of ligand–receptor affinity or availability of either factor. Phenotypic changes driven by inherent, stable expression of Bcr-Abl, reflected in part by promoting VE-cadherin expression as one downstream consequence in subpopulations of Ph+ ALL (Wang et al., 2007) define a point of convergence between the tumor cell and the marrow microenvironment that is likely to contribute to the maintenance of the tumor population.

Bcr-Abl As a Contributor to Ph+ LSC Transformation: Is It Sufficient?

It is generally hypothesized that prolonged cell survival affords leukemic cells the opportunity to acquire sequential genetic insults that facilitate acute transformation of CML-CP. In agreement with this hypothesis, ectopic expression of the anti-apoptotic protein Bcl-2 in p185/p190 Bcr-Abl transformed 32D hematopoietic cells confers leukemogenesis, even in the presence of p185ΔBCR mutant that is not typically competent to generate leukemia (Cirinna et al., 2000). In addition, hMRP8p210 Bcr-Abl transgenic mice arrested in the latent myeloproliferative (MPD) stage crossed with hMRP8p210 mice expressing hMRPBcl-2 have induction of acute myeloid leukemias (Jaiswal et al., 2003). These findings support the assertion that Bcr-Abl, together with a second "hit,", is necessary to induce acute transformation of CML-CP. Interestingly, subsequent investigation identified Bcl-2 as a direct target gene of Bcr-Abl oncogenic signaling (Dai et al., 2004). Indeed, many Bcl-2 family anti-apoptotic proteins including Mcl-1 (Aichberger et al., 2005a; Li et al., 2007b), survivin (Wang et al., 2005; Carter et al., 2006; Brauer et al., 2007), Bcl-2-interacting mediator (Bim) (Aichberger et al., 2005b), or programmed cell death 4 (PCD4) (Carayol et al., 2008) are directly up- or down-regulated by Bcr-Abl kinase. Among a plethora of proteins that impact survival, PI3K/Akt signaling also plays an essential role in regulation of leukemic cell apoptosis. It appears that 32D Bcr-Abl-expressing cells require additional genetic changes that stimulate Akt, independent of Bcr-Abl, for progressive leukemogenic signaling (Nieborowska-Skorska et al., 2000). This observation is in contrast to the ability of Bcr-Abl to directly activate the PI3K/Akt/mTOR signaling pathway (Mayerhofer et al., 2002; Kim et al., 2005b).

Additional studies of factors that may influence cell phenotype in a Ph+ setting have described a role for p53, critical to molecular decisions in cell cycle progression or arrest associated with DNA double-strand breaks. Ectopic expression of the a3b2 p210 form of Bcr-Abl induces transformation of p53−/− bone marrow cells, in which stringent check point control is lost (Skorski et al., 1996). Furthermore, mating of p210 Bcr-Abl transgenic mice with p53+/− heterozygous mice confirms the role of loss of p53 in transformation of CML-CP (Honda et al., 2000). Consistent with the complexity of function previously noted, Bcr-Abl kinase can also impact on p53 through promotion of MDM2 mRNA translation (Trotta et al., 2003), a negative regulator that targets p53 for phosphorylation, ubiquitination, and promotes its proteosome-mediated degradation (Asher et al., 2005; Itahana et al., 2007; Vousden and Lane, 2007).

Constitutive kinase activity can also synergize with cytokine signaling. Bcr-Abl and IL-3 promote hematopoietic cell proliferation and survival (Parada et al., 2001) with oncogenic transformation of 3T3 fibroblasts by Bcr-Abl requiring co-expression of the IL-3 receptor (Tao et al., 2008). However, Bcr-Abl alone can induce CML-like disease in IL-3Rβ chain knockout hematopoietic cells, suggesting IL-3 signaling is dispensable in some circumstances (Wong et al., 2003). The convergence of Bcr-Abl as a "first hit" with additional mutations, or response to soluble factors such as IL-3, may exert their influence over disease progression through their collective support of a tumor stem cell phenotype.

Tumor Stem Cells; Anatomical Organization and Origin

Cancer stem cells are a unique subpopulation of tumor cells characterized by self-renewal and differentiation capacity analogous to their normal stem cell counterparts (Bjerkvig et al., 2005; Lobo et al., 2007). A growing body of literature indicates that some cancer stem cells may derive from partially differentiated precursor cells.

LSCs of acute myeloid leukemia (AML) transformed from CML-CP have characteristics that suggest they are derived from granulocyte–macrophage progenitors (Jamieson et al., 2004; Michor, 2007), while B-lineage Ph+ ALL LSCs exhibit a phenotype with markers of a committed B progenitor (Wang et al., 2007; Castor et al., 2005). Observations are not limited to hematological malignancies, with breast cancer initiated from committed mammary progenitors (Li et al., 2007d; Polyak, 2007). Analyses of other tissue types have also identified stem cell fractions of solid tumors with acquired self-renewal property (Vescovi et al., 2006; Ricci-Vitiani et al., 2007; Kim et al., 2005a; Li et al., 2007a). One of many lessons gleaned from stem cell biology is that all adult stem cells rely on a supportive microenvironment for self-renewal and differentiation. Therefore, it is not surprising that the environment influences their neoplastic counterparts. Dysregulated expression or activity of adhesion molecules, subsequent to constitutive Bcr-Abl activity, may aid in organizing heterogeneous populations of leukemic cells within anatomically and functionally distinct microenvironment niches.

While characteristics of both the endosteal fibroblastic or sinusoidal endothelial niches of hematopoietic stem cells have become better understood in recent years (Zhang et al., 2003; Calvi et al., 2003; Kiel et al., 2005), less is known about the architecture of stem cell organization itself within these marrow niches. In *Drosophila melanogaster*, hematopoiesis occurs in the specialized lymph gland (Jung et al., 2005). Insights into the architecture of the hematopoietic organ of the fruit fly reveal structural features that are highly conserved among vertebrates across approximately 550 million years of evolution (Evans et al., 2003). The lymph gland is characterized by three distinct functional zones. These include a medullary zone compromising the quiescent, self-renewing pro-hemocytes, a cortical zone consisting of maturing hemocytes, and a posterior signaling center (PSC), composed of stromal cells that direct the development of hematopoietic cells. Intriguingly, cell surface markers are also differentially expressed in each zone. Markers expressed on medullary prohemocytes are lost on cortical hemocytes and cells expressing specific differentiation markers are not found in the medullary zone. The *Drosophila* equivalent of E-cadherin, DE-cadherin, is only expressed at the medullary zone, and plays a pivotal role in anchoring, sorting, and regulating the undifferentiated, slow-cycling prohemocytes (Jung et al., 2005). The maturing, cortical zone cells are progressively derived from the quiescent prohemocytes, coincident with gradual down-regulation of DE-cadherin (Jung et al., 2005). The PSC, which serves as the stem cell niche compromising predominantly the stromal cell population, instructs the hematopoietic process via the Hedgehog and Jak-Stat2 signaling pathways (Lebestky et al., 2003; Mandal et al., 2007). This anatomical, functional division has been strikingly conserved in regulation of stem development as well as in the context of hematopoietic tumor cells with a stem cell phenotype.

In mammals, hemogenic endothelium resides in the mouse aorta and gives rise to hematopoietic progenitors in a budding manner (Smith and Glomski, 1982). Aggregates of undifferentiated cells tethered to the ventral luminal wall of the abdominal aorta cluster to form bud-like structures that have been observed among Mongolian gerbil, mouse, pig, and human embryos (Smith and Glomski, 1982).

These budding cells have many characteristics in common with the primitive hematopoietic stem cells located at the yolk sac blood islands (Smith and Glomski, 1982). Further analysis reveals that the mouse E11.5 embryonic aorta region contains VE-cadherin$^+$PECAM-1^{high}CD45$^+$ cells that cluster predominantly to the luminal surface of the endothelial lining of the dorsal aorta (Taoudi and Medvinsky, 2007). Imaging studies have shown that murine bone marrow contains specific anatomic regions comprised of E-selectin positive endothelial cells that form specific microdomains (Sipkins et al., 2005). Interestingly, homing and engraftment of Nalm-6 human ALL leukemic cells to marrow niches are defined by discrete cell aggregates tethered to endothelial vessel walls (Sipkins et al., 2005). These observations establish that endothelial vascular niches are likely to direct organization HSCs, and perhaps LSCs, in a manner similar to that seen in Drosophila lymph gland (Jung et al., 2005) and also observed along the walls of the mammalian aorta (Smith and Glomski, 1982; Taoudi and Medvinsky, 2007).

The structural features of LSC organization that have been observed in vitro in the presence of bone marrow stroma is surprisingly similar to that seen in the Drosophila lymph gland and the mouse embryonic dorsal aorta described above (Wang et al., 2007). Ph+ ALL cells with a stem cell phenotype are hierarchically organized in a flame-like, finger-shaped hematopoietic cord (Wang et al., 2007). The periphery of the hematopoietic cord is dominated by maturing leukemic cells that are VE-cadherin^{Lo}Oct-4$^+$CD133$^-$ with the core column compromised by cells that are VE-cadherin^{hi}Oct-4$^-$CD133$^+$ (Wang et al., 2007). This heterogeneous population of leukemic cells is maintained on a monolayer of VCAM-1+ stromal cells and has the capacity to support tri-lineage hematopoiesis in vivo and in vitro when bone marrow stromal cells are available (unpublished data). These findings support the notion that Ph+ LSCs recapitulate the growth characteristics of normal hematopoietic tissues (Jung et al., 2005; Smith and Glomski, 1982; Taoudi and Medvinsky, 2007) and further hint that Bcr-Abl kinase activity may provide intrinsic signals that modulate adhesion molecule expression (such as VE-cadherin), whereas microenvironmental niches offer important extrinsic cues to support tumor stem cells.

Competition for Space in the Niche

Although Bcr-Abl induces expression of a variety of genes involved in cell adhesion (Juric et al., 2007), not all adhesion molecules are qualified for steady anchorage to the marrow niches due to the phenomenon termed "niche competition" (Colvin et al., 2004; Czechowicz et al., 2007; Kiel and Morrison, 2008). Stromal cell numbers are tightly regulated by bone morphogenetic proteins (BMPs) (Zhou et al., 1997), TGF-β (Ogata et al., 2007), and Notch signaling (Calvi et al., 2003). Because the number of resident structural cells is limited, the available niche space for HSC implantation during homing and engraftment of HSCs, or circulating leukemic progenitors, is correspondingly limited. This is evidenced by the observation that optimal allogenic HSCT engraftment requires pre-conditioning and that the HSC-depleting monoclonal antibody ACK2 increases the efficiency of HSC transplantation (Czechowicz et al., 2007). While niche availability for endogenous and exogenous normal HSCs appears equally opportunistic, the competition between tumor and normal stem cells is biased (Yamashita, 2008). In *Drosophila* ovary, differentiation-defective germline stem cells outcompete for niche occupancy via up-regulation of E-cadherin (Jin, 2008). As such, you can speculate that inherent changes in tumor cells, with Bcr-Abl expression as the example in the current chapter, may position a cell to be particularly competitive for niche occupancy as one contributing factor to the nature of Ph+ malignancies.

Theoretically, "constitutive adhesion" mediated by homotypic N-cadherin or VE-cadherin interactions (Hewat et al., 2007; Pokutta and Weis, 2007) might be preferentially supported by marrow stromal cells subsequently influencing niche competency. Diverse evidences support the concept that marrow niche cells preferentially support a subset of VE- or N-cadherin+/Ph+ leukemic cells for acute transformation. Marrow endosteal osteoblasts or sinusoidal endothelium expression of N-cadherin+ (Zhang et al., 2003; Calvi et al., 2003) or VE-cadherin (Kiel et al., 2005; Taoudi and Medvinsky, 2007) positions them to efficiently support homotypic interactions. Secondly, normal hematopoietic stem cells express VE-cadherin (Taoudi and Medvinsky, 2007), N-cadherin (Haug et al., 2008; Arai et al., 2004), or DE-cadherin (Jung et al., 2005) resulting in their "match" to an appropriate developmental site. Microenvironment cells also employ cadherins for classifying, sorting, and morphogenesis during embryonic development (Lien et al., 2006; Halbleib and Nelson, 2006). Additionally, tumor-like stem cells compete for niche spaces using DE-cadherin (Jin, 2007). Thus, evolution of LSCs may be under the selection of the marrow microenvironment based, in part, on the possibility that a leukemic subset that best "fits" the microenvironment is supported.

Microenvironment Cues and Bcr-Abl Converge on Stabilization of Tumor Cell VE-Cadherin

As noted earlier, in Ph+ ALL, Bcr-Abl drives a subset of leukemic progenitor cells to constitutively express VE- or N-cadherin (Zhang et al., 2007; Wang et al., 2007). Homotypic interactions of cadherins are critical for stabilizing these proteins on cell surface (Yap et al., 2007; Leckband and Prakasam, 2006). When unengaged, constitutive endocytosis can occur for newly synthesized VE-cadherin and N-cadherin (Pokutta and Weis, 2007; Lien et al., 2006) although in specific circumstances growth factors or neurotransmitters also induce VE- or N-cadherin internalization (Xiao et al., 2005; Tai et al., 2007). Internalized VE-cadherin or N-cadherin may then be subjected to a lysosome-dependent degradation (Xiao et al., 2003; Davis et al., 2003; Dejana, 2004). In contrast, stabilization of VE-cadherin via cell–cell contact sequesters its intracellular binding partner, β-catenin in both Ph+/VE-cadherin+ LSCs (Zhang et al., 2007; Wang et al., 2007) and in normal vascular endothelial cells (Pokutta and Weis, 2007; Lien et al., 2006; Yamada et al., 2005). Consistent with VE-cadherin, β-catenin levels are tightly regulated by opposing forces of stabilization and degradation. Newly synthesized β-catenin is subjected to Axin-APC-Gsk3β mediated serine/threonine phosphorylation and subsequent ubiquitin–proteosome dependent degradation. Wnt signaling antagonizes this process and promotes β-catenin nuclear translocation and association with the transcriptional co-activator TCF/LEF to drive target gene expression (Clevers, 2006; Reya and Clevers, 2005). Wnt/β-catenin signaling plays an essential role in regulating Ph+ LSC pluripotency as loss of β-catenin impairs the self-renewal of both normal and CML stem cells in vivo (Zhao et al., 2007). In Ph+ ALL LSCs, stabilization and accumulation of β-catenin via VE-cadherin retention in the cytoplasm alone is not sufficient to confer activation of β-catenin. The release of β-catenin from the VE-cadherin/β-catenin/actin adhesion complexes requires Bcr-Abl (Wang et al., 2007; Coluccia et al., 2007), Src (Coluccia et al., 2006), or FLT3 (Kajiguchi et al., 2007) dependent tyrosine phosphorylation. Thus, Bcr-Abl-driven VE-cadherin expression and microenvironmental stabilization of VE-cadherin via enhanced cell–cell adhesion, cooperatively circumvent the requirement of exogenous Wnt ligands for stabilizing intracellular β-catenin. In this unique context, sustained activation of β-catenin downstream of VE-cadherin stabilization contributes to the self-renewal capacity of Ph+ ALL leukemic stem cells.

VE-cadherin expressed by any cell type, whether normal or transformed, can be impacted on by several bone marrow-derived factors, with VEGF as one representative example. VEGF rapidly induces tyrosine phosphorylation of VE-cadherin following VEGF receptor-2 (Flk-1/KDR) occupancy, with subsequent induction of Src activation (Esser et al., 1998; Wallez et al., 2007). Src-dependent VE-cadherin or N-cadherin phosphorylation disassociates and releases β-catenin from its intracellular domain during endothelial migration, spreading, and angiogenesis (Potter et al., 2005; Lambeng et al., 2005; Lin et al., 2003; Qi et al., 2006). Disassociation of β-catenin from the cadherin–catenin–actin complexes promotes its serine/threonine phosphorylation and ubiquitin–proteosome-mediated degradation (Yap et al., 2007; Pokutta and Weis, 2007; Lien et al., 2006; Dejana, 2004). In bone marrow sinusoidal niches, frequent disruption and detachment of VE-cadherin+ ALL cells from the niches would be expected due, in part, to the relatively high concentration of local VEGF, elevated Src kinase activity, and VE-cadherin tyrosine phosphorylation. This allows microenvironmental cues to impose stringent selection on VE-cadherin+ leukemic cells in this site.

Src family kinases are often activated in the presence of constitutively expressed Bcr-Abl, independent of soluble growth factors (Wong and Witte, 2004; Goss et al., 2006). Integrin engagement with fibronectin/VCAM-1 in marrow matrix also activates Src kinase (Rias-Salgado et al., 2003; Shattil, 2005; Wang et al., 2006). These effects collectively attenuate the anchorage of VE-cadherin+ leukemic cells to the microenvironment via VE-cadherin tyrosine phosphorylation, and dissociation of the cadherin–catenin–actin complexes. Unexpectedly, VE-cadherin expressed on Ph+ ALL LSCs in our model was not tyrosine phosphorylated (Wang et al., 2007). The mechanisms underlying dephosphorylation of VE-cadherin in Ph+/VE-cadherin+ LSCs remain somewhat poorly understood. Accumulating evidences suggest that either the protein tyrosine phosphatases (PTPs) or, in particular, overexpression of PTP1B induced by Bcr-Abl kinase, is partially responsible for dephosphorylation of VE-cadherin (Tonks, 2006). Elevated PTP1B expression has been reported in cell lines ectopically expressing Bcr-Abl, or leukemic cells collected from patients with CML (LaMontagne, Jr. et al., 1998a; LaMontagne, Jr. et al., 1998b). Further analysis revealed that Bcr-Abl-induced PTP1B expression via the Y-Box binding protein, YB-1 transcriptional factor (Fukada and Tonks, 2003). PTP1B serves as a negative regulator of VEGF/Src signal transduction by dephosphorylation of tyrosine phosphorylated VE-cadherin and VEGFR-2 (Nakamura et al., 2008; Nawroth et al., 2002; McLachlan and Yap, 2007). Deregulation of PTP1B, driven by receptor tyrosine kinases (such as Erb) or non-RTK (such as Bcr-Abl) defines potential targets for therapy in a variety of cancers (Tonks and Muthuswamy, 2007). Thus, selection of a Ph+/VE-cadherin+ ALL leukemic progenitor for LSC transformation may be synergistically achieved by niche stabilization of VE-cadherin through homotypic interactions and Bcr-Abl upregulation of PTP1B and dephosphorylation of VE-cadherin. Potentially, activation of VEGFR-2/Src and VE-cadherin phosphorylation may promote leukemic cell proliferation, while stabilization of VE-cadherin and its dephosphorylation confer LSC quiescence.

VE-Cadherin, Smads, and the TGF-β Signaling Pathway in Hematological Tumors

Stromal cell-derived TGF-β warrants individual consideration based on its ability to affect normal hematopoietic cells, tumor cells, and elements of the marrow microenvironment. The inhibitory effects of TGF-β family of proteins on normal hematopoietic progenitors are well established (Cheng et al., 2001; Massague et al., 2000; Schmierer and Hill, 2007). Additional observations define a tumor suppressor role for the TGF-β pathway in human hematologic malignancies (Dong and Blobe, 2006; Kim and Letterio, 2003). Evidence also indicates that the TGF-β/Smad signaling pathway is involved in modulating normal (Langer et al., 2004) and leukemic stem cell self-renewal and maintenance (Mishra et al., 2005; Akhurst and Derynck, 2001; Derynck et al., 2001). TGF-β is a multipotent growth factor with a prominent role in modeling angiogenesis and vasculogenesis during development (Ten and Arthur, 2007). The pro-angiogenic activity of TGF-β appears to require the endothelial-specific accessory receptor endoglin (Lebrin et al., 2004; Lebrin and Mummery, 2008), which promotes endothelial-restricted marker expression, cell sorting, and endothelial tube formation, independent of VEGF signaling (Ten and Arthur, 2007; Jakowlew, 2006). In Ph+ ALL LSCs, TGF-β1 was demonstrated to up-regulate VE-cadherin expression (Wang et al., 2007).

VE-cadherin physically interacts with components of the TGF-β signaling complex, including TGF-β receptor II, endoglin, ALK-1, and ALK-5 (Rudini et al., 2008). VE-cadherin clustering recruits TGFβRII/TGFβRI complexes and induces downstream Smad phosphorylation (Rudini et al., 2008), suggesting that VE-cadherin is an endothelial regulator of TGF-β signaling. In advanced stage breast cancer cells, VE-cadherin promotes the formation of cord-like invasive structures, analogous to the hematopoietic cord of LSCs grown on stromal cells (Wang et al., 2007; Labelle et al., 2008). Importantly, VE-cadherin promotes TGF-β-initiated Smad2 phosphorylation and expression of target genes (Labelle et al., 2008). Notably, VE-cadherin modulation of TGF-β signaling converges on elevated Smad phosphorylation and activation (Rudini et al., 2008; Labelle et al., 2008), which are involved with hematopoietic stem cell self-renewal (Karlsson et al., 2007; Jian et al., 2006; McReynolds et al., 2007). These findings collectively establish VE-cadherin as a direct modulator of TGF-β signaling, with TGF-β made available to tumors in the marrow from a variety of sources, including bone marrow stromal cells. As such, Bcr-Abl expression may ultimately position tumors to respond to TGF-β through unique signaling pathways.

Increasing the Vulnerability of Tumor Cells by Interrupting Their Connection to the Microenvironment

Recent studies on the molecular targeting of Bcr-Abl oncoprotein demonstrate that Imatinib efficiently eliminates most leukemic progenitors, but does not deplete leukemic stem cells (Neering et al., 2007; Michor et al., 2005). Total body irradiation selectively impairs the quiescent hematopoietic stem cell re-population, while sparing the Ph+ LSC subset (Neering et al., 2007). These clinically relevant observations suggest that additional protective mechanisms underlie preferential survival of primitive LSCs. In contrast, parthenolide and TDZD-8 selectively induce apoptosis of leukemic stem and progenitor cells, without impact on normal hematopoietic cells (Michor et al., 2005; Guzman et al., 2005, 2007), indicating a promising strategy for achieving curative therapy with enhanced drug selectivity and specificity. However, it remains to be determined whether these treatments truly eradicate tumor stem cells from the bone marrow.

It has been assumed that the LSC fraction in mobilized peripheral blood contributes to relapse of CML following autologous hematopoietic stem cell transplantation (auto-HSCT). However, the molecular basis underlying the homing and engrafting of LSCs to marrow is poorly understood. Recently, CD44, the cognate ligand for endothelial adhesion receptor E-Selectin (Katayama et al., 2005), was shown to play an important role in directing homing and seeding of the mobilized LSCs in peripheral blood into the marrow microenvironment (Krause et al., 2006). CD44 is dispensable for induction of acute B-lymphoblastic leukemia by Bcr-Abl but required for AML LSCs (Krause et al., 2006). Monoclonal antibody specifically targeted to CD44 disrupts the connection between leukemic stem cells and the microenvironment and eradicates human AML LSCs from the bone marrow (Krause et al., 2006; Jin et al., 2006). In contrast to CD44 which is expressed on normal and malignant hematopoietic cells, CD96, an adhesion molecule of the Ig gene superfamily, is uniquely expressed by AML LSCs (Hosen et al., 2007). CD96-negative human AML LSCs fail to repopulate Rag–/– SCID mice in the marrow, suggesting anti-CD96 targeted therapies may have clinical utility (Hosen et al., 2007).

The Rho GTPases Rac1 and Rac2 are also regulators of normal HSC adhesion to marrow niches (Gu et al., 2003), and knockout of both Rac1 and Rac2 results in egress of HSCs into the periphery, whereas Rac2–/– HSCs fail to engraft in the bone marrow of irradiated recipient mice (Gu et al., 2003). In Bcr-Abl+ CML-BC, elevated Rac1/2 activity is frequently detected (Thomas et al., 2008) with Rac1 activation leading to nuclear translocation of β-catenin and enhanced LSC self-renewal (Wu et al., 2008). Consistently, targeted deletion of Rac1/2, or chemical inhibition of Rac1/2 activity with NSC23766, abrogates Bcr-Abl-induced MPD in the bone marrow (Thomas et al., 2007). These observations collectively support the concept that interruption of the tumor niche interaction may underlie novel therapeutic approaches.

It is well documented that, in addition to physical contact, soluble growth factors and cytokines are also important for LSC survival and maintenance in the bone marrow (Williams et al., 2007; Kaushansky, 2006; Metcalf, 2008). Antibody cocktails against the non-adhesive HSC biomarkers LSK (Lin-Sca1+Kit+) induce cycling in the HSC side population cells and diminish their ability to engraft in the marrow-irradiated mice, resulting in accumulation of relatively mature hematopoietic progenitors in the peripheral blood (Gilner et al., 2007). The neutralizing antibody ACK2, which blocks the stem cell factor (SCF) receptor c-Kit, was shown to deplete the marrow niche of up to the 95% of LSCs (Czechowicz et al., 2007). Because tumor stem cells in which differentiation is dysregulated can outcompete normal stem cells for niche occupancy (Jin, 2007), it can be speculated that transformed stem cells may represent the majority of the stem cell subpopulation at advanced stages of hematopoietic disease. Antibody neutralization or growth factor stimulation, that promotes the release of LSCs from the marrow microenvironment may offer a strategy to partially recover normal niche balance. In agreement with this speculation, G-CSF/GM-CSF stimulation of Imatinib-resistant CML-BC leukemic cells reduces the residual, non-dividing LSC population and enhances Imatinib chemosensitivity (Holtz et al., 2007).

Conclusions

Despite considerable efforts, and advances in recent decades, expression of the Bcr-Abl kinase in ALL/AML remains an independent high-risk factor associated with poor prognosis (Schultz et al., 2007; Mancini et al., 2005). Drug resistance remains a clinically challenging problem with persistence of Bcr-Abl expression correlated with failure of drug treatment and relapse of disease (Pui and Evans, 2006; Tallman et al., 2005; Hunter, 2007). It is widely recognized that leukemic stem cells present a major hurdle for disease eradication. However, our understanding of LSC biology and development of strategies to specifically target LSC subpopulations remain to be optimized. The tyrosine kinase inhibitor Imatinib, mentioned throughout this chapter, represents the first molecularly targeted therapy for Ph+ leukemia (Noble et al., 2004; Tibes et al., 2005), with second generation inhibitors such as Dasatinib (Porkka et al., 2008; Hantschel et al., 2008) that target both Bcr-Abl and Src serving as just one example of attempts to improve treatment as our understanding of the signaling pathways of importance has evolved. However, malignant clones of quiescent, primitive Ph+ LSCs often persist after treatment, even when apparently complete remissions are achieved (Graham et al., 2002; Bhatia et al., 2003). This observation suggests that cell signaling resulting from inherent, "hard-wired" modifications, combined with response to microenvironment cues, collectively define the challenge of tumor cell eradication. Creative strategies, potentially targeting a subset of tumor stem cells, will benefit from increased understanding of the communication between genetically altered tumor cells and their unique ability to respond to supportive microenvironment niches (Bissell and Labarge, 2005; Rubin, 2003).

Acknowledgments Supported by the National Institutes of Health Grant No. R01HL056888 (LFG), R01CA134573 (LFG), and P20 RR016440 (LFG). The authors thank Ms. Stephanie Rellick for critical reading of the manuscript and Dr. Brett Hall for contributing to artwork shown in Fig. 18.1.

References

Aichberger KJ, Mayerhofer M, Krauth MT, Skvara H, Florian S, Sonneck K, Akgul C, Derdak S, Pickl WF, Wacheck V, Selzer E, Monia BP, Moriggl R, Valent P, Sillaber C (2005a) Identification of mcl-1 as a BCR/ABL-dependent target in chronic myeloid leukemia (CML): Evidence for cooperative antileukemic effects of imatinib and mcl-1 antisense oligonucleotides. Blood 105:3303–3311.

Aichberger KJ, Mayerhofer M, Krauth MT, Vales A, Kondo R, Derdak S, Pickl WF, Selzer E, Deininger M, Druker BJ, Sillaber C, Esterbauer H, Valent P (2005b) Low-level expression of proapoptotic Bcl-2-interacting mediator in leukemic cells in patients with chronic myeloid leukemia: role of BCR/ABL, characterization of underlying signaling pathways, and reexpression by novel pharmacologic compounds. Cancer Res 65:9436–9444.

Akhurst RJ and Derynck R (2001) TGF-beta signaling in cancer–a double-edged sword. Trends Cell Biol 11:S44–S51.

Arai F, Hirao A, Ohmura M, Sato H, Matsuoka S, Takubo K, Ito K, Koh GY, Suda T (2004) Tie2/angiopoietin-1 signaling regulates hematopoietic stem cell quiescence in the bone marrow niche. Cell 118:149–161.

Asher G, Tsvetkov P, Kahana C, Shaul Y (2005) A mechanism of ubiquitin-independent proteasomal degradation of the tumor suppressors p53 and p73. Genes Dev 19:316–321.

Bazzoni G, Carlesso N, Griffin JD, Hemler ME (1996) Bcr/Abl expression stimulates integrin function in hematopoietic cell lines. J Clin Invest 98:521–528.

Bhatia R and Verfaillie CM (1998) Inhibition of BCR-ABL expression with antisense oligodeoxynucleotides restores beta1 integrin-mediated adhesion and proliferation inhibition in chronic myelogenous leukemia hematopoietic progenitors. Blood 91:3414–3422.

Bhatia R, McGlave PB, Verfaillie CM (1995) Treatment of marrow stroma with interferon-alpha restores normal beta 1 integrin-dependent adhesion of chronic myelogenous leukemia hematopoietic progenitors. Role of MIP-1 alpha. J Clin Invest 96:931–939.

Bhatia R, McCarthy JB, Verfaillie CM (1996) Interferon-alpha restores normal beta 1 integrin-mediated inhibition of hematopoietic progenitor proliferation by the marrow microenvironment in chronic myelogenous leukemia. Blood 87:3883–3891.

Bhatia R, Holtz M, Niu N, Gray R, Snyder DS, Sawyers CL, Arber DA, Slovak ML, Forman SJ (2003) Persistence of malignant hematopoietic progenitors in chronic myelogenous leukemia patients in complete cytogenetic remission following imatinib mesylate treatment. Blood 101:4701–4707.

Bissell MJ and Labarge MA (2005) Context, tissue plasticity, and cancer: are tumor stem cells also regulated by the microenvironment? Cancer Cell 7:17–23.

Bjerkvig R, Tysnes BB, Aboody KS, Najbauer J, Terzis AJ (2005) Opinion: the origin of the cancer stem cell: Current controversies and new insights. Nat Rev Cancer 5:899–904.

Brauer KM, Werth D, von SK, Bringmann A, Kanz L, Grunebach F, Brossart P (2007) BCR-ABL activity is critical for the immunogenicity of chronic myelogenous leukemia cells. Cancer Res 67:5489–5497.

Calvi LM, Adams GB, Weibrecht KW, Weber JM, Olson DP, Knight MC, Martin RP, Schipani E, Divieti P, Bringhurst FR, Milner LA, Kronenberg HM, Scadden DT (2003) Osteoblastic cells regulate the haematopoietic stem cell niche. Nature 425:841–846.

Carayol N, Katsoulidis E, Sassano A, Altman JK, Druker BJ, Platanias LC (2008) Suppression of programmed cell death 4 (PDCD4) protein expression by BCR-ABL-regulated engagement of the mTOR/p70 S6 kinase pathway. J Biol Chem 283:8601–8610.

Carter BZ, Mak DH, Schober WD, Cabreira-Hansen M, Beran M, McQueen T, Chen W, Andreeff M (2006) Regulation of survivin expression through Bcr-Abl/MAPK cascade: targeting survivin overcomes imatinib resistance and increases imatinib sensitivity in imatinib-responsive CML cells. Blood 107:1555–1563.

Castor A, Nilsson L, strand-Grundstrom I, Buitenhuis M, Ramirez C, Anderson K, Strombeck B, Garwicz S, Bekassy AN, Schmiegelow K, Lausen B, Hokland P, Lehmann S, Juliusson G, Johansson B, Jacobsen SE (2005) Distinct patterns of hematopoietic stem cell involvement in acute lymphoblastic leukemia. Nat Med 11:630–637.

Chen YY, Malik M, Tomkowicz BE, Collman RG, Ptasznik A (2008) BCR-ABL1 alters SDF-1alpha-mediated adhesive responses through the beta2 integrin LFA-1 in leukemia cells. Blood 111:5182–5186.

Cheng T, Shen H, Rodrigues N, Stier S, Scadden DT (2001) Transforming growth factor beta 1 mediates cell-cycle arrest of primitive hematopoietic cells independent of p21(Cip1/Waf1) or p27(Kip1). Blood 98:3643–3649.

Cirinna M, Trotta R, Salomoni P, Kossev P, Wasik M, Perrotti D, Calabretta B (2000) Bcl-2 expression restores the leukemogenic potential of a BCR/ABL mutant defective in transformation. Blood 96:3915–3921.

Clevers H (2006) Wnt/beta-catenin signaling in development and disease. Cell 127:469–480.

Coluccia AM, Benati D, Dekhil H, De FA, Lan C, Gambacorti-Passerini C (2006) SKI-606 decreases growth and motility of colorectal cancer cells by preventing pp60(c-Src)-dependent tyrosine phosphorylation of beta-catenin and its nuclear signaling. Cancer Res 66:2279–2286.

Coluccia AM, Vacca A, Dunach M, Mologni L, Redaelli S, Bustos VH, Benati D, Pinna LA, Gambacorti-Passerini C (2007) Bcr-Abl stabilizes beta-catenin in chronic myeloid leukemia through its tyrosine phosphorylation. EMBO J 26:1456–1466.

Colvin GA, Lambert JF, Abedi M, Hsieh CC, Carlson JE, Stewart FM, Quesenberry PJ (2004) Murine marrow cellularity and the concept of stem cell competition: geographic and quantitative determinants in stem cell biology. Leukemia 18:575–583.

Czechowicz A, Kraft D, Weissman IL, Bhattacharya D (2007) Efficient transplantation via antibody-based clearance of hematopoietic stem cell niches. Science 318:1296–1299.

Dai Y, Rahmani M, Corey SJ, Dent P, Grant S (2004) A Bcr/Abl-independent, Lyn-dependent form of imatinib mesylate (STI-571) resistance is associated with altered expression of Bcl-2. J Biol Chem 279:34227–34239.

Davis MA, Ireton RC, Reynolds AB (2003) A core function for p120-catenin in cadherin turnover. J Cell Biol 163:525–534.

Deininger MW, Goldman JM, Melo JV (2000a) The molecular biology of chronic myeloid leukemia. Blood 96:3343–3356.

Deininger MW, Vieira S, Mendiola R, Schultheis B, Goldman JM, Melo JV (2000b) BCR-ABL tyrosine kinase activity regulates the expression of multiple genes implicated in the pathogenesis of chronic myeloid leukemia. Cancer Res 60:2049–2055.

Dejana E (2004) Endothelial cell–cell junctions: happy together. Nat Rev Mol Cell Biol 5:261–270.

Derynck R, Akhurst RJ, Balmain A (2001) TGF-beta signaling in tumor suppression and cancer progression. Nat Genet 29:117–129.

Dierov J, Dierova R, Carroll M (2004) BCR/ABL translocates to the nucleus and disrupts an ATR-dependent intra-S phase checkpoint. Cancer Cell 5:275–285.

Dong M and Blobe GC (2006) Role of transforming growth factor-beta in hematologic malignancies. Blood 107:4589–4596.

Esser S, Lampugnani MG, Corada M, Dejana E, Risau W (1998) Vascular endothelial growth factor induces VE-cadherin tyrosine phosphorylation in endothelial cells. J Cell Sci 111(Pt 13):1853–1865.

Evans CJ, Hartenstein V, Banerjee U (2003) Thicker than blood: Conserved mechanisms in Drosophila and vertebrate hematopoiesis. Dev Cell 5:673–690.

Fan PD, Cong F, Goff SP (2003) Homo- and hetero-oligomerization of the c-Abl kinase and Abelson-interactor-1. Cancer Res 63:873–877.

Fang B, Zheng C, Liao L, Han Q, Sun Z, Jiang X, Zhao RC (2005) Identification of human chronic myelogenous leukemia progenitor cells with hemangioblastic characteristics. Blood 105: 2733–2740.

Fierro FA, Taubenberger A, Puech PH, Ehninger G, Bornhauser M, Muller DJ, Illmer T (2008) BCR/ABL expression of myeloid progenitors increases beta1-integrin mediated adhesion to stromal cells. J Mol Biol 377:1082–1093.

Frasca F, Vigneri P, Vella V, Vigneri R, Wang JY (2001) Tyrosine kinase inhibitor STI571 enhances thyroid cancer cell motile response to hepatocyte growth factor. Oncogene 20:3845–3856.

Fukada T and Tonks NK (2003) Identification of YB-1 as a regulator of PTP1B expression: implications for regulation of insulin and cytokine signaling. EMBO J 22:479–493.

Gavert N, Sheffer M, Raveh S, Spaderna S, Shtutman M, Brabletz T, Barany F, Paty P, Notterman D, Domany E, Ben-Ze'ev A (2007) Expression of L1-CAM and ADAM10 in human colon cancer cells induces metastasis. Cancer Res 67:7703–7712.

Geay JF, Buet D, Zhang Y, Foudi A, Jarrier P, Berthebaud M, Turhan AG, Vainchenker W, Louache F (2005) p210BCR-ABL inhibits SDF-1 chemotactic response via alteration of CXCR4 signaling and down-regulation of CXCR4 expression. Cancer Res 65:2676–2683.

Gilner JB, Walton WG, Gush K, Kirby SL (2007) Antibodies to stem cell marker antigens reduce engraftment of hematopoietic stem cells. Stem Cells 25:279–288.

Gordon MY, Dowding CR, Riley GP, Goldman JM, Greaves MF (1987) Altered adhesive interactions with marrow stroma of haematopoietic progenitor cells in chronic myeloid leukaemia. Nature 328:342–344.

Goss VL, Lee KA, Moritz A, Nardone J, Spek EJ, MacNeill J, Rush J, Comb MJ, Polakiewicz RD (2006) A common phosphotyrosine signature for the Bcr-Abl kinase. Blood 107: 4888–4897.

Graham SM, Jorgensen HG, Allan E, Pearson C, Alcorn MJ, Richmond L, Holyoake TL (2002) Primitive, quiescent, Philadelphia-positive stem cells from patients with chronic myeloid leukemia are insensitive to STI571 in vitro. Blood 99:319–325.

Gu Y, Filippi MD, Cancelas JA, Siefring JE, Williams EP, Jasti AC, Harris CE, Lee AW, Prabhakar R, Atkinson SJ, Kwiatkowski DJ, Williams DA (2003) Hematopoietic cell regulation by Rac1 and Rac2 guanosine triphosphatases. Science 302:445–449.

Gunsilius E, Duba HC, Petzer AL, Kahler CM, Grunewald K, Stockhammer G, Gabl C, Dirnhofer S, Clausen J, Gastl G (2000) Evidence from a leukaemia model for maintenance of vascular endothelium by bone-marrow-derived endothelial cells. Lancet 355:1688–1691.

Guzman ML, Rossi RM, Karnischky L, Li X, Peterson DR, Howard DS, Jordan CT (2005) The sesquiterpene lactone parthenolide induces apoptosis of human acute myelogenous leukemia stem and progenitor cells. Blood 105:4163–4169.

Guzman ML, Rossi RM, Neelakantan S, Li X, Corbett CA, Hassane DC, Becker MW, Bennett JM, Sullivan E, Lachowicz JL, Vaughan A, Sweeney CJ, Matthews W, Carroll M, Liesveld JL, Crooks PA, Jordan CT (2007) An orally bioavailable parthenolide analog selectively eradicates acute myelogenous leukemia stem and progenitor cells. Blood 110:4427–4435.

Halbleib JM and Nelson WJ (2006) Cadherins in development: Cell adhesion, sorting, and tissue morphogenesis. Genes Dev 20:3199–3214.

Hantschel O and Superti-Furga G (2004) Regulation of the c-Abl and Bcr-Abl tyrosine kinases. Nat Rev Mol Cell Biol 5:33–44.

Hantschel O, Rix U, Superti-Furga G (2008) Target spectrum of the BCR-ABL inhibitors imatinib, nilotinib and dasatinib. Leuk Lymphoma 49:615–619.

Haug JS, He XC, Grindley JC, Wunderlich JP, Gaudenz K, Ross JT, Paulson A, Wagner KP, Xie Y, Zhu R, Yin T, Perry JM, Hembree MJ, Redenbaugh EP, Radice GL, Seidel C, Li L (2008) N-cadherin expression level distinguishes reserved versus primed states of hematopoietic stem cells. Cell Stem Cell 2:367–379.

He Y, Wertheim JA, Xu L, Miller JP, Karnell FG, Choi JK, Ren R, Pear WS (2002) The coiled-coil domain and Tyr177 of bcr are required to induce a murine chronic myelogenous leukemia-like disease by bcr/abl. Blood 99:2957–2968.

Heisterkamp N, Voncken JW, Senadheera D, Gonzalez-Gomez I, Reichert A, Haataja L, Reinikainen A, Pattengale PK, Groffen J (2000) Reduced oncogenicity of p190 Bcr/Abl F-actin-binding domain mutants. Blood 96:2226–2232.

Hendrix MJ, Seftor EA, Hess AR, Seftor RE (2003) Molecular plasticity of human melanoma cells. Oncogene 22:3070–3075.

Hendrix MJ, Seftor EA, Meltzer PS, Gardner LM, Hess AR, Kirschmann DA, Schatteman GC, Seftor RE (2001) Expression and functional significance of VE-cadherin in aggressive human melanoma cells: Role in vasculogenic mimicry. Proc Natl Acad Sci U S A 98:8018–8023.

Hernandez SE, Krishnaswami M, Miller AL, Koleske AJ (2004) How do Abl family kinases regulate cell shape and movement? Trends Cell Biol 14:36–44.

Hess AR, Seftor EA, Gruman LM, Kinch MS, Seftor RE, Hendrix MJ (2006) VE-cadherin regulates EphA2 in aggressive melanoma cells through a novel signaling pathway: implications for vasculogenic mimicry. Cancer Biol Ther 5:228–233.

Hewat EA, Durmort C, Jacquamet L, Concord E, Gulino-Debrac D (2007) Architecture of the VE-cadherin hexamer. J Mol Biol 365:744–751.

Holtz M, Forman SJ, Bhatia R (2007) Growth factor stimulation reduces residual quiescent chronic myelogenous leukemia progenitors remaining after imatinib treatment. Cancer Res 67: 1113–1120.

Honda H, Ushijima T, Wakazono K, Oda H, Tanaka Y, Aizawa S, Ishikawa T, Yazaki Y, Hirai H (2000) Acquired loss of p53 induces blastic transformation in p210(bcr/abl)-expressing hematopoietic cells: A transgenic study for blast crisis of human CML. Blood 95: 1144–1150.

Hosen N, Park CY, Tatsumi N, Oji Y, Sugiyama H, Gramatzki M, Krensky AM, Weissman IL (2007) CD96 is a leukemic stem cell-specific marker in human acute myeloid leukemia. Proc Natl Acad Sci U S A 104:11008–11013.

Hunter T (2007) Treatment for chronic myelogenous leukemia: The long road to imatinib. J Clin Invest 117:2036–2043.

Iotti G, Ferrari-Amorotti G, Rosafio C, Corradini F, Lidonnici MR, Ronchetti M, Bardini M, Zhang Y, Martinez R, Blasi F, Calabretta B (2007) Expression of CCL9/MIP-1gamma is repressed by BCR/ABL and its restoration suppresses in vivo leukemogenesis of 32D-BCR/ABL cells. Oncogene 26:3482–3491.

Itahana K, Mao H, Jin A, Itahana Y, Clegg HV, Lindstrom MS, Bhat KP, Godfrey VL, Evan GI, Zhang Y (2007) Targeted inactivation of Mdm2 RING finger E3 ubiquitin ligase activity in the mouse reveals mechanistic insights into p53 regulation. Cancer Cell 12:355–366.

Jaiswal S, Traver D, Miyamoto T, Akashi K, Lagasse E, Weissman IL (2003) Expression of BCR/ABL and BCL-2 in myeloid progenitors leads to myeloid leukemias. Proc Natl Acad Sci U S A 100:10002–10007.

Jakowlew SB (2006) Transforming growth factor-beta in cancer and metastasis. Cancer Metastasis Rev 25:435–457.

Jamieson CH, Ailles LE, Dylla SJ, Muijtjens M, Jones C, Zehnder JL, Gotlib J, Li K, Manz MG, Keating A, Sawyers CL, Weissman IL (2004) Granulocyte–macrophage progenitors as candidate leukemic stem cells in blast-crisis CML. N Engl J Med 351:657–667.

Jian H, Shen X, Liu I, Semenov M, He X, Wang XF (2006) Smad3-dependent nuclear translocation of beta-catenin is required for TGF-beta1-induced proliferation of bone marrow-derived adult human mesenchymal stem cells. Genes Dev 20:666–674.

Jin Z (2008) Differentiation-Defective Stem Cells Outcompete Normal Stem Cells for Niche Occupancy in the Drosophila Ovary. Cell Stem Cell Vol 2, Issue 1 39–49.

Jin L, Hope KJ, Zhai Q, Smadja-Joffe F, Dick JE (2006) Targeting of CD44 eradicates human acute myeloid leukemic stem cells. Nat Med 12:1167–1174.

Jongen-Lavrencic M, Salesse S, Delwel R, Verfaillie CM (2005) BCR/ABL-mediated downregulation of genes implicated in cell adhesion and motility leads to impaired migration toward CCR7 ligands CCL19 and CCL21 in primary BCR/ABL-positive cells. Leukemia 19:373–380.

Jung SH, Evans CJ, Uemura C, Banerjee U (2005) The Drosophila lymph gland as a developmental model of hematopoiesis. Development 132:2521–2533.

Juric D, Lacayo NJ, Ramsey MC, Racevskis J, Wiernik PH, Rowe JM, Goldstone AH, O'Dwyer PJ, Paietta E, Sikic BI (2007) Differential gene expression patterns and interaction networks in BCR-ABL-positive and -negative adult acute lymphoblastic leukemias. J Clin Oncol 25: 1341–1349.

Kain KH and Klemke RL (2001) Inhibition of cell migration by Abl family tyrosine kinases through uncoupling of Crk-CAS complexes. J Biol Chem 276:16185–16192.

Kajiguchi T, Chung EJ, Lee S, Stine A, Kiyoi H, Naoe T, Levis MJ, Neckers L, Trepel JB (2007) FLT3 regulates beta-catenin tyrosine phosphorylation, nuclear localization, and transcriptional activity in acute myeloid leukemia cells. Leukemia 21:2476–2484.

Karlsson G, Blank U, Moody JL, Ehinger M, Singbrant S, Deng CX, Karlsson S (2007) Smad4 is critical for self-renewal of hematopoietic stem cells. J Exp Med 204:467–474.

Katayama Y, Hidalgo A, Chang J, Peired A, Frenette PS (2005) CD44 is a physiological E-selectin ligand on neutrophils. J Exp Med 201:1183–1189.

Kaushansky K (2006) Lineage-specific hematopoietic growth factors. N Engl J Med 354: 2034–2045.

Khuntia D, Brown P, Li J, Mehta MP (2006) Whole-brain radiotherapy in the management of brain metastasis. J Clin Oncol 24:1295–1304.

Kiel MJ and Morrison SJ (2008) Uncertainty in the niches that maintain haematopoietic stem cells. Nat Rev Immunol 8:290–301.

Kiel MJ, Yilmaz OH, Iwashita T, Yilmaz OH, Terhorst C, Morrison SJ (2005) SLAM family receptors distinguish hematopoietic stem and progenitor cells and reveal endothelial niches for stem cells. Cell 121:1109–1121.

Kim SJ and Letterio J (2003) Transforming growth factor-beta signaling in normal and malignant hematopoiesis. Leukemia 17:1731–1737.

Kim CF, Jackson EL, Woolfenden AE, Lawrence S, Babar I, Vogel S, Crowley D, Bronson RT, Jacks T (2005a) Identification of bronchioalveolar stem cells in normal lung and lung cancer. Cell 121:823–835.

Kim JH, Chu SC, Gramlich JL, Pride YB, Babendreier E, Chauhan D, Salgia R, Podar K, Griffin JD, Sattler M (2005b) Activation of the PI3K/mTOR pathway by BCR-ABL contributes to increased production of reactive oxygen species. Blood 105:1717–1723.

Koretzky GA (2007) The legacy of the Philadelphia chromosome. J Clin Invest 117: 2030–2032.

Krause DS, Lazarides K, von Andrian UH, Van Etten RA (2006) Requirement for CD44 in homing and engraftment of BCR-ABL-expressing leukemic stem cells. Nat Med 12: 1175–1180.

Kronenwett R, Butterweck U, Steidl U, Kliszewski S, Neumann F, Bork S, Blanco ED, Roes N, Graf T, Brors B, Eils R, Maercker C, Kobbe G, Gattermann N, Haas R (2005) Distinct molecular phenotype of malignant CD34(+) hematopoietic stem and progenitor cells in chronic myelogenous leukemia. Oncogene 24:5313–5324.

Labelle M, Schnittler HJ, Aust DE, Friedrich K, Baretton G, Vestweber D, Breier G (2008) Vascular endothelial cadherin promotes breast cancer progression via transforming growth factor beta signaling. Cancer Res 68:1388–1397.

Lambeng N, Wallez Y, Rampon C, Cand F, Christe G, Gulino-Debrac D, Vilgrain I, Huber P (2005) Vascular endothelial-cadherin tyrosine phosphorylation in angiogenic and quiescent adult tissues. Circ Res 96:384–391.

LaMontagne KR, Jr., Flint AJ, Franza BR, Jr., Pandergast AM, Tonks NK (1998a) Protein tyrosine phosphatase 1B antagonizes signalling by oncoprotein tyrosine kinase p210 bcr-abl in vivo. Mol Cell Biol 18:2965–2975.

LaMontagne KR, Jr., Hannon G, Tonks NK (1998b) Protein tyrosine phosphatase PTP1B suppresses p210 bcr-abl-induced transformation of rat-1 fibroblasts and promotes differentiation of K562 cells. Proc Natl Acad Sci U S A 95:14094–14099.

Langer JC, Henckaerts E, Orenstein J, Snoeck HW (2004) Quantitative trait analysis reveals transforming growth factor-beta2 as a positive regulator of early hematopoietic progenitor and stem cell function. J Exp Med 199:5–14.

Lebestky T, Jung SH, Banerjee U (2003) A Serrate-expressing signaling center controls Drosophila hematopoiesis. Genes Dev 17:348–353.

Lebrin F, Goumans MJ, Jonker L, Carvalho RL, Valdimarsdottir G, Thorikay M, Mummery C, Arthur HM, ten DP (2004) Endoglin promotes endothelial cell proliferation and TGF-beta/ALK1 signal transduction. EMBO J 23:4018–4028.

Lebrin F and Mummery CL (2008) Endoglin-mediated vascular remodeling: mechanisms underlying hereditary hemorrhagic telangiectasia. Trends Cardiovasc Med 18:25–32.

Leckband D and Prakasam A (2006) Mechanism and dynamics of cadherin adhesion. Annu Rev Biomed Eng 8:259–287.

Li C, Heidt DG, Dalerba P, Burant CF, Zhang L, Adsay V, Wicha M, Clarke MF, Simeone DM (2007a) Identification of pancreatic cancer stem cells. Cancer Res 67:1030–1037.

Li QF, Huang WR, Duan HF, Wang H, Wu CT, Wang LS (2007b) Sphingosine kinase-1 mediates BCR/ABL-induced upregulation of Mcl-1 in chronic myeloid leukemia cells. Oncogene 26:7904–7908.

Li Y, Clough N, Sun X, Yu W, Abbott BL, Hogan CJ, Dai Z (2007c) Bcr-Abl induces abnormal cytoskeleton remodeling, beta1 integrin clustering and increased cell adhesion to fibronectin through the Abl interactor 1 pathway. J Cell Sci 120:1436–1446.

Li Z, Tognon CE, Godinho FJ, Yasaitis L, Hock H, Herschkowitz JI, Lannon CL, Cho E, Kim SJ, Bronson RT, Perou CM, Sorensen PH, Orkin SH (2007d) ETV6-NTRK3 fusion oncogene initiates breast cancer from committed mammary progenitors via activation of AP1 complex. Cancer Cell 12:542–558.

Lien WH, Klezovitch O, Vasioukhin V (2006) Cadherin–catenin proteins in vertebrate development. Curr Opin Cell Biol 18:499–506.

Lin MT, Yen ML, Lin CY, Kuo ML (2003) Inhibition of vascular endothelial growth factor-induced angiogenesis by resveratrol through interruption of Src-dependent vascular endothelial cadherin tyrosine phosphorylation. Mol Pharmacol 64:1029–1036.

Lobo NA, Shimono Y, Qian D, Clarke MF (2007) The biology of cancer stem cells. Annu Rev Cell Dev Biol 23:675–699.

Lundell BI, McCarthy JB, Kovach NL, Verfaillie CM (1996) Activation-dependent alpha5beta1 integrin-mediated adhesion to fibronectin decreases proliferation of chronic myelogenous leukemia progenitors and K562 cells. Blood 87:2450–2458.

Luo Y and Radice GL (2005) N-cadherin acts upstream of VE-cadherin in controlling vascular morphogenesis. J Cell Biol 169:29–34.

Mancini M, Scappaticci D, Cimino G, Nanni M, Derme V, Elia L, Tafuri A, Vignetti M, Vitale A, Cuneo A, Castoldi G, Saglio G, Pane F, Mecucci C, Camera A, Specchia G, Tedeschi A,

Di RF, Fioritoni G, Fabbiano F, Marmont F, Ferrara F, Cascavilla N, Todeschini G, Nobile F, Kropp MG, Leoni P, Tabilio A, Luppi M, Annino L, Mandelli F, Foa R (2005) A comprehensive genetic classification of adult acute lymphoblastic leukemia (ALL): Analysis of the GIMEMA 0496 protocol. Blood 105:3434–3441.

Mandal L, Martinez-Agosto JA, Evans CJ, Hartenstein V, Banerjee U (2007) A Hedgehog- and Antennapedia-dependent niche maintains Drosophila haematopoietic precursors. Nature 446:320–324.

Massague J, Blain SW, Lo RS (2000) TGFbeta signaling in growth control, cancer, and heritable disorders. Cell 103:295–309.

Mayerhofer M, Valent P, Sperr WR, Griffin JD, Sillaber C (2002) BCR/ABL induces expression of vascular endothelial growth factor and its transcriptional activator, hypoxia inducible factor-1alpha, through a pathway involving phosphoinositide 3-kinase and the mammalian target of rapamycin. Blood 100:3767–3775.

McLachlan RW and Yap AS (2007) Not so simple: the complexity of phosphotyrosine signaling at cadherin adhesive contacts. J Mol Med 85:545–554.

McReynolds LJ, Gupta S, Figueroa ME, Mullins MC, Evans T (2007) Smad1 and Smad5 differentially regulate embryonic hematopoiesis. Blood 110:3881–3890.

Melo JV and Barnes DJ (2007) Chronic myeloid leukaemia as a model of disease evolution in human cancer. Nat Rev Cancer 7:441–453.

Metcalf D (2008) Hematopoietic cytokines. Blood 111:485–491.

Michor F (2007) Chronic myeloid leukemia blast crisis arises from progenitors. Stem Cells 25:1114–1118.

Michor F, Hughes TP, Iwasa Y, Branford S, Shah NP, Sawyers CL, Nowak MA (2005) Dynamics of chronic myeloid leukaemia. Nature 435:1267–1270.

Mishra L, Derynck R, Mishra B (2005) Transforming growth factor-beta signaling in stem cells and cancer. Science 310:68–71.

Najy AJ, Day KC, Day ML (2008) The ectodomain shedding of E-cadherin by ADAM15 supports ErbB receptor activation. J Biol Chem 283:18393–18401.

Nakamura Y, Patrushev N, Inomata H, Mehta D, Urao N, Kim HW, Razvi M, Kini V, Mahadev K, Goldstein BJ, McKinney R, Fukai T, Ushio-Fukai M (2008) Role of protein tyrosine phosphatase 1B in vascular endothelial growth factor signaling and cell–cell adhesions in endothelial cells. Circ Res 102:1182–1191.

Navarro P, Ruco L, Dejana E (1998) Differential localization of VE- and N-cadherins in human endothelial cells: VE-cadherin competes with N-cadherin for junctional localization. J Cell Biol 140:1475–1484.

Nawroth R, Poell G, Ranft A, Kloep S, Samulowitz U, Fachinger G, Golding M, Shima DT, Deutsch U, Vestweber D (2002) VE-PTP and VE-cadherin ectodomains interact to facilitate regulation of phosphorylation and cell contacts. EMBO J 21:4885–4895.

Neering SJ, Bushnell T, Sozer S, Ashton J, Rossi RM, Wang PY, Bell DR, Heinrich D, Bottaro A, Jordan CT (2007) Leukemia stem cells in a genetically defined murine model of blast-crisis CML. Blood 110:2578–2585.

Nieborowska-Skorska M, Slupianek A, Skorski T (2000) Progressive changes in the leukemogenic signaling in BCR/ABL-transformed cells. Oncogene 19:4117–4124.

Noble ME, Endicott JA, Johnson LN (2004) Protein kinase inhibitors: insights into drug design from structure. Science 303:1800–1805.

Nowell PC (2007) Discovery of the Philadelphia chromosome: a personal perspective. J Clin Invest 117:2033–2035.

Ogata S, Morokuma J, Hayata T, Kolle G, Niehrs C, Ueno N, Cho KW (2007) TGF-beta signaling-mediated morphogenesis: modulation of cell adhesion via cadherin endocytosis. Genes Dev 21:1817–1831.

Parada Y, Banerji L, Glassford J, Lea NC, Collado M, Rivas C, Lewis JL, Gordon MY, Thomas NS, Lam EW (2001) BCR-ABL and interleukin 3 promote haematopoietic cell proliferation and survival through modulation of cyclin D2 and p27Kip1 expression. J Biol Chem 276: 23572–23580.

Pelletier SD, Hong DS, Hu Y, Liu Y, Li S (2004) Lack of the adhesion molecules P-selectin and intercellular adhesion molecule-1 accelerate the development of BCR/ABL-induced chronic myeloid leukemia-like myeloproliferative disease in mice. Blood 104:2163–2171.

Pesce M, Anastassiadis K, Scholer HR (1999) Oct-4: Lessons of totipotency from embryonic stem cells. Cells Tissues Organs 165:144–152.

Pokutta S and Weis WI (2007) Structure and mechanism of cadherins and catenins in cell–cell contacts. Annu Rev Cell Dev Biol 23:237–261.

Polyak K (2007) Breast cancer: Origins and evolution. J Clin Invest 117:3155–3163.

Porkka K, Koskenvesa P, Lundan T, Rimpilainen J, Mustjoki S, Smykla R, Wild R, Luo R, Arnan M, Brethon B, Eccersley L, Hjorth-Hansen H, Hoglund M, Klamova H, Knutsen H, Parikh S, Raffoux E, Gruber F, Brito-Babapulle F, Dombret H, Duarte RF, Elonen E, Paquette R, Zwaan CM, Lee FY (2008) Dasatinib crosses the blood-brain barrier and is an efficient therapy for central nervous system Philadelphia chromosome-positive leukemia. Blood Aug 15:112 (4): 1005–12.

Potter MD, Barbero S, Cheresh DA (2005) Tyrosine phosphorylation of VE-cadherin prevents binding of p120- and beta-catenin and maintains the cellular mesenchymal state. J Biol Chem 280:31906–31912.

Ptasznik A, Urbanowska E, Chinta S, Costa MA, Katz BA, Stanislaus MA, Demir G, Linnekin D, Pan ZK, Gewirtz AM (2002) Crosstalk between BCR/ABL oncoprotein and CXCR4 signaling through a Src family kinase in human leukemia cells. J Exp Med 196:667–678.

Pui CH and Evans WE (2006) Treatment of acute lymphoblastic leukemia. N Engl J Med 354: 166–178.

Qi J, Wang J, Romanyuk O, Siu CH (2006) Involvement of Src family kinases in N-cadherin phosphorylation and beta-catenin dissociation during transendothelial migration of melanoma cells. Mol Biol Cell 17:1261–1272.

Ramaraj P, Singh H, Niu N, Chu S, Holtz M, Yee JK, Bhatia R (2004) Effect of mutational inactivation of tyrosine kinase activity on BCR/ABL-induced abnormalities in cell growth and adhesion in human hematopoietic progenitors. Cancer Res 64:5322–5331.

Reiss K, Maretzky T, Ludwig A, Tousseyn T, de SB, Hartmann D, Saftig P (2005) ADAM10 cleavage of N-cadherin and regulation of cell–cell adhesion and beta-catenin nuclear signalling. EMBO J 24:742–752.

Reiss K, Maretzky T, Haas IG, Schulte M, Ludwig A, Frank M, Saftig P (2006) Regulated ADAM10-dependent ectodomain shedding of gamma-protocadherin C3 modulates cell–cell adhesion. J Biol Chem 281:21735–21744.

Renshaw MW, McWhirter JR, Wang JY (1995) The human leukemia oncogene bcr-abl abrogates the anchorage requirement but not the growth factor requirement for proliferation. Mol Cell Biol 15:1286–1293.

Reya T and Clevers H (2005) Wnt signalling in stem cells and cancer. Nature 434:843–850.

Rias-Salgado EG, Lizano S, Sarkar S, Brugge JS, Ginsberg MH, Shattil SJ (2003) Src kinase activation by direct interaction with the integrin beta cytoplasmic domain. Proc Natl Acad Sci U S A 100:13298–13302.

Ricci-Vitiani L, Lombardi DG, Pilozzi E, Biffoni M, Todaro M, Peschle C, De MR (2007) Identification and expansion of human colon-cancer-initiating cells. Nature 445: 111–115.

Rubin H (2003) Microenvironmental regulation of the initiated cell. Adv Cancer Res 90:1–62.

Rudini N, Felici A, Giampietro C, Lampugnani M, Corada M, Swirsding K, Garre M, Liebner S, Letarte M, ten DP, Dejana E (2008) VE-cadherin is a critical endothelial regulator of TGF-beta signalling. EMBO J 27:993–1004.

Rustin GJ, Newlands ES, Begent RH, Dent J, Bagshawe KD (1989) Weekly alternating etoposide, methotrexate, and actinomycin/vincristine and cyclophosphamide chemotherapy for the treatment of CNS metastases of choriocarcinoma. J Clin Oncol 7:900–903.

Salgia R, Li JL, Ewaniuk DS, Pear W, Pisick E, Burky SA, Ernst T, Sattler M, Chen LB, Griffin JD (1997) BCR/ABL induces multiple abnormalities of cytoskeletal function. J Clin Invest 100:46–57.

Salgia R, Quackenbush E, Lin J, Souchkova N, Sattler M, Ewaniuk DS, Klucher KM, Daley GQ, Kraeft SK, Sackstein R, Alyea EP, von Andrian UH, Chen LB, Gutierrez-Ramos JC, Pendergast AM, Griffin JD (1999) The BCR/ABL oncogene alters the chemotactic response to stromal-derived factor-1alpha. Blood 94:4233–4246.

Savona M and Talpaz M (2008) Getting to the stem of chronic myeloid leukaemia. Nat Rev Cancer 8:341–350.

Schmierer B and Hill CS (2007) TGFbeta-SMAD signal transduction: molecular specificity and functional flexibility. Nat Rev Mol Cell Biol 8:970–982.

Schultz KR, Pullen DJ, Sather HN, Shuster JJ, Devidas M, Borowitz MJ, Carroll AJ, Heerema NA, Rubnitz JE, Loh ML, Raetz EA, Winick NJ, Hunger SP, Carroll WL, Gaynon PS, Camitta BM (2007) Risk- and response-based classification of childhood B-precursor acute lymphoblastic leukemia: a combined analysis of prognostic markers from the Pediatric Oncology Group (POG) and Children's Cancer Group (CCG). Blood 109:926–935.

Schulz B, Pruessmeyer J, Maretzky T, Ludwig A, Blobel CP, Saftig P, Reiss K (2008) ADAM10 regulates endothelial permeability and T-Cell transmigration by proteolysis of vascular endothelial cadherin. Circ Res 102:1192–1201.

Shattil SJ (2005) Integrins and Src: Dynamic duo of adhesion signaling. Trends Cell Biol 15: 399–403.

Shoval I, Ludwig A, Kalcheim C (2007) Antagonistic roles of full-length N-cadherin and its soluble BMP cleavage product in neural crest delamination. Development 134:491–501.

Sipkins DA, Wei X, Wu JW, Runnels JM, Cote D, Means TK, Luster AD, Scadden DT, Lin CP (2005) In vivo imaging of specialized bone marrow endothelial microdomains for tumour engraftment. Nature 435:969–973.

Skorski T, Nieborowska-Skorska M, Wlodarski P, Perrotti D, Martinez R, Wasik MA, Calabretta B (1996) Blastic transformation of p53-deficient bone marrow cells by p210bcr/abl tyrosine kinase. Proc Natl Acad Sci U S A 93:13137–13142.

Smith RA and Glomski CA (1982) "Hemogenic endothelium" of the embryonic aorta: Does it exist? Dev Comp Immunol 6:359–368.

Soper JT (1990) Gestational trophoblastic neoplasia. Curr Opin Obstet Gynecol 2:92–97.

Stoklosa T, Poplawski T, Koptyra M, Nieborowska-Skorska M, Basak G, Slupianek A, Rayevskaya M, Seferynska I, Herrera L, Blasiak J, Skorski T (2008) BCR/ABL inhibits mismatch repair to protect from apoptosis and induce point mutations. Cancer Res 68:2576–2580.

Sun X, Li Y, Yu W, Wang B, Tao Y, Dai Z (2008) MT1-MMP as a downstream target of BCR-ABL/ABL interactor 1 signaling: polarized distribution and involvement in BCR-ABL-stimulated leukemic cell migration. Leukemia 22:1053–1056.

Symowicz J, Adley BP, Gleason KJ, Johnson JJ, Ghosh S, Fishman DA, Hudson LG, Stack MS (2007) Engagement of collagen-binding integrins promotes matrix metalloproteinase-9-dependent E-cadherin ectodomain shedding in ovarian carcinoma cells. Cancer Res 67: 2030–2039.

Tai CY, Mysore SP, Chiu C, Schuman EM (2007) Activity-regulated N-cadherin endocytosis. Neuron 54:771–785.

Tallman MS, Gilliland DG, Rowe JM (2005) Drug therapy for acute myeloid leukemia. Blood 106:1154–1163.

Tao WJ, Lin H, Sun T, Samanta AK, Arlinghaus R (2008) BCR-ABL oncogenic transformation of NIH 3T3 fibroblasts requires the IL-3 receptor. Oncogene 27:3194–3200.

Taoudi S and Medvinsky A (2007) Functional identification of the hematopoietic stem cell niche in the ventral domain of the embryonic dorsal aorta. Proc Natl Acad Sci U S A 104: 9399–9403.

Tauchi T, Miyazawa K, Feng GS, Broxmeyer HE, Toyama K (1997) A coiled-coil tetramerization domain of BCR-ABL is essential for the interactions of SH2-containing signal transduction molecules. J Biol Chem 272:1389–1394.

Ten DP and Arthur HM (2007) Extracellular control of TGFbeta signalling in vascular development and disease. Nat Rev Mol Cell Biol 8:857–869.

Thomas EK, Cancelas JA, Chae HD, Cox AD, Keller PJ, Perrotti D, Neviani P, Druker BJ, Setchell KD, Zheng Y, Harris CE, Williams DA (2007) Rac guanosine triphosphatases represent integrating molecular therapeutic targets for BCR-ABL-induced myeloproliferative disease. Cancer Cell 12:467–478.

Thomas EK, Cancelas JA, Zheng Y, Williams DA (2008) Rac GTPases as key regulators of p210-BCR-ABL-dependent leukemogenesis. Leukemia 22:898–904.

Tibes R, Trent J, Kurzrock R (2005) Tyrosine kinase inhibitors and the dawn of molecular cancer therapeutics. Annu Rev Pharmacol Toxicol 45:357–384.

Tonks NK (2006) Protein tyrosine phosphatases: From genes, to function, to disease. Nat Rev Mol Cell Biol 7:833–846.

Tonks NK and Muthuswamy SK (2007) A brake becomes an accelerator: PTP1B–a new therapeutic target for breast cancer. Cancer Cell 11:214–216.

Trotta R, Vignudelli T, Candini O, Intine RV, Pecorari L, Guerzoni C, Santilli G, Byrom MW, Goldoni S, Ford LP, Caligiuri MA, Maraia RJ, Perrotti D, Calabretta B (2003) BCR/ABL activates mdm2 mRNA translation via the La antigen. Cancer Cell 3:145–160.

Vescovi AL, Galli R, Reynolds BA (2006) Brain tumour stem cells. Nat Rev Cancer 6: 425–436.

Vousden KH and Lane DP (2007) p53 in health and disease. Nat Rev Mol Cell Biol 8: 275–283.

Vrekoussis T, Stathopoulos EN, De GU, Kafousi M, Pavlaki K, Kalogeraki A, Chrysos E, Fiorentini G, Zoras O (2006) Modulation of vascular endothelium by imatinib: A study on the EA.hy 926 endothelial cell line. J Chemother 18:56–65.

Wallez Y, Cand F, Cruzalegui F, Wernstedt C, Souchelnytskyi S, Vilgrain I, Huber P (2007) Src kinase phosphorylates vascular endothelial-cadherin in response to vascular endothelial growth factor: Identification of tyrosine 685 as the unique target site. Oncogene 26:1067–1077.

Wang Y, Jin G, Miao H, Li JY, Usami S, Chien S (2006) Integrins regulate VE-cadherin and catenins: dependence of this regulation on Src, but not on Ras. Proc Natl Acad Sci U S A 103:1774–1779.

Wang L, O'Leary H, Fortney J, Gibson LF (2007) Ph+/VE-cadherin+ identifies a stem cell like population of acute lymphoblastic leukemia sustained by bone marrow niche cells. Blood 110:3334–3344.

Wang Z, Sampath J, Fukuda S, Pelus LM (2005) Disruption of the inhibitor of apoptosis protein survivin sensitizes Bcr-abl-positive cells to STI571-induced apoptosis. Cancer Res 65: 8224–8232.

Wertheim JA, Forsythe K, Druker BJ, Hammer D, Boettiger D, Pear WS (2002a) BCR-ABL-induced adhesion defects are tyrosine kinase-independent. Blood 99:4122–4130.

Wertheim JA, Miller JP, Xu L, He Y, Pear WS (2002b) The biology of chronic myelogenous leukemia: Mouse models and cell adhesion. Oncogene 21:8612–8628.

Wertheim JA, Perera SA, Hammer DA, Ren R, Boettiger D, Pear WS (2003) Localization of BCR-ABL to F-actin regulates cell adhesion but does not attenuate CML development. Blood 102:2220–2228.

Williams RT, den BW, Sherr CJ (2007) Cytokine-dependent imatinib resistance in mouse BCR-ABL+, Arf-null lymphoblastic leukemia. Genes Dev 21:2283–2287.

Wong S and Witte ON (2004) The BCR-ABL story: bench to bedside and back. Annu Rev Immunol 22:247–306.

Wong S, McLaughlin J, Cheng D, Shannon K, Robb L, Witte ON (2003) IL-3 receptor signaling is dispensable for BCR-ABL-induced myeloproliferative disease. Proc Natl Acad Sci U S A 100:11630–11635.

Wu X, Tu X, Joeng KS, Hilton MJ, Williams DA, Long F (2008) Rac1 activation controls nuclear localization of beta-catenin during canonical Wnt signaling. Cell 133:340–353.

Xiao K, Allison DF, Kottke MD, Summers S, Sorescu GP, Faundez V, Kowalczyk AP (2003) Mechanisms of VE-cadherin processing and degradation in microvascular endothelial cells. J Biol Chem 278:19199–19208.

Xiao K, Garner J, Buckley KM, Vincent PA, Chiasson CM, Dejana E, Faundez V, Kowalczyk AP (2005) p120-Catenin regulates clathrin-dependent endocytosis of VE-cadherin. Mol Biol Cell 16:5141–5151.

Yamada S, Pokutta S, Drees F, Weis WI, Nelson WJ (2005) Deconstructing the cadherin–catenin–actin complex. Cell 123:889–901.

Yamashita YM (2008) Selfish stem cells compete with each other. Cell Stem Cell 2:3–4.

Yap AS, Crampton MS, Hardin J (2007) Making and breaking contacts: the cellular biology of cadherin regulation. Curr Opin Cell Biol 19:508–514.

Zhang J, Niu C, Ye L, Huang H, He X, Tong WG, Ross J, Haug J, Johnson T, Feng JQ, Harris S, Wiedemann LM, Mishina Y, Li L (2003) Identification of the haematopoietic stem cell niche and control of the niche size. Nature 425:836–841.

Zhang B, Groffen J, Heisterkamp N (2007) Increased resistance to a farnesyltransferase inhibitor by N-cadherin expression in Bcr/Abl-P190 lymphoblastic leukemia cells. Leukemia 21: 1189–1197.

Zhao RC, Jiang Y, Verfaillie CM (2001) A model of human p210(bcr/ABL)-mediated chronic myelogenous leukemia by transduction of primary normal human CD34(+) cells with a BCR/ABL-containing retroviral vector. Blood 97:2406–2412.

Zhao C, Blum J, Chen A, Kwon HY, Jung SH, Cook JM, Lagoo A, Reya T (2007) Loss of beta-catenin impairs the renewal of normal and CML stem cells in vivo. Cancer Cell 12:528–541.

Zhou Y, Fisher SJ, Janatpour M, Genbacev O, Dejana E, Wheelock M, Damsky CH (1997) Human cytotrophoblasts adopt a vascular phenotype as they differentiate. A strategy for successful endovascular invasion? J Clin Invest 99:2139–2151.

Part VI
Putting It All Together

Chapter 19
Melanoma: Mutations in Multiple Pathways at the Tumor–Stroma Interface

Himabindu Gaddipati and Meenhard Herlyn

Cast of Characters

The preceding chapters catalog mutations in cancer genes that affect tumor microenvironment. From the signaling standpoint, most of them could be mapped to several key pathways known to play an important role in cancer (Vogelstein and Kinzler, 2004): (1.) The receptor tyrosine kinase (RTK) pathway involving cognate soluble ligands (**HGF**, **PDGF**, etc.), RTKs themselves (**c-Met, IGF-R, PDFG-R**, c-Kit, etc), **Ras**-family members (Ki,- Ha-, and N-), small GTPases (e.g., **RhoH**), and their downstream effectors c-Raf and MAP kinases; (2.) The p53 pathway, controlled to a large extent by the **ink4a** locus; (3.) The **HIF1** pathway, including the **VHL** tumor suppressor; (4.) The APC pathway, including the **cadherin/catenin** axis and **c-Myc;** (5.) The **TFGβ** pathway; and last but not least (6.) The PI3K pathway, including the key enzymes **AKT** and **PTEN**.

While individual mutations in these genes can profoundly alter tumor milieu, the naturally occurring tumors often bear mutations in multiple pathways, malignant melanoma being an illuminating case study (Table 19.1, modified from Dahl and Guldberg (2007). The nature of some of these mutations (in particular those underlined in the table) and the interplay between them are reviewed in detail below.

Introduction

Over the past few decades the incidence of melanoma has been steadily rising. Among skin cancers, melanoma has the highest mortality rate and the worst prognosis. Despite this alarming trend, patients with advanced stage melanoma continue to have virtually no effective treatment options. Research in recent times has contributed greatly to our understanding of the complex and diverse mechanisms that regulate melanomagenesis. Both germline and somatic mutations contribute to

M. Herlyn (✉)
The Wistar Institute, Philadelphia, PA, USA
e-mail: herlynm@wistar.org

A. Thomas-Tikhonenko (ed.), *Cancer Genome and Tumor Microenvironment*,
DOI 10.1007/978-1-4419-0711-0_19, © Springer Science+Business Media, LLC 2010

Table 19.1 Genetic alteration in melanoma with known cell-extrinsic effects

Genes with known influence over TME	Gene	Most frequent type of alteration	Frequency(%)
Proto-oncogenes	*KIT*	Mutation	2–10
	NRAS	Mutation	15–25
	BRAF	Mutation	50–70
	CTNNB	Mutation	2–23
	PIK3CA	Mutation	<5
	AKT3	Amplification	40–60
Tumor-suppressor genes	*INK4A*	Deletion, mutation	40–87
	ARF	Deletion, mutation	40–70
	PTEN	Deletion, mutation	5–40
	TP53	Mutation	0–25

the initiation and progression of melanoma. Additionally, complex and dynamic interactions between the tumor and the tumor microenvironment and various growth factors signaling pathways also play essential roles in tumorigenesis. Insights into key regulatory pathways, such as RTK and PI3K-Akt, have recently presented us with opportunities to evaluate potential new therapeutic targets.

The RTK/RAS/MAPK Pathway

Pathway Overview

The MAPK signal transduction pathway has been demonstrated to play a key role in the pathogenesis of melanoma. The MAPK pathway comprises a series of protein kinases such as RAF-MEK-ERK which are sequentially activated by phosphorylation (Widlund and Fisher, 2003). Ligand binding to cell surface RTKs initially activates RAS, which can now bind to effector proteins such as RAF or PI3K. The downstream effector ERK then phosphorylates cytoplasmic and nuclear targets (Kohno and Pouyssegur, 2006; Sridhar et al., 2005). Besides melanoma, deregulation of this cascade is a common occurrence in a number of other cancers such as colorectal, ovarian, thyroid, lung, and cholangiocarcinoma (Houben et al., 2004).

The RTK pathway can be activated in melanoma cell by a variety of ligands and their cognate receptors (Fig. 19.1). As detailed in the preceding chapters, many of them, when constitutively activated, have profound cell-extrinsic effects. Some of these activation events primarily occur by epigenetic (integrin binding, HSF/Met interaction, etc.) and some (c-Kit) – by genetic means.

HGF/SF

Stromal cells are the primary source of the HGF/SCF (hepatocyte growth factor/scatter factor) cytokine (Nakamura et al., 1997; Stoker et al., 1987). HGF

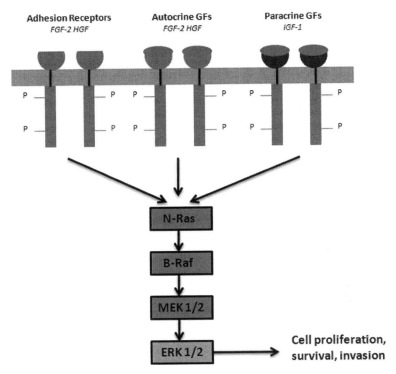

Fig. 19.1 Activation of the RTK pathway by various ligands. Original artwork by Kathryn Simmermon, MHA/MHE

interacts with its tyrosine kinase receptor c-Met to stimulate multiple signal transduction pathways and increase cellular proliferation and motility. *CMET* has been demonstrated to be inappropriately expressed in melanoma and a number of other cancers such as breast cancer and hepatoma. Recio and Merlino (2002) demonstrated that HGF/SCF promotes cellular proliferation by increasing *CMET* expression via activation of multiple kinases in MAPK, AKT, SAPK/JNK pathways. The effects were found to be mediated through upregulation of cyclin D1 and the ATF-2. While c-Met is not known to be mutated in melanomas, mutations have been discovered in the closely related c-Kit receptor.

c-Kit Receptor

c-Kit is a transmembrane growth factor receptor, which belongs to the type III receptor tyrosine kinase family. The *KIT* gene was identified as a viral oncogene in the Hardy–Zuckerman IV feline sarcoma virus (Besmer et al., 1986). Steel factor or stem cell factor, SCF is the ligand for c-Kit and is thought to mediate growth and survival through the activation of the MAPK pathway. Mutations in the murine locus for SCF ligand and its receptor c-Kit predispose to a variety of defects in melanocyte migration and homing to the basal epidermis, gametogenesis, or hematopoesis (Chabot et al., 1988; Geissler et al., 1988). In humans, the *KIT* gene maps to chromosome 4 (4q11–q12), which is in close proximity to the PDGFα receptor (d'Auriol et al., 1988; Stenman et al., 1989). Gastrointestinal-stromal tumors (GIST) are known to have activating mutations of *CKIT* and imitinib a potent c-Kit antagonist has been demonstrated to be an efficacious therapeutic agent. Activating events include missense mutations, small insertions and deletions (Sattler and Salgia, 2004). The majority of the mutations occur in the intracellular juxtamembrane domain in exon 11 in about 2–6% of melanomas (Went et al., 2004; Willmore-Payne et al., 2005, 2006). However, the extracellular dimerization domain (exon 9) and the kinase domain (exon 13) are also frequent mutational targets. *KIT* mutations are also found less frequently in other malignancies such as adult mastocytosis, small cell lung cancer, colon cancer, thyroid and testicular cancer. Interestingly, fluorescent in situ hybridization for *KIT* demonstrated selective loss of the normal alleles in all of the 3 L576 mutation-positive melanoma cases.

Activation of the c-Kit receptor results in activation of the classical RTK/RAS/MAPK pathway as well as activation of many other signaling molecules such as Src kinase family, PI3K family, and JAK/STAT. In the RTK pathway, the Grb2/SOS complex recruits RAS to form an active moiety, which in turn recruits RAF kinase to the plasma membrane. Interestingly, *BRAF/NRAS* gene mutations rarely occur in melanomas on mucosal surfaces, acral skin, and chronic sun-damaged skin. Seven percent of cases in these subtypes had *BRAF* mutations compared to 56% of cases in the intermittent sun-exposed category. In these tumors, alternative mechanisms ought to account for upregulation of the MAPK pathway. Indeed, the *KIT* oncogene was found to be mutated with much higher frequency, up to 30% of cases in a series of 102 primary melanomas encompassing these subtypes (Curtin et al., 2006).

In contrast, previous studies that were carried out in melanoma cell lines derived from intermittently sun-exposed skin with frequent *BRAF* mutations demonstrate either a complete absence of *KIT* mutations or a mutation frequency in the range of 2% (Went et al., 2004; Willmore-Payne et al., 2005, 2006). In some of these lines, *KIT* was shown to be either downregulated or even inhibiting tumor growth (Huang et al., 1996; Lassam and Bickford, 1992; Montone et al., 1997).

Finally, in some cases KIT and BRAF mutations coexist. For example, melanomas with the K642E mutation showed a copy number increase in *KIT* or a concurrent *BRAF* mutation. Mutational status or copy number increase correlated with increased protein expression in more than 60% of cases. Activating mutations in both KIT (in L576) and BRAF were also detected in a subset of malignant melanomas by Willmore-Payne et al (2006). Activating mutations in both c-Kit and BRAF might result in autonomous functioning of their respective pathways. Alexeev et al. demonstrated that constitutive activation of c-Kit RTK enhanced only migration but not proliferation of melanocytic cells. They also demonstrated that in order to escape from epidermal boundaries cells must lose c-Kit expression (Alexeev and Yoon, 2006). The importance of c-Kit mutations in specific subtypes of melanoma is clearly apparent from the recently reported dramatic response to imatinib therapy that was achieved in a patient with metastatic rectal melanoma (Hodi et al., 2008).

NRAS Mutations

RAS gene family members include *HRAS, NRAS and KRAS*. They encode 21 kDa proteins with GTPase activity (Meier et al., 2005).

Although *KRAS* mutations are more common in colon cancer, *NRAS* isoform mutations are predominant in melanoma (Keller et al., 2007; Whitwam et al., 2007). Besides downstream activation of the MAPK pathway, RAS also binds and activates the PI3K-AKT pathway. Additionally *RAS* interacts with p16 and p53.Oncogenic activating mutations in *RAS* often trigger a p53 and p16-mediated premature senescence response in melanoma, which block further steps in tumor progression (Serrano et al., 1997). Subsequent inactivating mutations in p16 or p53 tumor-suppressor genes may allow the premalignant cells to bypass the senescence response.

NRAS isoform mutations are found in approximately 15% of melanomas (Ball et al., 1994). They are typically located in exons 1 and 2 of the *RAS* gene. Most *NRAS* mutations entail the replacement of glutamine at residue 61 with amino acids like arginine, lysine, or leucine. This results in impaired GTP hydrolysis and subsequent sustained constitutive activation of the gene, which is independent of ligand-mediated activation of receptors on the cell surface. RAS remains in an activated GTP-bound state, RAF is continually recruited to the plasma membrane, and persistent phosphorylation-mediated activation of the RAF-MEK-ERK pathway ensues.

BRAF Mutations

BRAF is a serine/threonine-specific protein kinase that in melanomas is a key downstream mediator of RAS. Activating somatic missense mutations of the *BRAF* gene have been identified in 50–70% of malignant melanomas. All the mutations occur within the kinase domain, and a single amino acid substitution (V600E) accounts for approximately 80% of the mutations (Brose et al., 2002; Curtin et al., 2005; Davies et al., 2002; Pollock et al., 2003). V600E mutation is caused by a T-to-A substitution at nucleotide 1796 in exon 15 (Davies et al., 2002). Constitutive activation of *BRAF* is most likely facilitated by the switch from a small hydrophobic residue to a large hydrophilic moiety, which then enables the activation site to become continuously available for interaction (Houben et al., 2004). Additional point mutations occur at exons 11 and 1 (Kumar et al., 2003). V600E *BRAF* mutant has 10-fold greater kinase activity than the wild-type *BRAF*. Additionally, Lin et al. (2008) demonstrated by genomic analysis that the mutated *BRAF* gene may be amplified to low levels in melanoma. Willmore-Payne et al. (2006) demonstrated amplification in 2% of cases and chromosome 7 polysomy in 16.2% of mutant allele-positive tumors.

Both *BRAF* and *NRAS* mutations are commonly found in benign nevi. Therefore it is unlikely that they are the primary initiating factor in melanoma formation (Bauer et al., 2007; Pollock et al., 2003). Likely additional events involving synergistic mechanisms and pathways are required to facilitate progression to cancer. With rare exceptions the presence of *NRAS* and *BRAF* mutations were found to be mutually exclusive in multiple cohorts of melanoma samples (Davies et al., 2002; Houben et al., 2004).

Although adverse characteristics do not correlate significantly with mutational status in early phase VGP tumors, the presence of *NRAS/BRAF* mutations was associated with a significantly poorer prognosis and shortened overall survival in metastatic lesions (Houben et al., 2004). In this study *NRAS/BRAF* mutations were found in 66.3% of metastatic melanomas when compared to 50.9% of primary melanomas. This suggests that activating mutations of this nature facilitate melanoma progression and metastasis (Dong et al., 2003). Similar to TGF-β, which has been implicated in both tumor suppression and progression, BRAF may have a contrary role in tumor initiation: to help suppress genomic instability and induce senescence or growth arrest via upregulation of p53, p21Cip1, or p16 (Kerkhoff and Rapp, 1998; Lin et al., 1998). However, as the tumor progresses to metastasis with additional genetic mutations and insults, the unfavorable characteristics tend to become predominant. Interestingly, Kumat et al. noted in their cohort of patients a more favorable response to therapy and longer progression free survival in cases with *BRAF/NRAS* mutations when compared to mutation-free tumor samples (Houben et al., 2004).

Downstream of BRAF

MAPK pathway activation may also occur independently of BRAF/NRAS mutations. In one series of patients constitutive activation of *ERK* has been discovered in up to 43% of cases without *BRAF/NRAF* activation (Houben et al., 2004). It is know that PTEN negatively regulates the MAPK pathway. Therefore it is postulated that PTEN alterations and autocrine secretion of growth factors may contribute to *ERK* activation in a subset of tumors (Smalley, 2003; Wu et al., 2003). Additionally metastatic melanoma cell lines possess constitutively phosphorylated ERK1 and 2 (Satyamoorthy et al., 2001). This would lend credence to the hypothesis that multiple concurrent mechanisms may be at play in driving tumor progression and heterogeneity.

The PI3K/AKT Pathway

Pathway Overview

The PI3K-AKT signaling pathway plays an important role in mediating cell growth and survival in melanoma (Stahl et al., 2004). The pathway is activated through ligand-RTK (receptor tyrosine kinase) binding at the cell surface, which leads to activation of PI3K. PI3K activation converts PIP2 (phosphatidylinositol bisphosphate) at the plasma membrane to PIP3 (phosphatidylinositol (3,4,5)-trisphosphate). AKT kinase is then phosphorylated and activated. Several downstream members of the cascade are then phosphorylated and enabled to activate transcription factors. Activation of the AKT pathway also results in inhibition of GSK-3β and stabilization of β-catenin. Interestingly, point mutations of β-catenin resulting in constitutively stabilized protein have been detected in melanoma (Rubinfeld et al., 1997). β-catenin activation may also be mediated through the N-cadherin adhesion molecule. N-cadherin on the surface of VGP melanomas may facilitate gap junction cross talk with fibroblasts allowing for intimate interaction with the stromal microenvironment. PI3K/AKT pathway activation may also be mediated through RAS.

AKT Mutations

AKT (a.k.a. protein kinase B) has in fact three distinct isoforms AKT1, AKT2, and AKT3, which share a great degree of structural homology (Brazil et al., 2002; Nicholson and Anderson, 2002). Stahl et al. (2003) demonstrated that selective activation of AKT3 occurs as a result of overexpression and copy number increases of the *AKT3* gene, reduction in the PTEN activity due to haploinsufficiency, or loss of the PTEN gene. Copy number increases in the region of the chromosome 1q43–44 containing the *AKT3* gene have been described in the melanoma literature (Bastian et al., 1998; Thompson et al., 1995). Inhibition of AKT3 resulted in increased apoptosis of tumor cells and delayed tumor progression. The study also showed that although AKT activity was present in common nevi progressively higher levels of the protein were detected by immunohistochemical staining in sequential steps of melanoma progression (dysplastic nevi to metastatic melanomas). Therefore AKT3 levels appear to correlate with steps in tumor progression and confer a specific survival advantage in tumor microenvironment. Expression of AKT3 has been strongly correlated with melanoma progression, and inhibition results in apoptosis and a decline in xenograft growth (Stahl et al., 2004).

PTEN Mutations

Phosphatase and *ten*sin homolog deleted in chromosome 10 or *PTEN* is a known tumor-suppressor gene that is mutated somatically in up to 40% of melanomas. *PTEN* augments apoptosis by upregulating key proapoptosis factors such as caspases and BID while downregulating anti-apoptotic proteins such as Bcl2 (Wu et al., 2003). It is also inhibitory to growth factor-mediated activation of the MAPK pathway. Therefore alterations in the *PTEN* gene mediate cell survival, loss of adhesion and migration. Mutations have also been noted in a wide variety of cancers such as glioblastomas, endometrial, breast, thyroid, and prostate cancers.

The PTEN protein has both lipid phosphatase and protein phosphatase activity. The lipid phosphatase activity inhibits the AKT pathway activity by dephosphorylating PIP_3(phospatidylinosital triphosphate) (Birck et al., 2000; Guldberg et al., 1997; Tsao et al., 1998). Subsequent overactivation of the PI3K-AKT pathway has been demonstrated to contribute to melanomagenesis. About 30–40% of malignant melanoma cell lines and 5–15% of uncultured tumor samples harbor either homozygous deletions or inactivating nonsense or missense PTEN mutations (Guldberg et al., 1997). *PTEN* loss is rare in primary melanomas when compared to metastatic melanomas indicating that it may influence the later steps in tumorigenesis. However, since less than 40% of melanomas harbor *PTEN* mutations, alternate mechanisms of AKT/PI3K activation must exist (Birck et al., 2000; Guldberg et al., 1997; Tsao et al., 1998).

Interestingly *NRAS* and *PTEN* mutations have been found to be mutually exclusive (as are *NRAS* and *BRAF* mutations). On the other hand *BRAF* and *PTEN* mutations coexist in > 20% of melanomas (Tsao et al., 2000, 2004). This would lend credence to the hypothesis that *RAS* mutations are sufficient to activate both the MAPK and AKT pathways while separate mutations in the individual pathways are required to achieve the same outcome. Mutations in the catalytic subunit of PI3K (PIK3CA) rarely occur in melanoma (<5%) but have significant prevalence in a number of other human malignancies (Samuels et al., 2004).

Melanoma Pathways in the Context of Tumor Microenvironment

Solid human tumors such as melanoma are composed of diverse cellular elements in addition to the malignant cells. Stromal fibroblasts are influenced by tumor secreted chemokines and in turn "activated" fibroblasts produce paracrine stimulants and growth factors. Non neoplastic cells such as endothelial, immune, and smooth muscle cells also contribute to the cellular heterogeneity and the tumorigenic process by secreting various growth factors.

The IGF1/IGF-1R Axis

IGF1 has been shown to mediate important roles in melanoma progression in survival, growth, and motility through activation of the MAPK and the PI3K/AKT pathways. IGF-1 is only produced by fibroblasts and not by melanocytes. However, PDGF produced by melanoma cells stimulates fibroblasts to produce IGF1 (Herlyn and Shih, 1994). IGF1 then interacts with the IGF-1R receptor on the melanoma cell surface and mediates its effects through the activation of the MAPK and AKT/PI3K pathways.

However, activation of melanoma cells by IGF1 is restricted to the early radial growth phase (RGP) of tumor progression. In RGP primary melanoma cells require both IGF1 and bFGF (Rodeck et al., 1987). RGP melanoma cells are unable to grow anchorage independently and undergo apoptosis; however, the cells are rescued by

IGF-1 likely through stimulation of the PKB/AKT pathway and stabilization of β-catenin. Once cells invade the dermis they have autonomously activated survival pathways and constitutively produce bFGF. At this stage neither exogenous bFGF nor IGF-1 can stimulate aggressive melanoma cells (Herlyn et al., 1990). Oncogene-mediated transformation fails to occur in the absence of the IGF-1R. Reduction or total absence of growth was demonstrated in human glioblastoma, breast carcinoma, small cell lung carcinoma cells; melanoma and mouse melanoma cell lines by anti-sense strategies (Yeh et al., 2006). Yeh et al. successfully proved that *BRAF* or *NRAS* mutations do not render cells refractory to IGF1R targeting.

NOTCH Signaling Pathway in Melanoma

The Notch signaling pathway in mammalian cells has been implicated in diverse cellular processes that influence differentiation, cell fate, homeostasis, survival, proliferation, and angiogenesis (Artavanis-Tsakonas et al., 1999). The pathway is comprised of four transmembrane Notch receptors (Notch 1 to 4). The receptors are activated by at least five ligands (Delta 1,3,4 and Jagged 1,2). The activated receptor is subjected to two rounds of proteolytic cleavage by metalloprotease- and γ-secretase which results in release of the active intracellular domain (N^{IC}) from the plasma membrane which subsequently translocates to the nucleus to form a large transcriptional activation complex with mastermind-like (MAML) protein and CSL (CBF1/RBP-Jk, suppressor of hairless, LAG-1). This complex then mediates the transcription of target genes including the basic helix-loop-helix (bHLH) family of transcription factors such as members of the Hairy/Enhancer of split (HES) gene and Hairy/E (spl)-related with YRPW (Hey) gene families (Pinnix and Herlyn, 2007).

Deregulation of this cascade has also been implicated in neoplastic transformation. It is intriguing to note that depending on the cellular milieu notch pathway activation can result in both oncogenetic and tumor suppressive effects. Notch has been demonstrated to inhibit tumorigenesis in mouse basal and squamous cell carcinoma models. In B cell development, Notch 1 induces growth arrest and apoptosis (Morimura et al., 2000), while constitutive activation of the signaling pathway as a result of chromosomal translocation mediates tumorigenesis in T-cell acute lymphoblastic leukemia (Ellisen et al., 1991). Activating mutations in the *NOTCH1* gene have been demonstrated in greater than half of all T-ALL cases (Weng et al., 2004). Likewise activation contributes to oncogenesis in mouse mammary tumors (Sriuranpong et al., 2001) and transformed kidney epithelial cells (Capobianco et al., 1997), while a tumor-suppressor function has been delineated in small cell lung cancer (Sriuranpong et al., 2001), hepatocellular cancer (Qi et al., 2003), and prostate cancer (Shou et al., 2001).

In normal melanocytes the Notch pathway helps to promote the survival of the melancocyte precursor cells, melanoblasts, as well as melanocyte stem cells (Moriyama et al., 2006), most likely through the inhibition of apoptosis. Furthermore, Balint et al. demonstrated a likely stage-specific oncogenic role for *NOTCH* in Melanoma by showing preferential activation of *NOTCH* in 66% of melanoma samples in comparison to 7% of nevus samples (Balint et al., 2005). Specific Notch pathway inhibition by γ-secretase and DAPT significantly impacted tumor progression in primary melanoma, more so than in metastatic tumor cells. Therefore the Notch pathway was thought to play a more critical role in stimulating primary melanoma. Overexpression of N^{IC} resulted in greater tumor progression in vivo and increased levels of β-catenin were demonstrated (Balint et al., 2005). In a subsequent study Liu et al. demonstrated that Notch signaling upregulates both the MAPK and PI3K-Akt pathways by a post-transcriptional mechanism that is mediated through MAML (Liu et al., 2006). Consequently, inhibition of the MAPK or PI3K-Akt pathways inhibited the Notch-induced cell growth. Additionally, activation of the Notch pathway appears to play a role in the advancement of primary melanoma through upregulation of β-catenin (see above).

β3 Integrin-Mediated Effects

Integrins are a family of cell-adhesion receptors, which are composed of heterdimers of α and β subunits. Diversity of the α subunits and β subunits accounts for at least 20 types of integrins. Individual integrins can bind to different ligands by recognizing the specific amino acid sequence Arg-Gly-Asp (RGD) present on extracellular matrix like vitronectin, fibronectin, and von-Willebrand factor. They mediate both cell-extracellular matrix and cell–cell adhesion. More recently they have been shown to be involved in numerous malignant processes such as signaling pathways (Hynes, 1987), cell proliferation (Morino et al., 1995), apoptosis (Meredith and Schwartz, 1997), anoikis (Frisch and Ruoslahti, 1997), invasion and metastasis (Guan and Shalloway, 1992), and angiogenesis (Varner and Cheresh, 1996).

$\alpha_v\beta_3$ integrin is present on the surface of endothelial cells and tumor cells. In Melanoma $\alpha_v\beta_3$ integrin can activate MMP-2 on the cell surface to mediate invasion by collagen degradation (Brooks et al., 1996). $\alpha_v\beta_3$ integrin binds to the vitronectin ligand to bring about a change in morphology and migratory ability. Increased expression of the β_3 subunit has been shown to correlate with invasion in melanoma cells (Hsu et al., 1998).

Importantly, the onset of β_3-integrin expression can be correlated with transition from the noninvasive radial growth phase of melanoma to the invasive vertical growth phase in a 3D skin reconstruct model (Hsu et al., 1998). $\alpha_v\beta_3$ integrin is also involved in angiogenesis and tumor metastasis. A novel $\alpha_v\beta_3$-blocking disintegrin has been shown to inhibit bFGF-induced angiogenesis and metastasis in a mouse lung colonization model (Ramos et al., 2008).

Conclusions

The multiple pathways and mechanisms involved in the biology of melanoma demonstrate the complexity and diversity of the tumorigenic process. The numerous genetic means to achieve MAPK pathway activation, in collaboration with adjunct pathways, such as PI3K-Akt, Notch, c-Kit, have been delineated in this chapter. This serves to highlight the complicated network of regulation involved and the challenges we must face in overcoming the key drivers and the inherent redundancies in malignant processes.

References

Alexeev V and Yoon K. 2006. Distinctive role of the cKit receptor tyrosine kinase signaling in mammalian melanocytes. J Invest Dermatol 126:1102–1110.

Artavanis-Tsakonas S, Rand MD, Lake RJ. 1999. Notch signaling: cell fate control and signal integration in development. Science 284:770–776.

Balint K, Xiao M, Pinnix CC, Soma A, Veres I, Juhasz I, Brown EJ, Capobianco AJ, Herlyn M, Liu ZJ. 2005. Activation of Notch1 signaling is required for beta-catenin-mediated human primary melanoma progression. J Clin Invest 115:3166–3176.

Ball NJ, Yohn JJ, Morelli JG, Norris DA, Golitz LE, Hoeffler JP. 1994. Ras mutations in human melanoma: a marker of malignant progression. J Invest Dermatol 102:285–290.

Bastian BC, LeBoit PE, Hamm H, Brocker EB, Pinkel D. 1998. Chromosomal gains and losses in primary cutaneous melanomas detected by comparative genomic hybridization. Cancer Res 58:2170–2175.

Bauer J, Curtin JA, Pinkel D, Bastian BC. 2007. Congenital melanocytic nevi frequently harbor NRAS mutations but no BRAF mutations. J Invest Dermatol 127:179–182.

Besmer P, Murphy JE, George PC, Qiu FH, Bergold PJ, Lederman L, Snyder HW, Jr., Brodeur D, Zuckerman EE, Hardy WD. 1986. A new acute transforming feline retrovirus and relationship of its oncogene v-kit with the protein kinase gene family. Nature 320:415–421.

Birck A, Ahrenkiel V, Zeuthen J, Hou-Jensen K, Guldberg P. 2000. Mutation and allelic loss of the PTEN/MMAC1 gene in primary and metastatic melanoma biopsies. J Invest Dermatol 114:277–280.

Brazil DP, Park J, Hemmings BA. 2002. PKB binding proteins. Getting in on the Akt. Cell 111:293–303.

Brooks PC, Stromblad S, Sanders LC, von Schalscha TL, Aimes RT, Stetler-Stevenson WG, Quigley JP, Cheresh DA. 1996. Localization of matrix metalloproteinase MMP-2 to the surface of invasive cells by interaction with integrin alpha v beta 3. Cell 85:683–693.

Brose MS, Volpe P, Feldman M, Kumar M, Rishi I, Gerrero R, Einhorn E, Herlyn M, Minna J, Nicholson A, Roth JA, Albelda SM, Davies H, Cox C, Brignell G, Stephens P, Futreal PA, Wooster R, Stratton MR, Weber BL. 2002. BRAF and RAS mutations in human lung cancer and melanoma. Cancer Res 62:6997–7000.

Capobianco AJ, Zagouras P, Blaumueller CM, Artavanis-Tsakonas S, Bishop JM. 1997. Neoplastic transformation by truncated alleles of human NOTCH1/TAN1 and NOTCH2. Mol Cell Biol 17:6265–6273.

Chabot B, Stephenson DA, Chapman VM, Besmer P, Bernstein A. 1988. The proto-oncogene c-kit encoding a transmembrane tyrosine kinase receptor maps to the mouse W locus. Nature 335:88–89.

Curtin JA, Fridlyand J, Kageshita T, Patel HN, Busam KJ, Kutzner H, Cho KH, Aiba S, Brocker EB, LeBoit PE, Pinkel D, Bastian BC. 2005. Distinct sets of genetic alterations in melanoma. N Engl J Med 353:2135–2147.

Curtin JA, Busam K, Pinkel D, Bastian BC. 2006. Somatic activation of KIT in distinct subtypes of melanoma. J Clin Oncol 24:4340–4346.

Dahl C and Guldberg P. 2007. The genome and epigenome of malignant melanoma. Apmis 115:1161–1176.

d'Auriol L, Mattei MG, Andre C, Galibert F. 1988. Localization of the human c-kit protooncogene on the q11–q12 region of chromosome 4. Hum Genet 78:374–376.

Davies H, Bignell GR, Cox C, Stephens P, Edkins S, Clegg S, Teague J, Woffendin H, Garnett MJ, Bottomley W, Davis N, Dicks E, Ewing R, Floyd Y, Gray K, Hall S, Hawes R, Hughes J, Kosmidou V, Menzies A, Mould C, Parker A, Stevens C, Watt S, Hooper S, Wilson R, Jayatilake H, Gusterson BA, Cooper C, Shipley J, Hargrave D, Pritchard-Jones K, Maitland N, Chenevix-Trench G, Riggins GJ, Bigner DD, Palmieri G, Cossu A, Flanagan A, Nicholson A, Ho JW, Leung SY, Yuen ST, Weber BL, Seigler HF, Darrow TL, Paterson H, Marais R, Marshall CJ, Wooster R, Stratton MR, Futreal PA. 2002. Mutations of the BRAF gene in human cancer. Nature 417:949–954.

Dong J, Phelps RG, Qiao R, Yao S, Benard O, Ronai Z, Aaronson SA. 2003. BRAF oncogenic mutations correlate with progression rather than initiation of human melanoma. Cancer Res 63:3883–3885.

Ellisen LW, Bird J, West DC, Soreng AL, Reynolds TC, Smith SD, Sklar J. 1991. TAN-1, the human homolog of the Drosophila notch gene, is broken by chromosomal translocations in T lymphoblastic neoplasms. Cell 66:649–661.

Frisch SM and Ruoslahti E. 1997. Integrins and anoikis. Curr Opin Cell Biol 9:701–706.

Geissler EN, Ryan MA, Housman DE. 1988. The dominant-white spotting (W) locus of the mouse encodes the c-kit proto-oncogene. Cell 55:185–192.

Guan JL and Shalloway D. 1992. Regulation of focal adhesion-associated protein tyrosine kinase by both cellular adhesion and oncogenic transformation. Nature 358:690–692.

Guldberg P, thor Straten P, Birck A, Ahrenkiel V, Kirkin AF, Zeuthen J. 1997. Disruption of the MMAC1/PTEN gene by deletion or mutation is a frequent event in malignant melanoma. Cancer Res 57:3660–3663.

Herlyn M and Shih IM. 1994. Interactions of melanocytes and melanoma cells with the microenvironment. Pigment Cell Res 7:81–88.

Herlyn M, Kath R, Williams N, Valyi-Nagy I, Rodeck U. 1990. Growth-regulatory factors for normal, premalignant, and malignant human cells in vitro. Adv Cancer Res 54:213–234.

Hodi FS, Friedlander P, Corless CL, Heinrich MC, Mac Rae S, Kruse A, Jagannathan J, Van den Abbeele AD, Velazquez EF, Demetri GD, Fisher DE. 2008. Major response to imatinib mesylate in KIT-mutated melanoma. J Clin Oncol 26:2046–2051.

Houben R, Becker JC, Kappel A, Terheyden P, Brocker EB, Goetz R, Rapp UR. 2004. Constitutive activation of the Ras-Raf signaling pathway in metastatic melanoma is associated with poor prognosis. J Carcinog 3:6.

Hsu MY, Shih DT, Meier FE, Van Belle P, Hsu JY, Elder DE, Buck CA, Herlyn M. 1998. Adenoviral gene transfer of beta3 integrin subunit induces conversion from radial to vertical growth phase in primary human melanoma. Am J Pathol 153:1435–1442.

Huang S, Luca M, Gutman M, McConkey DJ, Langley KE, Lyman SD, Bar-Eli M. 1996. Enforced c-KIT expression renders highly metastatic human melanoma cells susceptible to stem cell factor-induced apoptosis and inhibits their tumorigenic and metastatic potential. Oncogene 13:2339–2347.

Hynes RO. 1987. Integrins: a family of cell surface receptors. Cell 48:549–554.

Keller JW, Franklin JL, Graves-Deal R, Friedman DB, Whitwell CW, Coffey RJ. 2007. Oncogenic KRAS provides a uniquely powerful and variable oncogenic contribution among RAS family members in the colonic epithelium. J Cell Physiol 210:740–749.

Kerkhoff E and Rapp UR. 1998. High-intensity Raf signals convert mitotic cell cycling into cellular growth. Cancer Res 58:1636–1640.

Kohno M and Pouyssegur J. 2006. Targeting the ERK signaling pathway in cancer therapy. Ann Med 38:200–211.

Kumar R, Angelini S, Czene K, Sauroja I, Hahka-Kemppinen M, Pyrhonen S, Hemminki K. 2003. BRAF mutations in metastatic melanoma: a possible association with clinical outcome. Clin Cancer Res 9:3362–3368.

Lassam N and Bickford S. 1992. Loss of c-kit expression in cultured melanoma cells. Oncogene 7:51–56.

Lin AW, Barradas M, Stone JC, van Aelst L, Serrano M, Lowe SW. 1998. Premature senescence involving p53 and p16 is activated in response to constitutive MEK/MAPK mitogenic signaling. Genes Dev 12:3008–3019.

Lin WM, Baker AC, Beroukhim R, Winckler W, Feng W, Marmion JM, Laine E, Greulich H, Tseng H, Gates C, Hodi FS, Dranoff G, Sellers WR, Thomas RK, Meyerson M, Golub TR, Dummer R, Herlyn M, Getz G, Garraway LA. 2008. Modeling genomic diversity and tumor dependency in malignant melanoma. Cancer Res 68:664–673.

Liu ZJ, Xiao M, Balint K, Smalley KS, Brafford P, Qiu R, Pinnix CC, Li X, Herlyn M. 2006. Notch1 signaling promotes primary melanoma progression by activating mitogen-activated protein kinase/phosphatidylinositol 3-kinase-Akt pathways and up-regulating N-cadherin expression. Cancer Res 66:4182–4190.

Meier F, Schittek B, Busch S, Garbe C, Smalley K, Satyamoorthy K, Li G, Herlyn M. 2005. The RAS/RAF/MEK/ERK and PI3K/AKT signaling pathways present molecular targets for the effective treatment of advanced melanoma. Front Biosci 10:2986–3001.

Meredith JE, Jr. and Schwartz MA. 1997. Integrins, adhesion and apoptosis. Trends Cell Biol 7:146–150.

Montone KT, van Belle P, Elenitsas R, Elder DE. 1997. Proto-oncogene c-kit expression in malignant melanoma: protein loss with tumor progression. Mod Pathol 10:939–944.

Morimura T, Goitsuka R, Zhang Y, Saito I, Reth M, Kitamura D. 2000. Cell cycle arrest and apoptosis induced by Notch1 in B cells. J Biol Chem 275:36523–36531.

Morino N, Mimura T, Hamasaki K, Tobe K, Ueki K, Kikuchi K, Takehara K, Kadowaki T, Yazaki Y, Nojima Y. 1995. Matrix/integrin interaction activates the mitogen-activated protein kinase, p44erk-1 and p42erk-2. J Biol Chem 270:269–273.

Moriyama M, Osawa M, Mak SS, Ohtsuka T, Yamamoto N, Han H, Delmas V, Kageyama R, Beermann F, Larue L, Nishikawa S. 2006. Notch signaling via Hes1 transcription factor maintains survival of melanoblasts and melanocyte stem cells. J Cell Biol 173:333–339.

Nakamura T, Matsumoto K, Kiritoshi A, Tano Y. 1997. Induction of hepatocyte growth factor in fibroblasts by tumor-derived factors affects invasive growth of tumor cells: in vitro analysis of tumor-stromal interactions. Cancer Res 57:3305–3313.

Nicholson KM and Anderson NG. 2002. The protein kinase B/Akt signalling pathway in human malignancy. Cell Signal 14:381–395.

Pinnix CC and Herlyn M. 2007. The many faces of Notch signaling in skin-derived cells. Pigment Cell Res 20:458–465.

Pollock PM, Harper UL, Hansen KS, Yudt LM, Stark M, Robbins CM, Moses TY, Hostetter G, Wagner U, Kakareka J, Salem G, Pohida T, Heenan P, Duray P, Kallioniemi O, Hayward NK, Trent JM, Meltzer PS. 2003. High frequency of BRAF mutations in nevi. Nat Genet 33:19–20.

Qi R, An H, Yu Y, Zhang M, Liu S, Xu H, Guo Z, Cheng T, Cao X. 2003. Notch1 signaling inhibits growth of human hepatocellular carcinoma through induction of cell cycle arrest and apoptosis. Cancer Res 63:8323–8329.

Ramos OH, Kauskot A, Cominetti MR, Bechyne I, Salla Pontes CL, Chareyre F, Manent J, Vassy R, Giovannini M, Legrand C, Selistre-de-Araujo HS, Crepin M, Bonnefoy A. 2008. A novel alpha(v)beta (3)-blocking disintegrin containing the RGD motive, DisBa-01, inhibits bFGF-induced angiogenesis and melanoma metastasis. Clin Exp Metastasis 25:53–64.

Recio JA and Merlino G. 2002. Hepatocyte growth factor/scatter factor activates proliferation in melanoma cells through p38 MAPK, ATF-2 and cyclin D1. Oncogene 21:1000–1008.

Rodeck U, Herlyn M, Menssen HD, Furlanetto RW, Koprowsk H. 1987. Metastatic but not primary melanoma cell lines grow in vitro independently of exogenous growth factors. Int J Cancer 40:687–690.

Rubinfeld B, Robbins P, El-Gamil M, Albert I, Porfiri E, Polakis P (1997) Stabilization of beta-catenin by genetic defects in melanoma cell lines. Science 275:1790–1792.

Samuels Y, Wang Z, Bardelli A, Silliman N, Ptak J, Szabo S, Yan H, Gazdar A, Powell SM, Riggins GJ, Willson JK, Markowitz S, Kinzler KW, Vogelstein B, Velculescu VE. 2004. High frequency of mutations of the PIK3CA gene in human cancers. Science 304:554.

Sattler M and Salgia R. 2004. Targeting c-Kit mutations: basic science to novel therapies. Leuk Res 28 Suppl 1:S11–20.

Satyamoorthy K, Li G, Vaidya B, Patel D, Herlyn M. 2001. Insulin-like growth factor-1 induces survival and growth of biologically early melanoma cells through both the mitogen-activated protein kinase and beta-catenin pathways. Cancer Res 61:7318–7324.

Serrano M, Lin AW, McCurrach ME, Beach D, Lowe SW. 1997. Oncogenic ras provokes premature cell senescence associated with accumulation of p53 and p16INK4a. Cell 88:593–602.

Shou J, Ross S, Koeppen H, de Sauvage FJ, Gao WQ. 2001. Dynamics of notch expression during murine prostate development and tumorigenesis. Cancer Res 61:7291–7297.

Smalley KS. 2003. A pivotal role for ERK in the oncogenic behaviour of malignant melanoma? Int J Cancer 104:527–532.

Sridhar SS, Hedley D, Siu LL. 2005. Raf kinase as a target for anticancer therapeutics. Mol Cancer Ther 4:677–685.

Sriuranpong V, Borges MW, Ravi RK, Arnold DR, Nelkin BD, Baylin SB, Ball DW. 2001. Notch signaling induces cell cycle arrest in small cell lung cancer cells. Cancer Res 61: 3200–3205.

Stahl JM, Cheung M, Sharma A, Trivedi NR, Shanmugam S, Robertson GP. 2003. Loss of PTEN promotes tumor development in malignant melanoma. Cancer Res 63:2881–2890.

Stahl JM, Sharma A, Cheung M, Zimmerman M, Cheng JQ, Bosenberg MW, Kester M, Sandirasegarane L, Robertson GP. 2004. Deregulated Akt3 activity promotes development of malignant melanoma. Cancer Res 64:7002–7010.

Stenman G, Eriksson A, Claesson-Welsh L. 1989. Human PDGFA receptor gene maps to the same region on chromosome 4 as the KIT oncogene. Genes Chromosomes Cancer 1:155–158.

Stoker M, Gherardi E, Perryman M, Gray J. 1987. Scatter factor is a fibroblast-derived modulator of epithelial cell mobility. Nature 327:239–242.

Thompson FH, Emerson J, Olson S, Weinstein R, Leavitt SA, Leong SP, Emerson S, Trent JM, Nelson MA, Salmon SE, et al. 1995. Cytogenetics of 158 patients with regional or disseminated melanoma. Subset analysis of near-diploid and simple karyotypes. Cancer Genet Cytogenet 83:93–104.

Tsao H, Zhang X, Benoit E, Haluska FG. 1998. Identification of PTEN/MMAC1 alterations in uncultured melanomas and melanoma cell lines. Oncogene 16:3397–3402.

Tsao H, Zhang X, Fowlkes K, Haluska FG. 2000. Relative reciprocity of NRAS and PTEN/MMAC1 alterations in cutaneous melanoma cell lines. Cancer Res 60:1800–1804.

Tsao H, Goel V, Wu H, Yang G, Haluska FG. 2004. Genetic interaction between NRAS and BRAF mutations and PTEN/MMAC1 inactivation in melanoma. J Invest Dermatol 122:337–341.

Varner JA and Cheresh DA. 1996. Integrins and cancer. Curr Opin Cell Biol 8:724–730.

Vogelstein B and Kinzler KW (2004) Cancer genes and the pathways they control. Nat Med 10:789–799

Weng AP, Ferrando AA, Lee W, Morris JPt, Silverman LB, Sanchez-Irizarry C, Blacklow SC, Look AT, Aster JC. 2004. Activating mutations of NOTCH1 in human T cell acute lymphoblastic leukemia. Science 306:269–271.

Went PT, Dirnhofer S, Bundi M, Mirlacher M, Schraml P, Mangialaio S, Dimitrijevic S, Kononen J, Lugli A, Simon R, Sauter G. 2004. Prevalence of KIT expression in human tumors. J Clin Oncol 22:4514–4522.

Whitwam T, Vanbrocklin MW, Russo ME, Haak PT, Bilgili D, Resau JH, Koo HM, Holmen SL. 2007. Differential oncogenic potential of activated RAS isoforms in melanocytes. Oncogene 26:4563–4570.

Widlund HR and Fisher DE. 2003. Microphthalamia-associated transcription factor: a critical regulator of pigment cell development and survival. Oncogene 22:3035–3041.

Willmore-Payne C, Holden JA, Tripp S, Layfield LJ. 2005. Human malignant melanoma: detection of BRAF- and c-kit-activating mutations by high-resolution amplicon melting analysis. Hum Pathol 36:486–493.

Willmore-Payne C, Holden JA, Hirschowitz S, Layfield LJ. 2006. BRAF and c-kit gene copy number in mutation-positive malignant melanoma. Hum Pathol 37:520–527.

Wu H, Goel V, Haluska FG. 2003. PTEN signaling pathways in melanoma. Oncogene 22: 3113–3122.

Yeh AH, Bohula EA, Macaulay VM. 2006. Human melanoma cells expressing V600E B-RAF are susceptible to IGF1R targeting by small interfering RNAs. Oncogene 25:6574–6581.

Chapter 20
Cooperation and Cancer

Kathleen Sprouffske and Carlo C. Maley

Cast of Characters

The preceding chapters detail how mutations in genes such as *PDGFB*, *CDH1*, *TGFBR1*, and *KRAS* shape tumor microenvironment. Chapter 19 further demonstrates that multiple mutations targeting parallel pathways readily occur in the same tumor. Do they arise and function independently or do they interact, coevolve, and influence tumor progression in concert? Some answers to this broad question could be found in the concluding chapter of the volume.

Introduction

Evolution is traditionally studied at the scales of millions of years and organisms in a process that selects for a population adapted to its environment. At this scale, the process of evolution effectively reduces the frequency of childhood-onset cancers, because childhood cancer susceptibility alleles are removed from the gene pool before reproduction. However, evolution acts at many levels, even within the cells of our bodies during our lifetimes. Over 30 years ago, Cairns and Nowell recognized that this form of somatic natural selection was a liability in that mutant cells, such as neoplastic cells, with a survival or reproductive advantage may expand in a tissue and somatic evolution can lead to malignancy (Cairns 1975; Nowell 1976). Here, we explore the relationship between neoplastic cells and the microenvironment from an evolutionary and ecological perspective of tumorigenesis.

Evolution and the Microenvironment in Cancer

Evolution in Cancer

Neoplastic cells have the necessary and sufficient ingredients for natural selection (Merlo et al. 2006) – specifically heritable traits that vary across the population of

C.C. Maley (✉)
Department of Cellular and Molecular Oncology, Wister Institute, Philadelphia, PA, USA
e-mail: cmaley@alum.mit.edu

A. Thomas-Tikhonenko (ed.), *Cancer Genome and Tumor Microenvironment*, DOI 10.1007/978-1-4419-0711-0_20, © Springer Science+Business Media, LLC 2010

somatic cells and affect their fitness (survival and proliferation). The genetic heterogeneity of cells within neoplasms has long been known (Heppner et al. 1980; Murphy et al. 1995; Barrett et al. 1999; Tsao et al. 2000; González-García et al. 2002; Harada et al. 2002; Castro et al. 2005). Epigenetic changes have more recently been recognized as another mechanism to transmit fitness modifications across generations of cells (Jones and Takai 2001; Bird 2002; Feinberg 2007). These genetic and epigenetic variants may be used to identify and study interactions between cells. A clone with higher rates of reproduction and/or survival than its neighbor is said to be more fit or competitive.

The problem of somatic evolution and cancer is as old as multicellular organisms. During evolution from single-celled to multicellular organisms, there was selection at the organismal level for cooperation between single cells to increase the fitness of the organism (Buss 1987; Smith and Szathmáry, 1997). In cooperating, each cell gave up its individual reproductive interests to better propagate its shared genetic material. Cancer happens when somatic cells stop cooperating and instead maximize their own fitness. At short timescales, these cells are successful. Ultimately, their host organism perishes and the neoplastic cells die. Thus, there is conflict between somatic evolution and organismal evolution. Constraints on somatic evolution to suppress cancer have evolved along with multicellularity (Cairns 1975; Pepper et al. 2007) (e.g., tumor suppressor gene products and adult tissue stem cells). Though cells still compete and neoplasms still develop, the constraints on somatic evolution result in cancers that typically develop only late in life, after our prime reproductive years.

Microenvironment in Cancer

New somatic mutations occur in this multicellular context and their fitness is affected by their particular microenvironment. To appreciate this process, we will first characterize the microenvironment and then provide several examples that exemplify the relationship between the microenvironment, new mutant cells, and fitness. The microenvironment, from a cellular perspective, can include other cells, the extracellular matrix, cytokines, oxygen, and other nutrients like glucose. In short, any cell or molecule that comes into contact with the cell can affect its fitness and shape the evolutionary process. Strikingly, a neoplastic state can be induced or suppressed by changing a cell's environment (Tlsty 2001).

The fitness effects of the hallmarks of cancer (Hanahan and Weinberg 2000) depend on the context of the microenvironment. A simple example is the gain of a mutation that allows constitutive secretion of angiogenic factors (neoangiogenesis). In a well-oxygenated neoplasm, this may have no effect, while the release of the same factors in a hypoxic neoplasm would facilitate the expansion of the angiogenic clone (and any neighbors). The acquisition of a novel mutation conferring insensitivity to antigrowth signals, such as downregulation of transforming growth factor-beta (TGF-β) receptors, is beneficial only for cells encountering TGF-β. Cells that acquire a mutation to overexpress growth factor receptors, for example, the platelet-derived growth factor ($PDGF$) receptor, are more competitive than their wild-type neighbors if the microenvironmental concentration of *PDGF* is limiting. Similarly, clones gaining oncogene-activating mutations may only have a competitive advantage over normal cells in a microenvironment low in growth factors. This may explain why there are few oncogenic mutations found in Barrett's esophagus (BE) (Maley 2007). Repeated wound healing responses due to acid reflux lead to chronic inflammation and probably high levels of progrowth signals. Thus, oncogenic mutations that allow independent growth are unlikely to provide a fitness advantage over normal cells in this environment.

In ecology, the environment is frequently divided into biotic (organisms) and abiotic (everything else) effectors. Within the neoplastic context, many of the abiotic factors are produced or regulated by other cells. Thus, abiotic factors in the microenviroment, such as cytokines and the extracellular matrix, may be seen as media through which cells may interact. Cellular interactions can be studied between populations of clones using ecological theory, such as commensalism, predation, and parasitism, or between individual cells from clones using evolutionary and game theory (see West et al. 2007 for more about the distinction). Here, we focus on the interactions between individuals involving competition and cooperation. In particular, we emphasize the understudied possibilities for cooperative interactions between individual cells.

Competition

Competition occurs between cells in the microenvironment due to limits in space and nutrients (e.g., oxygen and glucose). A nice example of competition in cancer is that of aerobic glycolysis (Gatenby and Gillies 2004). As neoplastic cells increase in number and are displaced further from blood vessels, they encounter the diffusion limit of oxygen. Those cells that constitutively activate anaerobic glucose metabolism via glycolysis have a competitive advantage over cells dependent on oxidative phosphorylation. Due to the increased glycolysis, acid builds up in the microenvironment and selects for cells that are able to adapt to acidosis. These glycolytic, acid-generating, and acid-tolerating neoplastic cells modify their environment and can outcompete normal aerobic cells, even in the presence of oxygen. This elegant example of competition within neoplasms is known as the "Warburg effect" (Gillies and Gatenby 2007). Each new hallmark of cancer (Hanahan and Weinberg 2000) acquired by a clone is accompanied by a concomitant competitive advantage, within the right microenvironment. Most cancer research has implicitly focused on competition, but cooperation is an equally important form of interaction with potentially dramatic implications for neoplastic progression and therapy.

Cooperation in Cancer

Cooperation is a mutually beneficial interaction between cells. The concept of cooperation takes into account the interactive role of the other cells in the microenvironment as well as the possible outcomes of the interaction for both of their fitnesses (see West et al. 2006 for a microorganism-focused review, see also Queller 1985;

Effect on recipient

Effect on actor		Positive	Negative
	Positive	Mutual Benefit	Selfishness
	Negative	Altruism	Spite

Taylor and Frank 1996; Frank 1998; Sachs et al. 2004; Foster and Wenseleers 2006; West et al. 2007). Assume that there are only two cells interacting, which we will call the actor and the recipient, and the recipient benefits from the actor's behavior. This action can be further classified as altruism if the actor's fitness is reduced or mutual benefit if the actor as well as the recipient benefits. Figure 20.1 shows the complete set of possible interactions. Cooperation occurs when the actor's behavior is selected, in part, due to its benefit on the recipient (West et al. 2007).

In cooperative systems, like multicellular organisms, the strategy of defection and cheating is an important concern. There are a number of ways cells can cheat. For example, they can passively reap the benefits from the cooperators without providing any benefit to the cooperators in return. Cells can also cheat by signaling to the cooperators, stimulating them to create extra factors in the microenvironment that act as public goods. The latter type of cheater occurs in bacterial populations of *Pseudomonas aeruginosa* (Diggle et al. 2007). In a quorum-sensing cooperative environment, a cheating strain refrained from contributing to the public goods. At the same time, it encouraged the cooperators to contribute public goods by secreting the signal the cooperators use to trigger contribution.

Cheating disrupts the organization of the group, though it is possible for mixed populations consisting of cooperators and defectors to coexist indefinitely. For this to occur, however, the strategies that cells take to boost their fitness must be stable to invasion by new mutants (known as "evolutionary stable strategies") (Axelrod and Hamilton 1981; Frank 1998; Gatenby and Vincent 2003). In the case of cancer, it is unclear whether the question of long-term stability is relevant. We already know that an equilibrium is not reached between the tumorigenic cheaters and the normal tissue cooperators because the outcome is physiologically unsustainable at the organismal level. However, one potential goal of therapy might be to drive the neoplasm into an evolutionary stable strategy that does not lead to the collapse of the system and thereby transforms cancer into a chronic illness.

Within a multicellular organism, the cells of the body cooperate together and thus are susceptible to cheating. In the simplest case, neoplastic cells increase their proliferation, decrease their contributions to the organisms, and thereby outcompete normal cells. In more complicated cases, tumor cells and their stroma cooperate together in the carcinogenic process of cheating from the normal functions of the body. While the context is different, the models of cooperation apply to both the organismal and the cellular dynamics. In the examples below, we will make clear whether we are discussing cheating between clones within the neoplasm or cheating in the multicellular organism because the neoplastic (cheater) cells are no longer cooperating with the normal cells.

Existing well-studied models of cooperation (Hamilton 1964b; Hamilton 1964a; Trivers 1971; Axelrod and Hamilton 1981; Taylor and Frank 1996; Sachs et al. 2004; Lehmann and Keller 2006; Nowak 2006; West et al. 2007) are applicable to analyzing both cooperation of cells within neoplasms and cooperation of cells within multicellular organisms. There are two primary differences between the models we introduce: (1) the relatedness of the interacting clones and (2) whether they have specific properties (e.g., a marker that serves to uniquely identify a cell type or reduced individual fitness due to cooperating). Relatedness between clones is highly variable (Kim and Shibata 2004; Salipante et al. 2008; Wasserstrom et al. 2008) even in the context of a multicellular organism where the common ancestor of all cells is the zygote.

We briefly introduce four models of cooperation before covering them in further detail below. The two kin selection strategies, specifically kin choice and kin fidelity, require that the clones share the allele that causes cooperation. Further, clones using the kin choice strategy need some unique identifier or marker in order to recognize cells carrying the cooperation allele. On the other hand, clones using the kin fidelity strategy only need to be in a microenvironment such that cooperation with neighbors is likely to result in cooperation between close relatives. The other two cooperation models, by-product mutualism and directed reciprocity, are used to analyze clones that have different alleles driving their fitness-enhancing phenotypes. Both strategies involve cooperation; however, individuals using the strategy of by-product mutualism have no individual fitness costs, while individuals using the directed reciprocity strategy do so at a cost of reduced individual fitness.

Closely Related Clones

Cells that are closely related, in that they share the alleles for "cooperative" phenotypes, may evolve cooperation through kin choice and kin fidelity. In both scenarios, a cell contributes to a cooperator's fitness at a cost to itself, a strategy that is stable only because the related cell passes on the shared alleles for cooperation. Formally, Hamilton's rule (Hamilton 1964a,b) says that this is a stable strategy when the fitness lost by the donor (c) is less than the product of the degree of relatedness between the donor and the recipient (r) and the fitness gained by the recipient (b), i.e., $c < rb$. Here, relatedness is 1 if the cells share the cooperation allele and 0 if they do not. The rate of genetic alterations (the mutation rate) alone modifies the probability that cells share the cooperation allele. (Normally this rule is applied to sexually reproducing organisms where siblings and other relatives may or may not share a gene due to segregation and sexual recombination.) In short, even if a cell helps its close relatives so much that it can no longer divide, it can still be a favorable strategy to propagate its genetic makeup by natural selection. We now turn to the details of two strategies for cooperation by closely related clones, those of kin choice and kin fidelity.

Kin Choice

Cells using the kin choice strategy need to somehow recognize cells that share the cooperation allele before committing to the cooperative interaction. This has been called the green-beard effect, in that all cells with the cooperation allele must have some signature phenotype (e.g., green beards) (Dawkins 1976; Hamilton 1964a,b; Dawkins 1976) so that they can easily recognize each other. Creating partnerships with cells based upon a unique, extracellular phenotype seems at first to be an intuitive and parsimonious strategy. However, imposters can easily exploit the cooperators by mimicking the kin recognition cues and passing themselves off as relatives (Sachs et al. 2004). In tumorigenesis, cooperators can consist of either host cells or neoplastic cells. Host cells cooperate to do the work of the multicellular organism and neoplastic cells cheat. Alternatively, neoplastic cells may cooperate to exploit the host, leaving them vulnerable to exploitation by newly arising neoplastic mutants. Instances of cooperation between neoplastic clones have been predicted by theory (Axelrod et al. 2006), while instances of cheating between neoplastic clones would be a novel observation.

In the multicellular context, a potential candidate for a human green-beard gene and a nice example of the strategy of kin choice is the cadherin family of calcium-dependent cell adhesion molecules. Cadherins are known to have a significant role in tumor progression; the level of accessible E-cadherin is inversely correlated with cell motility and migration (Larue and Bellacosa 2005), an important step in tumor progression. Cadherins are transmembrane proteins that symmetrically homodimer-ize, anchoring neighboring cells via at least one so-called extracellular cadherin domain (Patel et al. 2006). Swapping this recognition domain between different members of a cadherin family is sufficient to change a cell's self-recognition (Patel et al. 2006). It is also known that homophilic binding between E-cadherin molecules is sufficient to inhibit growth in normal cells (Perrais et al. 2007), mediated by β-catenin signaling. All together, this suggests that a cell altruistically reduces its fitness (via a decreased growth rate) when it abuts its neighbor. It has been suggested that these cadherin–catenin complexes may act as biosensors of their microenvironment (Lien et al. 2006), allowing cells to monitor their neighbors and respond accordingly in true green-beard fashion. Cells in normal tissue express E-cadherin and cooperate with similar cells by slowing their growth to maintain a beneficial density. Many primary epithelial cancers defect from the cooperation by not producing E-cadherin. (The framework to analyze this action will be introduced in the next section.) However, E-cadherin expression is reestablished in metastases from these primary tumors (Lien and Vasioukhin 2008). An explanation consistent with these observations and kin choice entails the emergence of cheating cells that, contrary to the cooperators, neither synthesize E-cadherin nor limit their growth. In the short term at least, these cells may be able to utilize the shared resources to divide more frequently than the cooperators. Finally, the metastatic cells may be faking the green beard; they express E-cadherin and cause any surrounding host cells to limit their growth. Presumably, these metastatic cells no longer suppress their own proliferation in response to E-cadherin activation, though this remains to be shown.

Kin Fidelity

Instead of using a form of green beard to recognize kin, during cooperation by kin fidelity, the donor cell provides benefits to cells in its neighborhood, regardless of their genotypes. In order for its cooperation genotype to be propagated, a cell must be in a relatively immobile microenvironment, so its neighbors are likely to be its relatives. However, the most proximal neighbors are also subject to competition for resources so that the fitness benefit that arises from kin fidelity can be limited by the cost associated with increased competition between relatives (Taylor 1992; Griffin et al. 2004) Thus, there is a conflict between maximizing an individual's fitness within a group and maximizing the fitness of the group in competition with other groups (Frank 1998, 2007). Kin fidelity suggests that the evolution of cooperation reaches a compromise between the within-group fitness (cooperation is not favored) and the between-group fitness (cooperation is favored). Thus, kin fidelity is important when the clones within a neoplasm are more similar to each other than they are to the surrounding normal tissue, as would occur in solid tumors composed of immobile cells. This should be true of all clonal neoplasms. Finally, cheaters simply need to be in the right location at the right time. A new mutant that uses the public goods without making any contribution would have a competitive advantage over the cooperators.

The potential for cooperation by kin fidelity in tumorigenesis is supported by recent evidence from cell lineage analysis in mouse lymphoma that confirms, at least in this case, that neoplastic cells within a tumor are more related to each other than to the surrounding normal tissue (Frumkin et al. 2008). In this situation, then, the neoplastic cells may evolve to cooperate with each other by kin fidelity in order to cheat on the host tissue.

Once cooperating neoplastic clones exist, kin fidelity can suggest an explanation for a low-level prevalence of motility, including the epithelial–mesenchymal transition (EMT) and the amoeboid motility. In EMT, epithelial cells take on characteristics of mesenchymal cells, thus increasing their motility (Larue and Bellacosa 2005; Larue 2008). By instead using amoeboid motility, cells can move at an even faster rate (Sahai 2005). It is assumed that migrating cells outcompete the other cooperative (Merlo et al. 2006), immobile neoplastic cells since they can move to regions with high oxygen and nutrient content (Wyckoff et al. 2000; Condeelis et al. 2005). However, tumors with a high proportion of cheaters are less able to compete against the host tissue and so there is selection to maintain low frequencies of migratory cheaters within the neoplasm, which is thought to be the case (Turley et al. 2008). This can explain how low levels of motile cells within a tumor can be a stable strategy, at least until disrupted by a new mutation.

Distantly Related Clones

While all somatic cells derive from the zygote, genetic instability during neoplastic progression can lead to the genetic divergence of clones (Maley et al. 2006). We now examine clones with an "ancient" common ancestor (though not before the zygote) that work together to escape the shackles of multicellularity. We do this through analysis with by-product mutualism and directed reciprocity strategies – the appropriate analysis depends on how much the clones paid, in terms of lost individual fitness, in order to cooperate. By-product mutualism is free for both clones. In contrast, in the case of directed reciprocity, both clones sacrifice some individual fitness in exchange for a net gain of fitness from the cooperation.

By-Product Mutualism

By-product mutualism, sometimes called direct benefits, occurs when a cell positively affects another at no cost to itself (Lehmann and Keller 2006; West et al. 2007). The positive interaction is not conditional on the cooperating cell recognizing or responding to specific actions of their partners. For example, a cell that releases some fitness-increasing growth factor will have a positive effect on all the members of the tissue within range, including itself. If its neighbors are also cooperators via by-product mutualism, they may release additional growth factors that increase both their own and the other cell's fitness. Several proposed examples of cooperation via by-product mutualism involving growth factors are described below. In another possible scenario, one clone could release matrix metalloproteinases (MMPs), promoting movement or angiogenesis for all of its neighbors, while the other clone could acquire the ability to stimulate angiogenesis (even more than the by-product of MMP degradation) to supply nutrients to the angiogenic clone as well as its neighbors; the neoplasm as a whole receives a fitness benefit from the combination of the cooperating clones. This example, though hypothetical, is not so far-fetched. We know that MMPs are synthesized and secreted into the extracellular milieu by a variety of tissues and cell types, including carcinoma and glioma cells (Mancini and Di Battista 2006). We also know that *VEGF* can exist as both free and sequestered forms (stored in the extracellular matrix for release by *MMP-9*) (Hicklin and Ellis 2005). This positive feedback loop of mutual benefits discourages cheating, since helping a neighboring cell only serves to sustain the benefits received from it. If a cell no longer helps its neighbors, it indirectly harms itself.

Directed Reciprocity

In contrast to by-product mutualism, directed reciprocity may evolve in the context of repeated interactions between two clones with indefinite duration. In this situation, formally captured by the prisoner's dilemma game, clones may evolve to donate a fitness advantage to their neighbor at a fitness cost to themselves. The prisoner's dilemma has been explored in much more detail elsewhere (Trivers 1971; Axelrod and Hamilton 1981; Bull and Rice 1991; Frank 1998; Sachs et al. 2004; Nowak 2006) and it embodies the inherent problem in cooperation – for an individual in a single interaction, cheating is often more profitable than cooperating.

In short, the directed reciprocity is an interaction in which mutual cooperation has higher fitness than mutual cheating, but if one individual cooperates and the other cheats, the cheater attains the maximal fitness and the cooperator receives the minimal fitness. A robust strategy in this environment is reciprocity (a.k.a., "tit for tat"), in which the individual simply mimics the most recent action taken by the other individual. Under certain conditions, this strategy can evolve (Axelrod and Hamilton 1981), despite the fact that for any one game, an individual could increase its fitness by cheating. These rules apply to cell–cell interactions, particularly in relatively immotile tissue so that cells can interact with their neighbors over extended periods of time.

Examples

Within tumorigenesis, we have yet to experimentally distinguish between by-product mutualism and directed reciprocity, and so we present all of the examples together. Measuring the fitness gains and losses between the clones before and after cooperation would be one method to distinguish these types of cooperation in future experiments.

We again turn to one of the hallmarks of cancer (Hanahan and Weinberg 2000) that is nicely positioned for participation in cooperative endeavors, angiogenesis. Any clone that induces the growth of new blood vessels necessarily benefits all nearby cells. Clones that in turn improve the fitness of the angiogenesis-promoting clone are cooperating partners in by-product mutualism or directed reciprocity. For example, one clone might induce the growth of new blood vessels by downregulating the expression of thrombospondin-1 (*TSP-1*), thus increasing angiogenesis by overexpressing *MMP-9*, which in turn increases the amount of stored *VEGF* freed from the extracellular matrix (Ren et al. 2006). Another nearby clone might begin overexpressing *VEGF* and establish the positive feedback loop that is indicative of by-product mutualism. It is unclear if there are any fitness costs to producing these public goods.

Additional hallmarks that are likely to be affected by cooperation are those that deal with growth, specifically antigrowth insensitivity and growth sufficiency. Any autonomous growth-enhancing process that also benefits heterotypic clones is poised for cooperation. For example, in breast cancer in mice, reciprocal interactions at the level of gene expression have been identified between the tumor and the stroma (Montel et al. 2006). Further, it is well established that modifications to the stroma can have an effect on neoplastic cells, sometimes permanently (Tlsty 2001). For example, grafts of carcinoma-associated fibroblasts (CAFs) from human prostate fibroblasts and epithelial cells from immortalized human cell lines showed that the fibroblasts had a very strong growth effect on the epithelial cells (Tlsty 2001). All that remains to prove cooperation in this case is to show that the neoplastic cells in turn can affect reproduction or survival of the fibroblasts.

Another potential example of cooperative growth effects was found in cocultures of mesenchymal stem cells and the breast cancer cell line MCF7/Ras (Karnoub et al. 2007). Upon injection into immunocompromised mice, the cocultured MCF7/Ras cancer cells and mesenchymal stem cells had significantly greater growth kinetics compared to injection of breast cancer cells alone. It remains to be determined whether both clones benefit from this interaction, and if so, the mechanism of the interaction.

In another example, breast cancer cells that have metastasized to the bone produce paracrine factors such as tumor necrosis factor-alpha (*TNF-α*) and insulin-like growth factor II (*IGF-II*) (Pederson et al. 1999). The factors induce osteoclasts to differentiate and degrade the bone matrix, which in turn liberates *TGF-β*. The final step in this positive feedback loop is the stimulation of tumor cell growth by *TGF-β* (Bussard et al. 2008). The positive feedback loop initiated by the breast cancers cells increased their fitness, but the fitness effect on osteoclasts determines if this is mutualism or exploitation. Although differentiation probably reduces their reproductive fitness, *TGF-β* increases osteoclast survival (Chambers 2000) and thus increases their fitness. Interestingly, it has been observed in vitro that osteoclast differentiation by TNF-α is significantly enhanced by *TGF-β* (Chambers 2000).

Examples showing conclusive cooperation between clones are as yet incomplete. Frequently, only one-half of the experiment has been done. There are, however, many promising examples of that one half, where a clone secretes some factors that benefit all clones in the neighborhood. For example, transcription growth factor-alpha (*TGF-α*), a member of the EGF family, can be expressed in a wide variety of adult tissues (Lee et al. 1995) and was also shown to be overexpressed in colon tumors (Tanaka et al. 1991) and colon cell lines (Coffey et al. 1987). In normal tissue, *TGF-α* activates the *EGF* receptor, which in turn stimulates growth. While aberrant *TGF-α* expression alone does not appear to be oncogenic in vivo, the resulting growth abnormalities allow these clones to participate in cooperative tumorigenesis (Lee et al. 1995).

Another potential example of clones cooperating has been identified in prostate cancer where cancer cells induce macrophages to promote angiogenesis (rather than lyse the cancer cells). Specifically, in normal wound healing, monocytes from the vascular system follow chemokine signals to the injured tissue and differentiate into a variety of macrophages, depending on the signals received from the injured tissue. The macrophages can then remove the tumor or the invading cell causing the injury by lysing it, identifying it to the T cells for future monitoring, and secreting cytokines that serve to amplify the response (reviewed in Lewis and Pollard 2006).

This would be an example of cooperation by the macrophages to remove dangers to the multicellular organism. Alternative signals may exploit the cooperative nature of the host macrophages to instead aid tumor cells. In this example, prostate cancer cells secrete the chemokine *CCL2* (also called monocyte chemoattractant protein-1, *MCP-1*) which recruits macrophages to the tumor. Rather than lysing the tumor cells, these macrophages increase prostate cells' fitness by promoting angiogenesis (Loberg et al. 2007), possibly in response to the hypoxic microenvironment (Lewis and Pollard 2006). As it is unknown if the macrophages have increased proliferation or survival due to their interactions with the prostate cancer cell, we cannot know if this interaction is cooperative or coercive.

Cervical cancer cells take advantage of the cooperative nature of fibroblasts in their host. Specifically, secretion of the platelet-derived growth factor (*PDGF*) by cervical cancer cells stimulates stromal fibroblast cells to produce fibroblast growth factor-2 (*FGF-2*) in a mouse model. *FGF-2* stimulates angiogenesis which benefits both cell populations (Pietras et al. 2008). Thus, the neoplastic cells exploit a property of fibroblasts, using their cooperative nature to cheat from the multicellular organism. Here, the fibroblasts may eventually transform into active cooperators. If *PDGF* stimulates proliferation or survival of the fibroblasts, then this would be a clear example of cooperation.

In another single-sided example, the deformation of the matrix by invading CAFs is sufficient to enable invasion by squamous cell carcinoma (SCC) cells. Here, SCC cells or normal keratinocytes alone were unable to invade, while either carcinoma cells with mesenchymal characteristics or an admixture of SCC and fibroblast cells could (Gaggioli et al. 2007). Thus, this may be a case of by-product mutualism because the activated fibroblasts (or mesenchymal-like carcinoma cells) benefit both themselves and the SCC cells that follow in their tracks. We are unable to confirm that this relationship is cooperative until we know if the leading cells also benefit from the presence of the carcinoma cells.

Conclusions

Cooperation is an important but understudied dynamic in the microenvironment of neoplasms. These interactions could increase the rate of progression to malignancy if two clones may independently acquire different hallmarks of cancer rather than waiting for one clone to accumulate all the hallmarks itself (Axelrod et al. 2006). Cells that participate in paracrine and heterotypic signaling are obvious places to begin the study of cooperation in neoplasia. Even more promising are the cells that have co-opted their neighbors to provide them with fitness-enhancing benefits. It may not be long before the neighbors acquire a mutation that benefits the neoplastic cell, thus establishing a positive feedback loop, such as in by-product mutualism. If normal cells are also acquiring genetic or epigenetic lesions, they may be coevolving with the neoplastic cells, though this remains an open question. Finally, it is likely that neoplasms with polyclonal origins (Novelli et al. 1996; Merritt et al. 1997; Newton 2006) collaborated or coevolved together *from initiation* to escape the restraints of multicellularity.

Analyzing tumorigenesis from an evolutionary and ecological perspective allows us to leverage decades of theory and knowledge acquired in other systems. This is particularly important in the pursuit of novel therapies. Cooperation allows a neoplasm to evolve the hallmarks of cancer, without requiring that they all occur within the same clone (Axelrod et al. 2006). This may both increase the rate of neoplastic progression and provide targets for cancer prevention by interfering with the cooperation. There is much research in microbiology and virology that may be directly applicable. For example, in experimental bacterial systems, interruption of spatial heterogeneity prevents adaptive radiation and the evolution of new clones (Rainey and Travisano 1998). We predict that decreasing the heterogeneity of the tumor environment will slow the evolution of new clones and the opportunities for tumorigenesis via cheating and cooperation. Also, theory has been developed to identify evolutionary stable strategies in which multiple clonal populations can stably coexist. This may be used to turn cancer into a long-term, chronic disease if we can force the neoplastic cells to coexist with normal cells (Gatenby and Vincent 2003), though the mechanism for achieving this is an open question.

The focus on tumorigenesis as a cell autonomous process emanating from neoplastic cells is obviously oversimplistic. While providing us hints of the richness of cooperative interactions, our focus on one-way paracrine interactions, such as signals by the tumor used to recruit coconspirators and signals by stromal cells used to activate tumor cells, still misses the full story. In these cases, our focus is inherently on the competitive effects between the neoplasm and the surrounding cells. We must expand our focus to feedback between cell types, particularly focusing on determining the fitness effects of neoplastic cells on the other cells in their microenvironment.

References

Axelrod R and Hamilton WD. 1981. The evolution of cooperation. Science 211:1390–1396.

Axelrod R, Axelrod DE, Pienta KJ. 2006. Evolution of cooperation among tumor cells. Proc Natl Acad Sci U S A 103:13474–13479.

Barrett MT, Sanchez CA, Prevo LJ, Wong DJ, Galipeau PC, Paulson TG, Rabinovitch PS, Reid BJ. 1999. Evolution of neoplastic cell lineages in Barrett oesophagus. Nat Genet 22:106–109.

Bird A. 2002. DNA methylation patterns and epigenetic memory. Genes Dev 16:6–21.

Bull JJ and Rice WR. 1991. Distinguishing mechanisms for the evolution of co-operation. J Theor Biol 149:63–74.

Buss LW. 1987. The Evolution of Individuality. Princeton University Press, Princeton NJ

Bussard KM, Gay CV, Mastro AM. 2008. The bone microenvironment in metastasis; what is special about bone? Cancer Metastasis Rev 27:41–55.

Cairns J. 1975. Mutation selection and the natural history of cancer. Nature 255:197–200.

Castro MA, Onsten TT, de Almeida RM, Moreira JC. 2005. Profiling cytogenetic diversity with entropy-based karyotypic analysis. J Theor Biol 234:487–495.

Chambers TJ. 2000. Regulation of the differentiation and function of osteoclasts. J Pathol 192:4–13.

Coffey RJ Jr, Goustin AS, Soderquist AM, Shipley GD, Wolfshohl J, Carpenter G, Moses HL. 1987. Transforming growth factor alpha and beta expression in human colon cancer lines: Implications for an autocrine model. Cancer Res 47:4590–4594.

Condeelis J, Singer RH, Segall JE. 2005. The great escape: When cancer cells hijack the genes for chemotaxis and motility. Annu Rev Cell Dev Biol 21:695–718.

Dawkins R. 1976. The Selfish Gene. Oxford: Oxford University Press.

Diggle SP, Griffin AS, Campbell GS, West SA. 2007. Cooperation and conflict in quorum-sensing bacterial populations. Nature 450:411–414.

Feinberg AP. 2007. Phenotypic plasticity and the epigenetics of human disease. Nature 447: 433–440.

Foster KR and Wenseleers T. 2006. A general model for the evolution of mutualisms. J Evol Biol 19:1283–1293.

Frank SA. 1998. Foundations of Social Evolution. Princeton University Press, Princeton, NJ 268

Frank SA. 2007. All of life is social. Curr Biol 17:R648–650.

Frumkin D, Wasserstrom A, Itzkovitz S, Stern T, Harmelin A, Eilam R, Rechavi G, Shapiro E. 2008. Cell Lineage Analysis of a Mouse Tumor. Cancer Res 68:5924–5931.

Gaggioli C, Hooper S, Hidalgo-Carcedo C, Grosse R, Marshall JF, Harrington K, Sahai E. 2007. Fibroblast-led collective invasion of carcinoma cells with differing roles for RhoGTPases in leading and following cells. Nature Cell Biology 9:1392–1400.

Gatenby RA and Gillies RJ. 2004. Why do cancers have high aerobic glycolysis? Nat Rev Cancer 4:891–899.

Gatenby RA and Vincent TL. 2003. Application of quantitative models from population biology and evolutionary game theory to tumor therapeutic strategies. Mol Cancer Ther 2: 919–927.

Gillies RJ and Gatenby RA. 2007. Adaptive landscapes and emergent phenotypes: Why do cancers have high glycolysis? J Bioenerg Biomembr 39:251–257.

González-García I, Solé RV, Costa J. 2002. Metapopulation dynamics and spatial heterogeneity in cancer. Proc Natl Acad Sci U S A 99:13085–13089.

Griffin AS, West SA, Buckling A. 2004. Cooperation and competition in pathogenic bacteria. Nature 430:1024–1027.

Hamilton WD. 1964a. The genetical evolution of social behaviour. I. J Theor Biol 7:1–16.

Hamilton WD. 1964b. The genetical evolution of social behaviour. II. J Theor Biol 7:17–52.

Hanahan D and Weinberg RA. 2000. The hallmarks of cancer. Cell 100:57–70.

Harada T, Okita K, Shiraishi K, Kusano N, Kondoh S, Sasaki K. 2002. Interglandular cytogenetic heterogeneity detected by comparative genomic hybridization in pancreatic cancer. Cancer Res 62:835–839.

Heppner G, Miller B, Cooper D, Miller FR. 1980. Growth interactions between mammary tumor cells. Cell Biology of Breast Cancer:161–172.

Hicklin DJ and Ellis LM. 2005. Role of the vascular endothelial growth factor pathway in tumor growth and angiogenesis. J Clin Oncol 23:1011–1027.

Jones PA and Takai D. 2001. The role of DNA methylation in mammalian epigenetics. Science 293:1068–1070.

Karnoub AE, Dash AB, Vo AP, Sullivan A, Brooks MW, Bell GW, Richardson AL, Polyak K, Tubo R, Weinberg RA. 2007. Mesenchymal stem cells within tumour stroma promote breast cancer metastasis. Nature 449:557–563.

Kim K and Shibata D. 2004. Tracing ancestry with methylation patterns: Most crypts appear distantly related in normal adult human colon. BMC Gastroenterol 4:8.

Larue L. 2008. P13K/AKT pathway and Epithelial–mesenchymal Transition This Volume.

Larue L and Bellacosa A. 2005. Epithelial–mesenchymal transition in development and cancer: Role of phosphatidylinositol 3' kinase/AKT pathways. Oncogene 24:7443–7454.

Lee DC, Fenton SE, Berkowitz EA, Hissong MA. 1995. Transforming growth factor alpha: Expression, regulation, and biological activities. Pharmacol Rev 47:51–85.

Lehmann L and Keller L. 2006. The evolution of cooperation and altruism–a general framework and a classification of models. J Evol Biol 19:1365–1376.

Lewis CE and Pollard JW. 2006. Distinct role of macrophages in different tumor microenvironments. Cancer Res 66:605–612.

Lien W-H and Vasioukhin V. 2008. Cadherin–catenin complexes in tumor progression. This Volume

Lien WH, Klezovitch O, Vasioukhin V. 2006. Cadherin–catenin proteins in vertebrate development. Curr Opin Cell Biol 18:499–506.

Loberg RD, Ying C, Craig M, Day LL, Sargent E, Neeley C, Wojno K, Snyder LA, Yan L, Pienta KJ. 2007. Targeting CCL2 with systemic delivery of neutralizing antibodies induces prostate cancer tumor regression in vivo. Cancer Res 67:9417–9424.

Maley CC. 2007. Multistage carcinogenesis in Barrett's esophagus. Cancer Lett 245: 22–32.

Maley CC, Galipeau PC, Finley JC, Wongsurawat VJ, Li X, Sanchez CA, Paulson TG, Blount PL, Risques RA, Rabinovitch PS, Reid BJ. 2006. Genetic clonal diversity predicts progression to esophageal adenocarcinoma. Nat Genet 38:468–473.

Mancini A and Di Battista JA. 2006. Transcriptional regulation of matrix metalloprotease gene expression in health and disease. Front Biosci 11:423–446.

Merlo LMF, Pepper JW, Reid BJ, Maley CC. 2006. Cancer as an evolutionary and ecological process. Nat Rev Cancer 6:924–935.

Merritt AJ, Gould KA, Dove WF. 1997. Polyclonal structure of intestinal adenomas in ApcMin/+ mice with concomitant loss of Apc+ from all tumor lineages. Proc Natl Acad Sci U S A 94:13927–13931.

Montel V, Mose E, Tarin D. 2006. Tumor-stromal interactions reciprocally modulate gene expression patterns during carcinogenesis and metastasis. Int J Cancer 119:251–263.

Murphy DS, Hoare SF, Going JJ, Mallon EE, George WD, Kaye SB, Brown R, Black DM, Keith WN. 1995. Characterization of extensive genetic alterations in ductal carcinoma in situ by fluorescence in situ hybridization and molecular analysis. J Natl Cancer Inst 87: 1694–1704.

Newton MA. 2006. On estimating the polyclonal fraction in lineage-marker studies of tumor origin. Biostatistics 7:503–514.

Novelli MR, Williamson JA, Tomlinson IP, Elia G, Hodgson SV, Talbot IC, Bodmer WF, Wright NA. 1996. Polyclonal origin of colonic adenomas in an XO/XY patient with FAP. Science 272:1187–1190.

Nowak MA. 2006. Evolutionary Dynamics. The Belknap Press of Harvard University Press, Cambridge, MA

Nowell PC. 1976. The clonal evolution of tumor cell populations. Science 194:23–28.

Patel SD, Ciatto C, Chen CP, Bahna F, Rajebhosale M, Arkus N, Schieren I, Jessell TM, Honig B, Price SR, Shapiro L. 2006. Type II cadherin ectodomain structures: Implications for classical cadherin specificity. Cell 124:1255–1268.

Pederson L, Winding B, Foged NT, Spelsberg TC, Oursler MJ. 1999. Identification of breast cancer cell line-derived paracrine factors that stimulate osteoclast activity. Cancer Res 59:5849–5855.

Pepper JW, Sprouffske K, Maley CC. 2007. Animal Cell Differentiation Patterns Suppress Somatic Evolution. PLoS Comput Biol 3:e250.

Perrais M, Chen X, Perez-Moreno M, Gumbiner BM. 2007. E-cadherin homophilic ligation inhibits cell growth and epidermal growth factor receptor signaling independently of other cell interactions. Mol Biol Cell 18:2013–2025.

Pietras K, Pahler J, Bergers G, Hanahan D. 2008. Functions of paracrine PDGF signaling in the proangiogenic tumor stroma revealed by pharmacological targeting. PLoS Med 5:e19

Queller DC. 1985. Kinship, reciprocity and synergism in the evolution of social behaviour. Nature 318:366–367.

Rainey PB and Travisano M. 1998. Adaptive radiation in a heterogeneous environment. Nature 394:69–72.

Ren B, Yee KO, Lawler J, Khosravi-Far R. 2006. Regulation of tumor angiogenesis by thrombospondin-1. Biochim Biophys Acta 1765:178–188.

Sachs JL, Mueller UG, Wilcox TP, Bull JJ. 2004. The evolution of cooperation. The Quarterly Review of Biology 79:135–160.

Sahai E. 2005. Mechanisms of cancer cell invasion. Curr Opin Genet Dev 15:87–96.

Salipante SJ, Thompson JM, Horwitz MS. 2008. Phylogenetic fate mapping: Theoretical and experimental studies applied to the development of mouse. . . . Genetics 178: 967–977.

Smith JA and Szathmáry E. 1997. The Major Transitions in Evolution. books.google.com

Tanaka S, Imanishi K, Yoshihara M, Haruma K, Sumii K, Kajiyama G, Akamatsu S. 1991. Immunoreactive transforming growth factor alpha is commonly present in colorectal neoplasia. Am J Pathol 139:123–129.

Taylor PD. 1992. Altruism in viscous populations—an inclusive fitness model. Evolutionary Ecology 6: 352–356.

Taylor PD and Frank SA. 1996. How to make a kin selection model. J Theor Biol 180:27–37.

Tlsty TD. 2001. Stromal cells can contribute oncogenic signals. Semin Cancer Biol 11: 97–104.

Trivers RL. 1971. The Evolution of Reciprocal Altruism. The Quarterly Review of Biology 46: 35–57.

Tsao JL, Yatabe Y, Salovaara R, Järvinen HJ, Mecklin JP, Aaltonen LA, Tavaré S, Shibata D. 2000. Genetic reconstruction of individual colorectal tumor histories. Proc Natl Acad Sci U S A 97:1236–1241.

Turley E, Veiseh M, Radisky D, Bissell M. 2008. Mechanisms of disease: Epithelial–mesenchymal transition–does cellular plasticity fuel neoplastic progression? Nat Clin Prac Oncol 5:280–290.

Wasserstrom A, Frumkin D, Adar R, Itzkovitz S, Stern T, Kaplan S, Shefer G, Shur I, Zangi L, Reizel Y, Harmelin A, Dor Y, Dekel N, Reisner Y, Benayahu D, Tzahor E, Segal E, Shapiro E. 2008. Estimating cell depth from somatic mutations. PLoS Comput Biol 4:e1000058.

West SA, Griffin AS, Gardner A. 2007. Social semantics: Altruism, cooperation, mutualism, strong reciprocity and group selection. J Evol Biol 20:415–432.

West SA, Griffin AS, Gardner A, Diggle SP. 2006. Social evolution theory for microorganisms. Nat Rev Microbiol 4:597–607.

Wyckoff JB, Jones JG, Condeelis JS, Segall JE. 2000. A critical step in metastasis: In vivo analysis of intravasation at the primary tumor. Cancer Res 60:2504–2511.

Index

A. Thomas-Tikhonenko (ed.), *Cancer Genome and Tumor Microenvironment*,
DOI 10.1007/978-1-4419-0711-0, © Springer Science+Business Media, LLC 2010